Infections and Pregnancy: A Clinical Approach

Infections and Pregnancy: A Clinical Approach

Editor: Marina Fox

MURPHY & MOORE
www.murphy-moorepublishing.com

www.murphy-moorepublishing.com

MURPHY & MOORE

Cataloging-in-Publication Data

Infections and pregnancy : a clinical approach / edited by Marina Fox.
p. cm.
Includes bibliographical references and index.
ISBN 978-1-63987-768-3
1. Pregnancy--Complications. 2. Pregnancy--Complications--Treatment.
3. Generative organs, Female--Infections. 4. Communicable diseases in pregnancy.
I. Fox, Marina.
RG572 .I54 2023
618.3--dc23

Murphy & Moore Publishing
1 Rockefeller Plaza,
New York City,
NY 10020, USA

ISBN 978-1-63987-768-3

Contents

Preface

Pregnancy refers to a period when one or more offsprings grow inside a woman's womb. It usually happens through sexual intercourse but it can also happen through assisted reproductive technology procedures. A combination of immunological and physiological changes during pregnancy increase the risk and severity of specific infections. If a woman contracts a serious infection during this period, it can endanger the mother as well as the child. It can also lead to complications such as preterm birth and low birth weight babies. Parasitic infections are common in pregnant women due to decreased body immunity and thus can impact physiological systems. Malaria and ameba infections have been linked to a higher risk of unfavorable pregnancy complications and outcomes. If a mother has a parasitic infection during pregnancy, this can alter immune responses in the fetus and infant. These immunological alterations may affect the way a child reacts to the same infection later in life. This book contains some path-breaking studies on the relationship between infections and pregnancy. It will serve as a reference to a broad spectrum of readers.

This book is a comprehensive compilation of works of different researchers from varied parts of the world. It includes valuable experiences of the researchers with the sole objective of providing the readers (learners) with a proper knowledge of the concerned field. This book will be beneficial in evoking inspiration and enhancing the knowledge of the interested readers.

In the end, I would like to extend my heartiest thanks to the authors who worked with great determination on their chapters. I also appreciate the publisher's support in the course of the book. I would also like to deeply acknowledge my family who stood by me as a source of inspiration during the project.

Editor

1

Malaria and Early Life Immunity: Competence in Context

Perri C. Callaway[1,2]*, Lila A. Farrington*[2] *and Margaret E. Feeney*[2,3]*

[1] *Infectious Diseases and Immunity Graduate Group, University of California, Berkeley, Berkeley, CA, United States,* [2] *Department of Medicine, University of California, San Francisco, San Francisco, CA, United States,* [3] *Department of Pediatrics, University of California, San Francisco, San Francisco, CA, United States*

***Correspondence:**
Margaret E. Feeney
margaret.feeney@ucsf.edu

Childhood vaccines have been the cornerstone tool of public health over the past century. A major barrier to neonatal vaccination is the "immaturity" of the infant immune system and the inefficiency of conventional vaccine approaches at inducing immunity at birth. While much of the literature on fetal and neonatal immunity has focused on the early life propensity toward immune tolerance, recent studies indicate that the fetus is more immunologically capable than previously thought, and can, in some circumstances, mount adaptive B and T cell responses to perinatal pathogens *in utero*. Although significant hurdles remain before these findings can be translated into vaccines and other protective strategies, they should lend optimism to the prospect that neonatal and even fetal vaccination is achievable. Next steps toward this goal should include efforts to define the conditions for optimal stimulation of infant immune responses, including antigen timing, dose, and route of delivery, as well as antigen presentation pathways and co-stimulatory requirements. A better understanding of these factors will enable optimal deployment of vaccines against malaria and other pathogens to protect infants during their period of greatest vulnerability.

Keywords: fetal immunity, neonatal immunity, malaria, plasmodium, neonatal vaccination

NEITHER MAN NOR MOUSE: IMMUNE COMPETENCE IN THE INFANT

The human infant has long been considered immunologically immature, or deficient, when judged against the yardstick of the adult immune system. Indeed, the fetus and newborn are vulnerable to severe disease and high morbidity from numerous pathogens that cause only mild disease in older hosts. It had previously been believed, based largely on extrapolation from mouse models of immune development, that the tolerogenic intrauterine environment is incompatible with the priming of fetal T cells or results in marked polarization of CD4 T cells toward a Th2 response over a Th1 response. However, it is now appreciated that human fetal immune development differs quite markedly from that of the mouse. Neonatal mice are profoundly immunodeficient—indeed, migration of murine T cells from the thymus begins only after birth. In contrast, during human gestation, T cells appear in the fetal liver at week 10 and T cell zones can be seen in the spleen during week 18 (1). The recent development of single-cell analysis tools has led to a remarkable burst of progress in the study of fetal and infant immune cell populations, and has revealed a surprising degree of immune competence at, and even before, full-term gestation (2–5).

Placental malaria offers a valuable model to examine the response to pathogen-derived antigens *in utero*, and findings from this model bear relevance to other parasitic pathogens. Annually, more than 125 million pregnancies occur in areas where malaria is endemic (6), and 25% of pregnancies in sub-Saharan Africa are complicated by malaria (7). While true congenital infection with malaria parasites is rare, malaria antigens gain access to the fetal circulation after crossing the placenta, and studies of cord blood from malaria-exposed neonates have demonstrated an impact on numerous immune cell populations (2, 8, 9). Thus, understanding the immunological implications of placental malaria exposure is of paramount importance to public health.

LEARNING TO ADAPT: T AND B CELLS

Not surprisingly, most T and B cells in umbilical cord blood are naïve in phenotype, reflecting the relative lack of antigen experience during intrauterine life. During early and mid-gestation, human fetal T cells are inclined toward tolerance, as has been reviewed elsewhere (10, 11). Upon encounter with non-self-antigens, naïve CD4 T cells in the mid-gestation fetus preferentially differentiate into FoxP3+ regulatory T-cells that, along with other regulatory populations, can actively suppress T cell activation and cytokine production (12–14). However, as the fetus approaches term, it must balance the demands of maternal tolerance with the need to mount an effector T cell response against potential pathogens encountered after birth. It was recently shown that even in the absence of intrauterine pathogen exposure, a sizeable subset of CD4 T cells in cord blood exhibit effector-memory differentiation and can produce both Th1 and Th2 cytokines (15). Indeed, TNFα and IFNγ production by fetal T cells that are alloreactive to maternal antigens may contribute to preterm labor (16). Whether fetal Th1 responses to pathogens such as malaria may contribute to preterm birth or poor growth *in utero* has not been adequately investigated.

Until recently, relatively few studies have applied single-cell analysis techniques to characterize the human T cell response to pathogen-derived antigens encountered *in utero*. In aggregate, these studies suggest that despite the numerous mechanisms enforcing fetal and neonatal tolerance, the fetus is capable of mounting robust T cell responses under particular conditions. Congenital viral infections such as CMV result in expansion and differentiation of virus-specific CD8 T cells that produce IFNγ, TNFα, and perform perforin-mediated cytolysis (17). Recently, we showed that in the setting of placental malaria, CD4 and CD8 T cells primed *in utero* demonstrate effector-memory differentiation, inflammatory cytokine production, and robust malaria antigen-specific T cell proliferation. These effector populations were associated with protection from both *P. falciparum* infection and symptomatic malaria during the first 2 years of life (2). The most profound effector T cell differentiation was observed in infants born to mothers with active placental malaria at the time of birth, possibly suggesting late gestation exposure (2). However, T cell responses were not observed in all exposed infants in this study, and other investigators have observed that *in utero P. falciparum* exposure tolerized fetal T cells in a subset of exposed infants (18). The timing, duration, and quantity of malaria antigen exposure (influenced by intermittent preventive therapy with antimalarials), as well as the degree of associated placental inflammation, may play a large role in influencing the balance between fetal T cell tolerance vs. effector differentiation.

Some evidence indicates that fetal B cells can also be primed *in utero*. Malaria-specific antibodies of the IgM class (which cannot cross the placenta) have been detected in the cord blood of malaria-exposed infants as early as 22 weeks gestation (8, 9, 19) and surprisingly, class-switching of malaria-specific B cells from IgM to IgG occurs in some infants prior to delivery (8). These findings raise the possibility that fetal B cells could be sensitized by maternal malaria vaccination, as has been reported with maternal tetanus and influenza vaccination (20, 21).

Together, these data indicate that the essential machinery for generation of robust T and B cell responses to pathogen-derived antigens is present during fetal life. They further suggest that the mechanisms that curb T cell inflammation *in utero* are not entirely cell-intrinsic, but also relate to extrinsic factors such as a lack of sufficient activating or co-stimulatory signals from antigen presenting cells (APCs) or from a tolerogenic cytokine environment. A better understanding of the conditions (e.g., timing, antigen load) that foster the priming and development of functionally competent pathogen-specific T cells (while avoiding induction of pathogen tolerance) could be of fundamental importance for efforts to develop vaccines that are optimally immunogenic in infancy.

APCs: PRESENTATION MATTERS

The maternal and fetal blood supply are separated by a single multinucleated cell layer termed the syncytiotrophoblast. Once malaria antigens or immune complexes cross the syncytiotrophoblast barrier, it is not clear where, how, and by "whom" (i.e., what cell type) they are taken up, processed, and presented to lymphocytes (**Figure 1**). This is a critical question, as APCs are key orchestrators of the immune response and play a paramount role in the initiation and regulation of adaptive immune responses through priming of antigen-specific T cells. Murine data indicate that neonatal T cells are extremely sensitive to the conditions of antigen presentation at priming, and small differences in the dose of antigen (22), type of APC (22, 23), and intensity of costimulation (22–24) strongly influence the efficacy of the ensuing T cell response. Given the many shortcomings of the neonatal mouse model (25), further studies are needed to confirm the relevance of these findings in human infants.

In adults, myeloid-lineage cells such as dendritic cells (DCs) and monocytes play a principal role in antigen presentation, although activated CD4 T and B cells also upregulate HLA-DR and can present antigen (26–28). In the fetus and neonate, dendritic cells and monocytes are both relatively inefficient in their ability to prime adaptive immune responses due to their reduced expression of MHC-II, co-stimulatory molecules, and Th1-polarizing cytokines (29–31). In particular, neonatal DC production of IL-12p70, the key cytokine required for Th1 polarization, is markedly reduced due to epigenetic regulation of the gene encoding its p35 subunit (29, 31–33). Th1 cytokine production by fetal DCs may be further inhibited by expression

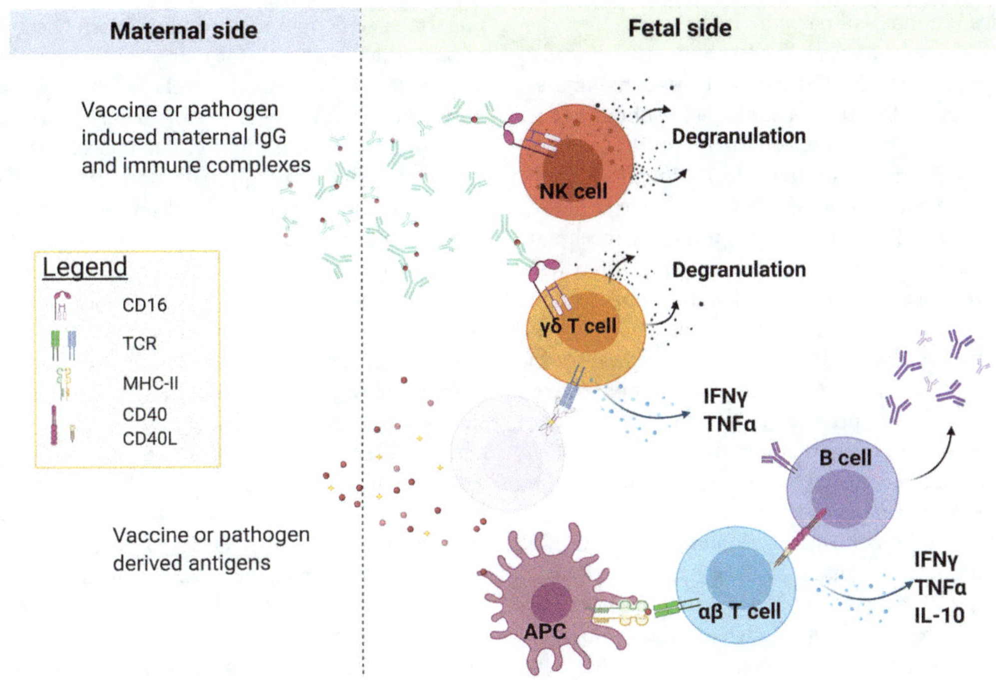

FIGURE 1 | Maternal-origin IgG is transported across the syncytiotrophoblast barrier of the placenta to the fetus via FcRn, possibly in the form of immune complexes. In areas of placental villous denudement or necrosis, unbound plasmodial antigen may also cross into the fetal circulation. *P. falciparum* antigens have been shown to prime fetal αβ T cells and B cells, the location and identity of the antigen-presenting cells remain unknown, but could include fetal Hofbauer cells, dendritic cells, or γδ T cells. Semi-innate Vγ9Vδ2 T cells can be directly activated by plasmodial-derived phosphoantigens via butyrophilin2a1 and butyrophilin3a1, even in the absence of prior antigen exposure. In addition, fetal lymphocytes expressing CD16/FcRγIIIa, including NK cells and possibly γδ T cells, may be activated by maternal IgG bound to antigen. Created with BioRender.com.

of arginase-2 (4). Fetal monocytes are also inefficient in their upregulation of costimulatory and antigen presentation machinery in response to IFNγ (34) despite enhanced sensitivity to inflammatory cytokines and increased expression of the IL6 receptor. Instead, inflammatory cytokines activate non-canonical signaling pathways in fetal monocytes, leading to upregulation of genes involved in the primitive antimicrobial response (34). This is likely a strategy to prevent activation of a potentially harmful anti-maternal adaptive response, which may trigger preterm labor and fetal expulsion (16).

It is possible that alternative cell populations may play a particularly important role in antigen presentation during fetal life. Macrophages termed Hofbauer cells reside within the placental villous stroma and express multiple Fc receptors, making them well-suited to a role in immune surveillance. Hofbauer cells are increased in placental malaria (35), but whether they play a role in antigen uptake is unclear. In an *ex vivo* human placental perfusion model, upon transplacental transfer immune-complexed MSP-1 was observed in the fetal villous stroma where it predominantly co-localized with fetal endothelial cells, not Hofbauer cells (36). Moreover, a recent and very detailed phenotypic analysis by Thomas et al. found that fetal-origin macrophages do not express HLA-DR (37). It is possible that non-myeloid cells, including non-classical lymphocytes, contribute to the induction of adaptive immune responses *in utero*. In adults, the Vγ9Vδ2 subset of γδ T cells (discussed in detail below) exhibit robust antigen presentation capabilities upon activation (38, 39) and can induce proliferation and differentiation of naïve αβ T cells comparable to that of mature DCs. Vγ9Vδ2 cells are highly prevalent during the second trimester (40), and their potential role in antigen presentation during fetal life merits further investigation.

INNATE ABILITY: NK CELLS AND NON-CLASSICAL LYMPHOCYTES

Innate immune populations may play a particularly important role in protecting the fetus and infant when little or no immunologic memory exists. In particular, semi-innate γδ T cells have several qualities that make them uniquely suited to protection of the fetus and infant. Unlike conventional αβ T cells, γδ T cells recognize conserved ligands and exhibit rapid, innate-like effector functions, including degranulation and cytokine production (41). This effector response is not dependent on prior antigen exposure nor on priming by dendritic cells, which are functionally immature in the fetus. γδ T cells are highly conserved across vertebrate species and are the first T cells to develop in the human fetus. It has been hypothesized that the primary selective advantage driving their remarkable conservation is their role in neonatal protection (39). Supporting this hypothesis, γδ T cells are required for protection of young, but not mature, mice in models of parasitic infection (42).

During malaria infection, a specialized subset of γδ T cells, defined by use of the δ2 and γ9 TCR chains, can act as innate-like effectors that can indirectly recognize phosphoantigens that are produced by the *Plasmodium* apicoplast (43). These Vγ9Vδ2 T cells exhibit intrinsic reactivity to *Plasmodium*, with rapid degranulation and production of IFNγ and TNFα, even in malaria-naïve individuals (44). They are able to kill extracellular merozoites via release of granulysin and inhibit parasite growth *in vitro* (45). Moreover, they have been associated with protection from malaria in human clinical trials (46, 47). In the fetus, this subset has been shown to dominate the γδ T cell repertoire in the second trimester (40). Following *in utero* malaria exposure, cord blood Vγ9Vδ2 T cells are preferentially activated, produce more IFNγ (48), and exhibit greater memory differentiation (49). Thus, Vγ9Vδ2 T cells may be poised to respond to *Plasmodium* infection in the fetus and neonate.

The role of NK cells and other innate lymphoid cells (ILCs) in the fetal and infant immune response to malaria has received little research attention. Fetal NK cells that develop early in gestation can respond robustly to antibody mediated and cytokine-induced stimulation, but respond weakly to HLA-devoid cells and are more susceptible to TGF-β mediated suppression (50). At birth, NK cells are highly responsive to immune complexes and exhibit robust antibody-dependent functions, including IFNγ production and degranulation (51). Higher cord blood frequencies of $CD56^{dim}CD16^{+}$ NK cells have been observed following maternal *P. falciparum* infection (52). In light of recent studies demonstrating an association between NK cell antibody dependent cellular cytotoxicity (ADCC) and malaria outcomes in children and adults (53), these findings raise the possibility that NK cells could play an important antimalarial role *in utero* and in the newborn through engagement of transplacentally acquired malaria-specific antibodies.

MATERNOFETAL ANTIBODY TRANSFER: PASSIVE AND AGGRESSIVE?

During gestation, maternal antibodies are transferred across the placenta to the fetus via an active transport mechanism mediated by FcRn, the neonatal Fc receptor. FcRn is expressed on syncytiotrophoblast cells beginning at approximately 13 weeks gestation (54), and selectively transfers IgG. Transfer of IgG increases as pregnancy progresses, rising sharply in the final month of gestation, such that full-term infants have IgG levels that generally exceed those of the mother (54, 55). FcRn-mediated transport is influenced by maternal IgG concentration and saturates in the setting of high total IgG levels.

Maternally derived antibodies are essential for infant protection from some pathogens that are commonly encountered during infancy. In the case of malaria, the importance of this passive maternal antibody transfer is not clear. It has been widely promulgated that transplacental transfer of antimalarial antibodies is responsible for the relatively low incidence of symptomatic malaria during the first 6 months of life. Yet, a thorough review of this literature found scant evidence to support a protective role in infancy, concluding instead that malaria-specific IgG in cord blood merely serves as a biomarker of maternal exposure (56). It should be noted, however, that most studies to address this relationship evaluated antibodies to only a very limited number of malaria antigens, and measured only total IgG, and not individual IgG subclasses.

IgG subclass and glycosylation can both greatly influence the efficiency of transplacental antibody transfer by FcRn (55). The overall transfer efficiency is highest for the IgG1 subclass, followed by IgG4, IgG3, and IgG2. It is notable that IgG3 is transferred to the fetus with low efficiency, as it is the strongest activator of complement via recruitment of C1q, and its potent opsonizing ability has been linked to clinical protection from malaria in adults and children (57–59). IgG3 also binds more strongly to FcγRIIIa, which is important in ADCC and other antibody-dependent functions, than other IgG subclasses (60). Interestingly, a polymorphism in the FcRn-binding domain of IgG3 (H435) has been associated with increased transplacental transfer of malaria-specific IgG3, increased half-life of IgG3 in the infant, and protection from clinical malaria during infancy (61). Given this evidence, it will be important to understand the IgG subclass profile of transplacentally-transferred IgG in malaria-endemic regions (62), as well as the significance of opsonized antigen, complement activation, and FcR-expressing fetal cells in infant protection from malaria. Furthermore, secondary glycan structures, which can vary across pathogen-specific antibody repertoires within an individual (51, 63, 64), have also been shown to modulate the efficiency of transplacental IgG transfer. For example, digalactosylated Fc-glycans bind more strongly to FcRn leading to increased transplacental transfer (51), and they also preferentially bind FcγRIIIa leading to better activation of neonatal NK cells (51). As vaccine adjuvants can influence antibody subclass and glycosylation (65) which in turn influence placental transfer of antibody (55), vaccine design should prioritize adjuvants that enable better transplacental transfer and activation of neonatal effector cells.

In addition to conferring passive immunity, maternofetal antibody transfer may play a role in conveying pathogens and pathogen-derived antigens to the fetus in the form of antigen-antibody complexes. While some malaria antigens may breach the maternofetal barrier due to focal denudement of the syncytiotrophoblast cell layer, the more common route of transfer is likely via FcRn-mediated active transport of antigen-antibody complexes (8, 36), as supported by experimental evidence from an *ex vivo* placental perfusion model (36). There is also some evidence that FcRn can facilitate congenital infection by mediating transfer of CMV and ZIKV virions in the form of immune complexes (66–68). Hence, maternal immunoglobulins can at times act as a Trojan horse, ferrying pathogen-derived antigens (or even intact pathogens) to the fetus.

IMPLICATIONS FOR VACCINATION IN PREGNANCY AND EARLY INFANCY

The ultimate goal of better understanding the components of the fetal, neonatal and pregnant immune systems is to enable the translation of this knowledge to vaccine development. Late stage trials are underway for vaccines to prevent placental malaria by inducing maternal antibodies against VAR2CSA, a pregnancy-specific adhesion ligand that is thought to be an important mediator of placental adherence (69). The goal of this vaccine approach is to stimulate maternal immunity and thus prevent placental malaria, sparing the infant from the clinical sequalae of placental insufficiency and inflammation, which include prematurity and poor growth. This distinguishes it from other vaccines targeting pregnant women, for which the rationale is to confer passive IgG-mediated immunity to the infant. Examples of this approach include vaccination against pertussis, influenza, and tetanus, all of which can be safely administered during pregnancy and induce high neutralizing titers of maternal antibodies that are transferred transplacentally and confer protection to the infant during the early months of life (70–73). Immunizing pregnant women against malaria (with RTS,S, whole sporozoites, or other vaccine candidates) could similarly induce transfer of malaria-specific IgG to the infant. However, whether this passive immunization approach would be of value hinges largely upon the still unanswered question of whether malaria-specific IgG antibodies, or a subclass thereof (e.g., IgG3), confer protection in infants. Moreover, it is important to note that maternal immunization can have adverse consequences by interfering with induction of antibodies in the infant. This has been most clearly demonstrated in the case of pertussis and viral pathogens such as measles, where maternal-origin IgG neutralizes vaccine antigen in the infant and thus preempts priming of infant B cells (74–77). However, even non-neutralizing antibodies can inhibit infant antibody production by mechanisms that may include masking of immunogenic epitopes, Fc-mediated engagement of inhibitory receptors, and/or clearance of maternal immune complexes; hence maternal antibody interference may be of concern for malaria. A recent meta-analysis estimated that maternal antibody inhibition results in a reduction of infant antibody responses to a broad range of antigens in common childhood vaccines (78). Interference by maternal-origin IgG has been hypothesized to contribute to the poor immunogenicity of RTS,S in infants (79). Ultimately such concerns may be mitigated by Fc engineering (currently being developed for monoclonal antibody therapies) and tailoring of adjuvants to induce antibodies of the desired subtype and glycosylation characteristics. As it is difficult to predict whether the benefits of maternal antibodies would outweigh the concern for antibody interference, the impact of maternal-origin IgG on infant vaccine responses should be an area of careful empiric investigation as malaria vaccine candidates enter field trials.

Mounting evidence that adaptive T and B cell responses can be primed *in utero* raises the additional question of whether *active immunization* of the fetus may indeed be possible. Such a strategy would be dependent upon delivery of antigen to the fetus in a context that favors priming of antigen-specific fetal T and/or B cells. The demonstration that fetal B and T cells are primed naturally in response to placental malaria in some infants (2, 8) should lend optimism to this prospect. Additionally, it has been shown that fetal T cells are primed in response to maternal influenza vaccination (20). While *in utero* vaccination may seem like a far horizon, these observations provide proof of concept that induction of protective immunity prior to birth may be possible. However, efforts toward fetal immunization would need to address the potential for induction of pathogen-specific tolerance *in utero*, which has been reported in some malaria-exposed infants (18, 80).

CONCLUSION

As pregnancy progresses, the fetal immune system gradually evolves from one that is skewed toward tolerance to one that is poised to fight foreign pathogens. The research agenda for translating recent advances in our understanding of fetal and neonatal immunology into vaccines that are safe and immunogenic when administered in early infancy is now coming into focus. Understanding how to best prime adaptive immune responses in the neonate is critical, due to both the increased susceptibility of newborns to infectious diseases and to the increased healthcare contact of this vulnerable population at the time of birth. This will be particularly important in the context of malaria vaccines, as the vast majority of malaria deaths occur in children under the age of five. Recent evidence from studies of infants exposed to perinatal pathogens indicates that fetal B and T cells can be primed and differentiate into effector cells *in utero*, providing grounds for optimism that they may respond to vaccination. In order to harness this intrinsic capability to engender durable antigen-specific memory in neonates, we will need to refine our understanding of which APCs are most able to prime fetal and neonatal immune responses and which adjuvants are best able to target and stimulate these APCs.

AUTHOR CONTRIBUTIONS

PC, LF, and MF wrote the manuscript. All authors contributed to the article and approved the submitted version.

REFERENCES

1. Haynes BF, Martin ME, Kay HH, Kurtzberg J. Early events in human T cell ontogeny. Phenotypic characterization and immunohistologic localization of T cell precursors in early human fetal tissues. *J Exp Med.* (1988) 168:1061–80. doi: 10.1084/jem.168.3.1061
2. Odorizzi PM, Jagannathan P, McIntyre TI, Budker R, Prahl M, Auma A, et al. In utero priming of highly functional effector T cell responses to human malaria. *Sci Transl Med.* (2018) 10:eaat6176. doi: 10.1126/scitranslmed.aat6176
3. Vermijlen D, Brouwer M, Donner C, Liesnard C, Tackoen M, Van Rysselberge M, et al. Human cytomegalovirus elicits fetal γδ T cell

responses in utero. *J Exp Med.* (2010) 207:807–21. doi: 10.1084/jem.20090348
4. McGovern N, Shin A, Low G, Low D, Duan K, Yao LJ, et al. Human fetal dendritic cells promote prenatal T-cell immune suppression through arginase-2. *Nature.* (2017) 546:662–6. doi: 10.1038/nature22795
5. Bunis D, Bronevetsky Y, Krow-Lucal E, Bhakta NR, Kim CC, Nerella S, et al. *Single-Cell Mapping of Progressive Fetal-to-Adult Transition in Human Hematopoiesis.* Rochester, NY: Social Science Research Network (2020). doi: 10.2139/ssrn.3569532
6. Dellicour S, Tatem AJ, Guerra CA, Snow RW, Kuile FO ter. Quantifying the number of pregnancies at risk of malaria in 2007: a demographic study. *PLoS Med.* (2010) 7:e1000221. doi: 10.1371/journal.pmed.1000221
7. Desai M, Kuile FO ter, Nosten F, McGready R, Asamoa K, Brabin B, et al. Epidemiology and burden of malaria in pregnancy. *Lancet Infect Dis.* (2007) 7:93–104. doi: 10.1016/S1473-3099(07)70021-X
8. Tassi Yunga S, Kayatani AK, Fogako J, Leke RJI, Leke RGF, Taylor DW. Timing of the human prenatal antibody response to *Plasmodium falciparum* antigens. *PLoS ONE.* (2017) 12:e0184571. doi: 10.1371/journal.pone.0184571
9. Metenou S, Suguitan AL, Long C, Leke RGF, Taylor DW. Fetal immune responses to *Plasmodium falciparum* antigens in a malaria-endemic region of Cameroon. *J Immunol.* (2007) 178:2770–7. doi: 10.4049/jimmunol.178.5.2770
10. Burt TD. Fetal regulatory t cells and peripheral immune tolerance *in utero*: implications for development and disease. *Am J Reprod Immunol.* (2013) 69:346–58. doi: 10.1111/aji.12083
11. Rackaityte E, Halkias J. Mechanisms of fetal T Cell tolerance and immune regulation. *Front Immunol.* (2020) 11:588. doi: 10.3389/fimmu.2020.00588
12. Elahi S, Ertelt JM, Kinder JM, Jiang TT, Zhang X, Xin L, et al. Immunosuppressive CD71+ erythroid cells compromise neonatal host defence against infection. *Nature.* (2013) 504:158–62. doi: 10.1038/nature12675
13. Gervassi A, Lejarcegui N, Dross S, Jacobson A, Itaya G, Kidzeru E, et al. Myeloid derived suppressor cells are present at high frequency in neonates and suppress *in vitro* T cell responses. *PLoS ONE.* (2014) 9:e107816. doi: 10.1371/journal.pone.0107816
14. Zhivaki D, Lemoine S, Lim A, Morva A, Vidalain P-O, Schandene L, et al. Respiratory syncytial virus infects regulatory B cells in human neonates via chemokine receptor CX3CR1 and promotes lung disease severity. *Immunity.* (2017) 46:301–14. doi: 10.1016/j.immuni.2017.01.010
15. Zhang X, Mozeleski B, Lemoine S, Dériaud E, Lim A, Zhivaki D, et al. CD4 T cells with effector memory phenotype and function develop in the sterile environment of the fetus. *Sci Transl Med.* (2014) 6:238ra72. doi: 10.1126/scitranslmed.3008748
16. Frascoli M, Coniglio L, Witt R, Jeanty C, Fleck-Derderian S, Myers DE, et al. Alloreactive fetal T cells promote uterine contractility in preterm labor via IFN-γ and TNF-α. *Sci Transl Med.* (2018) 10:eaan2263. doi: 10.1126/scitranslmed.aan2263
17. Marchant A, Appay V, van der Sande M, Dulphy N, Liesnard C, Kidd M, et al. Mature CD8+ T lymphocyte response to viral infection during fetal life. *J Clin Invest.* (2003) 111:1747–55. doi: 10.1172/JCI200317470
18. Malhotra I, Dent A, Mungai P, Wamachi A, Ouma JH, Narum DL, et al. Can prenatal malaria exposure produce an immune tolerant phenotype?: a prospective birth cohort study in Kenya. *PLoS Med.* (2009) 6:e1000116. doi: 10.1371/journal.pmed.1000116
19. King CL, Malhotra I, Wamachi A, Kioko J, Mungai P, Wahab SA, et al. Acquired immune responses to *Plasmodium falciparum* merozoite surface protein-1 in the human fetus. *J Immunol.* (2002) 168:356–64. doi: 10.4049/jimmunol.168.1.356
20. Rastogi D, Wang C, Mao X, Lendor C, Rothman PB, Miller RL. Antigen-specific immune responses to influenza vaccine in utero. *J Clin Invest.* (2007) 117:1637–46. doi: 10.1172/JCI29466
21. Englund JA, Mbawuike IN, Hammill H, Holleman MC, Baxter BD, Glezen WP. Maternal immunization with influenza or tetanus toxoid vaccine for passive antibody protection in young infants. *J Infect Dis.* (1993) 168:647–56. doi: 10.1093/infdis/168.3.647
22. Sarzotti M, Robbins DS, Hoffman PM. Induction of protective CTL responses in newborn mice by a murine retrovirus. *Science.* (1996) 271:1726–8. doi: 10.1126/science.271.5256.1726
23. Ridge JP, Fuchs EJ, Matzinger P. Neonatal tolerance revisited: turning on newborn T cells with dendritic cells. *Science.* (1996) 271:1723–6. doi: 10.1126/science.271.5256.1723
24. Forsthuber T, Yip HC, Lehmann PV. Induction of TH1 and TH2 immunity in neonatal mice. *Science.* (1996) 271:1728–30. doi: 10.1126/science.271.5256.1728
25. Adkins B, Leclerc C, Marshall-Clarke S. Neonatal adaptive immunity comes of age. *Nat Rev Immunol.* (2004) 4:553–64. doi: 10.1038/nri1394
26. Lanzavecchia A, Roosnek E, Gregory T, Berman P, Abrignani S. T cells can present antigens such as HIV gp120 targeted to their own surface molecules. *Nature.* (1988) 334:530–2. doi: 10.1038/334530a0
27. Barnaba V, Watts C, Boer M de, Lane P, Lanzavecchia A. Professional presentation of antigen by activated human T cells. *Eur J Immunol.* (1994) 24:71–5. doi: 10.1002/eji.1830240112
28. Cruz-Adalia A, Ramirez-Santiago G, Osuna-Pérez J, Torres-Torresano M, Zorita V, Martínez-Riaño A, et al. Conventional CD4+ T cells present bacterial antigens to induce cytotoxic and memory CD8+ T cell responses. *Nat Commun.* (2017) 8:1591. doi: 10.1038/s41467-017-01661-7
29. Goriely S. A defect in nucleosome remodeling prevents IL-12(p35) gene transcription in neonatal dendritic cells. *J Exp Med.* (2004) 199:1011–6. doi: 10.1084/jem.20031272
30. Aksoy E, Albarani V, Nguyen M, Laes J-F, Ruelle J-L, De Wit D, et al. Interferon regulatory factor 3-dependent responses to lipopolysaccharide are selectively blunted in cord blood cells. *Blood.* (2007) 109:2887–93. doi: 10.1182/blood-2006-06-027862
31. Renneson J, Dutta B, Goriely S, Danis B, Lecomte S, Laes J-F, et al. IL-12 and type I IFN response of neonatal myeloid DC to human CMV infection. *Eur J Immunol.* (2009) 39:2789–99. doi: 10.1002/eji.200939414
32. Kollmann TR, Crabtree J, Rein-Weston A, Blimkie D, Thommai F, Wang XY, et al. Neonatal innate TLR-mediated responses are distinct from those of adults. *J Immunol.* (2009) 183:7150–60. doi: 10.4049/jimmunol.0901481
33. Upham JW, Lee PT, Holt BJ, Heaton T, Prescott SL, Sharp MJ, et al. Development of interleukin-12-producing capacity throughout childhood. *Infect Immun.* (2002) 70:6583–8. doi: 10.1128/IAI.70.12.6583-6588.2002
34. Krow-Lucal ER, Kim CC, Burt TD, McCune JM. Distinct functional programming of human fetal and adult monocytes. *Blood.* (2014) 123:1897–904. doi: 10.1182/blood-2013-11-536094
35. Gaw SL, Hromatka BS, Ngeleza S, Buarpung S, Ozarslan N, Tshefu A, et al. Differential activation of fetal hofbauer cells in primigravidas is associated with decreased birth weight in symptomatic placental malaria. *Malar Res Treat.* (2019) 2019:1378174. doi: 10.1155/2019/1378174
36. May K, Grube M, Malhotra I, Long CA, Singh S, Mandaliya K, et al. Antibody-dependent transplacental transfer of malaria blood-stage antigen using a human ex vivo placental perfusion model. *PLoS ONE.* (2009) 4:e7986. doi: 10.1371/journal.pone.0007986
37. Thomas JR, Appios A, Zhao X, Dutkiewicz R, Donde M, Lee CYC, et al. Phenotypic and functional characterization of first-trimester human placental macrophages, Hofbauer cells. *J Exp Med.* (2020) 218:e20200891. doi: 10.1084/jem.20200891
38. Brandes M, Willimann K, Moser B. Professional antigen-presentation function by human γδ T cells. *Science.* (2005) 309:264–8. doi: 10.1126/science.1110267
39. Vantourout P, Hayday A. Six-of-the-best: unique contributions of γδ T cells to immunology. *Nat Rev Immunol.* (2013) 13:88–100. doi: 10.1038/nri3384
40. Dimova T, Brouwer M, Gosselin F, Tassignon J, Leo O, Donner C, et al. Effector Vγ9Vδ2 T cells dominate the human fetal γδ T-cell repertoire. *PNAS.* (2015) 112:E556–65. doi: 10.1073/pnas.1412058112
41. Vermijlen D, Gatti D, Kouzeli A, Rus T, Eberl M. γδ T cell responses: How many ligands will it take till we know? *Semin Cell Dev Biol.* (2018) 84:75–86. doi: 10.1016/j.semcdb.2017.10.009
42. Ramsburg E, Tigelaar R, Craft J, Hayday A. Age-dependent requirement for γδ T cells in the primary but not secondary protective immune response against an intestinal parasite. *J Exp Med.* (2003) 198:1403–14. doi: 10.1084/jem.20030050
43. Behr C, Poupot R, Peyrat MA, Poquet Y, Constant P, Dubois P, et al. *Plasmodium falciparum* stimuli for human gammadelta T cells are related to phosphorylated antigens of mycobacteria. *Infect Immun.* (1996) 64:2892–6. doi: 10.1128/IAI.64.8.2892-2896.1996

44. Ho M, Webster HK, Tongtawe P, Pattanapanyasat K, Weidanz WP. Increased gamma delta T cells in acute *Plasmodium falciparum* malaria. *Immunol Lett.* (1990) 25:139–41. doi: 10.1016/0165-2478(90)90105-Y
45. Costa G, Loizon S, Guenot M, Mocan I, Halary F, Saint-Basile G de, et al. Control of *Plasmodium falciparum* erythrocytic cycle: γδ T cells target the red blood cell–invasive merozoites. *Blood.* (2011) 118:6952–62. doi: 10.1182/blood-2011-08-376111
46. Seder RA, Chang LJ, Enama ME, Zephir KL, Sarwar UN, Gordon IJ, et al. Protection against malaria by intravenous immunization with a nonreplicating sporozoite vaccine. *Science.* (2013) 341:1359–65. doi: 10.1126/science.1241800
47. Lyke KE, Ishizuka AS, Berry AA, Chakravarty S, DeZure A, Enama ME, et al. Attenuated PfSPZ Vaccine induces strain-transcending T cells and durable protection against heterologous controlled human malaria infection. *PNAS.* (2017) 114:2711–6. doi: 10.1073/pnas.1615324114
48. Engelmann I, Moeller U, Santamaria A, Kremsner PG, Luty AJ. Differing activation status and immune effector molecule expression profiles of neonatal and maternal lymphocytes in an African population. *Immunology.* (2006) 119:515–21. doi: 10.1111/j.1365-2567.2006.02466.x
49. Cairo C, Longinaker N, Cappelli G, Leke RGF, Ondo MM, Djokam R, et al. Cord blood Vγ2Vδ2 T cells provide a molecular marker for the influence of pregnancy-associated malaria on neonatal immunity. *J Infect Dis.* (2014) 209:1653–62. doi: 10.1093/infdis/jit802
50. Ivarsson MA, Loh L, Marquardt N, Kekäläinen E, Berglin L, Björkström NK, et al. Differentiation and functional regulation of human fetal NK cells. *J Clin Invest.* (2013) 123:3889–901. doi: 10.1172/JCI68989
51. Jennewein MF, Goldfarb I, Dolatshahi S, Cosgrove C, Noelette FJ, Krykbaeva M, et al. Fc glycan-mediated regulation of placental antibody transfer. *Cell.* (2019) 178:202–15.e14. doi: 10.1016/j.cell.2019.05.044
52. Nouatin O, Gbédandé K, Ibitokou S, Vianou B, Houngbegnon P, Ezinmegnon S, et al. Infants' peripheral blood lymphocyte composition reflects both maternal and post-natal infection with *Plasmodium falciparum. PLoS ONE.* (2015) 10:e0139606. doi: 10.1371/journal.pone.0139606
53. Hart GT, Tran TM, Theorell J, Schlums H, Arora G, Rajagopalan S, et al. Adaptive NK cells in people exposed to *Plasmodium falciparum* correlate with protection from malaria. *J Exp Med.* (2019) 216:1280–90. doi: 10.1084/jem.20181681
54. Jauniaux E, Jurkovic D, Gulbis B, Liesnard C, Lees C, Campbell S. Materno-fetal immunoglobulin transfer and passive immunity during the first trimester of human pregnancy. *Hum Reprod.* (1995) 10:3297–300. doi: 10.1093/oxfordjournals.humrep.a135906
55. Wilcox CR, Holder B, Jones CE. Factors affecting the FcRn-mediated transplacental transfer of antibodies and implications for vaccination in pregnancy. *Front Immunol.* (2017) 8:1294. doi: 10.3389/fimmu.2017.01294
56. Dobbs KR, Dent AE. Plasmodium malaria and antimalarial antibodies in the first year of life. *Parasitology.* (2016) 143:129–38. doi: 10.1017/S0031182015001626
57. Richards JS, Stanisic DI, Fowkes FJ, Tavul L, Dabod E, Thompson JK, et al. Association between naturally acquired antibodies to erythrocyte-binding antigens of *Plasmodium falciparum* and protection from malaria and high-density parasitemia. *Clin Infect Dis.* (2010) 51:e50–60. doi: 10.1086/656413
58. Boyle MJ, Reiling L, Feng G, Langer C, Osier FH, Aspeling-Jones H, et al. Human antibodies fix complement to inhibit *Plasmodium falciparum* invasion of erythrocytes and are associated with protection against malaria. *Immunity.* (2015) 42:580–90. doi: 10.1016/j.immuni.2015.02.012
59. Roussilhon C, Oeuvray C, Muller-Graf C, Tall A, Rogier C, Trape JF,et al. Long-term clinical protection from falciparum malaria is strongly associated with IgG3 antibodies to merozoite surface protein 3. *PLoS Med.* (2007) 4:e320. doi: 10.1371/journal.pmed.0040320
60. Bruhns P, Iannascoli B, England P, Mancardi DA, Fernandez N, Jorieux S, et al. Specificity and affinity of human Fcγ receptors and their polymorphic variants for human IgG subclasses. *Blood.* (2009) 113:3716–25. doi: 10.1182/blood-2008-09-179754
61. Dechavanne C, Dechavanne S, Sadissou I, Lokossou AG, Alvarado F, Dambrun M, et al. Associations between an IgG3 polymorphism in the binding domain for FcRn, transplacental transfer of malaria-specific IgG3, and protection against *Plasmodium falciparum* malaria during infancy: a birth cohort study in Benin. *PLoS Med.* (2017) 14:e1002403. doi: 10.1371/journal.pmed.1002403
62. Dobano C, Santano R, Vidal M, Jimenez A, Jairoce C, Ubillos I, et al. Differential patterns of IgG subclass responses to *Plasmodium falciparum* antigens in relation to malaria protection and RTS,S vaccination. *Front Immunol.* (2019) 10:439. doi: 10.3389/fimmu.2019.00439
63. Pou C, Nkulikiyimfura D, Henckel E, Olin A, Lakshmikanth T, Mikes J, et al. The repertoire of maternal anti-viral antibodies in human newborns. *Nat Med.* (2019) 25:591–6. doi: 10.1038/s41591-019-0392-8
64. Martinez DR, Fong Y, Li SH, Yang F, Jennewein MF, Weiner JA, et al. Fc characteristics mediate selective placental transfer of IgG in HIV-infected women. *Cell.* (2019) 178:190–201.e11. doi: 10.1016/j.cell.2019.05.046
65. Francica JR, Zak DE, Linde C, Siena E, Johnson C, Juraska M, et al. Innate transcriptional effects by adjuvants on the magnitude, quality, and durability of HIV envelope responses in NHPs. *Blood Adv.* (2017) 1:2329–42. doi: 10.1182/bloodadvances.2017011411
66. Maidji E, McDonagh S, Genbacev O, Tabata T, Pereira L. Maternal antibodies enhance or prevent cytomegalovirus infection in the placenta by neonatal Fc receptor-mediated transcytosis. *Am J Pathol.* (2006) 168:1210–26. doi: 10.2353/ajpath.2006.050482
67. Hermanns K, Göhner C, Kopp A, Schmidt A, Merz WM, Markert UR, et al. Zika virus infection in human placental tissue explants is enhanced in the presence of dengue virus antibodies in-vitro. *Emerg Microbes Infect.* (2018) 7:1–8. doi: 10.1038/s41426-018-0199-6
68. Zimmerman MG, Quicke KM, O'Neal JT, Arora N, Machiah D, Priyamvada L, et al. Cross-reactive dengue virus antibodies augment Zika virus infection of human placental macrophages. *Cell Host Microbe.* (2018) 24:731–42.e6. doi: 10.1016/j.chom.2018.10.008
69. Fried M, Duffy PE. Malaria during pregnancy. *Cold Spring Harb Perspect Med.* (2017) 7:a025551. doi: 10.1101/cshperspect.a025551
70. Winter K, Nickell S, Powell M, Harriman K. Effectiveness of prenatal versus postpartum tetanus, diphtheria, and a cellular pertussis vaccination in preventing infant pertussis. *Clin Infect Dis.* (2017) 64:3–8. doi: 10.1093/cid/ciw634
71. Healy CM, Munoz FM, Rench MA, Halasa N, Edwards KM, Baker CJ. Prevalence of pertussis antibodies in maternal delivery, cord, and infant serum. *J Infect Dis.* (2004) 190:335–40. doi: 10.1086/421033
72. Nunes MC, Cutland CL, Jones S, Hugo A, Madimabe R, Simões EAF, et al. Duration of infant protection against influenza illness conferred by maternal immunization: secondary analysis of a randomized clinical trial. *JAMA Pediatr.* (2016) 170:840. doi: 10.1001/jamapediatrics.2016.0921
73. Chen ST, Edsall G, Peel MM, Sinnathuray TA. Timing of antenatal tetanus immunization for effective protection of the neonate. *Bull World Health Organ.* (1983) 61:159–65.
74. Englund JA, Anderson EL, Reed GF, Decker MD, Edwards KM, Pichichero ME, et al. The effect of maternal antibody on the serologic response and the incidence of adverse reactions after primary immunization with acellular and whole-cell pertussis vaccines combined with diphtheria and tetanus toxoids. *Pediatrics.* (1995) 96:580–4.
75. Jones C, Pollock L, Barnett SM, Battersby A, Kampmann B. The relationship between concentration of specific antibody at birth and subsequent response to primary immunization. *Vaccine.* (2014) 32:996–1002. doi: 10.1016/j.vaccine.2013.11.104
76. Albrecht P, Ennis FA, Saltzman EJ, Krugman S. Persistence of maternal antibody in infants beyond 12 months: mechanism of measles vaccine failure. *J Pediatr.* (1977) 91:715–8. doi: 10.1016/S0022-3476(77)81021-4
77. Njie-Jobe J, Nyamweya S, Miles DJC, van der Sande M, Zaman S, Touray E, et al. Immunological impact of an additional early measles vaccine in Gambian children: responses to a boost at 3 years. *Vaccine.* (2012) 30:2543–50. doi: 10.1016/j.vaccine.2012.01.083
78. Voysey M, Kelly DF, Fanshawe TR, Sadarangani M, O'Brien KL, Perera R, et al. The influence of maternally derived antibody and infant age at vaccination on infant vaccine responses: an individual participant meta-analysis. *JAMA Pediatr.* (2017) 171:637. doi: 10.1001/jamapediatrics.2 017.0638
79. Rts T, Partnership (2014) SCT. Efficacy and safety of the RTS,S/AS01 malaria vaccine during 18 months after vaccination: a phase 3 randomized, controlled trial in children and young infants at 11 African sites. *PLoS Med.* (2014) 11:e1001685. doi: 10.1371/journal.pmed.1001685

80. Dent A, Malhotra I, Mungai P, Muchiri E, Crabb BS, Kazura JW, et al. Prenatal malaria immune experience affects acquisition of *Plasmodium falciparum* merozoite surface protein-1 invasion inhibitory antibodies during infancy. *J Immunol.* (2006) 177:7139–45. doi: 10.4049/jimmunol.177.10.7139

2

The Development, Fine Specificity, and Importance of High-Avidity Antibodies to VAR2CSA in Pregnant Cameroonian Women Living in Yaoundé, an Urban City

Koko Vanda[1], Naveen Bobbili[1], Masako Matsunaga[2], John J. Chen[2], Ali Salanti[3], Rose F. G. Leke[4] and Diane Wallace Taylor[1]*

[1] Department of Tropical Medicine, Medical Microbiology and Pharmacology, John A. Burns School of Medicine, University of Hawaii, Honolulu, HI, United States, [2] Department of Quantitative Health Sciences, John A. Burns School of Medicine, University of Hawaii, Honolulu, HI, United States, [3] Centre for Medical Parasitology, Department for Immunology and Microbiology, Faculty of Health and Medical Sciences, University of Copenhagen and Department of Infectious Disease, Copenhagen University Hospital, Copenhagen, Denmark, [4] Faculty of Medicine and Biomedical Research, The Biotechnology Center, University of Yaoundé 1, Yaoundé, Cameroon

***Correspondence:**
Diane Wallace Taylor
dwtaylor@hawaii.edu

Pregnant women infected with *Plasmodium falciparum* often produce antibodies (**Abs**) to VAR2CSA, a ligand that binds to placental chondroitin sulfate A causing placental malaria (**PM**). Antibodies to VAR2CSA are associated with improved pregnancy outcomes. Antibody avidity is a surrogate marker for the extent of maturation of the humoral immune response. Little is known about high avidity Abs to VAR2CSA for women living in urban African cities. Therefore, this study sought to determine: i) if high avidity Abs to full-length VAR2CSA (**FV2**) increase with gravidity in women in Yaoundé, Cameroon exposed to ~ 0.3-1.1 infectious mosquito bites per month, ii) if high avidity Abs to FV2 are directed against a specific region of VAR2CSA, and iii) if having high avidity Abs to FV2 improve pregnancy outcomes. Plasma samples collected at delivery from 695 women who had Abs to FV2 were evaluated. Ab levels and the Avidity Index (**AI**), defined as the percent Abs remaining bound to FV2 after incubation with 3M NH_4SCN, were determined. Similar Ab levels to FV2 were present in women of all gravidities (G1 through 6+; p=0.80), except significantly lower levels were detected in PM–negative (PM–) primigravidae (p <0.001). Median Ab avidities increased between gravidity 1 and 2 (p<0.001) and remained stable thereafter (G3-G6+: p=0.51). These results suggest that B cell clonal expansion began during the first pregnancy, with clonal selection primarily occurring during the second. However, the majority of women (84%) had AI <35, a level of high avidity Abs previously reported to be associated with improved pregnancy outcomes. When plasma from 107 Cameroonian women was tested against 8 different regions of FV2, high avidity Abs were predominately restricted to DBL5 with median AI of 50 compared to AI <25 for the other domains. The only significance influence of high avidity Abs on pregnancy outcome was that babies born to mothers with AI above the median were 104 g heavier than babies born to women with AI below the median (p=0.045). These results suggest that a vaccine that boosts maturation of the immune response to VAR2CSA may be beneficial for women residing in urban areas.

Keywords: ***Plasmodium falciparum*, pregnant women, placental malaria, VAR2CSA, antibody avidity, urban cities**

INTRODUCTION

Plasmodium falciparum infections during pregnancy may be harmful to both the mother and the developing fetus. Malaria-infected erythrocytes (**IE**) sequester in the intervillous space (**IVS**) of the placenta and stimulate an inflammatory response, thereby increasing the risk of maternal complications, stillbirths, premature deliveries, reduced infant birthweights, and low birthweight babies (1–4). Primigravidae are more susceptible to the effects of placental malaria (**PM**) than multigravida women. Sequestration is mediated primarily by an antigen expressed on the surface of IE called VAR2CSA that binds to chondroitin sulfate A (CSA) on syncytial trophoblasts lining the IVS (5, 6). Since CSA is only expressed in the placenta, IE expressing VAR2CSA are normally quickly eliminated in children and non-pregnant adults before an immune response is induced. However, when women are infected with *P. falciparum* for the first-time during pregnancy, they are exposed to VAR2CSA and a primary immune response is induced. The presence of antibodies (Abs) to VAR2CSA, especially in subsequent pregnancies, reduces the severity of PM and has been associated with increased infant birthweight, longer periods of pregnancy, reduced prevalence of PM, and reduced risk of low birthweight (LBW) babies (6–10) [reviewed in (11)]. Thus, immunity to PM and VAR2CSA is unique, in that it is pregnancy-associated and gravidity dependent.

Most studies assessing the benefits of Abs to VAR2CSA have been conducted in areas with high malaria transmission. The impact of Abs to VAR2CSA on pregnancy outcomes in urban settings with intermediate or low levels of transmission is less clear, in part, because a large sample size is needed to detect small changes. Currently, neither the amount, specificity nor immunological properties of Abs to VAR2CSA needed to improve pregnancy outcomes is known. In general, high Ab levels to VAR2CSA are associated with infection, not protection (11). Thus, many questions remain about the natural acquisition of Abs to VAR2CSA in pregnant women and their role in pregnancy outcomes in different transmission settings.

Antibody avidity, or functional affinity, is often listed as a functional assay, in that it measures the overall strength of binding of Abs circulating in plasma to an antigen (12). During affinity maturation, antigen is presented on follicular dendritic cells within germinal centers and B cells with B-cell receptors (sIg) that can outcompete circulating Abs and other maturing B cells for the antigen will be selected; thereby, increasing Ab avidity. Thus, Ab avidity is a marker for the extent of maturation of the humoral response against an antigen. Several studies have suggested that high avidity Abs to VAR2CSA might be beneficial to pregnant women residing in areas with intense malaria transmission. For example, pregnant women with high levels of high avidity Abs to VAR2CSA (i.e., >35% of Ab remained bound after treatment with 3M NH_4SCN) early in pregnancy, had a reduced risk of placental malaria at delivery; whereas, having high Ab levels to VAR2CSA *per se* was not associated with improved pregnancy outcome (13). A second study, designed to identify differences in the fine-specificity of Abs to VAR2CSA between PM -positive (**PM+**) and PM− multigravid women, found that the only significant difference was the presence of higher levels of high avidity Abs to full-length VAR2CSA (**FV2**) among the 21 assays studied using VAR2CSA-associated recombinant proteins (14). It remains unclear, however, if Ab avidity plays a direct role in enhancing inhibition or releasing IE bound to trophoblasts or if avidity is simply a marker of maturation of the overall immune response to VAR2CSA.

The role of Abs to VAR2CA in a low to intermediate transmission areas, such as the city of Yaoundé, Cameroon, where pregnant women were exposed to ~0.3 to 1.1 infectious mosquito bites per month, remains unclear (15, 16). Tutterrow et al., followed 50 women throughout pregnancy who were positive for *P. falciparum* (Pf) parasites either by microscopy or PCR early in the second trimester and reported that 60% of the women who were PM− at delivery, lacked Abs to FV2 (17). These data suggest that Abs to antigens other than VAR2CSA assist in clearing infected erythrocytes. Several studies have shown that Abs to other non-VAR2CSA *P. falciparum* antigens were associated with improved pregnancy outcomes in women residing in Yaoundé, Cameroon (8, 18). Thus, the prevalence, amount and importance of high avidity Abs to VAR2CSA in areas with relatively low malaria transmission remains to be determined.

The purpose of the current study was to determine if: i) high avidity Abs to full-length VAR2CSA (**FV2**) increased with gravidity in women in Yaoundé, Cameroon prior to implementation of intermittent preventive treatment (**IPTp**), ii) high avidity Abs to FV2 were directed against a specific region of FV2, and iii) having high avidity Abs to FV2 at delivery was associated with reduced prevalence of PM or improved infant birthweight.

MATERIALS AND METHODS

Ethical Approvals

The original study, conducted between 1995 and 2001, was approved by the National Ethics Committee, Cameroon and the IRB, Georgetown University (IRB#:1994-158) for collection of plasma, placental tissue and clinical information. Women participating in the study gave written informed consent. The use of the de-identified, archival plasma samples and clinical information in the current study were determined to be exempt from human subjects' research by the Committee on Human Subjects, University of Hawaii-Manoa (CHS#21891).

The Study Design

Clinical and Laboratory Data

Plasma used in this study were consecutively collected at delivery between 1995 and 2001 in Yaoundé, Cameroon, at the Biyem Assi District Hospital where care was provided to women living in the adjacent area and at the Central Maternity Hospital, a referral hospital for a diverse group of women (19). At the time of recruitment, information on the woman's pregnancy and malaria histories were recorded on a standardized questionnaire, a heparinized peripheral blood sample was drawn, and a biopsy of the placenta was excised. In the laboratory, thick and thin slides were prepared of maternal peripheral and placental IVS blood and impression smears were made using the excised placental tissue for detection of *P. falciparum* infected erythrocytes (**IE**). Histological sections of the placenta were also prepared to confirm infection. A woman was considered to be PM+ if parasites were detected in either the placental blood, impression smears or by histology. Maternal anaemia was assessed by determining the packed cell volume (**PCV**) (19). All data were maintained in a password-protected archival database. The deidentified plasma samples were stored at −80° C until used, except during transportation on dry ice from the Biotechnology Center, Cameroon to Georgetown University and later from the Georgetown University to the University of Hawaii. A total of 1,649 plasma samples and corresponding clinical information were available. An advantage of using the clinical data and plasma from this group is that the women were recruited before the implementation in 2004 of IPT; therefore, the women developed natural immunity to PM that aided in clearing their placental infections. Post-IPTp, placental parasitemia were either prevented or eliminated by sulfadoxine–pyrimethamine treatment, making it impossible to assess the role of Abs to VAR2CSA in naturally-acquired immunity. HIV status of the women was not determined, but the prevalence in pregnant women attending urban antenatal clinics at the time of sample collection was 7.1% (20).

Sample Selection

The current study on Ab avidity is an extension of a study conducted in 2017 that used data from the archival samples in statistical predictive models to identify the best combination of antigens associated with absence of PM (18). The study design, sample selection, and results of that study have been reported previously (8, 18). In the 2017 study, plasma samples from 341 PM+ women who delivered live babies ≥28 weeks of gestation, along with three times the number (n=1,036) of randomly-selected PM–negative (PM–) women were screened at a 1:200 dilution in a bead-based multiplex assay for Abs to 17 VAR2CSA-associated antigens (FV2, DBL 1-6 of the FCR3, 3D7 and 7G8 lines, ID1-ID2a (FCR3 and 3D7) and 11 antigens reported to be associated with immunity to *P. falciparum* (AMA-1, CSP, EBA-175, LSA1, MSP1, MSP2, MSP3, MSP11, Pf41, Pf70 and RESA) (18). In addition, plasma from 30 males of equivalent age residing in Yaoundé served as negative controls for the var antigens. The resulting database, consisting of over 74,000 Ab data points, allowed us to evaluate each sample for potential Ab deterioration due to long-term storage and to identify the samples with Abs to FV2. The cut-off for Ab-positivity was the mean + 2SD of the male controls. A total of 695 women were identified who were Ab+ for FV2. Thus, plasma and clinical information from the 695 Ab+ women, and plasma from 20 age-matched sympatric males, were evaluated in the avidity assay.

The Multiplex Assay for Measuring Ab Levels and Avidity to FV2

The multiplex-immunoassay for measuring Abs to FV2 and the avidity assay were detailed previously (13, 14). In brief, FV2 of the FCR3 line was produced in baculovirus as previously described (21). The antigen was covalently coupled at saturating concentrations to SeroMap beads (Luminex) overnight according to the manufacturer's directions. Beads were then blocked with PBS+1% bovine serum albumin (BSA) and resuspended to 2,000 beads/50µl. Ab levels and avidity were determined by combining 50µl of plasma diluted 1:300 in PBS +1% BSA (pH 7.2) with 50µl of coupled beads (total dilution of plasma =1:600) in duplicate in filter microtitre wells. Following incubation at room temperature (**RT**) on a rotary shaker for 1 hr., beads were washed twice with PBS+0.05% Tween 20 and once with 1% BSA in PBS. Then, one of the paired wells was incubated with 100µl of PBS and one well with 100µl of 3M NH_4SCN for 30 min are RT. After washing, beads were incubated with 100µl of secondary antibody (R-phycoerythrin-conjugated, Affinity Pure F $(ab')_2$ fragment, Goat anti-human IgG Fc fragment specific, Jackson Immunoresearch, West Grove, PA) diluted to 2µg/ml in PBS-1% BSA was added to each well and incubated in the dark on a rotary shaker for 1 hr. Beads were washed, re-suspended in 100µl PBS-1% BSA and 85µl of the microsphere suspension was analyzed using a Liquichip M100 reader (Qiagen, Valencia, CA). The reader was programmed to read a minimum of 100 beads per spectral address, DD Gate 7,500–15,000. Results for Ab levels were expressed as median fluorescence intensity (**MFI**), where the linear part of the MFI binding curve extended from ~1,000 to >25,000 MFI (r coefficient of >0.90 for Ab dilution versus MFI) (22). Results from the avidity assay are expressed as an avidity index (**AI**) that equals the percentage of Abs that remains bound to FV2 after treatment with the chaotrope, using the formula (AI = [MFI beads with salt]/[MFI beads with no salt] x100). The entire assay was repeated by two investigators (KV, NB). When inadequate bead counts were obtained, the samples were re-run. The MFI for the two replicates were averaged and used for data analysis. Samples with MFI greater than the mean + 2 SD for the negative male controls were considered to be Ab+.

Measuring Ab Avidity to Different VAR2CSA Domains

The following Duffy-binding like (**DBL**) domains of VAR2CSA were coupled to SeroMap beads as described above: DBL1 (3D7), and the FCR3 lines of 1D1-2a, DBL 1 + 2, DBL2, DBL3, DBL4, DBL5, DBL6, and FV2. Characteristics of the recombinant proteins have been detailed previously (23, 24). The recombinant proteins were covalently coupled at saturating amounts to beads with different spectral addresses and then pooled to create a 10-plex.

In establishing the assay, results from the 10-plex were compared with each of the antigens as a mono-plex to confirm that competition among the antigens did not occur. For the assay, 50μl of plasma diluted 1:300 was combined with 50μl of the 10-plex (2,000 beads of each antigen) for 60 min at RT. The remainder of the methods was the same as that described above. A total of 107 plasma samples with known MFI to FV2 were screened, including 20 sample with MFI of 5,000–10,000; 30 samples with 10,000–15,000; 28 samples with 15,000–20,000; and 29 samples with 20,000–25,000 MFI.

Statistical Analysis

Demographic, clinical, and parasitological characteristics were first summarized by descriptive statistics: frequencies and percentages for categorical variables, i.e., maternal anaemia status; means with standard deviations (SD) or medians with interquartile ranges (IQR) and 25th and 75th percentiles for continuous variables based on data distribution. To compare the groups (e.g., by PM status or AI status), t-tests (or Wilcoxon-Rank-Sum tests) and analysis of variance [ANOVA or Kruskal-Wallis tests (**KW**)] were used for continuous variables depending on distribution and number of the groups. Chi Square tests were used for categorical variables. Post-hoc comparison test was used, when overall significance was identified, to examine the difference between two specific gravidity groups or AI groups. The relationships between birthweight and AI, and between PM and AI after adjusting for age and gravidity were examined by multivariable linear and logistic regression models, respectively. The relationship between MFI and AI was also assessed using linear regression. Statistical significance was determined by $p<0.05$.

RESULTS

Description of the Study Population

Among the 695 women studied, 460 women were PM− and 235 were PM+ (**Table 1**). PM+ women were younger (24.4 vs 26.3 years; p<0.001); had fewer pregnancies (2 vs. 3; p<0.001); had lower hematocrits (31.3% vs 33.9% PCV; p<0.001); and were more likely to be anemic (28.7% vs. 18.9%; $p = 0.011$) than PM− women. A minor difference in length of gestation was found between PM+ and PM− pregnancies (39.3 vs. 40 weeks, p=0.019), but no differences were evident in percentage of premature deliveries or proportion of LBW babies (**Table 1**). However, singleton babies born to PM+ mothers were an estimated 138 gm lower in birthweight and singletons born full-term were 141 gm lighter ($p = 0.007$, $p = 0.002$, respectively). Thus, among women who had Abs to FV2, mothers with PM+ appeared to have lower birthweight babies than those without PM.

Antibody Levels to FV2 Were Lower in PM− Primigravidae, but Similar Among Other Women

Plasma samples collected at delivery from the 695 pregnant women and 20 age-equivalent males were screened for Abs to FV2 at a 1:300 dilution in the avidity assay. Overall, 644/695

TABLE 1 | Characteristics of women with antibodies to full-length VAR2CSA.

	PM− n = 460	PM+ n = 235	P value[a]
Age, Years [mean ± SD]	26.3 ± 5.6	24.4 ± 5.5	<0.001
Gravidity [median (IQR)]	3 (2,5)	2 (1,4)	<0.001
Placental parasitemia % [median (IQR)]	0	0.68 (0.16, 2.5)	NS
Maternal hematocrit, % PCV [mean ± SD][b]	33.9 ± 5.9	31.3 ± 5.6	<0.001
Maternal anemia status[c] [%]	18.9	28.7	0.011
Weeks of Gestation [median (IQR)][d]	40.0 (38.0, 41.0)	39.3 (38.0, 40.6)	0.019
Preterm deliveries [%][d,e]	19.9% (83/418)	21.6% (42/204)	0.915
Infant birth weight, g [mean ± SD][d]	3,131 ± 627	2,993 ± 600	0.007
Infant birthweight from term deliveries [mean ± SD][d]	3,297 ± 459	3,156 ± 482	0.002
Low-birthweight [%][d]	13.9	18.1	0.203

[a]*Statistical Tests: t-tests for age, maternal hematocrit, and infant birthweight; Wilcoxon-Rank-Sum tests for gravidity and weeks of gestation; Chi square tests of independence for anaemia, preterm delivery, and low birthweight.*
[b]*Analysis was performed on 569 subjects for whom data were available.*
[c]*Women with hematocrits <30% were defined as anemic.*
[d]*Twins were excluded from the analysis: n=622 women for weeks of gestation, preterm deliveries; n=648 for infant birthweight and low birthweight; n=493 for infant birthweight of full-term deliveries.*
[e]*Preterm delivery was defined as <37 weeks of delivery.*

(93%) women had MFI to FV2 greater than the mean+2 SD of the male controls; whereas, 51 women, who originally tested positive at a 1:200 dilution, had MFI below the cut-off at a 1:300 dilution. Thus, results from only 644 women were included in the analysis.

Ab levels to FV2 for women with different gravidity (G1 through ≥G6) were compared (**Figure 1**). A difference in median Ab levels was found among the groups (Kruskal-Wallis test (**KW**): $p = 0.002$) with an apparent up-ward trend from primigravidae (G1) through grand-multigravid mothers (≥G6) (**Figure 1**). However, *post hoc* pairwise comparisons showed that the only significant difference in Ab levels among the groups was between G1 and G2 ($p = 0.005$). There was no difference in Ab levels between G2 and G6+ women (KW: $p = 0.57$: dotted rectangle in **Figure 1**).

When Ab levels were evaluated based on presence/absence of PM, only PM− primigravidae had significantly lower Ab levels than women in the other groups (e.g., primigravidae PM− vs PM+ p<0.001; PM− primi- vs PM− secondi-gravidae; p<0.001) (**Figure 2**). No difference in Ab levels was found among the other PM− gravidity groups (KW: $p = 0.78$) or among PM+ women G1 though G6+ (KW: $p = 0.54$). Thus, the distribution of Ab levels to VAR2CSA was similar among all the gravidity groups ($p = 0.80$), except for lower Ab levels in first-time mothers who were PM− at delivery.

Antibody Avidity to FV2 Increased Between Gravidity 1 and Gravidity 2

A significant increase in median AI occurred between G1 and G2 ($p < 0.001$) and then AI leveled off thereafter (KW test: $p = 0.50$) (**Figure 3**). Thus, the predominant increase in AI occurred between women in their first and second pregnancies.

When stratified by placental-malaria status at delivery, AI values were significantly lower in PM− primigravidae than

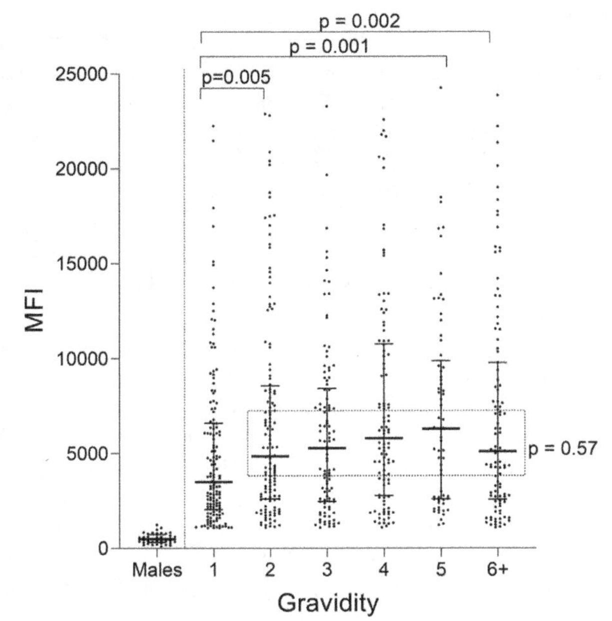

FIGURE 1 | Antibody levels to full-length FV2 at delivery in different gravidity groups. A significant difference in median Ab levels was detected among the six gravidity (G) groups (Kruskal-Wallis test: $p = 0.002$). Post hoc pairwise comparison showed that primigravidae (G1) had significantly lower Ab levels to FV2 than each of the other gravidity groups. Ab levels among groups shown in the rectangle did not differ significantly (Kruskal-Wallis test: $p = 0.57$). n = 644 women and 20 males (replicates shown, n=40 data points). Horizontal lines represent medians and IQR.

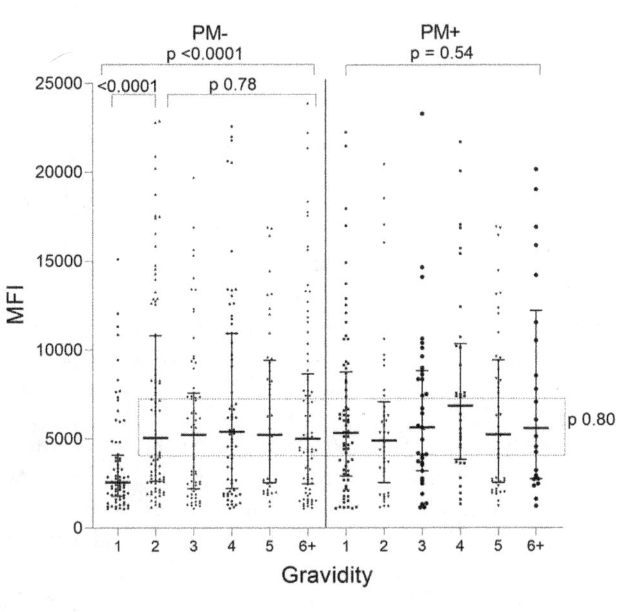

FIGURE 2 | Antibodies to FV2 at delivery in PM− and PM+ women. Antibody levels were significantly lower in PM− primigravidae (G1) than G2 (Mann-Whitney test: $p < 0.001$), but no significant difference was found among the gravidity groups shown in the rectangle (Kruskal-Wallis test: $p = 0.80$). n = 644 women. Horizontal lines represent medians and IQR.

secundigravidae ($p < 0.001$) and lower in PM+ primigravidae than G3 women ($p = 0.050$) (**Figure 4**). Thereafter, the AI leveled off (KW test: PM− $p = 0.60$; PM+ $p = 0.28$). Thus, median AI values were lower in both PM− and PM+ primigravidae, but significantly increased during the second pregnancy in PM− mothers and between the first and third pregnancy in PM+ women.

Overall, AI values were low with 48% of the women having AI <20 and 75% having AI <30 (**Figure 5**). Only 16% of women had AI ≥35; 9.5% had AI ≥40; and only 2.8% had AI ≥50. Thus, the majority of women did not produce significant amounts of high avidity Abs, and only 2.8% had AI >50, which is considered to be a high avidity response. In a high transmission area, women with AI >35 early in pregnancy were reported to have a decreased risk of PM at delivery (13). Only 16% of women in Yaoundé had this level of high avidity Abs at delivery.

Relationship Between MFI and AI was Similar in Secundigravidae and Above

During affinity maturation, B cell clonal expansion and selection occur, resulting in an increase in both Ab levels (MFI) and avidity (AI). To help determine when affinity maturation began, the relationship between MFI and AI was assessed (**Figure 6**). No relationship existed between MFI and AI in PM− primigravidae, indicating that Abs were produced, but significant clonal selection had not occurred ($p = 0.31$, i.e., regression line was not significantly different from zero) (**Figure 6A**). A moderate association (r = 0.552), however, was detected in PM+

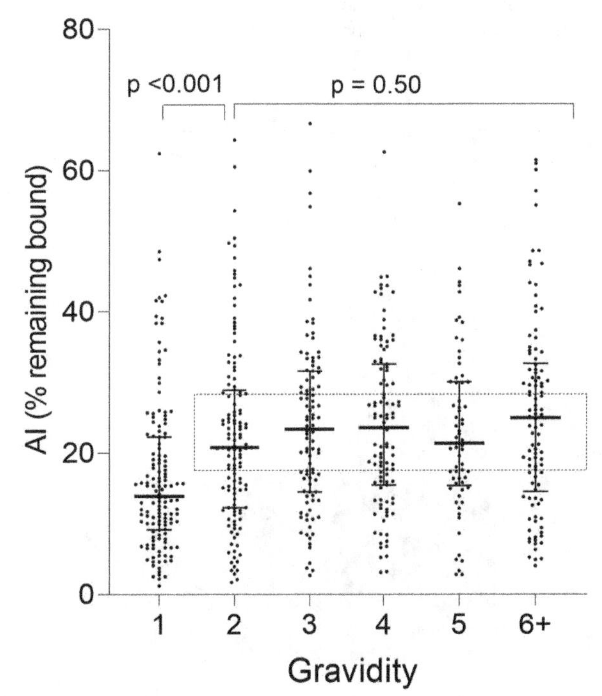

FIGURE 3 | Distribution of Ab avidity (AI) among pregnant women at delivery. AI were significantly lower in G1 than G2 ($p < 0.001$), but AI did not change thereafter (rectangle: Kruskal-Wallis test: G2 through G6+ $p = 0.50$). Horizontal lines represent medians and IQR.

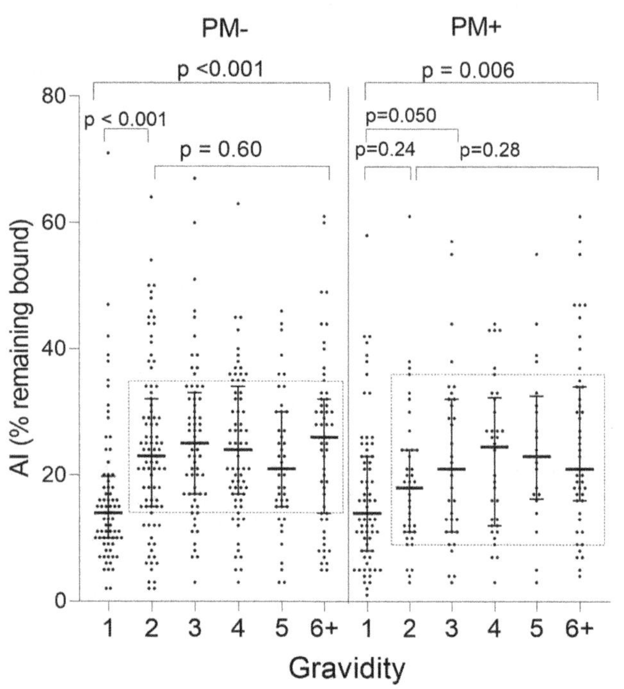

FIGURE 4 | Comparison of Ab avidity (AI) at delivery in PM− and PM+ women. A significant increase in AI occurred in PM− women between G1 and G2 women ($p < 0.001$) and between G1 and G3 in PM+ women ($p = 0.05$), but AI did not increase significantly thereafter (samples within rectangles for G2 through G6+: Kruskal-Wallis test: PM− $p = 0.60$; PM+ $p = 0.28$). Horizontal lines represent medians and IQR.

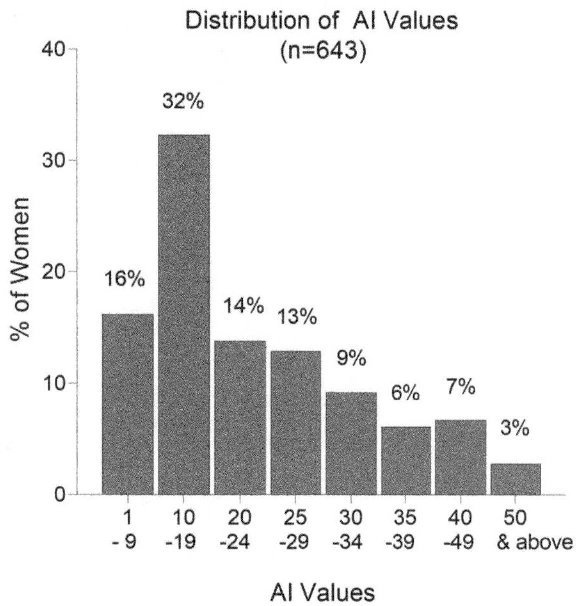

FIGURE 5 | Frequency distribution of Avidity Indices (AI). Numbers above each column are the percentage of samples in the AI category. n = 643 women.

primigravidae, suggesting that affinity maturation was occurring at term in some women (**Figure 6B**). A modest association was also seen in secundigravidae (G2) (**Figure 6C**), as well as in women gravidae G3 and above (n=373 women) (**Figure 6D**). Even among grand multi-gravid women (G6+), the association between MFI and AI still remained modest (r = 0.508). These data suggest that affinity maturation was occurring in some primigravidae who had PM at delivery, as well as in some women with prior pregnancies.

High Avidity Abs for Were Directed Mainly to DBL5

The extracellular part of VAR2CSA consists of six Duffy-binding-like domains (DBL) domains, a large intradomain (ID2) and a C-terminal region predicted to be intracellular (25). A total of 107 plasma samples with MFI to FV2 ranging from 5,000 to >20,000 were screened in the Ab avidity assay against the 6 DBL domains, ID1–ID2, and FV2 (**Figure 7**). The range of MFI for each domain, as well as the percentage of women who were Ab+, are shown in **Figure 7A**. Overall, 55% (e.g., DBL2) to 98% (e.g., DBL5) of the women had Abs to the DBL domains, with the highest Ab levels found for DBL5. Likewise, DBL5 had the highest AI compared to the other domains, in fact, the AI for DBL5 was significantly higher than the median AI to FV2 (median (25%,75% IQR): DBL5 52 (36,64) vs. FV2 24 (16,31); $p<0.001$). AI values for the other domains were much lower than to DBL5, with AI for the N-terminal domains DBL 1 through 3 having AI <20 and the more C-terminal domains, DBL 4 and DBL6 having slightly higher AI of 20 to 25. Thus, although most women had Abs to most of the domains, some regions of FV2 support affinity maturation better than others, with the majority of high avidity Abs induced by DBL5.

Mothers With High AI Appear to Have Higher Birthweight Babies

Since the frequency distribution of AI did not identify definable groups of women (**Figure 5**), the pregnant women were divided into two groups based on the median. Women in Group 1 had AI <20.5 and Group 2 had AI ≥20.5 (**Table 2**). Compared to Group 1, women in Group 2 were older (mean age: 26.4 vs. 24.9 years, p<0.001); had higher gravidities (median 3 vs 2, p<0.001); and higher hematocrits (mean PCV: 33.5% vs. 32.4%, $p=0.038$). Women with AI above the median appeared to have higher birthweight babies than those with AI below the median (average birthweight: 3,160 vs 3,020 g, $p=0.006$). After adjusting for age and gravidity, the difference remained statistically significant ($p=0.045$), with an average difference of 104 g. The percentage of women with PM at delivery was lower in Group than 2 than Group 1 (30% vs 39%; $p = 0.016$). However, after adjusting for age and gravidity, no significant association was found between AI and presence of PM. Likewise, no relationship between low and high AI and the distribution of placental parasitemia ($p = 0.45$) was found. Thus, these data suggest that having high avidity Abs to FV2 may be associated with increased infant birthweight, but additional factors could also influence the results.

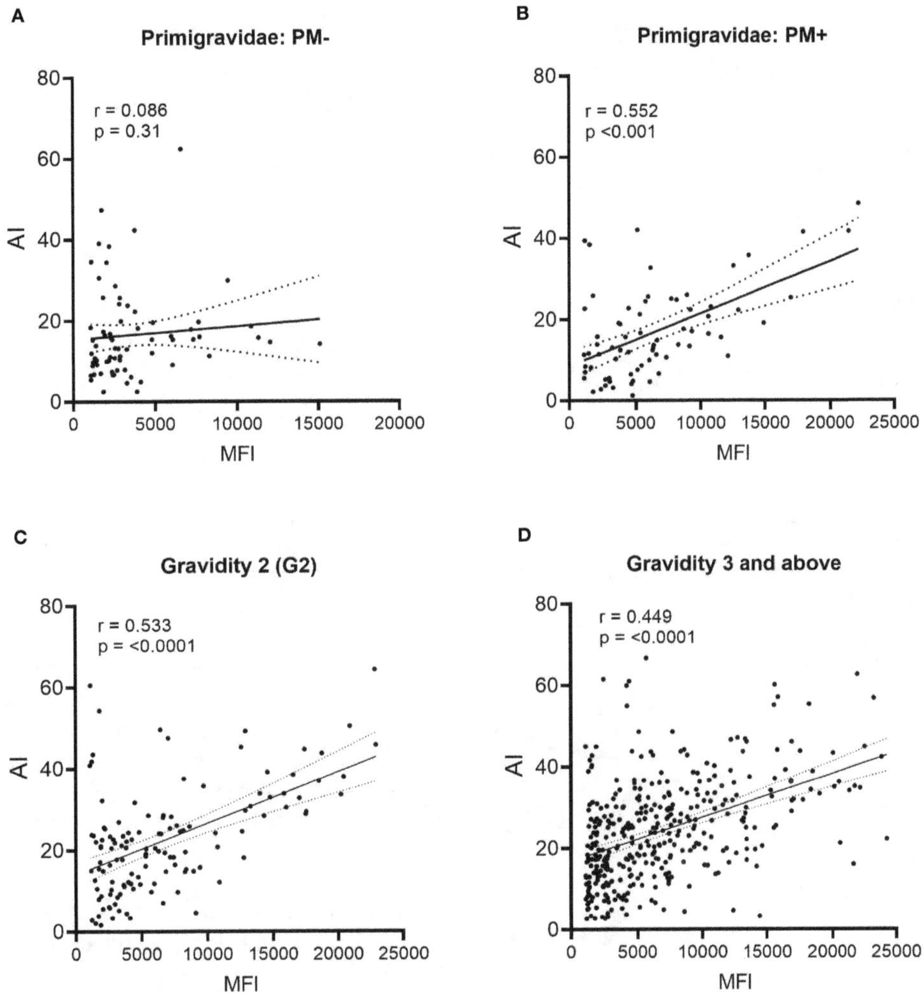

FIGURE 6 | Comparison of Ab levels (MFI) and avidity (AI) using linear regression. **(A)** Placental malaria-negative (PM−) primigravidae (n = 71), **(B)** Placental malaria-positive (PM+) primigravidae (n = 70); **(C)** all secundigravidae (G2) (n = 127); and **(D)** all women gravidity 3 (G3) and above (n = 373). Linear regression lines with 95% confidence bands are shown. P values indicate if the line is significantly different from zero.

DISCUSSION

The timing of affinity maturation resulting in production of higher affinity Abs to VAR2CSA is an important component in acquiring immunity to PM. Previous studies have shown that the Ab response to VAR2CSA is different in urban cities from that in high transmission areas. For example, in Cameroon, >90% of women living in the rural village of Ngali II, where they receive ~200 infectious mosquito bites during pregnancy, had Abs to FV2 at delivery (13, 26); whereas, in Yaoundé, only 39% of women (n=1,337) were Ab+ (8). In Yaoundé, approximately half of the women who had PM at term do not have Abs to FV2 (8, 17). Thus, infection is not always accompanied by Ab production to FV2 in an urban setting. Clearly, when pregnant women receive only a few infectious mosquito bites during a single pregnancy, the resulting humoral response is limited. Results from the current study on Ab avidity help create a picture about the natural acquisition of Abs to VAR2CSA in pregnant women residing in Yaoundé. Although the data from this study are open to interpretation, the following picture is consistent with the current data set and data from past studies.

Antibody-Levels to FV2 Remain Low in PM-Negative Primigravidae, Suggesting That Abs to Other Malarial Antigens Aid in Parasite Clearance

Primigravidae lack Abs to FV2 prior to pregnancy. Thus, primigravidae with Abs to FV2 at delivery who were PM− must have become infected early enough in pregnancy to mount an Ab-response and clear their placental infections prior to delivery. However, since Ab levels to FV2 were low, Abs to other antigens may have helped limit parasite replication and aided in parasite clearance **(Figure 1)**. This possibility is supported by results from a study that measured Ab levels in 1,377 women living in Yaoundé, (i.e., the same initial set of plasma samples used herein) to 17 VAR2CSA-associated antigens, including FV2, DBL-1-6 of the

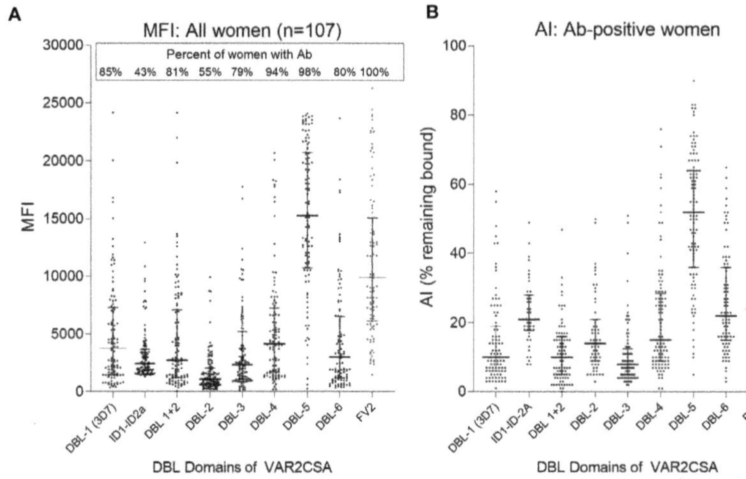

FIGURE 7 | Antibody MFI and AI to different regions of VAR2CSA. Plasma samples from 107 women were screened for Ab avidity against DBL1 (3D7 line), the FCR3 lines of ID1-ID2a, the DBL2 through DBL6, and FV2. **(A)** MFI for the 107 samples. Horizonal lines represent medians and IQR. **(B)** AI for women who had Ab against each of the domains (sample size: DBL1 n = 91; ID1-ID2a n = 46; DBL1+2 n = 87; DBL2 n= 59; DBL3 n = 84; DBL4 n = 101; DBL5 n = 105; DBL6 n = 86; FV2 n = 107). Horizontal lines represent medians and IQR.

TABLE 2 | Comparison of birth outcomes and AI to FV2.

	Group 1: AI <20.5 n = 319	Group 2AI: ≥20.5 n = 324	p-value[a]
Age, years [mean ± SD]	24.9 ± 6.0	26.4 ± 5.4	<0.001
Gravidity [median, (IQR)]	2 (1, 4)	3 (2, 5)	<0.001
Maternal hematocrit, % PCV [mean ± SD][b]	32.4 ± 6.0	33.5 ± 5.7	0.038
Maternal anaemia [%][b]	25.6 (69/270)	18.8 (48/256)	0.077
Weeks of gestation [median, (IQR)][c]	39.7 (37.8, 40.9)	39.9 (38.1, 40.9)	0.739
Infant birth weight, g [mean + SD][c]	3020 ± 633	3160 ± 615	0.006
Low birth weight babies [%][c]	16.9 (50/295)	13.2 (40/304)	0.236
Placental malaria-positive (%)	39.2 (125/319)	29.9 (97/324)	0.017

[a]*Statistical tests: t-tests for age, maternal hematocrit, and infant birthweight; Kruskal-Wallis tests for gravidity and weeks of gestation; Chi-square tests of independence for maternal anemia, placental malaria, and low birthweight.*

[b]*Analysis was performed on subjects for whom data were available, (n = 526).*

[c]*Only singleton deliveries were included: weeks of gestation (n = 576), infant birthweight and percent LBW (n = 599).*

FCR3, DBL, and 7G8 lines, IDI-ID2a (FCR3 and 3D7) and 11 non-VAR antigens associated with immunity to *P. falciparum* (AMA-1, CSP, EBA-175, LAS1, MSP1, MSP2, MSP3, MSP11, Pf41, Pf70, and RESA), and then used the data in seven statistical models to identify the combination of antigens that best correlated with absence of PM at term (18). A combination of Abs to AMA-1, MSP2, EBA-175, Pf41, and MSP11 was the best predictor of PM status. FV2 was among the top 10 individual predictors, but it did not improve the prediction when added to the combination. Likewise, in a parallel study, Abs to MSP3, EBA-175 and Pf41 were associated with reduced risk of high placental parasitemia and Abs to EBA-175 with reduced risk to premature deliveries in PM+ women (8). Thus, Abs to other malaria antigens, in conjunction with FV2, may play a significant role in improving pregnancy outcomes. Since Ab level were low (**Figure 2**) in PM− primigravidae and there was no evidence that affinity maturation had occurred (**Figures 3, 4**), initial exposure to low levels of FV2 may be sufficient to activate short-lived plasma cells, but insufficient to induce strong clonal expansion of B cells, long-lived plasma cells, memory B cells, or affinity maturation.

Antibody-Levels to FV2 Reached Maximal Levels in PM+ Primigravidae

The anti-VAR2CSA response was significantly stronger in primigravidae who had placental parasitemia at term (**Figure 2**), possibly due to longer exposure to higher amounts of the antigen. Interestingly, distribution and median MFI of anti-FV2 Abs were similar at term in PM+ primigravidae and all other gravidity groups regardless of placental malaria status (**Figure 2**). After the first exposure to a sufficient concentration of FV2, Ab data are consistent with the speculation that B cell clonal expansion is similar in primigravidae to that of multigravida women. Thus, in primigravidae, exposure to an adequate amount of FV2 may be sufficient to induce substantial clonal expansion, but insufficient to induce affinity maturation (**Figure 3**).

Affinity Maturation Takes Place Primarily During the Second Pregnancy

The change in the Avidity Index between primigravidae and secundigravidae (**Figures 3, 4**) is reminiscent of a primary and secondary Ab response. During second pregnancies (PM− women) and possibly into the third pregnancies (PM+ women), affinity maturation appeared to be occurring. At this time, women had both higher Ab levels and a higher proportion of higher avidity Abs (i.e., higher AI); however, the association between MFI and AI was only modest (r values ranging from 0.4 to 0.5) (**Figures 6B, C**). In general r values >0.7 are considered to be strong associations. From the scattergrams, data show that a few secundigravidae and ≥G3 had high MFI but low AI (below the line) and a group of women with low AI and high MFI (values above the line) (**Figures 6C, D**). Thus, the two processes may not always occur simultaneously. Neither the quantity nor quality of Abs to FV2 appears to increase following additional exposure to VAR2CSA-expressing IE beyond the second pregnancy. These results suggest that in low transmission areas, two pregnancies are required for women to achieve the naturally acquired humoral response to VAR2CSA. However, the ultimate response is much less robust than that obtained by women living in rural areas with high exposure to VAR2CSA during pregnancy.

High Avidity Abs Appear to be Restricted Primarily to DBL5 in this Urban Setting

In Yaounde, most women had detectable levels of Abs to the individual DBL domains, with the predominant Ab response to DBL5 (**Figure 7A**). That is, the median Ab level to DBL5 was 15,277 MFI; whereas, median Ab levels to the other domains were <4,000 MFI (**Figure 6**). In a high transmission village, the absence of PM at term was associated with women having high Ab levels to multiple domains and strains (lines) (17). Thus, the breadth of the Ab response to VAR2CSA is much higher in a rural, compared to the urban, site. Likewise, the median AI for DBL-5 was 52 compared to <25 for the other domains (**Figure 7B**). To our knowledge, similar data are not available on the avidity of Abs to DBL domains in women in high transmission areas. In summary, in Yaoundé the Ab response was similar to a primary Ab response when primigravidae are exposed to a new antigen and secundigravidae have a secondary exposure.

The above conclusions are based on the Ab response to the FCR3 line of *P. falciparum*. Like other malarial antigens, VAR2CSA is polymorphic with six DBL domains, each of which contains conserved and polymorphic sequences. Conserved epitopes on the molecular surface that bind Abs are most predominant in DBL5, thereby, inducing strain-transcending or cross-reactivity Abs (25). Among isolates, DBL5 domains average 86% amino acid identity, which may explain, in part, the high AIs to DBL5 (27). For a vaccine to VAR2CSA to be successful, the response must be against strain transcending epitopes. A limitation of the current study is the possibility that affinity maturation occurred to a few non-strain transcending epitopes that were not detected in this study. Likewise, this study used 3M NH_4SCN which is a very strong chaotrope for malarial antigens (22) and may efficiently remove Abs bound to more flexible epitopes. If a less stringent chaotrope had been used, additional evidence of affinity maturation may have been detected. Overall, these results suggest that in urban cities when women become infected only a few times during pregnancy, most high avidity Abs are directed against the DBL5 domain.

In high transmission areas, Abs to VAR2CSA have been reported to be associated with increase length of pregnancy, higher birthweight babies, lower placental parasitemia, and reduced prevalence of placental malaria at delivery (6, 7, 9, 10). The influence of Abs to VAR2CSA has been more difficult to assess in urban settings, in part, because a large sample size is need to detect small effects. Using data from 1,337 women, Abs to FV2 were found to be beneficial for PM+, but not PM–, women (8). That is, in PM+ women the presence of Abs to FV2 was associated with lower placental parasitemia and higher birth weight babies compared to PM+ women without Abs to FV2. In the current study, where all women had Abs to FV2, women whose AI to FV2 were above the median delivered higher birthweight babies compared to women whose AI was below the median (**Table 2**). The comparison remained significant after adjusting for age and gravidity. Thus, there is some evident that affinity maturation has a beneficial role in a low transmission setting; however, the increase of birthweight was only 104 g and may be of minimal clinical relevance. It remains unclear if Abs to FV2 with higher AI are better at blocking or reversing the attachment of infected erythrocytes to trophoblasts or if they are merely a surrogate marker for the overall maturation of the immune response to VAR2CSA.

The Ab response to VAR2CSA has been measured in other urban settings, e.g., Blantyre, (Malawi); Lambarene, Gabon; and Manjica, Mozambique (28–35). It is difficult to make direct comparisons between these cities and Yaoundé at the time the women were recruited, since factors that influence development of immunity differ among the cities, including time of the study, assays used, sample size, and range of intermediate malaria transmission. However, commonality among the results exist. In these urban cities, Ab levels in PM+ were higher than those in PM-primigravidae (28, 32, 36), Ab levels were higher in PM+ than PM – mothers at term, but there was no difference between PM+ and PM– multigravidae, regardless of the assay used to measure Abs to Var2CSA (18, 28, 33–35, 37). Similar to Yaoundé, Abs to FV2 were not associated with maternal peripheral parasitemia or percentage of LBW babies (29, 33); however, like higher avidity Abs, Abs that mediate phagocytosis of VAR2CSA-expressing IE were associated with increased infant birthweight (29). Abs, to a non-var antigen, AMA-1, were reported to contribute to improving infant birthweight (34). Thus, the results of this study may be applicable to other urban cities. With implementation of intervention strategies, such as IPT and insecticide treated bed nets, transmission of malaria is on the decline in many places (38). Today rural environments are becoming intermediate transmission areas similar to Yaoundé. Thus, the results reported herein are of both current and future interest.

AUTHORS CONTRIBUTIONS

The following were contributed by the authors: sample and data collection (RL), study design (NB and DT), conduction of the experiments (KV and NB), data analysis (MM and JC), provision of critical reagents and advice (AS), and manuscript preparation (RL, AS, and DT). All authors contributed to the article and approved the submitted version.

ACKNOWLEDGMENTS

We acknowledge the excellent research team at the Biotechnology Centre, Cameroon, for sample collection, clinical survey, and laboratory studies. We also want to thank all the women and families who participated in the study. Without their help, this study would not have been possible. We thank J. Smith and B. Gamain for providing recombinant proteins.

REFERENCES

1. Desai M, ter Kuile F, Nosten F, McGready R, Asamoa K, Brabin B, et al. Epidemiology and burden of malaria in pregnancy. *Lancet Infect Dis* (2007) 7:93–104. doi: 10.1016/S1473-3099(07)70021-X
2. Brabin BJ, Romagosa C, Abdelgalil S, Menéndez C, Verhoeff FH, McGready R, et al. The sick placenta - The role of malaria. *Placenta* (2004) 25:359–78. doi: 10.1016/j.placenta.2003.10.019
3. Moore KA, Simpson JA, Scoullar MJL, McGready R, Fowkes FJI. Quantification of the association between malaria in pregnancy and stillbirth: a systematic review and meta-analysis. *Lancet Glob Heal* (2017) 5: e1101–12. doi: 10.1016/S2214-109X(17)30340-6
4. Rogerson SJ, Hviid L, Duffy PE, Leke RF, Taylor DW. Malaria in pregnancy: pathogenesis and immunity. *Lancet Infect Dis* (2007) 7:105–17. doi: 10.1016/S1473-3099(07)70022-1
5. Fried M, Duffy PE. Adherence of *Plasmodium falciparum* to chondroitin sulfate A in the human placenta. *Science* (1996) 272:1502–4. doi: 10.1126/science.272.5267.1502
6. Salanti A, Dahlbäck M, Turner L, Nielsen MA, Barfod L, Magistrado P, et al. Evidence for the involvement of VAR2CSA in pregnancy-associated malaria. *J Exp Med* (2004) 200:1197–203. doi: 10.1084/jem.20041579
7. Duffy P, Fried M. Antibodies that inhibit *Plasmodium falciparum* adhesion to chondroitin sulfate A are associated with increased birth weight and gestational age of newborns. *Infect Immun* (2003) 71:6620–3. doi: 10.1128/IAI.71.11.6620-6623.2003
8. Lloyd YM, Fang R, Bobbili N, Vanda K, Ngati E, Sanchez-Quintero MJ, et al. Association of antibodies to VAR2CSA and merozoite antigens with pregnancy outcomes in women living in Yaoundé, Cameroon. *Infect Immun* (2018) 86(9):e00166–18. doi: 10.1128/IAI.00166-18
9. Staalsoe T, Shulman C, Bulmer J, Kawuondo K, Marsh M, Hviid L. Variant surface antigen-specific IgG and protection against clinical consequences of pregnancy-associated *Plasmodium falciparum* malaria. *Lancet* (2004) 363:283–9. doi: 10.1016/S0140-6736(03)15386-XTitle
10. Tuikue Ndam N, Denoeud-Ndam L, Doritchamou J, Viwami F, Salanti A, Nielsen MA, et al. Protective antibodies against placental malaria and poor outcomes during pregnancy, Benin. *Emerg Infect Dis* (2015) 21:813–23. doi: 10.3201/eid2105.141626
11. Cutts JC, Agius PA, Zaw L, Powell R, Moore K, Draper B, et al. Pregnancy-specific malarial immunity and risk of malaria in pregnancy and adverse birth outcomes: A systematic review. *BMC Med BMC Med* (2020) 18:1–21. doi: 10.1186/s12916-019-1467-6
12. Hedman K, Lappalainen M, Soderlund M, Hedman L. Avidity of IgG in serodiagnosis of infectious diseases. *Rev Med Microbiol* (1993) 4:123–9. doi: 10.1097/00013542-199307000-00001
13. Tutterrow YL, Salanti A, Avril M, Smith JD, Pagano IS, Ako S, et al. High avidity antibodies to full-length VAR2CSA correlate with absence of placental malaria. *PloS One* (2012) 7:e40049_. doi: 10.1371/journal.pone.0040049
14. Babakhanyan A, Fang R, Wey A, Salanti A, Sama G, Efundem C, et al. Comparison of the specificity of antibodies to VAR2CSA in Cameroonian multigravidae with and without placental malaria: A retrospective case-control study. *Malar J BioMed Cent* (2015) 14:1–10. doi: 10.1186/s12936-015-1023-6
15. Manga L, Robert V, Messi J, Desfontaine M, Carnevale P. Le pludisme urbain a Yaoundé, Cameroun. 1. Etude entomologique dans deux quartiers centraux. *Mem Soc r belge Ent* (1992) 35:155–62.
16. Fondjo E, Robert V, Le Goff G, Toto J, Carnevale P. Le paludisme urbain a Yaoundé (Cameroun) 2. Etude entomologique dans deux quartiers per urbanises. *Bull La Soc Pathol Exot* (1992) 85:57–63.
17. Tutterrow YL, Avril M, Singh K, Long CA, Leke RJ, Sama G, et al. High levels of antibodies to multiple domains and strains of VAR2CSA correlate with the absence of placental malaria in Cameroonian women living in an area of high *Plasmodium falciparum* transmission. *Infect Immun* (2012) 80:1479–90. doi: 10.1128/IAI.00071-12
18. Siriwardhana C, Fang R, Salanti A, Leke RGF, Bobbili N, Taylor DW, et al. Statistical prediction of immunity to placental malaria based on multi-assay antibody data for malarial antigens. *Malar J* (2017) 16:391. doi: 10.1186/s12936-017-2041-3
19. Tako EA, Zhou A, Lohoue J, Leke R, Taylor DW, Leke RFG. Risk factors for placental malaria and its effect on pregnancy outcome in Yaoundé, Cameroon. *Am J Trop Med Hyg* (2005) 72:236–42. doi: 10.4269/ajtmh.2005.72.236
20. UNAID/WHO. *Cameroon: epidemiological fact sheets on HIV/AIDS and sexually transmitted infections – 2004 update.* Geneva, Switz: WHO (2004).
21. Khunrae P, Dahlbäck M, Nielsen MA, Andersen G, Ditlev SB, Resende M, et al. Full-length recombinant *Plasmodium falciparum* VAR2CSA binds specifically to CSPG and induces potent parasite adhesion-blocking antibodies. *J Mol Biol* (2010) 397(3):826–34. doi: 10.1016/j.jmb.2010.01.040
22. Taylor DW, Bobbili N, Kayatani A, Tassi Yunga S, Kidima W, Leke RFG. Measuring antibody avidity to *Plasmodium falciparum* merozoite antigens using a multiplex immunoassay approach. *Malar J* (2020) 19(1):171. doi: 10.1186/s12936-020-03243-3
23. Nielsen MA, Pinto VV, Resende M, Dahlbäck M, Ditlev SB, Theander TG, et al. Induction of adhesion-inhibitory antibodies against placental *Plasmodium falciparum* parasites by using single domains of VAR2CSA. *Infect Immun* (2009) 77:2482–7. doi: 10.1128/IAI.00159-09
24. Clausen TM, Christoffersen S, Dahlbäck M, Langkilde AE, Jensen KE, Resende M, et al. Structural and functional insight into how the *Plasmodium falciparum* VAR2CSA protein mediates binding to chondroitin sulfate A in placental malaria. *J Biol Chem* (2012) 287:23332–45. doi: 10.1074/jbc.M112.348839
25. Andersen P, Nielsen MA, Resende M, Rask TS, Dahlbäck M, Theander T, et al. Structural insight into epitopes in the pregnancy-associated malaria protein VAR2CSA. *PloS Pathog* (2008) 4. 4(2):e42. doi: 10.1371/journal.ppat.0040042
26. Leke RFG, Bioga JD, Zhou J, Fouda GG, Leke RJI, Tchinda V, et al. Longitudinal studies of *Plasmodium falciparum* malaria in pregnant women living in a rural Cameroonian village with high perennial transmission. *Am J Trop Med Hyg* (2010) 83:996–1004. doi: 10.4269/ajtmh.2010.10-0249
27. Avril M, Cartwright MM, Hathaway MJ, Hommel M, Elliott SR, Williamson K, et al. Immunization with VAR2CSA-DBL5 recombinant protein elicits broadly cross-reactive antibodies to placental *Plasmodium falciparum*-infected erythrocytes. *Infect Immun* (2010) 78(5):2248–56. doi: 10.1128/IAI.00410-09
28. Ataíde R, Hasang W, Wilson DW, Beeson JG, Mwapasa V, Molyneux ME, et al. Using an improved phagocytosis assay to evaluate the effect of HIV on specific antibodies to pregnancy- associated malaria. *PloS One* (2010) 5(5): e10807. doi: 10.1371/journal.pone.0010807
29. Ataíde R, Mwapasa V, Molyneux ME, Meshnick SR, Rogerson SJ. Antibodies that induce phagocytosis of malaria infected erythrocytes: Effect of HIV infection and correlation with clinical outcomes. *PloS One* (2011) 6:1–6. doi: 10.1371/journal.pone.0022491
30. Feng G, Aitken E, Yosaatmadja Y, Kalilani L, Meshnick S, Jaworowski A, et al. Antibodies to variant surface antigens of *Plasmodium falciparum*-infected erythrocytes are associated with protection from treatment failure and the development of anemia in pregnancy. *J Infect Dis* (2009) 200(2):299–306. doi: 10.1086/599841
31. Hommel M, Chan JA, Umbers AJ, Langer C, Rogerson SJ, Smith JD, et al. Evaluating antibody functional activity and strain-specificity of vaccine candidates for malaria in pregnancy using in vitro phagocytosis assays. *Parasites Vectors Parasites Vectors* (2018) 11:1–7. doi: 10.1186/s13071-018-2653-7
32. Khattab A, Reinhardt C, Staalsoe T, Fievet N, Kremsner PG, Deloron P, et al. Analysis of IgG with specificity for variant surface antigens expressed by

placental *Plasmodium falciparum* isolates. *Mala J* (2004) 3(3):21. doi: 10.1186/1475-2875-3-21

33. Mayor A, Rovira-Vallbona E, Machevo S, Bassat Q, Aguilar R, Quinto L, et al. Parity and placental infection affect antibody responses against *Plasmodium falciparum* during pregnancy. *Infect Immun* (2011) 79(4):1654–9. doi: 10.1128/IAI.01000-10
34. Mayor A, Kumar U, Bardaji A, P. G, Jimenez A, Hamad A, et al. Improved pregnancy outcomes in women exposed to malaria with high antibody levels against *Plasmodium falciparum*. *J Infect Dis* (2013) 207(11):1664–74. doi: 10.1093/infdis/jit083
35. Serra-Casas E, Menéndez C, Bardají A, Quintó L, Dobaño C, Sigauque B, et al. The effect of intermittent preventive treatment during pregnancy on malarial antibodies depends on HIV status and is not associated with poor delivery outcomes. *J Infect Dis* (2010) 201(1):123–31. doi: 10.1086/648595
36. Hommel M, Elliott SR, Soma V, Kelly G, Fowkes FJI, Chesson JM, et al. Evaluation of the antigenic diversity of placenta-binding *Plasmodium falciparum* variants and the antibody repertoire among pregnant women. *Infect Immun* (2010) 78(5):1963–78. doi: 10.1128/IAI.01365-09
37. Beeson JG, Mann EJ, Elliott SR, Lema VM, Tadesse E, Molyneux ME, et al. Antibodies to variant surface antigens of *Plasmodium falciparum*-infected erythrocytes and adhesion inhibitory antibodies are associated with placental malaria and have overlapping and distinct targets. *J Infect Dis* (2004) 189(3):540–51. doi: 10.1086/381186
38. World Malaria Report. The World Health Organization (2019). ISBN: 978-92-4-156572-1. www.who.int/publications/i/item/9789241565721

3

The Role of microRNAs in the Infection by *T. gondii* in Humans

Geraldo Magela de Faria Junior[1†], *Fernando Henrique Antunes Murata*[2†], *Hernan Alejandro Lorenzi*[3†], *Bruno Bello Pede Castro*[4†], *Letícia Carolina Paraboli Assoni*[1], *Christiane Maria Ayo*[1†], *Cinara Cássia Brandão*[1†] *and Luiz Carlos de Mattos*[1*†]

[1] *Immunogenetics Laboratory, Molecular Biology Department, Faculdade de Medicina de São José do Rio Preto (FAMERP), São José do Rio Preto, Brazil,* [2] *Beltsville Agricultural Research Center, Animal Parasitic Diseases Laboratory, United States Department of Agriculture, Agricultural Research Service, Beltsville, MD, United States,* [3] *Department of Infectious Diseases, J. Craig Venter Institute, Rockville, MD, United States,* [4] *Department of Preventive Veterinary Medicine and Animal Health, Faculty of Veterinary Medicine, University of São Paulo, São Paulo, Brazil*

Correspondence:
Luiz Carlos de Mattos
luiz.demattos@edu.famerp.br

MicroRNAs are molecules belonging to an evolutionarily conserved family of small non-coding RNAs, which act on post-transcriptional gene regulation, causing messenger RNA (mRNA) degradation or inhibiting mRNA translation into proteins. These molecules represent potential biomarkers for diagnosis, non-invasive prognosis, and monitoring the development of the disease. Moreover, they may provide additional information on the pathophysiology of parasitic infections and guide strategies for treatment. The Apicomplexan parasite *Toxoplasma gondii* modifies the levels of microRNAs and mRNAs in infected host cells by modulating the innate and adaptive immune responses, facilitating its survival within the host. Some studies have shown that microRNAs are promising molecular markers for developing diagnostic tools for human toxoplasmosis. MicroRNAs can be detected in human specimens collected using non-invasive procedures. changes in the circulating host microRNAs have been associated with *T. gondii* infection in mice and ocular toxoplasmosis in humans. Besides, microRNAs can be amplified from samples using sensitive and molecular-specific approaches such as real-time PCR. This review presents recent findings of the role that microRNAs play during *T. gondii* infection and discuss their potential use of these small nuclei acid molecules to different approaches such as laboratory diagnosis, modulation of cell and tissue infected as other potential applications in human toxoplasmosis.

Keywords: microRNAs, immune system, *toxoplasma gondii*, communicable diseases, toxoplasmosis

INTRODUCTION

MicroRNAs are small non-coding RNAs acting on post-transcriptional regulation of gene expression, causing messenger RNA (mRNA) degradation or blocking mRNA translation (Glinge et al., 2017; Malla et al., 2019). Since microRNAs are present in serum and plasma (Chen et al., 2008' Chim et al., 2008; Gilad et al., 2008; Lawrie et al., 2008; Mitchell et al., 2008; McDonald et al., 2011), urine (Hanke et al., 2010; Gidlöf et al., 2011; Glinge et al., 2017), and other body fluids (Park et al., 2009; Weber et al., 2010; Glinge et al., 2017), the interest to explore them as potential biomarkers for diagnosis, non-invasive prognosis, and monitoring the development of the disease (Li et al., 2019).

Besides, they may provide additional information on the pathophysiology of disease and guide treatment strategies (Lu et al., 2005; Perron et al., 2007; Gilad et al., 2008; Wang et al., 2009; D'Alessandra et al., 2010; Tijsen et al., 2010; Wang et al., 2010; Glinge et al., 2017; Hu et al., 2018).

The expression of microRNAs has also been reported in infection by Apicomplexan microorganisms, mostly obligatory intracellular parasites infecting animals and humans and causing parasitic diseases of significant public health impact (Cavalier-Smith, 1993). Some of these parasitic diseases are caused by *Plasmodium falciparum*, *Plasmodium vivax*, *Cryptosporidium parvum*, and *Toxoplasma gondii* (Lüder and Gross, 2005; World Health Organization, 2015) which are commonly reported in outbreaks in Brazil (Judice et al., 2016). These parasites can hijack host gene expression, modulating immune response pathways, including those involved in apoptosis and cytokine production (Judice et al., 2016). Thus, the intracellular modulation of host gene expression improves the ability of Apicomplexans to infect and proliferate in target cells such as epithelial (Deng et al., 2004; Lüder and Gross, 2005; McDonald et al., 2013), liver (Prudêncio et al., 2006; Sturm et al., 2006), erythrocytes (Gazzinelli et al., 2014), and some immune cells (Leng et al., 2009).

Recently, it was demonstrated that the microRNAs miR-155-5p and miR-29c-3p are up-expressed, and the miR-21-5p and miR-125b-5p are down-expressed in acute ocular toxoplasmosis, in comparison to asymptomatic individuals (Pereira et al., 2019). These data open the opportunity to explore the up-and down-expression of microRNA as potential tools to investigate many aspects of this parasitic disease. The review discusses the importance of microRNAs in the infection by *T. gondii* and toxoplasmosis, a disease of significant concern to public health worldwide.

microRNA – DEFINITION, BIOGENESIS, AND FUNCTION

MicroRNAs are 18-22 nucleotides long non-coding RNAs that act on post-transcriptional gene regulation causing degradation of messenger RNA (mRNA) or inhibiting its translation into proteins (Glinge et al., 2017; Malla et al., 2019). MicroRNA influence many cellular processes, including cell proliferation, differentiation, migration, apoptosis, angiogenesis, and carcinogenesis (Malla et al., 2019).

The first microRNA described, named lin-4, was identified by Lee et al., 1993 in the nematode *Caenorhabditis elegans* (Lee et al., 1993). It was later described in eukaryotes, including humans (Tang et al., 2018). Subsequent studies identified 28,000 mature microRNAs by sequencing (Malla et al., 2019), and 2,500 were found in humans as sotirage in mirbase (http://www.mirbase.org/) (Glinge et al., 2017) of which 60% regulate protein-encoding genes (Friedman et al., 2009; Glinge et al., 2017). Details can be found in a recent review by Judice et al. (2016).

The study and processing of microRNAs as biomarkers requires attention since it's fragile structure and stability may be compromised depending on the methods and the biological material used (e.g., blood, serum, plasma, urine) (Wang et al., 2012; Rice et al., 2015; Glinge et al., 2017). Nevertheless, there are reports that microRNAs are stable in serum and plasma samples, and they are resistant to RNAse action, extreme pH, freezing and thawing conditions (Chen et al., 2008; Gilad et al., 2008; Mitchell et al., 2008; Glinge et al., 2017).

MicroRNA expression is complex and begins in the cell nucleus. The miRNA gene transcription by the action of RNA polymerase II results in the formation of a double-stranded primary miRNA (pri-miRNA) with a tail at its 5' end and a poly-A tail at the 3' end (Filella and Foj, 2017; Malla et al., 2019). Pri-miRNAs then give rise to a hairpin structure that mates with a microprocessor (500-650 kDa). This structure has an endonuclease RNAse III (Drosha) and an essential cofactor (DGCR8/Pasha), which combine and form the precursor miRNA (pre-miRNA) that is then transported to the cytoplasm by a nuclear export protein called Exportin-5 (exp5) and the Ran GTP cofactor (Malla et al., 2019). In the cytoplasm, the pre-miRNA is processed by the Dicer RNase, resulting in a double-stranded RNA of approximately 22 nucleotides. One strand becomes the mature microRNA, while the other, a microRNA-5p, is degraded (Filella and Foj, 2017; Malla et al., 2019). Subsequently, the mature microRNA binds to the Argonaut protein (AGO) and forms the RNA-induced silencer complex (RISC) (Chan et al., 2005; Murakami et al., 2006; Filella and Foj, 2017; Malla et al., 2019). Mature microRNAs are incorporated into RISC to regulate gene expression by mRNA degradation or translational repression (Murakami et al., 2006) (**Figure 1**).

Toxoplasma gondii INFECTION AND HOST IMMUNE RESPONSE

Toxoplasma gondii (T. gondii), the etiological agent for toxoplasmosis, is an intracellular parasite that infects nucleated cells from all warm-blooded animals (Li et al., 2019; Hou et al., 2019). It has three infectious stages known as tachyzoite, bradyzoite, and sporozoites (within oocysts) (Dubey et al., 1998). Tachyzoites are crescent-shaped, with a pointed end in the anterior region and rounded in the posterior region. This mobile stage can invade nucleated cells and multiply by repeated endodyogeny within parasitophorous vacuoles within any cell of the intermediate host and in non-intestinal epithelial cells of the definitive host (Robert-Gangneux and Dardé, 2012). Bradyzoites, also called cystozoites, is the form found in tissue cysts of intermediate hosts and multiply slowly within a tissue cyst (Dubey et al., 1998). Infected felines can eliminate unsporulated oocysts with faeces to the environment. Under ideal temperature and humidity conditions, oocysts sporulate, forming two sporocysts containing four sporozoites each. The oocyst wall is characterised by a multilayered structure protecting the parasite against physical and chemical damage, allowing the parasite to survive for long periods in the environment (Dubey et al., 1998; Robert-Gangneux and Dardé, 2012).

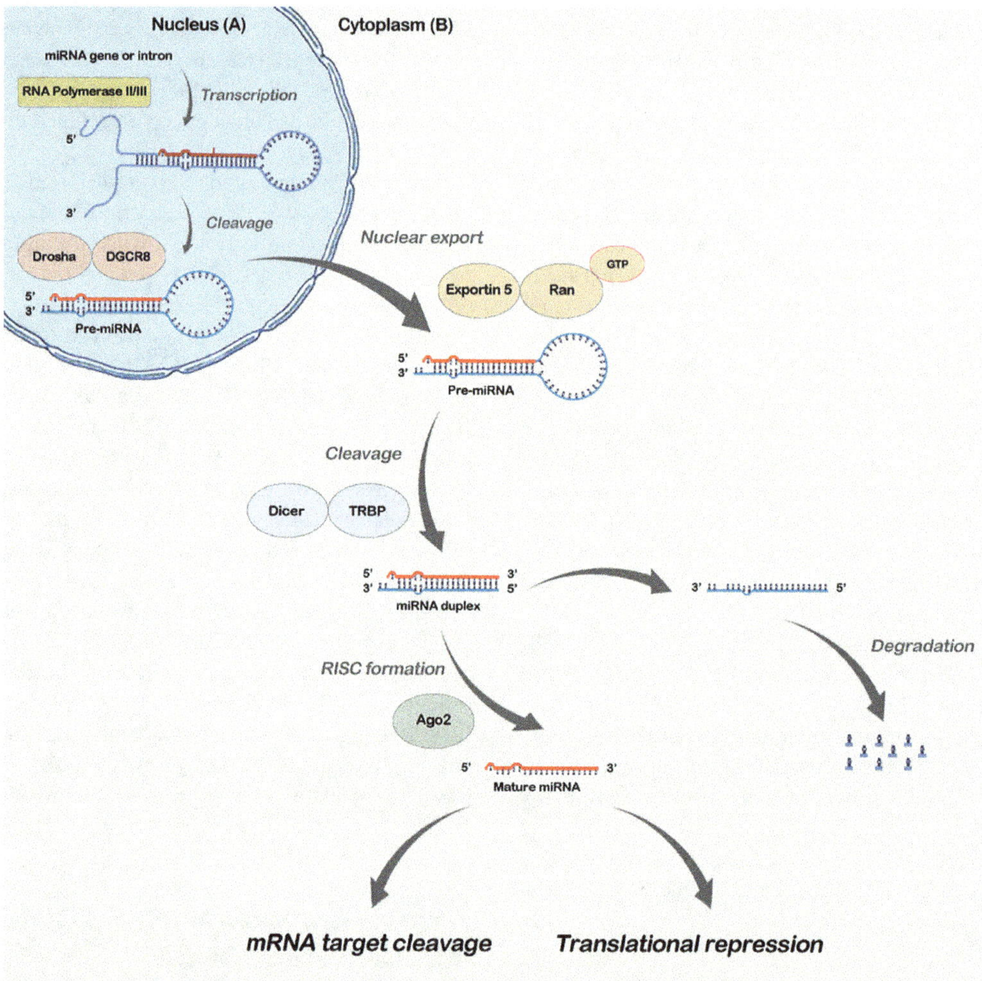

FIGURE 1 | microRNA Biogenesis Steps. In the nucleus, miRNA gene transcription occurs by RNA polymerase III, resulting in the primary double-stranded miRNA (pri73 miRNA). The miRNA precursor (pre-miRNA) formation occurs, which is transported to the cytoplasm through exp5 and the Ran GTP cofactor **(A)**. In the cytoplasm, pre miRNA is processed by Dicer RNAse, resulting in a double-stranded RNA, mature RNA and microRNA-5p. The second is degraded, and the mature microRNA binds to Argonaut protein (AGO) and forms the RNA-induced silencer complex (RISC). Mature microRNAs incorporate into RISC, regulating gene expression by mRNA degradation or transductional repression **(B)**.

T. gondii is horizontally transmitted by ingestion of contaminated water and food and vertically from mother to child during pregnancy (Robert-Gangneux and Dardé, 2012; Murata et al., 2016). In most cases, the infection by *T. gondii* is asymptomatic (Lima and Lodoen, 2019). However, the disease is commonly severe in immunocompromised individuals and neonates (Robert-Gangneux and Dardé, 2012). A small portion of immunocompetent individuals may also develop symptoms (Robert-Gangneux and Dardé, 2012). Immunosuppressed individuals commonly develop neurological symptoms and encephalitis. However, if the infection is acquired during pregnancy, it can result in severe or fatal toxoplasmosis (Robert-Gangneux and Dardé, 2012). The severity of the disease is associated with conditions such as the period of gestation, type of strain, dose and host immune system (Dubey et al., 2012; Murata et al., 2016), and congenital toxoplasmosis may lead to visual and hearing complications and cognitive impairments (Li et al., 2019).

The human immune response against *T. gondii* infection includes the production of IL-12 by neutrophils, dendritic cells and macrophages (Bliss et al., 1999; Aldebert et al., 2007). These cytokines are crucial for host resistance, blocking parasite replication and increasing the degradation of tryptophan (Pfefferkorn, 1984; Lima and Lodoen, 2019).

T. gondii uses sophisticated strategies to infect the host cell. The parasite releases proteins from organelles called rhoptries and dense granules, signalising host cells and their transcriptional responses (Lima and Lodoen, 2019; Tuladhar et al., 2019). By this mechanism, the parasite can manipulate host signalling pathways, modulating the release of cytokines and consequently compromising an effective host immune response against the parasite.

Three types of *T. gondii* strains called type I, type II and type III carrying different virulence factors were identified in mouse models. Studies have shown that the type I strain is the most virulent while type II and III strains are avirulent (Howe et al., 1996; Mordue et al., 2001). Type I strain can cause a lethal infection in mice at a dose of 1 parasite, while type II and III strains have a lethal media dose equal to or higher than 10^5 (Sibley and Boothroyd, 1992). An experimental study identified several characteristics that may correlate with virulence in a host, including phenotyping difference in growth, migration, and transmigration, with type I strain growing faster and with migration abilities greater than type II and III strains (Barragan and Sibley, 2003). The type I strain virulence correlates with the immune response inducing a more potent TH1-inflammatory response than Type II or III. Genetic studies have identified secretory proteins discharged from apical organelles, called rhoptries (ROPs), as the determinant of acute virulence in type 1 strain (Taylor et al., 2006; Saeij et al., 2007).

A study conducted by Saeji et al., 2006 showed that human and mouse cells response to parasite infection depends on *T. gondii* strain (e.g., types I, II and III). Types I and III (encoding ROP16 allele $ROP16_{I/III}$) cause direct and prolonged phosphorylation of host transcription factors STAT3 and STAT6 (Saeij et al., 2006). As a result, there is a decrease in the production of IL-12 in macrophages (Saeij et al., 2006; Saeij et al., 2007; Butcher et al., 2011; Cai and Shen, 2017; Lima and Lodoen, 2019; Tuladhar et al., 2019). Type II strains (carrying a $GRA15_{II}$ allele) activate the host transcription factor NF-kB, which leads to the production of pro-inflammatory cytokines in the host cell (Butcher et al., 2005; Lima and Lodoen, 2019; Tuladhar et al., 2019). These effects are caused by parasite rhoptry and dense granule proteins (Saeij et al., 2007; Ong et al., 2010; Yamamoto et al., 2012).

In humans and animals, the immune response mediated by IFN-γ is essential to control acute and chronic infections caused by the parasite (Suzuki et al., 1988; Suzuki et al., 1989). This cytokine can induce a vast transcriptional program (Platanias, 2005), and *T. gondii* infection blocks the positive regulation of many of those IFN-γ-controlled genes (Kim et al., 2007).

Studies in humans have shown that the three types of parasite strains described above can inhibit the transcriptional activity of the STAT1 protein through ROP16 or GRA15 proteins, which activate the NF-kB signalling pathway (Rosowski et al., 2011; Rosowski and Saeij, 2012; Lima and Lodoen, 2019). With the release of IFN-γ, signalling of the JAK/STAT pathway begins, allowing the displacement of the STAT1 homodimers to the cell nucleus, where it interacts with the gamma-activated sequence (GAS) in the DNA to initiate transcription (Sadzak et al., 2008). In response, *T. gondii* inhibits the expression of human genes that respond to IFN-γ, blocking the expression of the JAK/STAT pathway and consequently preventing the separation of STAT1 from the host nuclear DNA (Rosowski et al., 2014).

Studies conducted by Gray et al., 2016 and Olias et al., 2016 revealed two mechanisms used by the parasite to manipulate the host immune system: (i) the inhibitor of STAT1-dependent transcription (TgIST), which is a protein, binds to activated STAT1 dimers in the nucleus of IFN-γ-dependent cells, and (ii) the Mi2/NuRD complex, which can modify the chromatin of cells, blocking IFN-γ-dependent transcriptional mechanisms (Gray et al., 2015; Olias et al., 2016).

The NF-kB signalling pathway is another important pathway deregulated by *T. gondii*, which produces pro-inflammatory cytokines in host immunity (Lima and Lodoen, 2019). It was observed that in Human Foreskin Fibroblast (HFFs) infected with a type I strain of *T. gondii*, phosphorylation of the transcription factor p65/RelA was reduced, preventing translocation to the host cell nucleus and limiting the activation of the NF-kB pathway (Butcher et al., 2011). Besides, the same type I strain inhibited the production of IL-1β by human neutrophils, impairing the activity of the NF-kB pathway (Lima and Lodoen, 2019) (**Figure 2**).

HOST microRNAs DURING *Toxoplasma gondii* INFECTION

The microRNA blockade of mRNA is fundamental for protection against pathogenic virus and bacteria in plants, insects and animals (Hou et al., 2019). microRNAs interact mainly with the 3' untranslated region of their target mRNAs, controlling the translation or affecting the transcript stability favouring mRNA degradation (Hou et al., 2019). Some studies have shown that Apicomplexan parasites affect the host microRNA expression profile (Deng et al., 2004; McDonald et al., 2013; Hou et al., 2019). After cell invasion, these microorganisms regulate gene expression of host cells, including those cells of the immune system, such as macrophages and dendritic cells (Leng et al., 2009; Hou et al., 2019). This process contributes to parasite persistence and microbial growth (Blader et al., 2001; Hou et al., 2019).

T. gondii infection perturbs the expression of specific host microRNAs, which contributes to efficient parasite replication (Cong et al., 2017) by altering the signalling pathways involved in the defensive response of infected cells (Hakimi and Ménard, 2010). The infection by cysts and tachyzoites lead to altered microRNA expression in mouse brain (Xu et al., 2013) and spleen (He et al., 2016). However, it is unknown whether sporulated oocyst infections also modify the expression levels of microRNAs in animal brains during acute and chronic infection (Hu et al., 2018).

There is evidence that *T. gondii* modulates the expression of important microRNAs (Zeiner et al., 2010). With the activation state of NF-κB, 14% of the host microRNAs are altered in primary fibroblasts 24 hours post-infection (Shapira et al., 2002; Judice et al., 2016). In agreement with these observations, two studies showed that during infection, there is an increased expression of miR-17-92 and miR-106b-25, which regulate the progression of the mammalian cell cycle from G1 to the S phase influencing the apoptosis pathways (Xiao and Rajewsky, 2009; Cai and Shen, 2017) (**Table 1**).

The transcription factor NF-κB plays a fundamental role in *T. gondii* immunity, and it is believed that the parasite might use it

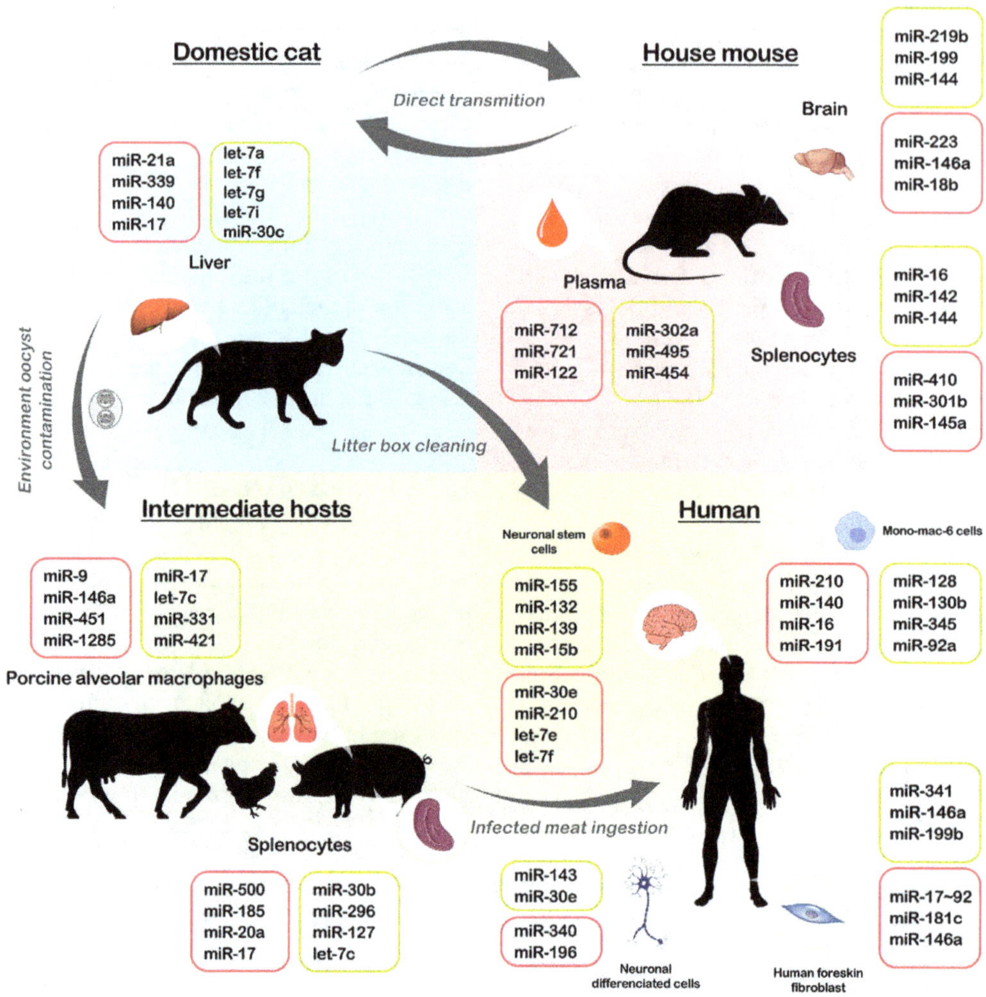

FIGURE 2 | Life cycle of Toxoplasma and host miRNA interaction. *T gondii* has a complex life cycle, in which the parasite can infect felids (domestic cats), farm animals, mice, and even humans. Felids are definitive hosts. Oocysts are released from infected cat faeces and become infected in the environment after sporulate. Infected felids present modifications in microRNA expressions. Humans become infected by ingestion of undercooked meat of infected animals or by the ingestion of soil, water or food contained sporulated oocysts derived from the environment. In the human host, the disease can affect various organs tissues such as skeletal muscle, brain (neuronally differentiated cells and neuronal stem cells) and myocardium, presenting modifications in microRNA expressions. Also, porcine alveolar macrophages and splenocytes samples from infected pigs have modified microRNA profiles. Mice are used mainly to study toxoplasmosis *in vivo* because they may naturally be infected by the parasite and affect multiple organs while changing their microRNA profile. These animals can also be having multiple organs affected by the infection, and it is known that the spleen, plasma, and brain have their miRNA profile altered during the infection. The colour box represents the increase (pink) and decreases (yellow) of miRNA expressions.

to modulate innate and adaptive immune responses of the host (Denkers et al., 2004; Mason et al., 2004). *T. gondii* can suppress NF-κB activation (Shapira et al., 2002) by inducing the expression of miR-146a in the host (Taganov et al., 2006). The activation of NF-κB signalling and *STAT3* gene up-regulates the expression of miRNAs miR-30c-1, miR-125b-2, miR-23b-27b-24-1 and miR-17-92 in response to *T. gondii* infection (Cai et al., 2013). (**Table 1**). The expression of the immunomodulatory microRNAs miR-146a and miR-155 was induced in the brains of mice infected with specific *T. gondii* strains (Cannella et al., 2014). Animals infected with a type II strain showed significant induction of miR-146a, an essential regulator of the inflammatory immune response (Taganov et al., 2006; Saba et al., 2014; Judice et al., 2016). It was also observed that the absence of miR-146a expression affects parasitic load, leading to significant differences in IFN-γ production and long-term survival of infected mice (Judice et al., 2016).

The microRNA miR-155 is highly expressed in human and animal Th17 cells (Hu et al., 2013; Escobar et al., 2014) (**Table 1**). Besides, this microRNA is critical for TH17 cell cytokine expression and Treg cell homeostasis. Studies in animals showed that miR-155 is associated with recruiting Treg and CD8+ cells in *T. gondii* infection (Cai and Shen, 2017). microRNAs can also modify innate immune response

TABLE 1 | The role of microRNAs in toxoplasmosis diseases.

microRNA	Disease/ Parasite	Effects	References
microRNA-17-92; microRNA-106b-25	Toxoplasma/ *T. gondii*	Apoptosis and G1/S cell cycle transition pathways.	(Xiao and Rajewsky, 2009; Cai and Shen, 2017)
microRNA-146a	Toxoplasma/ *T. gondii*	NF-κB signalling pathway	(Taganov et al., 2006)
microRNA-30c-1; microRNA-125b-2; microRNA-23b-27b-24-1; microRNA-17-92	Toxoplasma/ *T. gondii*	Associated with the anti-apoptosis responses of the host cells.	(Cai et al., 2013)
microRNA-146a	Toxoplasma/ *T. gondii*	Cellular response in the host to infection by *T. gondii* and inflammatory response regulator.	(Taganov et al., 2006; Cannella et al., 2014; Saba et al., 2014; Judice et al., 2016)
microRNA-155	Toxoplasma/ *T. gondii*	Cellular response in the host to infection by *T. gondii* and required for Cytokine expression by TH17 cells and Treg-Cell homeostasis.	(Cannella et al., 2014; Cai and Shen, 2017)
microRNA-132b	Toxoplasma/ *T. gondii*	Influence on *Toxoplasma* encephalopathy.	(Cai and Shen, 2017)
microRNA-712-3p; microRNA-511-5p; microRNA-217-5p	Toxoplasma/ *T. gondii*	Possible biomarkers of *T. gondii* infection	(Jia et al., 2014)

signalling through pathogen-aware receptors (Fabbri et al., 2013). An example is miR-132b, found in abundance in neural tissue cells and regulated by cyclic AMP-response element-binding (CREB). This microRNA is involved in neurological disorders such as schizophrenia, Alzheimer disease, Parkinson disease and is also involved in *T. gondii* encephalopathy (Miller et al., 2012; Cai and Shen, 2017) (**Table 1**).

Another study in mice by Cai et al. (2014) found three microRNAs (miR-712-3p, miR-511-5p, and miR-217-5p) at the beginning of the infection. According to these authors, the increase in these microRNAs is *T. gondii* specific, and these molecules are predominantly expressed in cells infected with RH and ME49 strains (Miller et al., 2012; Cai et al., 2014). Thus, the expression profile of these microRNAs suggests that they can be used as biomarkers of *T. gondii* infection. Furthermore, other pathogens such as *Plasmodium berghei*, *Plasmodium yoelii*, *Plasmodium chabaudi*, and *C. parvum* do not induce the expression of these microRNAs reinforces the use of microRNAs as potential *T. gondii* biomarkers (Judice et al., 2016). Therefore, the potential specific expression of miR-712-3p, miR-511-5p and miR-217-5p during *T. gondii* infection makes them excellent candidate biomarkers for diagnosis (Judice et al., 2016).

Recently, two studies carried out in Brazil evaluated the expression of microRNAs in ocular toxoplasmosis and cerebral toxoplasmosis in HIV patients (Pereira et al., 2019). In one of them, the authors reported that the microRNAs miR-155-5p and miR-29c-3p were up-expressed in ocular toxoplasmosis compared to asymptomatic individuals. They also observed that the miR-21-5p and miR-125b-5p were down-expressed in acute ocular toxoplasmosis compared to asymptomatic individuals (Pereira et al., 2019). The other one demonstrated that the miR-21-5p and miR-146a5p were up-expressed in HIV patients with cerebral toxoplasmosis compared with asymptomatic individuals and seronegative individuals. These authors observed that the plasma of HIV patients with cerebral toxoplasmosis CT/HIV and asymptomatic individuals expressed similar levels of miR-29c-3p, miR-155-5p and miR-125b-5p (Pereira et al., 2019). The data showed in these studies demonstrate some specific patterns of miRNAs as potential biomarkers for ocular toxoplasmosis and HIV cerebral toxoplasmosis patients. These findings may help understand the complex parasite-host interaction and diagnosis, prognosis, and therapeutic control in human toxoplasmosis.

microRNAs FOR DIAGNOSIS OF *T. gondii* INFECTION IN HUMANS

T. gondii infection is usually asymptomatic in healthy individuals. When symptomatic, most infected people develop non-specific symptoms such as fever or cervical lymphadenopathy that can be easily misdiagnosed as the common flu, mononucleosis, etc. (Robert-Gangneux and Dardé, 2012). Ocular toxoplasmosis is the most common complication caused by *T. gondii* infection. However, the infection can be severe or even fatal in immunocompromised individuals (e.g. HIV-infected, solid organs transplant recipients) and by transplacental transmission, the foetus may develop severe stages of the pulmonary disease disseminated and cerebral toxoplasmosis (Robert-Gangneux et al., 2018).

The diagnosis of toxoplasmosis is still based on serology and clinical evaluation (Villard et al., 2016). Serological tests are essential, and most can determine the stage of infection (Dhakal et al., 2015; Murata et al., 2016). It is crucial to monitor the serological status of pregnant women since the parasite can cross the placental barrier and infect the foetus leading in many cases to severe illness and abortion (Robert-Gangneux and Dardé, 2012). Anti-*T. gondii* IgM and IgG antibodies are common biomarkers for the diagnosis of toxoplasmosis. IgM is associated with recent infection and IgG with chronic infection. Although the evaluation of these antibodies differentiates acute from chronically infected patients, antibodies may be persistent or absent in some cases. Therefore, additional tests are necessary to confirm serological results, making the diagnose of *T. gondii* difficult and time-consuming (Goebel et al., 1999; Carmen et al., 2006; Cai and Shen, 2017). IgM antibodies usually appear one week after infection and may drop to undetectable levels within six months. However, in some cases, IgM can be detected for more than one year after infection (Goebel et al., 1999). The evaluation of other acute antibodies like IgA in conjunction with IgM can help diagnose acute toxoplasmosis, especially in neonates (Montoya, 2002; Murata et al., 2016; Pomares and Montoya, 2016). IgG antibodies usually appear within the first two weeks of infection and usually persist for a lifetime in low titres. The presence of these antibodies with the avidity of IgG can be an essential tool to determine the timing of infection (Montoya, 2002; Murata et al., 2016; Villard et al., 2016).

Molecular approaches can be used as a complement of serological tests when the diagnose is unclear by serology and can be used to detect *T. gondii* DNA in various samples (Okay et al., 2009; Robert-Gangneux and Dardé, 2012; Murata et al., 2017; Murata et al., 2020). The most used targets for *T. gondii* are the *B1* multi-copy gene and the 529 bp repeat element with 35 and 200-300 copies in the *T. gondii* genome, respectively (Homan et al., 2000; Ivović et al., 2012; Camilo et al., 2017; Nakashima et al., 2020; Murata et al., 2020). Although molecular tests for the diagnosis of toxoplasmosis are becoming more frequent, they are still controversial, and there is no agreement about the best method or target to be used (Garweg et al., 2011; Maenz et al., 2014; Greigert et al., 2019; Murata et al., 2020). Also, the concentration of *T. gondii* DNA during chronic infection is usually undetectable even when molecular sensitivity tests are performed (Ivović et al., 2012). Consequently, the diagnosis of *T. gondii* infection is still difficult and the development of novel methods with higher specificity and sensitivity is paramount.

Several studies have related the use of microRNAs as new biomarkers in several diseases such as cancer (Wang et al., 2020; Kooshkaki et al., 2020; Di et al., 2020), cardiovascular (Sun et al., 2020), and bacterial diseases (Jia et al., 2014), as well as a non-invasive diagnosis and monitoring method of parasitic disease progression (Hu et al., 2013). A study by Jia et al., 2014 used 60 BALB/c female mice intraperitoneally infected with 10^6 tachyzoites of RH or ME49 strain per mice to assess the feasibility of using microRNAs as biomarkers of early *T. gondii* infection. Seventy-two hours after infection, the presence of 414 murine microRNAs was evaluated on plasma RNA samples by real-time PCR. The results showed that microRNAs miR-712-3p, miR-511-5p, and miR-217-5p are significantly expressed in mice infected with either *T. gondii* strains (Jia et al., 2014). These authors also found that the up-regulation of these three microRNAs were *T. gondii* specific when compared to similar infections with *P. berghei*, *P. yoelii*, *P. chabaudi*, *C. parvum*, Mouse Hepatitis Virus, and *Staphylococcus aureus*. This observation has drawn attention to the use of microRNAs as early biomarkers of infection in parasitic diseases, which results in their usefulness in the laboratory diagnosis of acute infection, especially before the appearance of IgM antibodies.

The use of a test that could detect *T. gondii* infection in earlier stages would be ideal, mainly during pregnancy, as early treatment of infected mothers seems to decrease the risk of transmission and severity to the foetus improving clinical outcomes (Wallon et al., 2013; Begeman et al., 2017). Expression of microRNAs may precede IgM class antibodies in parasitic diseases since that IgM antibodies may eventually be undetected within the first weeks following infection (Murata et al., 2020). Furthermore, the microRNAs may be biomarkers of high sensitivity and specificity for diagnosis at different stages of infection.

Jia et al., 2014 have shown that three microRNAs were specific for *T. gondii* infection in mice, but there is no study to compare the expression of these biomarkers in humans. The main advantage of using microRNA to diagnose human toxoplasmosis is that they can be found in samples commonly acquired for the diagnosis of *T. gondii* infection such as peripheral blood, amniotic fluid, and aqueous humour, as well as in other types of specimens that can be collected using non-invasive methods like urine, saliva, and others. Also, real-time PCR for detecting specific microRNAs to diagnose human toxoplasmosis is likely the best approach since it usually has higher sensibility and specificity than conventional PCR (Ivović et al., 2012).

To our knowledge, few studies in the literature relate microRNAs to the diagnosis of toxoplasmosis in humans. Our research group investigates the use of four microRNAs (miR-712-3p, miR-511-5p, miR-217-5p, and miR-9-2) for the diagnosis of human ocular toxoplasmosis using blood samples. Our study may contribute to a better understanding of microRNAs' role during *T. gondii* infections in humans (**Table 1**).

FINAL CONSIDERATIONS

The data presented in this revision concerning microRNAs attract the attention for the potential use of these small nucleic acid molecules to explore at least four different aspects of human toxoplasmosis. One of them refers to laboratory diagnosis. Diagnosis methods based on early detection of microRNAs could be an essential tool, especially for detecting microRNA in peripheral blood before IgM antibodies appear. In this context, microRNAs could be explored as biological markers of infection, especially in the acute phase of the disease, allowing the early treatment of human acute toxoplasmosis. This strategy could reduce tissue inflammation and, consequently, the tissue damage in target organs such as the eye and brain.

Another potential application of the detection of microRNA in human toxoplasmosis refers to the tissue targeted by *T. gondii*. Investigations aiming to check if one or more specific microRNA might be expressed in some particular infected tissues would establish a correlation with the clinical form of human toxoplasmosis. Despite the parasite infecting any nucleated cell, it remains in a latent phase, and the majority of individuals remains asymptomatic. However, the human toxoplasmosis clinical manifestation occurs in some target organs and would be appropriate to understand the potential relation between the

T. gondii and the infected tissues. This strategy could favour the comprehension of new aspects of the host-parasite interaction in human toxoplasmosis.

The observations that some types of microRNA are up-regulated in ocular toxoplasmosis and cerebral toxoplasmosis in HIV patients open opportunity to investigate if this up- or down-regulation correlates specific strains. This strategy could be adding new information on how different *T. gondii* strains modulate the host cells affecting cell mobility through blood, neurological, and ocular barriers. Besides, it would be possible to verify microRNAs also correlates the different ways of *T. gondii* acquisition of the infection by placenta or acquired after birth.

Finally, exploring mi-RNA in the different clinical forms of human toxoplasmosis would clarify how host microRNAs modulate this parasite infection and how *T. gondii* interacts with human hosts.

AUTHOR CONTRIBUTIONS

GMFJr, CA, FM, and HL wrote the manuscript. LA and BC drew the table and figure in the manuscript. CB and LM revised the manuscript. All authors contributed to the article and approved the submitted version.

REFERENCES

1. Aldebert, D., Durand, F., Mercier, C., Brenier-Pinchart, M. P., Cesbron Delauw, M. F., and Pelloux, H. (2007). *Toxoplasma gondii* Triggers Secretion of Interleukin-12 But Low Level of Interleukin-10 From the THP-1 Human Monocytic Cell Line. *Cytokine* 37, 206–211. doi: 10.1016/j.cyto.2007.03.012
2. Barragan, A., and Sibley, L. D. (2003). Migration of *Toxoplasma gondii* Across Biological Barriers. *Trends Microbiol.* 11, 426–430. doi: 10.1016/s0966-842x (03)00205-1
3. Begeman, I. J., Lykins, J., Zhou, Y., Lai, B. S., Levigne, P., El Bissati, K., et al. (2017). Point-of-Care Testing for *Toxoplasma gondii* IgG/IgM Using Toxoplasma ICT IgG-IgM Test With Sera From the United States and Implications for Developing Countries. *PloS Negl. Trop. Dis.* 11, e0005670. doi: 10.1371/journal.pntd.0005670
4. Blader, I. J., Manger, I. D., and Boothroyd, J. C. (2001). Microarray Analysis Reveals Previously Unknown Changes in *Toxoplasma gondii*-Infected Human Cells. *J. Biol. Chem.* 276, 24223–24231. doi: 10.1074/jbc.M100951200
5. Bliss, S. K., Marshall, A. J., Zhang, Y., and Denkers, E. Y. (1999). Human Polymorphonuclear Leukocytesproduce IL-12,TNF-Alpha, and the Chemokines Macrophage-Inflammatory Protein-1 Alpha and–1 Beta in Response to *Toxoplasma gondii* Antigens. *J. Immunol.* 162, 7369–7375.
6. Butcher, B. A., Fox, B. A., Rommereim, L. M., Kim, S. G., Maurer, K. J., Yarovinsky, F., et al. (2011). *Toxoplasma gondii* Rhoptry Kinase ROP16 Activates STAT3 and STAT6 Resulting in Cytokine Inhibition and Arginase-1dependent Growth Control. *PloS Pathog.* 7, e1002236. doi: 10.1371/journal.ppat.1002236
7. Butcher, B. A., Kim, L., Panopoulos, A. D., Watowich, S. S., Murray, P. J., and Denkers, E. Y. (2005). IL-10-Independent STAT3 Activation by *Toxoplasma gondii* Mediates Suppression of IL-12 and TNF-Alpha in Host Macrophages. *J. Immunol.* 174,3148–3152. doi: 10.4049/jimmunol.174.6.3148
8. Cai, Y., Chen, H., Jin, L., You, Y., and Shen, J. (2013). STAT3-Dependent Transactivation of miRNA Genes Following *Toxoplasma gondii* Infection in Macrophage. *Parasit. Vectors* 6:356. doi: 10.1186/1756-3305-6-356
9. Cai, Y., Chen, H., Mo, X., Tang, Y., Xu, X., Zhang, A., et al. (2014). *Toxoplasma gondii* Inhibits Apoptosis Via a Novel STAT3-mir-17-92-Bim Pathway in Macrophages. *Cell. Signal.* 26, 1204–1212. doi: 10.1016/j.cellsig.2014.02.013
10. Cai, Y., and Shen, J. (2017). Modulation of Host Immune Responses to *Toxoplasma gondii* by microRNAs. *Parasite Immunol* 39, e12417. doi: 10.1111/pim.12417
11. Camilo, L. M., Pereira-Chioccola, V. L., Gava, R., Meira-Strejevitch, C. S., Vidal, J. E., de Mattos, C. C. B., et al. (2017). Molecular Diagnosis of Symptomatic Toxoplasmosis: A 9-Year Retrospective and Prospective Study in a Referral Laboratory in São Paulo, Brazil. *Braz. J. Infect. Dis.* 21, 638–647. doi: 10.1016/j.bjid.2017.07.003
12. Cannella, D., Brenier-Pinchart, M. P., Braun, L., van Rooyen, J. M., Bougdour, A., Bastien, O., et al. (2014). miR-146a and miR-155 Delineate a microRNA Fingerprint Associated With Toxoplasma Persistence in the Host Brain. *Cell Rep.* 6, 928–937. doi: 10.1016/j.celrep.2014.02.002
13. Carmen, J. C., Hardi, L., and Sinai, A. P. (2006). *Toxoplasma gondii* Inhibits Ultraviolet Light-Induced Apoptosis Through Multiple Interactions With the Mitochondrion-Dependent Programmed Cell Death Pathway. *Cell. Microbiol.* 8, 301–315. doi: 10.1111/j.1462-5822.2005.00622.x
14. Cavalier-Smith, T. (1993). Kingdom Protozoa and Its 18 Phyla. *Microbiol. Rev.* 57, 953–994. doi: 10.1128/MR.57.4.953-994.1993
15. Chan, J. A., Krichevsky, A. M., and Kosik, K. S. (2005). microRNA-21 is an Antiapoptotic Factor in Human Glioblastoma Cells. *Cancer Res.* 65, 6029–6033. doi: 10.1158/0008-5472.CAN-05-0137
16. Chen, X., Ba, Y., Ma, L., Cai, X., Yin, Y., Wang, K., et al. (2008). Characterisation of microRNAs in Serum: A Novel Class of Biomarkers for Diagnosis of Cancer and Other Diseases. *Cell Res.* 18, 997–1006. doi: 10.1038/cr.2008.282
17. Chim, S. S., Shing, T. K., Hung, E. C., Leung, T. Y., Lau, T. K., Chiu, R. W., et al. (2008). Detection and Characterisation of Placental microRNAs in Maternal Plasma. *Clin. Chem.* 54, 482–490. doi: 10.1373/clinchem.2007.097972
18. Cong, W., Zhang, X. X., He, J. J., Li, F. C., Elsheikha, H. M., and Zhu, X. Q. (2017). Global miRna Expression Profiling of Domestic Cat Livers Following Acute *Toxoplasma gondii* Infection. *Oncotarget* 8, 25599–25611. doi: 10.18632/oncotarget.16108
19. D'Alessandra, Y., Devanna, P., Limana, F., Straino, S., Di Carlo, A., Brambilla, P. G., et al. (2010). Circulating microRNAs are New and Sensitive Biomarkers of Myocardial Infarction. *Eur. Heart J.* 31, 2765–2773. doi: 10.1093/eurheartj/ehq167
20. Deng, M., Lancto, C. A., and Abrahamsen, M. S. (2004). *Cryptosporidium Parvum* Regulation of Human Epithelial Cell Gene Expression. *Int. J. Parasitol.* 34, 73–82. doi: 10.1016/j.ijpara.2003.10.001
21. Denkers, E. Y., Butcher, B. A., Del Rio, L., and Kim, L. (2004). Manipulation of Mitogen-Activated Protein Kinase/Nuclear Factor-Kappab-Signaling Cascades During Intracellular *Toxoplasma gondii* Infection. *Immunol. Rev.* 201, 191– 205. doi: 10.1111/j.0105-2896.2004.00180.x
22. Dhakal, R., Gajurel, K., Pomares, C., Talucod, J., Press, C. J., and Montoya, J. G. (2015). Significance of a Positive Toxoplasma Immunoglobulin M Test Result in the United States. *J. Clin. Microbiol.* 53, 3601–3605. doi: 10.1128/JCM.01663-15
23. Di, Z., Di, M., Fu, W., Tang, Q., Liu, Y., Lei, P., et al. (2020). Integrated Analysis Identifies a Nine-microRNA Signature Biomarker for Diagnosis and Prognosis in Colorectal Cancer. *Front. Genet.* 11:192. doi: 10.3389/fgene.2020.00192
24. Dubey, J. P., Lago, E. G., Gennari, S. M., Su, C., and Jones, J. L. (2012). Toxoplasmosis in Humans and Animals in Brazil: High Prevalence, High Burden of Disease, and Epidemiology. *Parasitology* 139, 1375–1424. doi: 10.1017/S0031182012000765
25. Dubey, J. P., Lindsay, D. S., and Speer, C. A. (1998). Structures of *Toxoplasma gondii* Tachyzoites, Bradyzoites, and Sporozoites and Biology and Development of Tissue Cysts. *Clin. Microbiol. Rev.* 11, 267–299. doi: 10.1128/CMR.11.2.267
26. Escobar, T. M., Kanellopoulou, C., Kugler, D. G., Kilaru, G., Nguyen, C. K., Nagarajan, V., et al. (2014). miR-155 Activates Cytokine Gene Expression in Th17 Cells by Regulating the DNA-Binding Protein Jarid2 to Relieve Polycomb-Mediated Repression. *Immunity* 40, 865–879. doi: 10.1016/ j.immuni.2014.03.014
27. Fabbri, M., Paone, A., Calore, F., Galli, R., and Croce, C. M. (2013). A New Role for microRNAs, as Ligands of Toll-Like Receptors. *RNA Biol.* 10, 169–174. doi: 10.4161/rna.23144
28. Filella, X., and Foj, L. (2017). miRNAs as Novel Biomarkers in the Management of Prostate Cancer. *Clin. Chem. Lab. Med.* 55, 715–736. doi: 10.1515/cclm-2015-1073 Friedman, R. C., Farh, K. K., Burge, C. B., and Bartel, D.

P. (2009). Most Mammalian miRNAs are Conserved Targets of microRNAs. *Genome Res.* 19, 92–105. doi: 10.1101/gr.082701
29. Garweg, J. G., de Groot-Mijnes, J. D. F., and Montoya, J. G. (2011). Diagnostic Approach to Ocular Toxoplasmosis. *Ocul. Immunol. Inflamm.* 19, 255–261. doi: 10.3109/09273948.2011.595872
30. Gazzinelli, R. T., Kalantari, P., Fitzgerald, K. A., and Golenbock, D. T. (2014). Innate Sensing of Malaria Parasites. *Nat. Rev. Immunol.* 14, 744–757. doi: 10.1038/nri3742
31. Gidlöf, O., Andersson, P., van der Pals, J., Götberg, M., and Erlinge, D. (2011). Cardiospecific microRNA Plasma Levels Correlate With Troponin and Cardiac Function in Patients With ST Elevation Myocardial Infarction, are Selectively Dependent on Renal Elimination, and Can Be Detected in Urine Samples. *Cardiology* 118, 217–226. doi: 10.1159/000328869
32. Gilad, S., Meiri, E., Yogev, Y., Benjamin, S., Lebanony, D., Yerushalmi, N., et al. (2008). Serum microRNAs are Promising Novel Biomarkers. *PloS One* 3, e3148. doi: 10.1371/journal.pone.0003148
33. Glinge, C., Clauss, S., Boddum, K., Jabbari, R., Jabbari, J., Risgaard, B., et al. (2017). Stability of Circulating Blood-Based microRNAs - Pre-Analytic Methodological Considerations. *PloS One* 12, e0167969. doi: 10.1371/journal.pone.0167969
34. Goebel, S., Lüder, C. G., and Gross, U. (1999). Invasion by *Toxoplasma gondii* Protects Human-Derived HL-60 Cells From Actinomycin D-Induced Apoptosis. *Med. Microbiol. Immunol.* 187, 221–226. doi: 10.1007/s004300050096
35. Gray, N. K., Hrabalkova, L., Scanlon, J. P., and Smith, R. W. (2015). Poly(a)- Binding Proteins and miRNA Localisation: Who Rules the Roost? *Biochem. Soc Trans.* 43, 1277–1284. doi: 10.1042/BST20150171
36. Greigert, V., Di Foggia, E., Filisetti, D., Villard, O., Pfaff, A. W., Sauer, A., et al. (2019). When Biology Supports Clinical Diagnosis: Review of Techniques to Diagnose Ocular Toxoplasmosis. *Br. J. Ophthalmol.* 103, 1008–1012. doi: 10.1136/bjophthalmol-2019-313884
37. Hakimi, M. A., and Menard, R. (2010). Do Apicomplexan Parasites Hijack the Host Cell microRNA Pathway for Their Intracellular Development? *F1000 Biol. Rep.* 2:42. doi: 10.3410/B2-42
38. Hanke, M., Hoefig, K., Merz, H., Feller, A. C., Kausch, I., Jocham, D., et al. (2010). A Robust Methodology to Study Urine microRNA as Tumor Marker: microRNA-126 and microRNA-182 are Related to Urinary Bladder Cancer. *Urol. Oncol.* 28, 655–661. doi: 10.1016/j.urolonc.2009.01.027
39. He, J. J., Ma, J., Wang, J. L., Xu, M. J., and Zhu, X. Q. (2016). Analysis of miRNA Expression Profiling in Mouse Spleen Affected by Acute *Toxoplasma gondii* Infection. *Infect. Genet. Evol.* 37, 137–142. doi: 10.1016/j.meegid.2015.11.005
40. Homan, W. L., Vercammen, M., Braekeleer, J., and Verschueren, H. (2000). Identification of a 200- to 300-Fold Repetitive 529 Bp DNA Fragment in *Toxoplasma gondii*, and Its Use for Diagnostic and Quantitative PCR. *Int. J. Parasitol.* 30, 69–75. doi: 10.1016/s0020-7519(99)00170-8
41. Hou, Z., Liu, D., Su, S., Wang, L., Zhao, Z., Ma, Y., et al. (2019). Comparison of Splenocyte microRNA Expression Profiles of Pigs During Acute and Chronic Toxoplasmosis. *BMC Genomics* 20, 97. doi: 10.1186/s12864-019-5458-y
42. Howe, D. K., Summers, B. C., and Sibley, L. D. (1996). Acute Virulence in Mice is Associated With Markers on Chromosome VIII in *Toxoplasma gondii*. *Infect. Immun.* 64, 5193–5198. doi: 10.1128/IAI.64.12.5193-5198.1996
43. Hu, R. S., He, J. J., Elsheikha, H. M., Zhang, F. K., Zou, Y., Zhao, G. H., et al. (2018). Differential Brain microRNA Expression Profiles After Acute and Chronic Infection of Mice With *Toxoplasma gondii* Oocysts. *Front. Microbiol.* 9, 2316. doi: 10.3389/fmicb.2018.02316
44. Hu, R., Huffaker, T. B., Kagele, D. A., Runtsch, M. C., Bake, E., Chaudhuri, A. A., et al. (2013). microRNA-155 Confers Encephalogenic Potential to Th17 Cells by Promoting Effector Gene Expression. *J. Immunol.* 190, 5972–5980. doi: 10.4049/jimmunol.1300351
45. Ivovic, V., Vujanic, M., Zivkovic, T., Klun, I., and Djurkovic-Djakovic, O. (2012). Molecular Detection and Genotyping of *Toxoplasma gondii* From Clinical Samples. *Intec.* 103–120. doi: 10.5772/50830
46. Jia, B., Chang, Z., Wei, X., Lu, H., Yin, J., Jiang, N., et al. (2014). Plasma microRNAs are Promising Novel Biomarkers for the Early Detection of *Toxoplasma gondii* Infection. *Parasit. Vectors* 7:433. doi: 10.1186/1756-3305-7-433
47. Judice, C. C., Bourgard, C., Kayano, A. C., Albrecht, L., and Costa, F. T. (2016). microRNAs in the Host-Apicomplexan Parasites Interactions: A Review of Immunopathological Aspects. *Front. Cell Infect. Microbiol.* 6, 5. doi: 10.3389/ fcimb.2016.00005
48. Kim, S. K., Foutus, A. E., and Boothroyd, J. C. (2007). *Toxoplasma gondii* Dysregulates IFN-G-Inducible Gene Expression in Human Fibroblasts: Insights From a Genome-Wide Transcriptional Profiling. *J. Immunol.* 178, 5154–5165. doi: 10.4049/jimmunol.178.8.5154
49. Kooshkaki, O., Rezaei, Z., Rahmati, M., Vahedi, P., Derakhshani, A., Brunetti, O., et al. (2020). Mir-144: A New Possible Therapeutic Target and Diagnostic/ Prognostic Tool in Cancers. *Int. J. Mol. Sci.* 21:2578. doi: 10.3390/ijms21072578
50. Lawrie, C. H., Gal, S., Dunlop, H. M., Pushkaran, B., Liggins, A. P., Pulford, K., et al. (2008). Detection of Elevated Levels of Tumour-Associated microRNAs in Serum of Patients With Diffuse Large B-Cell Lymphoma. *Br. J. Haematol.* 141, 672–675. doi: 10.1111/j.1365-2141.2008.07077.x
51. Lee, R. C., Feinbaum, R. L., and Ambros, V. (1993). The *C. Elegans* Heterochronic Gene *Lin-4* Encodes Small Rnas With Antisense Complementarity to Lin-14. *Cell* 75, 843–854. doi: 10.1016/0092-8674(93)90529-Y
52. Leng, J., Butcher, B. A., and Denkers, E. Y. (2009). Dysregulation of Macrophage Signal Transduction by *Toxoplasma gondii*: Past Progress and Recent Advances. *Parasite Immunol.* 31, 717–728. doi: 10.1111/j.1365-3024.2009.01122.x
53. Lima, T. S., and Lodoen, M. B. (2019). Mechanisms of Human Innate Immune Evasion by *Toxoplasma gondii*. *Front. Cell. Infect. Microbiol.* 9, 103. doi: 10.3389/fcimb.2019.00103
54. Li, S., Yang, J., Wang, L., Du, F., Zhao, J., and Fang, R. (2019). Expression Profile of microRNAs in Porcine Alveolar Macrophages After *Toxoplasma gondii* Infection. *Parasit. Vectors* 12, 65. doi: 10.1186/s13071-019-3297-y
55. Lüder, C. G., and Gross, U. (2005). Apoptosis and Its Modulation During Infection With *Toxoplasma gondii*: Molecular Mechanisms and Role in Pathogenesis. *Curr. Top. Microbiol. Immunol.* 289, 219–237. doi: 10.1007/3-540-27320-4_10
56. Lu, J., Getz, G., Miska, E. A., Alvarez-Saavedra, E., Lamb, J., Peck, D., et al. (2005). microRNA Expression Profiles Classify Human Cancers*Nature* 435, 834–838. doi: 10.1038/nature03702
57. Maenz, M., Schlüter, D., Liesenfeld, O., Schares, G., Gross, U., and Pleyer, U. (2014). Ocular Toxoplasmosis Past, Present and New Aspects of an Old Disease. *Prog. Retin. Eye Res.* 39, 77–106. doi: 10.1016/j.preteyeres.2013.12.005
58. Malla, R. R., Kumari, S., Gavara, M. M., Badana, A. K., Gugalavath, S., Kumar, D. K. G., et al. (2019). A Perspective on the Diagnostics, Prognostics, and Therapeutics of microRNAs of Triple-Negative Breast Cancer. *Biophys. Rev.* 11, 227–234. doi: 10.1007/s12551-019-00503-8
59. Mason, N. J., Artis, D., and Hunter, C. A. (2004). New Lessons From Old Pathogens: What Parasitic Infections Have Taught Us About the Role of Nuclear Factor-Kappab in the Regulation of Immunity. *Immunol. Rev.* 201, 48–56. doi: 10.1111/j.0105-2896.2004.00189.x
60. McDonald, V., Korbel, D. S., Barakat, F. M., Choudhry, N., and Petry, F. (2013). Innate Immune Responses Against *Cryptosporidium Parvum* Infection. *Parasite Immunol.* 35, 55–64. doi: 10.1111/pim.12020
61. McDonald, J. S., Milosevic, D., Reddi, H. V., Grebe, S. K., and Algeciras- Schimnich, A. (2011). Analysis of Circulating microRNA: Preanalytical and Analytical Challenges. *Clin. Chem.* 57, 833– 840. doi: 10.1373/ clinchem.2010.157198
62. Miller, B. H., Zeier, Z., Xi, L., Lanz, T. A., Deng, S., Strathmann, J., et al. (2012). microRNA-132 Dysregulation in Schizophrenia Has Implications for Both Neurodevelopment and Adult Brain Function. *Proc. Natl. Acad. Sci. U.S.A.* 109, 3125–3130. doi: 10.1073/pnas.1113793109
63. Mirbase. Available at: www.mirbase.org/ (Accessed June 20, 2020). Mitchell, P. S., Parkin, R. K., Kroh, E. M., Fritz, B. R., Wyman, S. K., Pogosova- Agadjanyan, E. L., et al. (2008). Circulating microRNAs as Stable Blood-Based Markers for Cancer Detection. *Proc. Natl. Acad. Sci. U. S. A.* 105, 10513–10518. doi: 10.1073/pnas.0804549105
64. Montoya, J. G. (2002). Laboratory Diagnosis of *Toxoplasma gondii* Infection and Toxoplasmosis. *J. Infect. Dis.* 185, S73–S82. doi: 10.1086/338827
65. Mordue, D. G., Monroy, F., Regina, M. L., Dinarello, C. A., and Sible, L. D. (2001). Acute Toxoplasmosis Leads to Lethal Overproduction of Th1 Cytokines. *J. Immunol.* 167, 4574–4584. doi: 10.4049/jimmunol.167.8.4574
66. Murakami, Y., Yasuda, T., Saigo, K., Urashima, T., Toyoda, H., Okanoue, T., et al. (2006). Comprehensive Analysis of microRNA Expression Patterns in Hepatocellular Carcinoma and Non-Tumorous Tissues. *Oncogene* 25, 2537– 2545. doi: 10.1038/sj.onc.1209283
67. Murata, F. H. A., Ferreira, M. N., Camargo, N. S., Santos, G. S., Spegiorin, L. C. J. F., Silveira-Carvalho, A. P., et al. (2016). Frequency of Anti-*Toxoplasma gondii* IgA,

IgM and IgG Antibodies in High-Risk Pregnancies, in Brazil. *Rev. Soc. Bras. Med. Trop.* 49, 512–514. doi: 10.1590/0037-8682-0046-2016
68. Murata, F. H. A., Ferreira, M. N., Pereira-Chioccola, V. L., Spegiorin, L. C. J. F., Meira-Strejevitch, C. S., Gava, R., et al. (2017). Evaluation of Serological and Molecular Tests Used to Identify *Toxoplasma gondii* Infection in Pregnant Women Attended in a Public Health Service in São Paulo State, Brazil. *Diagn. Microbiol. Infect. Dis.* 89, 13–19. doi: 10.1016/j.diagmicrobio.2017.06.004
69. Murata, F. H. A., Previato, M., Frederico, F. B., Barbosa, A. P., Nakashima, F., de Faria, G. M.Jr, et al. (2020). Evaluation of Serological and Molecular Tests Used for the Identification of *Toxoplasma gondii* Infection in Patients Treated in an Ophthalmology Clinic of a Public Health Service in São Paulo State, Brazil. *Front. Cell Infect. Microbiol.* 9, 472. doi: 10.3389/fcimb.2019.00472
70. Nakashima, F., Pardo, V. S., Miola, M. P., Murata, F. H. A., Paduan, N., Longo, S. M., et al. (2020). Serum IgG Anti-*Toxoplasma gondii* Antibody Concentrations Do Not Correlate Nested PCR Results in Blood Donors. *Front. Cell Infect. Microbiol* 9, 461. doi: 10.3389/fcimb.2019.00461
71. Okay, T. S., Yamamoto, L., Oliveira, L. C., Manuli, E. R., Andrade Junior, H. F., and Del Negro, G. M. (2009). Significant Performance Variation Among PCR Systems in Diagnosing Congenital Toxoplasmosis in São Paulo, Brazil: Analysis of 467 Amniotic Fluid Samples. *Clinics* 64, 171–176. doi: 10.1590/S1807-59322009000300004
72. Olias, P., Etheridge, R. D., Zhang, Y., Holtzman, M. J., and Sibley, L. D. (2016). Toxoplasma Effector Recruits the Mi-2/Nurd Complex to Repress STAT1 Transcription and Block IFN-G-Dependent Gene Expression. *Cell Host Microbe* 20, 72–82. doi: 10.1016/j.chom.2016.06.006
73. Ong, Y. C., Reese, M. L., and Boothroyd, J. C. (2010). *Toxoplasma* Rhoptry Protein 16 (ROP16) Subverts Host Function by Direct Tyrosine Phosphorylation of STAT6. *J. Biol. Chem.* 285, 28731–28740. doi: 10.1074/jbc.M110.112359
74. Park, N. J., Zhou, H., Elashoff, D., Henson, B. S., Kastratovic, D. A., Abemayor, E., et al. (2009). Salivary microRNA: Discovery, Characterisation, and Clinical Utility for Oral Cancer Detection. *Clin. Cancer Res.* 15, 5473–5477. doi: 10.1158/1078-0432.CCR-09-0736
75. Pereira, I. S., Maia, M. M., da Cruz, A. B., Telles, J. P. M., Vidal, J. E., Gava, R., et al. (2019). Plasma Extracellular microRNAs are Related to AIDS/Cerebral Toxoplasmosis Co-Infection. *Parasite Immunol.* 42, e12696. doi: 10.1111/pim.12696
76. Perron, M. P., Boissonneault, V., Gobeil, L. A., Ouellet, D. L., and Provost, P. (2007). Regulatory Rnas: Future Perspectives in Diagnosis, Prognosis, and Individualised Therapy. *Methods Mol. Biol.* 361, 311–326. doi: 10.1385/1-59745-208-4:311
77. Pfefferkorn, E. R. (1984). Interferon Gamma Blocks the Growth of *Toxoplasma gondii* in Human fibroblasts by Inducing the Host Cells to Degrade Tryptophan. *Proc. Natl. Acad. Sci. U.S.A.* 81, 908–912. doi: 10.1073/ pnas.81.3.908
78. Platanias, L. C. (2005). Mechanisms of Type-I and Type-II-Interferon-Mediated Signaling. *Nat. Rev. Immunol.* 5, 375–386. doi: 10.1038/nri1604
79. Pomares, C., and Montoya, J. G. (2016). Laboratory Diagnosis of Congenital Toxoplasmosis. *J. Clin. Microbiol.* 54, 2448–2454. doi: 10.1128/JCM.00487-16
80. Prudencio, M., Rodriguez, A., and Mota, M. M. (2006). The Silent Path to Thousands of Merozoites: The Plasmodium Liver Stage. *Nat. Rev. Microbiol.* 4, 849–856. doi: 10.1038/nrmicro1529
81. Rice, J., Roberts, H., Burton, J., Pan, J., States, V., Rai, S. N., et al. (2015). Assay Reproducibility in Clinical Studies of Plasma miRNA. *PloS One* 10, e0121948. doi: 10.1371/journal.pone.0121948
82. Robert-Gangneux, F., and Darde, M. L. (2012). Epidemiology of and Diagnostic Strategies for Toxoplasmosis. *Clin. Microbiol. Rev.* 25, 583. doi: 10.1128/CMR.05013-11
83. Robert-Gangneux, F., Meroni, V., Dupont, D., Botterel, F., Garcia, J. M. A., Brenier-Pinchart, M. P., et al. (2018). Toxoplasmosis in Transplant Recipients, Europe, 2010-2014. *Emerg. Infect. Dis.* 24, 1497–1504. doi: 10.3201/eid2408.180045
84. Rosowski, E. E., Lu, D., Julien, L., Rodda, L., Gaiser, R. A., Jensen, K. D., et al. (2011). Strain-Specific Activation of the NF-Kappab Pathway by GRA15, a Novel *Toxoplasma gondii* Dense Granule Protein. *J. Exp. Med.* 208, 195–212. doi: 10.1084/jem.20100717
85. Rosowski, E. E., Nguyen, Q. P., Camejo, A., Spooner, E., and Saeij, J. P. (2014). *Toxoplasma gondii* Inhibits Gamma Interferon (IFN-G)- and IFN-B Induced Host Cell STAT1 Transcriptional Activity by Increasing the Association of STAT1 With DNA. *Infect. Immun.* 82, 706–719. doi: 10.1128/IAI.01291-13
86. Rosowski, E. E., and Saeij, J. P. (2012). *Toxoplasma Gondii* Clonal Strains All Inhibit STAT1 Transcriptional Activity But Polymorphic Effectors Differentially Modulate Ifng Induced Gene Expression and STAT1 Phosphorylation. *PloS One* 7, e51448. doi: 10.1371/journal.pone.0051448
87. Saba, R., Sorensen, D. L., and Booth, S. A. (2014). microRNA-146a: A Dominant, Negative Regulator of the Innate Immune Response. *Front. Immunol.* 5:578. doi: 10.3389/fimmu.2014.00578
88. Sadzak, I., Schiff, M., Gattermeier, I., Glinitzer, R., Sauer, I., Saalmüller, A., et al. (2008). Recruitment of STAT1 to Chromatin is Required for Interferon-Induced Serine Phosphorylation of Stat1 Transactivation Domain. *Proc. Natl. Acad. Sci. U.S.A.* 105, 8944–8949. doi: 10.1073/pnas.0801794105
89. Saeij, J. P. J., Boyle, J. P., Coller, S., Taylor, S., Sibley, L. D., Brooke-Powell, E. T., et al. (2006). Polymorphic Secreted Kinases are Key Virulence Factors in Toxoplasmosis. *Science* 3145806, 1780–1783. doi: 10.1126/science.1133690
90. Saeij, J. P. J., Coller, S., Boyle, J. P., Jerome, M. E., White, M. W., and Boothroyd, J. C. (2007). Toxoplasma Co-Opts Host Gene Expression by Injection of a Polymorphic Kinase Homologue. *Nature* 445, 324–327. doi: 10.1038/nature05395
91. Shapira, S., Speirs, K., Gerstein, A., Caamano, J., and Hunter, C. A. (2002). Suppression of NF-Kappab Activation by Infection With *Toxoplasma gondii*. *J. Infect. Dis.* 185, S66–S72. doi: 10.1086/338000
92. Sibley, L. D., and Boothroyd, J. C. (1992). Virulent Strains of *Toxoplasma gondii* Comprise a Single Clonal Lineage. *Nature* 359, 82–85. doi: 10.1038/359082a0
93. Sturm, A., Amino, R., van de Sand, C., Regen, T., Retzlaff, S., Rennenberg, A., et al. (2006). Manipulation of Host Hepatocytes by the Malaria Parasite for Delivery Into Liver Sinusoids. *Science* 313, 1287–1290. doi: 10.1126/science.1129720
94. Sun, B., Meng, M., Wei, J., and Wang, S. (2020). Long Non-Coding RNA PVT1 Contributes to Vascular Endothelial Cell Proliferation Via Inhibition of Mir−190a−5p in Diagnostic Biomarker Evaluation of Chronic Heart Failure. *Exp. Ther. Med.* 19, 3348–3354. doi: 10.3892/etm.2020.8599
95. Suzuki, Y., Conley, F. K., and Remington, J. S. (1989). Importance of Endogenous IFN-Gamma for Prevention of Toxoplasmic Encephalitis in Mice. *J. Immunol.* 143, 2045–2050.
96. Suzuki, Y., Orellana, M. A., Schreiber, R. D., and Remington, J. S. (1988). Interferon-Gamma: The Major Mediator of Resistance Against *Toxoplasma gondii*. *Science* 240, 516–518. doi: 10.1126/science.3128869
97. Taganov, K. D., Boldin, M. P., Chang, K. J., and Baltimore, D. (2006). NF-KappaB- Dependent Induction of microRNA miR-146, an Inhibitor Targeted to Signaling Proteins of Innate Immune Responses. *Proc. Natl. Acad. Sci. U.S.A.* 103, 12481–12486. doi: 10.1073/pnas.0605298103
98. Tang, W., Xu, P., Wang, H., Niu, Z., Zhu, D., Lin, Q., et al. (2018). microRNA-150 Suppresses Triple-Negative Breast Cancer Metastasis Through Targeting HMGA2. *Onco. Targets Ther.* 24, 2319–2332. doi: 10.2147/OTT.S161996
99. Taylor, S., Barragan A, A., Su, C., Fux, B., Fentress, S. J., Tang, K., et al. (2006). A Secreted Serine-Threonine Kinase Determines Virulence in the Eukaryotic Pathogen. *Toxoplasma gondii. Sci.* 314, 1776–1780. doi: 10.1126/science.1133643
100. Tijsen, A. J., Creemers, E. E., Moerland, P. D., de Windt, L. J., van der Wal, A. C., Kok, W. E., et al. (2010). miR 423-5p as a Circulating Biomarker for Heart Failure. *Circ. Res.* 106, 1035–1039. doi: 10.1161/CIRCRESAHA.110.218297
101. Tuladhar, S., Kochanowsky, J. A., Bhaskara, A., Ghotmi, Y., Chandrasekaran, S., and Koshy, A. A. (2019). The ROP16III-Dependent Early Immune Response Determines the Subacute CNS Immune Response and Type III *Toxoplasma gondii* Survival. *PloS Pathog.* 15, e1007856. doi: 10.1371/journal.ppat.1007856
Villard, O., Cimon, B., L'Ollivier, C., Fricker-Hidalgo, H., Godineau, N., Houze, S., et al. (2016). Serological Diagnosis of *Toxoplasma gondii* Infection:
102. Recommendations From the French National Reference Center for Toxoplasmosis. *Diagn. Microbiol. Infect. Dis.* 84, 22–23. doi: 10.1016/j.diagmicrobio.2015.09.009
103. Wallon, M., Peyron, F., Cornu, C., Vinault, S., Abrahamowicz, M., Kopp, C. B., et al. (2013). Congenital Toxoplasma Infection: Monthly Prenatal Screening Decreases Transmission Rate and Improves Clinical Outcome At Age 3 Years. *Clin. Infect. Dis.* 56, 1223–1231. doi: 10.1093/cid/cit032
104. Wang, X., Kan, Y., Chen, L., Ge, P., Ding, T., Zhai, Q., et al. (2020). mir−150 is a Negative Independent Prognostic Biomarker for Primary Gastrointestinal Diffuse Large B−Cell Lymphoma. *Oncol. Lett.* 19, 3487–3494. doi: 10.3892/ol.2020.11452
105. Wang, K., Yuan, Y., Cho, J. H., McClarty, S., Baxter, D., and Galas, D. J. (2012). Comparing the Microrna Spectrum Between Serum and Plasma. *PloS One* 7, e41561. doi: 10.1371/journal.pone.0041561
106. Wang, K., Zhang, S., Marzolf, B., Troisch, P., Brightman, A., Hu, Z., et al. (2009). Circulating MmicroRNA, Potential Biomarkers for Drug-Induced Liver Injury. *Proc. Natl. Acad. Sci. U.S.A.* 106, 4402–4407. doi: 10.1073/pnas.0813371106
107. Wang, G. K., Zhu, J. Q., Zhang, J. T., Li, Q., Li, Y., He, J., et al. (2010). Circulating microRNA: A Novel Potential Biomarker for Early

4

Poor Birth Outcomes in Malaria in Pregnancy: Recent Insights into Mechanisms and Prevention Approaches

Caroline L. L. Chua[1], *Wina Hasang*[2], *Stephen J. Rogerson*[2*] *and Andrew Teo*[2,3*]

[1] *School of Biosciences, Taylor's University, Subang Jaya, Malaysia,* [2] *Department of Medicine at Royal Melbourne Hospital, Peter Doherty Institute, University of Melbourne, Melbourne, VIC, Australia,* [3] *Lee Kong Chian School of Medicine, Nanyang Technological University, Singapore, Singapore*

Correspondence:
Stephen J. Rogerson
sroger@unimelb.edu.au
Andrew Teo
andrewcc.teo@ntu.edu.sg

Pregnant women in malaria-endemic regions are susceptible to malaria in pregnancy, which has adverse consequences on birth outcomes, including having small for gestational age and preterm babies. These babies are likely to have low birthweights, which predisposes to infant mortality and lifelong morbidities. During malaria in pregnancy, *Plasmodium falciparum*-infected erythrocytes express a unique variant surface antigen, VAR2CSA, that mediates sequestration in the placenta. This process may initiate a range of host responses that contribute to placental inflammation and dysregulated placental development, which affects placental vasculogenesis, angiogenesis and nutrient transport. Collectively, these result in the impairment of placental functions, affecting fetal development. In this review, we provide an overview of malaria in pregnancy and the different pathological pathways leading to malaria in pregnancy-associated low birthweight. We also discuss current prevention and management strategies for malaria in pregnancy, and some potential therapeutic interventions that may improve birth outcomes. Lastly, we outline some priorities for future research that could bring us one step closer to reducing this health burden.

Keywords: low birthweight, preterm birth, small for gestational age, malaria, pregnancy, VAR2CSA

INTRODUCTION

Global efforts to combat malaria have resulted in declining malaria transmission in many regions over the last decade. Unfortunately, young children and pregnant women remain vulnerable, especially in areas with sustained transmission. Malaria, a disease caused by the *Plasmodium* spp. parasite, can result in severe morbidity and mortality. Worldwide, infection with *Plasmodium falciparum* contributes to the highest burden, and it will be the main focus of this review (1). Despite childhood exposure that leads to acquisition of immunity against malaria, first time pregnant mothers or primigravidas are again susceptible to the disease due to a combination of host and parasitic factors (2, 3). Malaria in pregnancy (MiP) results in placental infection, termed placental malaria (PM), which predisposes to placental injury and insufficiency. Placental insufficiency refers to poor placental function and is commonly observed in PM. It is also hypothesized to be a leading cause of low birthweight (LBW). A baby with LBW is defined as a live born who is <2,500 g regardless of gestational age (4). LBW deliveries can be due to preterm birth (live birth < 37 gestational weeks) or small for gestational age (SGA) (birthweight < 10th percentile for its gestational age). Of note, the precise mechanisms behind MiP-associated preterm birth and SGA remains unclear. *P. falciparum* infection can cause inflammation and potentially disrupt the fine immunological balance required to maintain pregnancy to term (5–7). On the other hand, SGA is often linked to placental insufficiency and there is also substantial evidence to suggest dysregulated placental development in mothers with MiP (8, 9). Interestingly, preterm birth does not commonly co-exist with SGA, further highlighting the complexity of MiP-associated birth outcomes (10).

LBW is an important indicator of infant mortality. MiP is estimated to cause approximately 900,000 LBW deliveries annually, with an estimated 100,000 MiP-related infant deaths (1, 11). Apart from high mortality risk, there is also increased morbidity in the surviving LBW infants, who are at elevated risk of poor cognitive and social development (12). LBW due to fetal growth restriction, the cause of SGA, is linked to increased incidence of adult diseases including type 2 diabetes and cardiovascular diseases (13). Hence, the prevention of MiP-associated LBW remains a priority in research. In this review, we discuss recent findings on the causes of LBW in *P. falciparum*-MiP and the different pathological pathways such as SGA and preterm birth in contributing to MiP-associated LBW. We also highlight existing gaps in our knowledge on the pathogenesis of LBW in MiP. Lastly, we review current interventions and provide suggestions for future work that allows us to better understand and manage MiP.

MALARIA IN PREGNANCY: AN OVERVIEW OF PATHOGENESIS AND IMMUNITY

Malaria in pregnancy threatens the well-being of the mother and her developing fetus, and an infected mother is likely to be an important reservoir of *Plasmodium* infection. One prominent feature of *P. falciparum*-infected erythrocytes (IEs) is their ability to adhere to endothelial and placental receptors. The latter allows them to sequester in the placenta, leading to placental infection and inflammation. Histological sections of *P. falciparum*-infected placentas reveal the presence of IEs, particularly at the surface of the syncytiotrophoblast, which is the main site of exchange for nutrient, waste and other metabolites between maternal and fetal circulations. Within the placental intervillous spaces, which are occupied by maternal blood, increased infiltrates of phagocytic cells with substantial amounts of ingested parasites can be observed; this is known as intervillositis (14, 15). The binding phenotype of IEs during pregnancy is mediated by their expression of variant surface antigens (VSA). Placental-binding parasites express VAR2CSA, a major VSA that is mainly expressed during pregnancy, and they bind specifically to the placental receptor known as chondroitin sulfate A (CSA) (16–19). Therefore, prior to pregnancy, antibodies against placental-binding IEs are uncommon, predisposing primigravidas to the adverse effects of PM (2, 20). In subsequent pregnancies, the protective anti-VAR2CSA antibodies can be naturally acquired in a gravidity-dependent manner and have been demonstrated to be effective against MiP and its consequences, thus preventing LBW (21). However, the specific antigenic targets and mechanisms of protection remain unclear. A recent systematic review showed that antibodies against different placental-binding antigens including VAR2CSA were associated with increased risk of PM and its consequences, suggesting that they may be markers of infection instead of correlates of protection (22). Nonetheless, it is likely that antibodies that are protective can inhibit binding of IEs to the placenta and/or facilitate clearance through opsonising phagocytosis, thus prevent placental inflammation and the subsequent adverse effects on fetal growth (**Figure 1**), and defining the characteristics of potentially protective antibodies remains a priority.

CAUSES OF MIP-ASSOCIATED LBW

The Link Between MiP, Dysregulated Placental Development and Small for Gestational Age Babies

Small for gestational age is commonly caused by fetal growth restriction. This condition significantly increases the risk of LBW, stillbirth, infant mortality and morbidity, and the risk of being diagnosed with chronic diseases in adulthood (13). Interestingly, SGA infants were two times more likely to experience *Plasmodium*-infection and clinical malaria by the age of 6 months, after adjusting for mosquito exposure (23). A recent study from an area of low malaria transmission reported several factors that were associated with increased odds of SGA during *P. falciparum*-related MiP, including symptomatic malaria and infection after 12–16 weeks' gestation (24), In addition, the risk of SGA was reported to increase by 1.13 times for every episode of infection during pregnancy (24). In contrast, in areas of high malaria transmission and particularly when pregnant women received anti-malarials in the form of intermittent preventive treatment in pregnancy (IPTp), there was no association between number of malaria episodes and SGA, suggesting that the timing of MiP may contribute to increased risk of SGA (25, 26). Indeed, placental pigment deposition (past-chronic infection) was associated with increased risk of SGA but not LBW or preterm birth, suggesting early chronic infection (usually outside of IPTp coverage) may drive SGA and not preterm labor (25, 27). Alterations in the downstream pathways of MiP such as growth factors and their regulators may further contribute to SGA. Recently, reduced plasma concentrations of placental growth factor in mid-pregnancy were associated with SGA and may indicate early placental insufficiency (9). MiP is known to be associated with reduced expression and bioavailability of placental growth factor, with the latter occurring through increased expression of their soluble inhibitor, soluble fms-like tyrosine kinase-1 (sFlt-1) (26, 28, 29). In addition, MiP leads to increased levels of asymmetric dimethylarginine, which is a competitive inhibitor of nitric oxide synthase (29). When nitric oxide synthase is inhibited, nitric oxide production is similarly affected, resulting in increased sFlt-1 levels and reduced levels of vascular endothelial growth factor (VEGF) family of proteins (30). This subsequently leads to

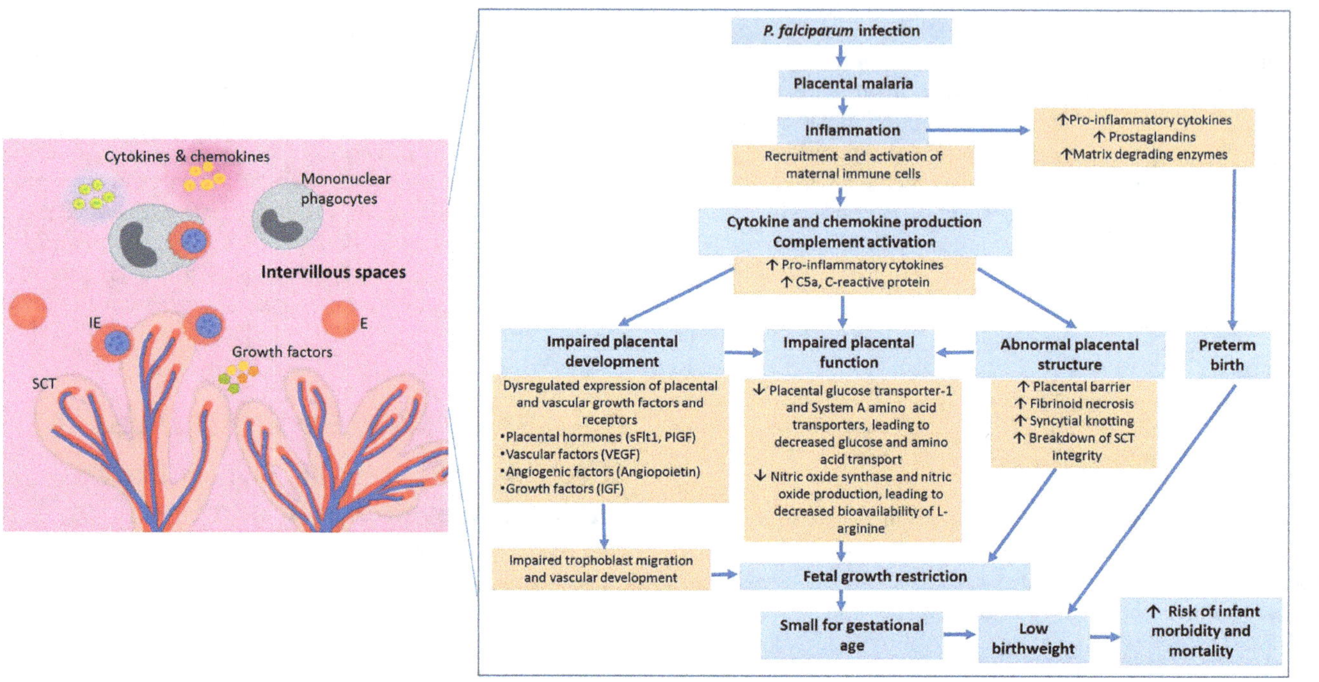

FIGURE 1 | Pathways leading to malaria in pregnancy-associated low birthweight. Infected erythrocytes express unique variant surface antigens that mediate binding to placental receptors. Sequestration leads to recruitment and activation of different immune cells that can result in a cascade of downstream inflammatory events. These inflammatory events include secretion of cytokines and chemokines that have been associated with poor pregnancy outcomes. The increased pro-inflammatory environment has been associated with – (1) dysregulated expression of growth hormones, vascular factors and angiopoietin-1 and -2; (2) abnormal placental development; and (3) reduced placental nutrient transport, overall contributing to placental insufficiency. Together, these factors contribute to malaria in pregnancy associated low birthweight which is the biggest predictor of infant morbidity and mortality globally and annually., ↑, increase; ↓, decrease; E, Erythrocytes; IE, Infected erythrocytes; SCT, Syncytiotrophoblast; IVS, Intervillous space; sFlt1, soluble fms-like tyrosine kinase-1; PIGF, Phosphatidylinositol-glycan biosynthesis class F protein; VEGF, Vascular endothelial growth factor; IGF, Insulin-like growth factor.

dysregulated placental vasculogenesis and angiogenesis that may affect placental functions, contributing to SGA.

The Link Between MiP, Inflammation and Preterm Babies

MiP is also associated with preterm birth, where these babies are usually born small and have increased risk of mortality due to complications such as brain hemorrhage, sepsis, acute respiratory illnesses and perinatal asphyxia (31). Surviving infants may develop life-long morbidities such as learning disabilities, which become obvious when the infant reaches school age (32). *Plasmodium* infection in both early and late pregnancies has been associated with preterm deliveries. A study from Malawi showed that earlier infection (before 24 weeks gestation) was associated with a higher risk of preterm delivery (26). In a Cameroon study, pregnant women who experienced MiP during the third trimester were four times more likely to have preterm deliveries (7). Similarly, in areas with low malaria transmission such as Southeast Asia, *P. falciparum* infection during late pregnancy was also associated with preterm delivery (24).

Studies on populations in malarious areas have identified several factors that significantly increase the risk of preterm birth, including PM, systemic inflammation (particularly CXCL9 and IL-1β), primigravidity, long-term iron supplementation and severe anemia (33–35). A recent systematic review found that maternal anemia in the first trimester, but not other trimesters, was associated with increased risk of preterm birth (36). Of note, the risk of MiP is highest during the first trimester, however, how severe maternal anemia contributes to preterm deliveries remains unclear. Interestingly, vertical parasite transmission, though uncommon, was also reported to contribute to preterm and LBW deliveries; this may partly be attributed to placental inflammation as higher complement activity was reported in cord blood infection (37, 38).

Several inflammatory mediators within the maternal peripheral circulation have also been associated with preterm delivery, but more investigations are required to understand whether they serve as biomarkers or play a pathological role. One of these markers is the soluble tumor necrosis factor receptor 2, which was found at increased levels in HIV positive women with MiP. Women who had elevated levels of this receptor throughout pregnancy also had preterm deliveries (6). Another study reported that in Papua New Guinean women who received one dose of IPTp with sulfadoxine-pyrimethamine (SP) and chloroquine, maternal serum levels of the acute phase protein α1-acid glycoprotein (AGP), an inflammatory marker, at delivery were positively correlated with several birth parameters including LBW, preterm and SGA deliveries (9). In the same study, women with two or more doses of IPTp with SP and azithromycin (SPAZ) were observed to have reduced levels of AGP at delivery, suggesting that SPAZ may reduce inflammation thus preventing deleterious pregnancy outcomes (9). The levels of AGP were previously shown to be increased in *P. falciparum*-infected children and adults with uncomplicated malaria illness (39, 40), while the role of AGP in MiP, especially in higher transmission areas, requires further investigation. Our understanding of the pathways leading to preterm birth in MiP is still rather limited, although placental inflammation is likely to be a main contributing factor. During the initiation of labor, a pro-inflammatory environment is generated through the activation of maternal immune cells and placental stromal cells, which subsequently produce high levels of pro-inflammatory cytokines, prostaglandins and matrix-degrading enzymes. These are associated with the triggering of uterine contraction, cervical ripening and membrane rupture, signaling the beginning of the birthing process. In MiP, particularly PM with intervillositis, the massive leukocyte infiltrates may trigger an inflammatory environment similar to the one observed in labor, leading to the premature initiation of parturition. Various cytokines that are implicated in the induction of preterm birth such as IL-1β, IL-6, macrophage migration inhibitory factor and CXCL1 have also been found at elevated levels during MiP (33, 41). Recently, in a murine model of MiP, dysregulated expression of placental ATP-binding cassette transporters was associated with preterm labor (42). Further studies are required to determine if a similar mechanism operates in the human disease.

POTENTIAL PATHWAYS LEADING TO MIP-ASSOCIATED LBW

Effects of MiP on Placental Development

The placenta is an important organ that acts as an interface between the mother and her fetus. Successful placental development requires a fine immunological balance to be achieved between maternal, placental and fetal immunity. PM can alter nitric oxide bioavailability, and it may lead to host inflammatory responses. Either of these processes may result in poor placental development, leading to placental insufficiency when the placenta is unable to fully support the growth of the developing baby (26, 29).

The first trimester is associated with the highest risk of *Plasmodium*-infection especially in primigravid women (43, 44). Critically, the timing of infection appears to determine the risks and severity of adverse birth outcomes. For MiP, early exposure (<15 gestational weeks) was associated with reduced volume of placental transport villi and smaller surface areas for diffusion across the villi (45). Other abnormalities such as impaired development of placental vascular space, excessive syncytial knotting (aggregation of syncytiotrophoblast nuclei), increased fibrinoid necrosis areas and thickening of syncytiotrophoblast basal membrane have also been observed (46–48). The timing of infection that resulted in such placental pathologies, however, is unknown. Ultrastructural studies showed the breakdown of syncytiotrophoblast integrity in regions associated with IEs (49). These abnormal changes to the placenta were associated with decreased birth weight (45, 46, 49).

MiP and the subsequent immune activation are associated with placental pathologies that arise due to disruptions in placental tissue (trophoblast) and vascular development. An *in vitro* model demonstrated impaired trophoblast invasion and migration after incubation with sera from *P. falciparum*-infected women (50). In the same study, elevated levels of soluble factors that inhibit trophoblast invasion such as human chorionic gonadotropin and IL-10 were found in these sera. There was a corresponding decrease in the invasion stimulatory factors such as insulin-like growth factors and IL-8 (50). There are two main events in vascular development; vasculogenesis (formation of new blood vessels) and angiogenesis (development of blood vessels from existing vasculature). In a recent review, three main pathways that are associated with impaired vascular development and adverse birth outcomes in MiP were identified, including reduced bioavailability of L-arginine and nitric oxide, excessive complement activation and dysregulated hemoglobin-scavenging system due to increased intravascular haemolysis (51). In a Brazilian cohort, MiP altered the angiogenic profile of the placenta and was associated with increased placental barrier thickness, which is likely to affect nutrient and gas transfer (47). Often, *Plasmodium*-infected placentas become the foci of inflammation where maternal immune cells are recruited and retained. This concomitant inflammation generates various soluble inflammatory mediators including tumor necrosis factor-α, interferon-γ, complement C5a, and C-reactive protein (33, 37). In addition, higher levels of chemoattractant proteins such as macrophage inflammatory protein-1 (alpha and beta) and monocyte chemoattractant protein-1 were observed (41, 52). These inflammatory mediators and chemoattractants are known to regulate the levels of key placental growth factors and receptors, including insulin-like growth factors, angiopoietin (1 and 2), soluble endoglin, sFlt-1 and VEGF (8, 37), which in turn disturb the delicate balance required for normal placental development. All of these analytes have been associated with reduced birth weight and LBW deliveries (33, 53). Taken together, placental trophoblast development, vascular development pathways and inflammatory responses appear to be interdependent and may synergistically contribute to poor birth outcomes in MiP. However, it remains to be determined if inflammatory inhibitors and/or promoters of placental growth factors may alleviate the impact of MiP on placental development and birth outcome.

Intervillositis and Placental Insufficiency

Untreated *Plasmodium* infection during pregnancy increases the risk of intervillositis (inflammation in placental intervillous spaces). These spaces are occupied by maternal blood that surrounds the chorionic villi, serving as the materno-fetal exchange surface. Importantly, intervillositis, but not PM without intervillositis per se, was more commonly linked to adverse birth outcomes. This is particularly true in areas of high malaria transmission such as Tanzania and Malawi, where intervillositis was associated with abnormalities in the placenta and significantly higher rates of LBW (up to 50%)

(15, 54, 55). PM-associated intervillositis is characterized by the accumulation of mononuclear cells, predominantly monocytes/macrophages. The inflammatory foci serve as a physical barrier that may compromise placental transport function and cause hypoxia. These immune cells can also be activated to produce inflammatory molecules that affect various downstream signaling pathways in the placenta, leading to impairment of fetal growth.

Investigations on *Plasmodium*-infected placentas revealed that compromised nutrient transport is one of the molecular mechanisms contributing to growth restriction and reduced birth weight. In women with PM-associated intervillositis, reduced expression of glucose transporter isoform 1 (GLUT-1) on the syncytiotrophoblast basal membrane was reported (56). Transplacental glucose transport is primarily facilitated by GLUT-1 and its expression was positively correlated with birthweight. In addition, lower expression and activity of system A group of amino acid transporters were also found in PM-associated intervillositis. Maternal to cord blood ratios of several amino acids were lower in cases with intervillositis compared to uninfected controls and importantly, cord concentrations of amino acids were positively correlated with fetal/placental weight ratios (57). In a follow-up study, lower placental mammalian target of rapamycin (mTOR) activity was observed in infected placentas with intervillositis, which in turn is associated with reduced placental amino acid uptake and lower birthweight (58). Recently, increased placental autophagy was proposed as a possible mediator of placental insufficiency in PM and similarly, this has been reported in other non-infectious pregnancy complications such as preeclampsia and intrauterine growth restriction (59–61). The dysregulation of this process may negatively affect the uptake of amino acids by the placenta and future studies should further explore this association.

PREVENTION OF MIP-ASSOCIATED LBW: A PROSPECTIVE ON CURRENT AND FUTURE STRATEGIES

Insecticide-Treated Nets, Indoor Residual Spraying, and Intermittent Preventive Treatment

The World Health Organization recommends the prevention and management of MiP via the use insecticide-treated bed nets (ITN), IPTp and effective case management of malaria disease. Additionally, there are encouraging data to suggest that indoor residual spraying insecticide (IRS) may also be effective in reducing MiP and improving birth outcomes (62, 63). ITN and IRS, whether deployed individually or in combination, aim to reduce vector exposure and limit transmission, hence are likely to be beneficial (**Figure 2**). The use of ITN is a simple yet effective strategy to prevent *Plasmodium* infection and its consequences. There is substantial evidence from earlier studies suggesting that this strategy resulted in reduced prevalence of maternal parasitemia, improved birth weights and a 25% reduction in the risk of LBW deliveries (64–66). On the other hand, IRS, by decreasing vector contact, was associated with reduced risk of preterm birth, LBW delivery and fetal/neonatal deaths in both HIV-negative and HIV-infected women (62, 63).

Currently, all pregnant women residing in areas with high malaria transmission are recommended to receive three or more treatment courses of IPTp with SP, where each course should be administered at least one month apart, starting in the second trimester (67). This replaces the original recommendation of two doses of SP, following substantial data that demonstrated reduced risk of preterm birth and LBW as well as improved birth weight when three or more courses were administered (68–70). In mathematical modeling studies, it was estimated that three or more doses of IPTp-SP uptake would lead to a 30% relative reduction in LBW occurrence (70–73).

Despite these preventive strategies, the prevalence of PM and LBW remain a huge threat to pregnancies in malarious regions due to several reasons. Given that IPTp is only administered from the second trimester onwards, pregnant women are not protected during the first trimester and the later weeks of third trimester. This inadequate IPTp coverage throughout pregnancy, poor population coverage, development of drug and insecticide resistance, and the use of suboptimal drugs which results in the failure to clear submicroscopic infection, are likely to contribute to increased risk of preterm birth, SGA and LBW (26, 74, 75). Following reports on the increased prevalence of SP-resistant parasites, there are concerns regarding the future effectiveness of this prophylactic regimen in protecting against consequences of MiP (72, 76, 77). For this reason, other antimalarial drugs such as amodiaquine, mefloquine, chloroquine–azithromycin and dihydroartemisinin-piperaquine have been tested as potential alternatives to IPTp-SP (78, 79). Dihydroartemisinin-piperaquine appears to be a promising choice, as trial results showed that malaria burden including maternal parasitemia and PM was significantly lower in women who received this drug compared to those who received SP (80, 81). However, dihydroartemisinin-piperaquine did not lead to improved birth outcomes when compared with SP (81, 82). A recent systematic review showed that SP resistance decreased the effectiveness of IPTp especially in areas with high SP resistance, but this regimen is still associated with decreased cases of LBW (82).

The exact mechanisms by which SP leads to improved birth outcomes in the treated individuals remain elusive. In addition to malaria prevention, SP also serves as a broad-spectrum antibiotic that can resolve or prevent other infections of bacterial origin (sexually transmitted, reproductive tract and urinary tract infections) that have also been associated with adverse birth outcomes (69, 82). In addition, it was postulated that sulfadoxine can modulate bacterial microflora composition within the gut and vagina, which subsequently promotes weight gain (83) There is an ongoing study investigating the effect of SP on microbiota in the gut and/or vagina, in which the researchers proposed that higher birth weights following SP administration in pregnancy can be attributed to the modulation of these bacterial populations (84). To corroborate, antibiotic exposure during pregnancy led to increased gestational weight gain, which is an important predictor of birthweights (85). The overall reduction in malarial and other non-malarial infections during pregnancy is likely to

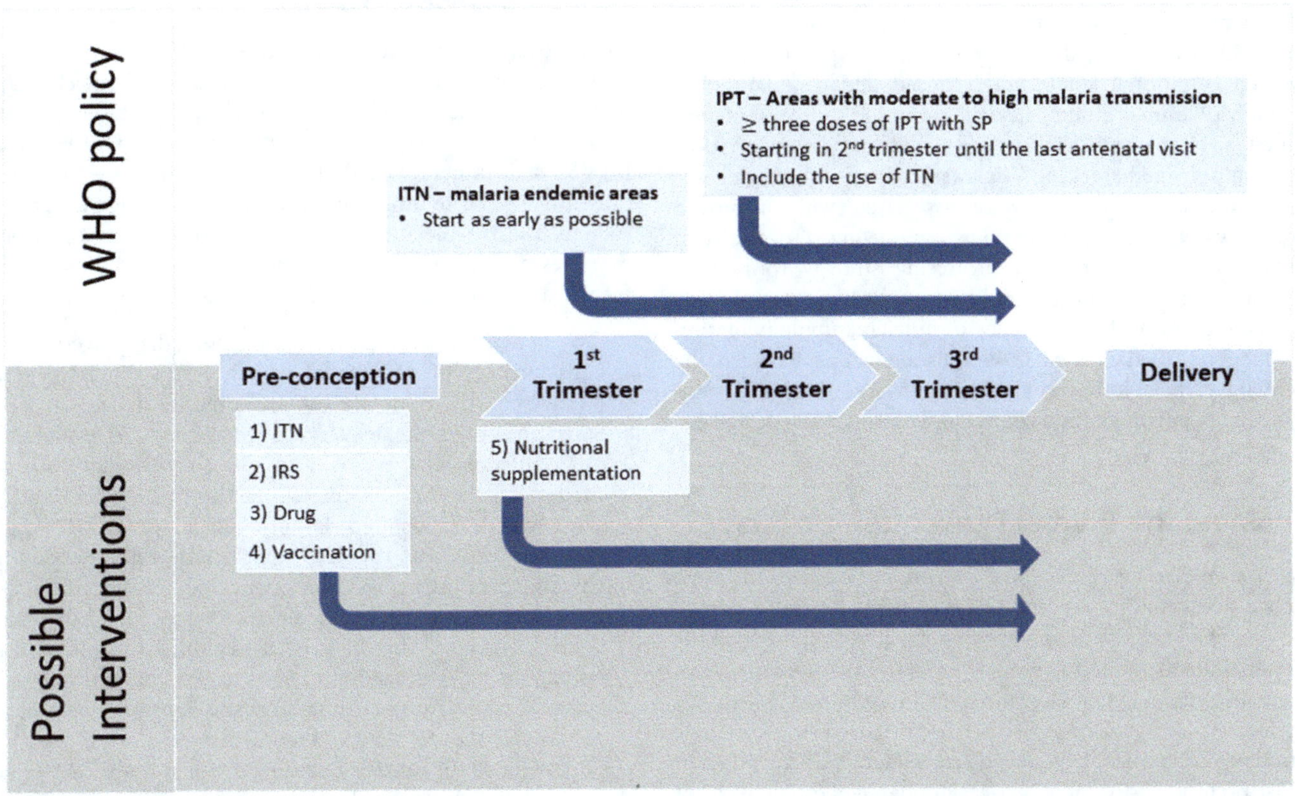

FIGURE 2 | Timeline of pregnancy events with WHO recommendations and possible interventions. Malaria in pregnancy (MiP) is preventable and the current WHO recommendations for Africa include three or more doses of intermittent preventive treatment during pregnancy (IPT) with sulfadoxine-pyrimethamine (SP) taken one month apart starting from fetus quickening. In addition, sleeping under insecticide treated nets (ITNs) has been shown to reduce parasite burden during pregnancy. Strong evidence indicates that MiP starts during the first trimester with irreversible damage and it is during this period of time that pregnant mothers are at the highest risk of parasitemia. Furthermore, recent evidence suggests that women often harbor parasites before conception, and these parasites may switch to a placental-binding phenotype, that is likely to contribute to placental inflammation, especially in women pregnant for the first time. We propose several potential interventions which may help to alleviate the harmful impact of MiP. (1) ITNs should be used from early pregnancy, or before conception, to reduce the risk of acquiring new infections. (2) Indoor residual spraying should be evaluated for its effectiveness against MiP. (3) Pre-pregnancy intermittent screening for malaria, with treatment by safe and effective drugs, should be considered. (4) Pregnant women need access to an effective vaccine that can induce protection against MiP. Currently, there are two vaccines that are in clinical trials. (5) The nutritional status of the mother should be optimized during pregnancy with appropriate micro- or macronutrient supplements to ensure optimal placental development and thus better birth outcomes.

minimize chronic maternal inflammation, thus improving birth outcomes (9, 82).

Given the limitations associated with current drugs, there is an urgent need to evaluate the safety and efficacy of new antimalarials or a combination of preventive strategies that are suitable for wider coverage and at earlier time points in pregnancy to protect against MiP in the first trimester.

Nutritional Interventions a Viable but Under-Interventions: Approach

Another major contributor to LBW is maternal undernutrition, a condition that is also highly prevalent in many areas with high malaria transmission. There is a growing number of studies suggesting that malaria and maternal undernutrition may worsen pregnancy outcomes (86, 87). Malnourishment during pregnancy, indicated by low body mass index and smaller mid-upper arm circumference, was associated with lower levels of antibodies to placental-binding IE and increased parasite load in the placenta (88). The impaired development of protective antibodies may reduce the host's ability to clear infection, thus prolonged infection is likely to result in chronic inflammation in the placenta. In addition, undernutrition during pregnancy may also affect placental size and its functional capacity, given that maternal weight and gestational weight gain are both mediators of placental weight. All three factors were positively correlated to birthweight (89). Furthermore, both MiP and maternal undernourishment have been reported to impair trophoblast invasion and migration, as well as increase uterine artery resistance (50, 90, 91). In recent studies, MiP and undernourishment during pregnancy were observed to affect the levels of L-arginine-nitric oxide biogenesis; this pathway is essential for placental vascular development (29, 92).

In a comprehensive study that analyzed 23 systematic reviews on nutritional interventions during pregnancy, a few factors including provision of vitamin A, low-dose calcium, zinc and multiple micronutrients were shown to be associated with reduced risk of LBW (93). Similarly, several earlier macronutrient supplementation studies in malarious regions such as Sub-Saharan Africa provided evidence of improved birthweight, increased gestational length and reduced odds of LBW (94). Using a MiP animal model, dietary L-arginine supplementation resulted in improved fetal weights, reduced levels of pro-inflammatory mediators and increased levels of angiogenic factors, the last of which were associated with improved placental vascular development and remodeling (29). Nutrient intervention appears to be a promising strategy to prevent LBW, hence more studies should be carried out to evaluate the effectiveness of different types of nutrient supplementation in reducing MiP-associated LBW. Distinguishing between the potential beneficial impacts of malaria prevention with IPTp and of nutrient supplementation will require careful study designs.

Vaccines: the Pivotal Prevention Strategy

Efficacious malaria vaccines could potentially be one of the most effective strategies to prevent LBW in MiP. Previous studies have described the requirements of an effective vaccine for MiP, which include the ability to induce protective antibodies against placental-binding IEs to prevent their binding to CSA in the placenta *via* the parasites' VAR2CSA protein. These binding-inhibition antibodies have been associated with protection against preterm birth, increased gestational age, the delivery of heavier infants and importantly, reduced risk of LBW delivery (21). Furthermore, these binding-inhibition antibodies against whole parasites were demonstrated to be strain-independent, raising the possibility that targeting an immunogenically-conserved subunit or domain of VAR2CSA, which is a large (~350 kDa) multidomain protein, could be effective (95). Given its large size, later studies then identified a minimal binding region on the VAR2CSA protein that binds with high affinity to CSA. Antibodies in the sera collected from malaria-exposed pregnant women were able to bind to recombinant VAR2CSA and purified antibodies against this protein exhibited binding-inhibitory activity (96–99). Importantly, a study from Benin then demonstrated strong antibody responses against the VAR2CSA N-terminal region of DBL3X to be associated with protection against SGA and reduced prevalence of both LBW babies and placental infection at delivery, possibly by reducing parasite burden and thus lowering the risk of placental insufficiency (97). However, recent studies have identified distinct pathogenicity among the parasite variants and diversity in functional antibodies against different placental binding variants, suggesting that a polyvalent VAR2CSA-based vaccine may provide better protection (100, 101). To corroborate, two isoforms of VAR2CSA subunit protein that recently completed phase 1 clinical trial, ID1-ID2a (PAMVAC) and DBL1x-DBL2x (PRIMVAC), only demonstrated binding-inhibition activities against homologous parasite variants and the duration of immune responses is unknown (102, 103). Critically, the duration of immune responses and whether vaccination translates to clinical protection remains to be determined.

FUTURE DIRECTIONS

Great advances have been made over the last two decades in understanding and reducing MiP, especially with effective anti-malarials and the use of ITNs during pregnancy. Despite this, our understanding of factors that contribute to LBW during MiP is still rather limited. In addition, with the increasing pressure of parasite resistance against existing drugs, alternatives such as a viable vaccine will be crucial to combat MiP. Hence, more research efforts should be channeled toward these areas of investigation. Herein, some areas of future research are proposed.

1. To better understand and manage the adverse birth consequences of MiP, there is a need to differentiate the relative contributions of SGA and preterm delivery to LBW. SGA and preterm delivery in MiP may be initiated by different molecular events, and hence may require different modes of interventions. In resource-limited malaria endemic areas where ultrasound is unavailable, pregnancy dating is based on recall of last menstrual period, abdominal palpation, or newborn assessments, all of which may be inaccurate. In addition, the reference curve for birth weights is based on those that have been established in the Western populations. Several studies have created population-specific charts detailing mean birth weights and percentiles at different gestational ages to have a better representation of their own populations (10, 104). In addition, a global healthcare project has developed standards and tools for assessing newborn weight, length and head circumference by gestational age and sex (105). These can lead to more accurate classifications of birth outcomes in MiP and studies on their effectiveness in differentiating SGA and preterm birth can be done.
2. Changes to the placenta in PM are only studied upon delivery, given the invasive nature of sampling placental blood or biopsies during pregnancy. However, this rarely captures the whole picture of placental events that occurred throughout pregnancy, limiting our interpretation of how placental changes during gestation can lead to LBW. Although the use of animal models may address this challenge, there are concerns regarding the relevance and transferability of the findings to human disease (106). One way to better understand the placental pathophysiology during MiP is to employ the use of Doppler ultrasound to investigate utero-and feto-placental blood flow and resistance. In earlier studies, MiP in the first half of gestation was associated with altered uteroplacental blood flow, suggesting the possibility of vascular deficiency (90, 107). This technique, together with measurement of various maternal analytes in the peripheral blood, may provide a clearer picture of the events in the placenta during MiP.
3. Our current understanding on inflammation in PM focuses on the roles of monocytes and macrophages as the main contributors of inflammatory mediators associated with LBW. However, there are recent studies suggesting that neutrophils, which are the most abundant leukocytes in the peripheral blood, may also play a role in orchestrating the inflammation (108, 109). Their role in MiP requires further clarification.

4. Our current understanding of protective antibodies in MiP is that these antibodies should be able to inhibit IEs binding to the placenta and promote opsonic phagocytosis (21). However, their importance and relative contribution to protection through other immune effector mechanisms such as antibody-dependent respiratory burst and antibody-dependent cellular cytotoxicity are less well-understood. This knowledge will be important in vaccine design and the evaluation of vaccine efficacy.
5. Early studies in The Gambia and Nigeria demonstrated that passive transfer of anti-malarial antibodies resolved malaria (110, 111). Currently, there are existing clinical trials that are investigating the protective efficacy of monoclonal antibodies as anti-infective agents (ClinicalTrials.gov Identifier: NCT04327310 and NCT04206332). Therefore, monoclonal antibodies, targeting either the domains of VAR2CSA or the circumsporozoite protein to prevent establishment of infection can be further developed as therapeutics for MiP.
6. In terms of improving vaccine design, there is a need to identify conserved subdomains of VAR2CSA that can induce protective antibodies, against the different parasite variants.
7. SP may be less efficacious in areas with high SP-resistant parasites. Moreover, SP is only given at the start of second trimester, but there is substantial evidence showing that infection during the first trimester can also greatly impact birth outcomes (24, 26). Hence new antimalarial drug combinations that can be administered in the first trimester need to be evaluated in future clinical trials.
8. SP, a broad-spectrum antibiotic, may be effective against sexually transmitted and reproductive tract infections (highly prevalent in malaria endemic regions), thus it may resolve infections other than malaria to improve adverse birth outcomes (69). Future studies to explore the use of effective antimalarials coupled with SP may be beneficial.
9. Malnutrition is an important contributor to LBW, and nutrient supplementations during pregnancy appear to be an attractive and feasible intervention to minimize the risk of LBW deliveries. However, the beneficial effect of nutrient supplementation may be masked if administered together with IPTp, thus undermining its impact on birth outcomes. Hence, future trials of nutrient supplementations require careful study designs such as having intermittent-screening and treatment with nutrient supplementations, or choosing a trial site in a lower transmission setting where IPTp is not a first line policy.

CONCLUSION

As of 2019, 38 countries and territories were granted the "malaria-free" status by WHO, while transmission continues in other regions. Hence, pregnant women remain at risk of MiP, which leads to increased mortality and morbidity in both the mother and her infant. MiP-associated LBW is preventable, but there needs to be a concerted effort in the adoption and implementation of current prevention strategies in malarious areas. Continuous efforts in research are needed, to better understand the molecular mechanisms associated with poor birth outcomes, and ultimately to enable design of specific targeted approaches for improving birth outcomes. In the face of increased parasite resistance, the effectiveness of IPT with SP in preventing this health burden may be at threat in the near future. Therefore, there is an urgent need to design and evaluate other therapeutic options that can be used to protect against MiP and its deleterious consequences.

AUTHOR CONTRIBUTIONS

All authors listed have made a substantial, direct and intellectual contribution to the work, and approved it for publication.

REFERENCES

1. World Health Organization. *World Malaria Report 2019*. Geneva: World Health Organization (2019).
2. Salanti A, Staalsoe T, Lavstsen T, Jensen ATR, Sowa MPK, Arnot DE, et al. Selective upregulation of a single distinctly structured var gene in chondroitin sulphate A-adhering *Plasmodium falciparum* involved in pregnancy-associated malaria. *Mol Microbiol.* (2003) 49:179–91. doi: 10.1046/j.1365-2958.2003.03570.x
3. Veenstra van Nieuwenhoven AL, Heineman MJ, Faas MM. The immunology of successful pregnancy. *Hum Reprod Update.* (2003) 9:347–57. doi: 10.1093/humupd/dmg026
4. World Health Organization. *Low Birthweight: Country, Regional and Global Esitmates*. Geneva: World Health Organization (2004).
5. Sykes L, MacIntyre DA, Yap XJ, Teoh TG, Bennett PR. The Th1:th2 dichotomy of pregnancy and preterm labour. *Mediators Inflamm.* (2012) 2012:967629. doi: 10.1155/2012/967629
6. McDonald CR, Weckman AM, Conroy AL, Olwoch P, Natureeba P, Kamya MR, et al. Systemic inflammation is associated with malaria and preterm birth in women living with HIV on antiretrovirals and co-trimoxazole. *Sci Rep.* (2019) 9:6758. doi: 10.1038/s41598-019-43191-w
7. Nkwabong E, Mayane DN, Meka E, Essiben F. Malaria in the third trimester and maternal-perinatal outcome. *Int J Gynaecol Obstet.* (2020) 8:13261. doi: 10.1002/ijgo.13261
8. Umbers AJ, Boeuf P, Clapham C, Stanisic DI, Baiwog F, Mueller I, et al. Placental malaria-associated inflammation disturbs the insulin-like growth factor axis of fetal growth regulation. *J Infect Dis.* (2011) 203:561–9. doi: 10.1093/infdis/jiq080
9. Unger HW, Hansa AP, Buffet C, Hasang W, Teo A, Randall L, et al. Sulphadoxine-pyrimethamine plus azithromycin may improve birth outcomes through impacts on inflammation and placental angiogenesis independent of malarial infection. *Sci Rep.* (2019) 9:2260. doi: 10.1038/s41598-019-38821-2
10. Rijken MJ, De Livera AM, Lee SJ, Boel ME, Rungwilailaekhiri S, Wiladphaingern J, et al. Quantifying low birth weight, preterm birth and small-for-gestational-age effects of malaria in pregnancy: a population cohort study. *PLoS ONE.* (2014) 9:e100247. doi: 10.1371/journal.pone.0100247
11. Desai M, ter Kuile FO, Nosten F, McGready R, Asamoa K, Brabin B, et al. Epidemiology and burden of malaria in pregnancy. *Lancet Infect Dis.* (2007) 7:93–104. doi: 10.1016/S1473-3099(07)70021-X
12. Upadhyay RP, Naik G, Choudhary TS, Chowdhury R, Taneja S, Bhandari

N, et al. Cognitive and motor outcomes in children born low birth weight: a systematic review and meta-analysis of studies from South Asia. *BMC Pediatr.* (2019) 19:35. doi: 10.1186/s12887-019-1408-8
13. Knop MR, Geng TT, Gorny AW, Ding R, Li C, Ley SH, et al. Birth weight and risk of type 2 diabetes mellitus, cardiovascular disease, and hypertension in adults: a meta-analysis of 7 646 267 participants from 135 studies. *J Am Heart Assoc.* (2018) 7:e008870. doi: 10.1161/JAHA.118.008870
14. Rogerson SJ, Mkundika P, Kanjala MK. Diagnosis of *Plasmodium falciparum* malaria at delivery: comparison of blood film preparation methods and of blood films with histology. *J Clin Microbiol.* (2003) 41:1370–4. doi: 10.1128/JCM.41.4.1370-1374.2003
15. Muehlenbachs A, Fried M, McGready R, Harrington WE, Mutabingwa TK, Nosten F, et al. A novel histological grading scheme for placental malaria applied in areas of high and low malaria transmission. *J Infect Dis.* (2010) 202:1608–16. doi: 10.1086/656723
16. Rogerson SJ, Chaiyaroj SC, Ng K, Reeder JC, Brown GV. Chondroitin sulfate A is a cell surface receptor for *Plasmodium falciparum*-infected erythrocytes. *J Exp Med.* (1995) 182:15–20. doi: 10.1084/jem.182.1.15
17. Tuikue Ndam NG, Salanti A, Bertin G, Dahlbäck M, Fievet N, Turner L, et al. High level of var2csa transcription by *Plasmodium falciparum* isolated from the placenta. *J Infect Dis.* (2005) 192:331–5. doi: 10.1086/430933
18. Yosaatmadja F, Andrews KT, Duffy MF, Brown GV, Beeson JG, Rogerson SJ. Characterization of VAR2CSA-deficient *Plasmodium falciparum*-infected erythrocytes selected for adhesion to the BeWo placental cell line. *Malar J.* (2008) 7:51. doi: 10.1186/1475-2875-7-51
19. Dorin-Semblat D, Tétard M, Claës A, Semblat JP, Dechavanne S, Fourati Z, et al. Phosphorylation of the VAR2CSA extracellular region is associated with enhanced adhesive properties to the placental receptor CSA. *PLoS Biol.* (2019) 17:e3000308. doi: 10.1371/journal.pbio.3000308
20. Fodjo BA, Atemnkeng N, Esemu L, Yuosembom EK, Quakyi IA, Tchinda VH, et al. Antibody responses to the full-length VAR2CSA and its DBL domains in Cameroonian children and teenagers. *Malar J.* (2016) 15:532. doi: 10.1186/s12936-016-1585-y
21. Teo A, Feng G, Brown GV, Beeson JG, Rogerson SJ. functional antibodies and protection against blood-stage malaria. *Trends Parasitol.* (2016) 32:887–98. doi: 10.1016/j.pt.2016.07.003
22. Cutts JC, Agius PA, Zaw L, Powell R, Moore K, Draper B, et al. Pregnancy-specific malarial immunity and risk of malaria in pregnancy and adverse birth outcomes: a systematic review. *BMC Med.* (2020) 18:14. doi: 10.1186/s12916-019-1467-6
23. Agbota G, Accrombessi M, Cottrell G, Martin-Prével Y, Milet J, Ouédraogo S, et al. Increased risk of malaria during the first year of life in small-for-gestational-age infants: a longitudinal study in Benin. *J Infect Dis.* (2018) 219:1642–51. doi: 10.1093/infdis/jiy699
24. Moore KA, Simpson JA, Wiladphaingern J, Min AM, Pimanpanarak M, Paw MK, et al. Influence of the number and timing of malaria episodes during pregnancy on prematurity and small-for-gestational-age in an area of low transmission. *BMC Med.* (2017) 15:117. doi: 10.1186/s12916-017-0877-6
25. Kalilani-Phiri L, Thesing PC, Nyirenda OM, Mawindo P, Madanitsa M, Membe G, et al. Timing of malaria infection during pregnancy has characteristic maternal, infant and placental outcomes. *PLoS ONE.* (2013) 8:e74643. doi: 10.1371/journal.pone.0074643
26. Elphinstone RE, Weckman AM, McDonald CR, Tran V, Zhong K, Madanitsa M, et al. Early malaria infection, dysregulation of angiogenesis, metabolism and inflammation across pregnancy, and risk of preterm birth in Malawi: a cohort study. *PLoS Med.* (2019) 16:e1002914. doi: 10.1371/journal.pmed.1002914
27. Ategeka J, Kakuru A, Kajubi R, Wasswa R, Ochokoru H, Arinaitwe E, et al. Relationships between measures of malaria at delivery and adverse birth outcomes in a high-transmission area of Uganda. *J Infect Dis.* (2020) 222:863–70. doi: 10.1093/infdis/jiaa156
28. Karumanchi SA, Haig D. Flt1, pregnancy, and malaria: evolution of a complex interaction. *Proc Natl Acad Sci USA.* (2008) 105:14243–4. doi: 10.1073/pnas.0807932105
29. McDonald CR, Cahill LS, Gamble JL, Elphinstone R, Gazdzinski LM, Zhong KJY, et al. Malaria in pregnancy alters l-arginine bioavailability and placental vascular development. *Sci Transl Med.* (2018) 10:eaan6007. doi: 10.1126/scitranslmed.aan6007
30. Krause BJ, Hanson MA, Casanello P. Role of nitric oxide in placental vascular development and function. *Placenta.* (2011) 32:797–805. doi: 10.1016/j.placenta.2011.06.025
31. Saigal S, Doyle LW. An overview of mortality and sequelae of preterm birth from infancy to adulthood. *Lancet.* (2008) 371:261–9. doi: 10.1016/S0140-6736(08)60136-1
32. Brydges CR, Landes JK, Reid CL, Campbell C, French N, Anderson M. Cognitive outcomes in children and adolescents born very preterm: a meta-analysis. *Dev Med Child Neurol.* (2018) 60:452–68. doi: 10.1111/dmcn.13685
33. Fried M, Kurtis JD, Swihart B, Pond-Tor S, Barry A, Sidibe Y, et al. Systemic inflammatory response to malaria during pregnancy is associated with pregnancy loss and preterm delivery. *Clin Infect Dis.* (2017) 65:1729–35. doi: 10.1093/cid/cix623
34. Brabin B, Gies S, Roberts SA, Diallo S, Lompo OM, Kazienga A, et al. Excess risk of preterm birth with periconceptional iron supplementation in a malaria endemic area: analysis of secondary data on birth outcomes in a double blind randomized controlled safety trial in Burkina Faso. *Malar J.* (2019) 18:161. doi: 10.1186/s12936-019-2797-8
35. Mikomangwa WP, Oms M, Aklillu E, Kamuhabwa AAR. Adverse birth outcomes among mothers who received intermittent preventive treatment with Sulphadoxine-Pyrimethamine in the low malaria transmission region. *BMC Pregnancy Childbirth.* (2019) 19:236. doi: 10.1186/s12884-019-2397-1
36. Rahmati S, Azami M, Badfar G, Parizad N, Sayehmiri K. The relationship between maternal anemia during pregnancy with preterm birth: a systematic review and meta-analysis. *J Matern Fetal Neonatal Med.* (2020) 33:2679–89. doi: 10.1080/14767058.2018.1555811
37. Conroy AL, Silver KL, Zhong K, Rennie M, Ward P, Sarma JV, et al. Complement activation and the resulting placental vascular insufficiency drives fetal growth restriction associated with placental malaria. *Cell Host Microbe.* (2013) 13:215–26. doi: 10.1016/j.chom.2013.01.010
38. Mahamat O, Gisele Ndum K, Laurentine S, Ngum Helen N. Cord malaria infection, complement activation, oxidative stress, gestational age, and birth weight, characterized by high *Plasmodium falciparum* prevalence in Bamenda, Cameroon. *J Trop Med.* (2020) 2020:7209542. doi: 10.1155/2020/7209542
39. Mansor SM, Molyneux ME, Taylor TE, Ward SA, Wirima JJ, Edwards G. Effect of *Plasmodium falciparum* malaria infection on the plasma concentration of alpha 1-acid glycoprotein and the binding of quinine in Malawian children. *Br J Clin Pharmacol.* (1991) 32:317–21. doi: 10.1111/j.1365-2125.1991.tb03905.x
40. Silamut K, Molunto P, Ho M, Davis TM, White NJ. Alpha 1-acid glycoprotein (orosomucoid) and plasma protein binding of quinine in falciparum malaria. *Br J Clin Pharmacol.* (1991) 32:311–5. doi: 10.1111/j.1365-2125.1991.tb03904.x
41. Abrams ET, Brown H, Chensue SW, Turner GDH, Tadesse E, Lema VM, et al. Host response to malaria during pregnancy: placental monocyte recruitment is associated with elevated β chemokine expression. *J Immunol.* (2003) 170:2759–64. doi: 10.4049/jimmunol.170.5.2759
42. Fontes KN, Reginatto MW, Silva NL, Andrade CBV, Bloise FF, Monteiro VRS, et al. Dysregulation of placental ABC transporters in a murine model of malaria-induced preterm labor. *Sci Rep.* (2019) 9:11488. doi: 10.1038/s41598-019-47865-3
43. Tuikue Ndam N, Tornyigah B, Dossou AY, Escriou G, Nielsen MA, Salanti A, et al. Persistent *Plasmodium falciparum* infection in women with an intent to become pregnant as a risk factor for pregnancy-associated malaria. *Clin Infect Dis.* (2018) 67:1890–6. doi: 10.1093/cid/ciy380
44. Hounkonnou CPA, Briand V, Fievet N, Accrombessi M, Yovo E, Mama A, et al. Dynamics of submicroscopic *Plasmodium falciparum* infections throughout pregnancy: a preconception cohort study in Benin. *Clin Infect Dis.* (2019) 71:166–74. doi: 10.1093/cid/ciz748
45. Moeller SL, Nyengaard JR, Larsen LG, Nielsen K, Bygbjerg IC, Msemo OA, et al. Malaria in early pregnancy and the development of the placental vasculature. *J Infect Dis.* (2019) 220:1425–34. doi: 10.1093/infdis/jiy735
46. Crocker IP, Tanner OM, Myers JE, Bulmer JN, Walraven G, Baker PN. Syncytiotrophoblast degradation and the pathophysiology of the malaria-infected placenta. *Placenta.* (2004) 25:273–82. doi: 10.1016/j.placenta.2003.09.010

47. Ataíde R, Murillo O, Dombrowski JG, Souza RM, Lima FA, Lima GF, et al. Malaria in pregnancy interacts with and alters the angiogenic profiles of the placenta. *PLoS Negl Trop Dis.* (2015) 9:e0003824. doi: 10.1371/journal.pntd.0003824
48. Ahenkorah J, Tetteh-Quarcoo PB, Nuamah MA, Kwansa-Bentum B, Nuamah HG, Hottor B, et al. The impact of Plasmodium infection on placental histomorphology: a stereological preliminary study. *Infect Dis Obstet Gynecol.* (2019) 2019:2094560. doi: 10.1155/2019/2094560
49. Kidima WB. Syncytiotrophoblast functions and fetal growth restriction during placental malaria: updates and implication for future interventions. *Biomed Res Int.* (2015) 2015:451735. doi: 10.1155/2015/451735
50. Umbers AJ, Stanisic DI, Ome M, Wangnapi R, Hanieh S, Unger HW, et al. Does malaria affect placental development? Evidence from in vitro models. *PLoS ONE.* (2013) 8:e55269. doi: 10.1371/annotation/4faa7351-837e-4531-a513-0ea80277017f
51. Ngai M, Weckman AM, Erice C, McDonald CR, Cahill LS, Sled JG, et al. Malaria in pregnancy and adverse birth outcomes: new mechanisms and therapeutic opportunities. *Trends Parasitol.* (2020) 36:127–37. doi: 10.1016/j.pt.2019.12.005
52. Sampaio NG, Eriksson EM, Schofield L. *Plasmodium falciparum* PfEMP1 modulates monocyte/macrophage transcription factor activation and cytokine and chemokine responses. *Infect Immun.* (2018) 86:00447–17. doi: 10.1128/IAI.00447-17
53. Silver KL, Zhong K, Leke RGF, Taylor DW, Kain KC. Dysregulation of angiopoietins is associated with placental malaria and low birth weight. *PLoS ONE.* (2010) 5:e9481. doi: 10.1371/journal.pone.0009481
54. Ordi J, Ismail MR, Ventura PJ, Kahigwa E, Hirt R, Cardesa A, et al. Massive chronic intervillositis of the placenta associated with malaria infection. *Am J Surg Pathol.* (1998) 22:1006–11. doi: 10.1097/00000478-199808000-00011
55. Rogerson SJ, Pollina E, Getachew A, Tadesse E, Lema VM, Molyneux ME. Placental monocyte infiltrates in response to *Plasmodium falciparum* malaria infection and their association with adverse pregnancy outcomes. *Am J Trop Med Hyg.* (2003) 68:115–9. doi: 10.4269/ajtmh.2003.68.1.0680115
56. Chandrasiri UP, Chua CL, Umbers AJ, Chaluluka E, Glazier JD, Rogerson SJ, et al. Insight into the pathogenesis of fetal growth restriction in placental malaria: decreased placental glucose transporter isoform 1 expression. *J Infect Dis.* (2014) 209:1663–7. doi: 10.1093/infdis/jit803
57. Boeuf P, Aitken EH, Chandrasiri U, Chua CL, McInerney B, McQuade L, et al. *Plasmodium falciparum* malaria elicits inflammatory responses that dysregulate placental amino acid transport. *PLoS Pathog.* (2013) 9:e1003153. doi: 10.1371/journal.ppat.1003153
58. Dimasuay KG, Aitken EH, Rosario F, Njie M, Glazier J, Rogerson SJ, et al. Inhibition of placental mTOR signaling provides a link between placental malaria and reduced birthweight. *BMC Med.* (2017) 15:1. doi: 10.1186/s12916-016-0759-3
59. Dimasuay KG, Gong L, Rosario F, McBryde E, Spelman T, Glazier J, et al. Impaired placental autophagy in placental malaria. *PLoS ONE.* (2017) 12:e0187291. doi: 10.1371/journal.pone.0187291
60. Lima FA, Barateiro A, Dombrowski JG, de Souza RM, Costa DS, Murillo O, et al. *Plasmodium falciparum* infection dysregulates placental autophagy. *PLoS ONE.* (2019) 14:e0226117. doi: 10.1371/journal.pone.0226117
61. Nakashima A, Tsuda S, Kusabiraki T, Aoki A, Ushijima A, Shima T, et al. Current understanding of autophagy in pregnancy. *Int J Mol Sci.* (2019) 20:2342. doi: 10.3390/ijms20092342
62. Muhindo MK, Kakuru A, Natureeba P, Awori P, Olwoch P, Ategeka J, et al. Reductions in malaria in pregnancy and adverse birth outcomes following indoor residual spraying of insecticide in Uganda. *Malar J.* (2016) 15:437. doi: 10.1186/s12936-016-1489-x
63. Roh ME, Shiboski S, Natureeba P, Kakuru A, Muhindo M, Ochieng T, et al. Protective effect of indoor residual spraying of insecticide on preterm birth among pregnant women with HIV infection in Uganda: a secondary data analysis. *J Infect Dis.* (2017) 216:1541–9. doi: 10.1093/infdis/jix533
64. Gamble C, Ekwaru JP, ter Kuile FO. Insecticide-treated nets for preventing malaria in pregnancy. *Cochrane Database Syst Rev.* (2006) 19:CD003755. doi: 10.1002/14651858.CD003755.pub2
65. Feng G, Simpson JA, Chaluluka E, Molyneux ME, Rogerson SJ. Decreasing burden of malaria in pregnancy in Malawian women and its relationship to use of intermittent preventive therapy or bed nets. *PLoS ONE.* (2010) 5:e12012. doi: 10.1371/journal.pone.0012012
66. Eisele TP, Larsen DA, Anglewicz PA, Keating J, Yukich J, Bennett A, et al. Malaria prevention in pregnancy, birthweight, and neonatal mortality: a meta-analysis of 32 national cross-sectional datasets in Africa. *Lancet Infect Dis.* (2012) 12:942–9. doi: 10.1016/S1473-3099(12)70222-0
67. World Health Organization. *WHO Policy Brief for the Implementation of Intermittent Preventive Treatment of Malaria in Pregnancy Using Sulfadoxine-Pyrimethamine (IPTp-SP).* Geneva: World Health Organization (2013).
68. Kayentao K, Garner P, van Eijk AM, Naidoo I, Roper C, Mulokozi A, et al. Intermittent preventive therapy for malaria during pregnancy using 2 vs 3 or more doses of sulfadoxine-pyrimethamine and risk of low birth weight in Africa: systematic review and meta-analysis. *JAMA.* (2013) 309:594–604. doi: 10.1001/jama.2012.216231
69. Chico RM, Chaponda EB, Ariti C, Chandramohan D. Sulfadoxine-pyrimethamine exhibits dose-response protection against adverse birth outcomes related to malaria and sexually transmitted and reproductive tract infections. *Clin Infect Dis.* (2017) 64:1043–51. doi: 10.1093/cid/cix026
70. Quakyi I, Tornyigah B, Houze P, Kusi KA, Coleman N, Escriou G, et al. High uptake of intermittent preventive treatment of malaria in pregnancy is associated with improved birth weight among pregnant women in Ghana. *Sci Rep.* (2019) 9:19034. doi: 10.1038/s41598-019-55046-5
71. Cates JE, Westreich D, Unger HW, Bauserman M, Adair L, Cole SR, et al. Intermittent preventive therapy in pregnancy and incidence of low birth weight in malaria-endemic countries. *Am J Public Health.* (2018) 108:399–406. doi: 10.2105/AJPH.2017.304251
72. van Eijk AM, Larsen DA, Kayentao K, Koshy G, Slaughter DEC, Roper C, et al. Effect of *Plasmodium falciparum* sulfadoxine-pyrimethamine resistance on the effectiveness of intermittent preventive therapy for malaria in pregnancy in Africa: a systematic review and meta-analysis. *Lancet Infect Dis.* (2019) 19:546–56. doi: 10.1016/S1473-3099(18)30732-1
73. Mlugu EM, Minzi O, Asghar M, Färnert A, Kamuhabwa AAR, Aklillu E. Effectiveness of sulfadoxine-pyrimethamine for intermittent preventive treatment of malaria and adverse birth outcomes in pregnant women. *Pathogens.* (2020) 9:207. doi: 10.3390/pathogens9030207
74. Cottrell G, Moussiliou A, Luty AJ, Cot M, Fievet N, Massougbodji A, et al. Submicroscopic *Plasmodium falciparum* infections are associated with maternal anemia, premature births, and low birth weight. *Clin Infect Dis.* (2015) 60:1481–8. doi: 10.1093/cid/civ122
75. Hounkonnou CPA, Ndam NT, Fievet N, Accrombessi M, Yovo E, Mama A, et al. Sub-optimal intermittent preventive treatment in pregnancy (IPTp) is associated with an increased risk of submicroscopic *P. falciparum* infection in pregnant women: a prospective cohort study in Benin. *Clin Infect Dis.* (2020) 9:ciaa1355. doi: 10.1093/cid/ciaa1355
76. Fagbemi KA, Adebusuyi SA, Nderu D, Adedokun SA, Pallerla SR, Amoo AOJ, et al. Analysis of sulphadoxine-pyrimethamine resistance-associated mutations in *Plasmodium falciparum* isolates obtained from asymptomatic pregnant women in Ogun State, Southwest Nigeria. *Infect Genet Evol.* (2020) 85:104503. doi: 10.1016/j.meegid.2020.104503
77. Taylor SM, Levitt B, Freedman B, Madanitsa M, Thwai KL, Kalilani-Phiri L, et al. Interactions between antenatal sulfadoxine-pyrimethamine, drug-resistant *Plasmodium falciparum* parasites, and delivery outcomes in Malawi. *J Infect Dis.* (2020) 222:661–9. doi: 10.1093/infdis/jiaa145
78. Kimani J, Phiri K, Kamiza S, Duparc S, Ayoub A, Rojo R, et al. Efficacy and safety of azithromycin-chloroquine versus sulfadoxine-pyrimethamine for intermittent preventive treatment of *Plasmodium falciparum* malaria infection in pregnant women in Africa: an open-label, randomized trial. *PLoS ONE.* (2016) 11:e0157045. doi: 10.1371/journal.pone.0157045
79. González R, Pons-Duran C, Piqueras M, Aponte JJ, Ter Kuile FO, Menéndez C. Mefloquine for preventing malaria in pregnant women. *Cochrane Database Syst Rev.* (2018) 3:CD011444. doi: 10.1002/14651858.CD011444.pub3
80. Kakuru A, Jagannathan P, Muhindo MK, Natureeba P, Awori P, Nakalembe M, et al. Dihydroartemisinin-piperaquine for the prevention of malaria in pregnancy. *N Engl J Med.* (2016) 374:928–39. doi: 10.1056/NEJMoa1509150
81. Kajubi R, Ochieng T, Kakuru A, Jagannathan P, Nakalembe M, Ruel T, et al. Monthly sulfadoxine-pyrimethamine versus dihydroartemisinin-

piperaquine for intermittent preventive treatment of malaria in pregnancy: a double-blind, randomised, controlled, superiority trial. *Lancet.* (2019) 393:1428–39. doi: 10.1016/S0140-6736(18)32224-4

82. Roh ME, Ter Kuile FO, Rerolle F, Glymour MM, Shiboski S, Gosling R, et al. Overall, anti-malarial, and non-malarial effect of intermittent preventive treatment during pregnancy with sulfadoxine-pyrimethamine on birthweight: a mediation analysis. *Lancet Glob Health.* (2020) 8:e942–53. doi: 10.1016/S2214-109X(20)30119-4
83. Gutman J, Slutsker L. Intermittent preventive treatment with sulfadoxine-pyrimethamine: more than just an antimalarial? *Am J Trop Med Hyg.* (2017) 96:9–10. doi: 10.4269/ajtmh.16-0888
84. Meshnick SR, Carroll IM. *Sulfadoxine-Pyrimethamine IPTp in Malawi: Effects on the Gut and Vaginal Microbiomes.* (2016). Available online at: https://grantome.com/grant/NIH/R21-AI125800-02 (accessed February 2, 2021).
85. Unger HW, Wangnapi RA, Ome-Kaius M, Boeuf P, Karl S, Mueller I, et al. Azithromycin-containing intermittent preventive treatment in pregnancy affects gestational weight gain, an important predictor of birthweight in Papua New Guinea - an exploratory analysis. *Matern Child Nutr.* (2016) 12:699–712. doi: 10.1111/mcn.12215
86. Lovel HJ, Newby RM, Hillier VF. Severe placental malaria and maternal shortness, thinness, and small skeletal size in rural Congo: cohort study. *BMJ.* (2005) 331:1439–40. doi: 10.1136/bmj.331.7530.1439
87. Cates JE, Unger HW, Briand V, Fievet N, Valea I, Tinto H, et al. Malaria, malnutrition, and birthweight: a meta-analysis using individual participant data. *PLoS Med.* (2017) 14:e1002373. doi: 10.1371/journal.pmed.1002373
88. Chandrasiri UP, Fowkes FJ, Richards JS, Langer C, Fan YM, Taylor SM, et al. The impact of lipid-based nutrient supplementation on anti-malarial antibodies in pregnant women in a randomized controlled trial. *Malar J.* (2015) 14:193. doi: 10.1186/s12936-015-0707-2
89. Ashorn P, Hallamaa L, Allen LH, Ashorn U, Chandrasiri U, Deitchler M, et al. Co-causation of reduced newborn size by maternal undernutrition, infections, and inflammation. *Matern Child Nutr.* (2018) 14:e12585. doi: 10.1111/mcn.12585
90. Griffin JB, Lokomba V, Landis SH, Thorp JMJr, Herring AH, Tshefu AK, et al. Plasmodium falciparum parasitaemia in the first half of pregnancy, uterine and umbilical artery blood flow, and foetal growth: a longitudinal Doppler ultrasound study. *Malar J.* (2012) 11:319. doi: 10.1186/1475-2875-11-319
91. Baker BC, Hayes DJ, Jones RL. Effects of micronutrients on placental function: evidence from clinical studies to animal models. *Reproduction.* (2018) 156:R69–82. doi: 10.1530/REP-18-0130
92. Weckman AM, McDonald CR, Baxter JB, Fawzi WW, Conroy AL, Kain KC. Perspective: L-arginine and L-citrulline supplementation in pregnancy: a potential strategy to improve birth outcomes in low-resource settings. *Adv Nutr.* (2019) 10:765–77. doi: 10.1093/advances/nmz015
93. da Silva Lopes K, Ota E, Shakya P, Dagvadorj A, Balogun OO, Peña-Rosas JP, et al. Effects of nutrition interventions during pregnancy on low birth weight: an overview of systematic reviews. *BMJ Glob Health.* (2017) 2:e000389. doi: 10.1136/bmjgh-2017-000389
94. Unger HW, Ashorn P, Cates JE, Dewey KG, Rogerson SJ. Undernutrition and malaria in pregnancy - a dangerous dyad? *BMC Med.* (2016) 14:142. doi: 10.1186/s12916-016-0695-2
95. Fried M, Nosten F, Brockman A, Brabin BJ, Duffy PE. Maternal antibodies block malaria. *Nature.* (1998) 395:851–2. doi: 10.1038/27570
96. Clausen TM, Christoffersen S, Dahlback M, Langkilde AE, Jensen KE, Resende M, et al. Structural and functional insight into how the *Plasmodium falciparum* VAR2CSA protein mediates binding to chondroitin sulfate A in placental malaria. *J Biol Chem.* (2012) 287:23332–45. doi: 10.1074/jbc.M112.348839
97. Ndam NT, Denoeud-Ndam L, Doritchamou J, Viwami F, Salanti A, Nielsen MA, et al. Protective antibodies against placental malaria and poor outcomes during pregnancy, Benin. *Emerg Infect Dis.* (2015) 21:813–23. doi: 10.3201/eid2105.141626
98. Doritchamou JY, Herrera R, Aebig JA, Morrison R, Nguyen V, Reiter K, et al. VAR2CSA domain-specific analysis of naturally acquired functional antibodies to *Plasmodium falciparum* placental malaria. *J Infect Dis.* (2016) 214:577–86. doi: 10.1093/infdis/jiw197
99. Chêne A, Gangnard S, Dechavanne C, Dechavanne S, Srivastava A, Tétard M, et al. Down-selection of the VAR2CSA DBL1-2 expressed in *E. coli* as a lead antigen for placental malaria vaccine development. *NPJ Vaccines.* (2018) 3:28. doi: 10.1038/s41541-018-0064-6
100. Patel JC, Hathaway NJ, Parobek CM, Thwai KL, Madanitsa M, Khairallah C, et al. Increased risk of low birth weight in women with placental malaria associated with P. falciparum VAR2CSA clade. *Sci Rep.* (2017) 7:7768. doi: 10.1038/s41598-017-04737-y
101. Doritchamou J, Teo A, Morrison R, Arora G, Kwan J, Manzella-Lapeira J, et al. Functional antibodies against placental malaria parasites are variant dependent and differ by geographic region. *Infect Immun.* (2019) 87:00865-18. doi: 10.1128/IAI.00865-18
102. Mordmüller B, Sulyok M, Egger-Adam D, Resende M, de Jongh WA, Jensen MH, et al. First-in-human, randomized, double-blind clinical trial of differentially adjuvanted PAMVAC, A vaccine candidate to prevent pregnancy-associated malaria. *Clin Infect Dis.* (2019) 69:1509–16. doi: 10.1093/cid/ciy1140
103. Sirima SB, Richert L, Chêne A, Konate AT, Campion C, Dechavanne S, et al. PRIMVAC vaccine adjuvanted with Alhydrogel or GLA-SE to prevent placental malaria: a first-in-human, randomised, double-blind, placebo-controlled study. *Lancet Infect Dis.* (2020) 20:585–97. doi: 10.1016/S1473-3099(19)30739-X
104. Kemfang Ngowa JD, Domkam I, Ngassam A, Nguefack-Tsague G, Dobgima Pisoh W, Noa C, et al. References of birth weights for gestational age and sex from a large cohort of singleton births in cameroon. *Obstet Gynecol Int.* (2014) 2014:361451. doi: 10.1155/2014/361451
105. Villar J, Cheikh Ismail L, Victora CG, Ohuma EO, Bertino E, Altman DG, et al. International standards for newborn weight, length, and head circumference by gestational age and sex: the newborn cross-sectional study of the INTERGROWTH-21st project. *Lancet.* (2014) 384:857–68. doi: 10.1016/S0140-6736(14)60932-6
106. Doritchamou J, Teo A, Fried M, Duffy PE. Malaria in pregnancy: the relevance of animal models for vaccine development. *Lab Anim.* (2017) 46:388–98. doi: 10.1038/laban.1349
107. Ome-Kaius M, Karl S, Wangnapi RA, Bolnga JW, Mola G, Walker J, et al. Effects of *Plasmodium falciparum* infection on umbilical artery resistance and intrafetal blood flow distribution: a Doppler ultrasound study from Papua New Guinea. *Malar J.* (2017) 16:35. doi: 10.1186/s12936-017-1689-z
108. Chua CLL, Robinson LJ, Baiwog F, Stanisic DI, Hamilton JA, Brown GV, et al. High numbers of circulating pigmented polymorphonuclear neutrophils as a prognostic marker for decreased birth weight during malaria in pregnancy. *Int J Parasitol.* (2015) 45:107–11. doi: 10.1016/j.ijpara.2014.12.002
109. Aitken EH, Alemu A, Rogerson SJ. Neutrophils and malaria. *Front Immunol.* (2018) 9:3005. doi: 10.3389/fimmu.2018.03005
110. Cohen S, McGregor IA, Carrington S. Gamma-globulin and acquired immunity to human malaria. *Nature.* (1961) 192:733–7. doi: 10.1038/192733a0
111. Edozien JC, Gilles HM, Udeozo IOK. Adult and cord-blood gamma-globulin and immunity to malaria in Nigerians. *Lancet.* (1962) 280:951–5. doi: 10.1016/S0140-6736(62)90725-0

5

Fetal Cytokine Balance, Erythropoietin and Thalassemia but not Placental Malaria Contribute to Fetal Anemia Risk

Edward R. Kabyemela[1,2], Michal Fried[1,3], Jonathan D. Kurtis[4], Gwamaka Moses[1,5], J. Patrick Gorres[3], Atis Muehlenbachs[1] and Patrick E. Duffy[1,3]*

[1] Mother Offspring Malaria Studies (MOMS) Project, Seattle Biomedical Research Institute, Seattle, WA, United States, [2] School of Medicine, Muhimbili University of Health and Allied Sciences, Dar es Salaam, Tanzania, [3] Laboratory of Malaria Immunology and Vaccinology, National Institutes of Allergy and Infectious Diseases, National Institutes of Health (NIH), Bethesda, MD, United States, [4] Department of Pathology and Laboratory Medicine, Center for International Health Research, Rhode Island Hospital, Brown University, Providence, RI, United States, [5] Mbeya College of Health and Allied Sciences, University of Dar es Salaam, Mbeya, Tanzania

***Correspondence:**
Patrick E. Duffy
patrick.duffy@nih.gov

Fetal anemia is common in malaria-endemic areas and a risk factor for anemia as well as mortality during infancy. Placental malaria (PM) and red cell abnormalities have been proposed as possible etiologies, but the relationship between PM and fetal anemia has varied in earlier studies, and the role of red cell abnormalities has not been studied in malaria-endemic areas. In a Tanzanian birth cohort study designed to elucidate the pathogenesis of severe malaria in young infants, we performed a cross-sectional analysis of risk factors for fetal anemia. We determined PM status, newborn red cell abnormalities, and maternal and cord blood levels of iron regulatory proteins, erythropoietin (EPO), cytokines and cytokine receptors. We examined the relationship between these factors and fetal anemia. Fetal anemia was present in 46.2% of the neonates but was not related to PM. Maternal iron deficiency was common (81.6%), most frequent in multigravidae, and interacted with parity to modify risk of fetal anemia, but it was not directly related to risk. Among offspring of iron-deficient women, the odds of fetal anemia increased with fetal α^{+}-thalassemia, as well as these patterns of cord blood cytokines: increased cord IL-6, decreased TNF-RI, and decreased sTfR. The EPO response to fetal anemia was low or absent and EPO levels were significantly decreased in newborns with the most severe anemia. This study from an area of high malaria transmission provides evidence that 1) fetal α^{+}-thalassemia and cytokine balance, but not PM at delivery, are related to fetal anemia; 2) maternal iron deficiency increases the risk that other factors may cause fetal anemia; and 3) fetal anemia has a multifactorial etiology that may require a variety of interventions, although measures that reduce maternal iron deficiency may be generally beneficial.

Keywords: placental malaria, fetal anemia, thalassemia, cytokines, erythropoietin

INTRODUCTION

Fetal anemia can be the result of immune or non-immune insults. The most common immune etiology is maternal Rhesus (Rh) disease. If untreated, fetal anemia may lead to hydrops, multi-organ failure and fetal death (1, 2). In Malawi, fetal anemia at birth increased anemia risk during the first half of infancy, as well as shorter time to first illness, higher cumulative morbidity, and infant mortality (3, 4). In Kenya, anemia during infancy is a risk factor for infant mortality (5).

Fetal anemia, defined as cord blood hemoglobin less than 12.5g/dl, is common in areas where malaria is transmitted (6). Placental malaria (PM) and thalassemia are also common in areas of stable transmission, and have been proposed but not proven to explain the high incidence of fetal anemia in such areas (6). The association of fetal anemia and PM has varied in earlier studies with some showing association (7–9) but others reporting no association (10–12). In an area of high parasite resistance to sulfadoxine-pyrimethamine (SP) in Tanzania, the use of SP for intermittent preventive therapy (IPTp) to prevent PM and the parasite *dhps* c581 SP resistance allele are independently related to decreased levels of cord blood hemoglobin in the newborn (13).

α^+-thalassemia has not been examined as a cause of fetal anemia in areas of malaria transmission (6). Because malaria is rare in African newborns (14), hemolysis of infected red cells cannot explain fetal anemia, but other mechanisms related to malarial anemia could be involved. In older children and adults, malarial anemia has been associated with inflammatory cytokines like tumor necrosis factor-α (TNF-α) and interferon-γ (IFN-γ) that can inhibit erythropoiesis (15), cause dyserythropoiesis and promote erythrophagocytosis (16). Levels of the anti-inflammatory cytokine interleukin (IL)-10 (17) and the ratio of IL-10 to TNF-α (18) are significantly lower in African children during severe malarial anemia, and placental levels of TNF-α are significantly higher in African mothers with severe malarial anemia (19).

Iron deficiency is another major cause of anemia, is common among pregnant women living in resource-poor settings of both malarious and non-malarious countries, and is more common in multigravid than primigravid women (20, 21). Neonatal iron stores are influenced by maternal iron storage levels (22) and maternal iron deficiency anemia was found to be a risk factor for fetal anemia in Malawi (7). Transplacental transfer of iron from the mother is the only source of iron to the developing fetus. This is achieved through the formation of an iron-transferrin complex (Fe-Tf), with iron from maternal circulation binding to transferrin receptor 1 (TFR1) on the apical surface of the syncytiotrophoblast (23). This complex is endocytosed, then iron is released into the endosome through ferroportin on the basal side of the syncytiotrophoblast, and finally into fetal circulation (24).

Erythropoietin (EPO) is a major regulator of RBC production in the bone marrow. EPO binds to its receptor on the red blood cell (RBC) progenitor surface, inducing proliferation and terminal differentiation of erythroid precursor cells while also protecting against RBC precursor apoptosis (25). Several studies have reported increases in cord blood EPO concentration in response to fetal hypoxia caused by a variety of conditions including intrauterine growth restriction (26) and maternal smoking (27). Increased levels of EPO in blood or amniotic fluid have also been reported in neonates with severe anemia caused by hemolytic anemia (28) and Rh immunization (29).

In the present study, we searched for potential causes and mediators of fetal anemia in an area of Tanzania with intense malaria transmission. We determined PM status, iron status in mothers and newborns, and inherited red cell abnormalities in newborns. We measured plasma levels of inflammatory and anti-inflammatory cytokines that have been previously implicated in the pathogenesis of anemia (TNF-α and its receptors (soluble TNF-RI and TNF-RII), IFN-γ, IL-6, and IL-10) in cord blood. Levels of sTfR and erythropoietin (EPO) were also measured in these samples. We examined the relationship of all these factors to the risk of fetal anemia.

MATERIALS AND METHODS

Study Cohort and Laboratory Procedures

Mothers and newborns included in this analysis were participating in a birth cohort study known locally as the Mother-Offspring Malaria Studies (MOMS) Project at Muheza Designated District Hospital, Muheza, Tanga-Tanzania. The study protocols were approved by the Division of Microbiology and Infectious Diseases at the U.S. National Institutes of Health and by the institutional review boards of Seattle Biomedical Research Institute (contracted to the Western Institutional Review Board, Puyallup, WA, USA, now WCGH IRB) and the Medical Research Coordinating Committee in Tanzania. Written informed consent was obtained from each child's mother before participation for herself and her newborn. Clinical procedures for the MOMS Project have been previously described (30–38). Hemoglobin was measured using a Cell Dyne 1200 hematology analyzer (Abbot Diagnostics Division, Abbot Park, IL-60064, USA).

Maternal peripheral blood was obtained by venipuncture from women immediately after delivery and anticoagulated with citrate phosphate dextrose. Plasma was obtained by centrifugation at 3,000 *g* for 3 min and stored at -70°C until thawed on the day that assays were performed. Thick and thin smears were prepared; thin smears were fixed with methanol. Blood slides were stained for 10 minutes in 10% Giemsa, washed in tap water, air-dried, then examined using light microscopy at 100 × magnification. Ten thousand red cells were examined in the thin smear before concluding that a placental blood slide was negative.

Levels of ferritin, sTfR, EPO, cytokines and cytokine receptors were analyzed using a multiplexed, bead-based platform (BioPlex®, BioRad, Irvine, CA) and custom-made assay kits as previously described (39, 40). Detection limits for these assays were as follows: ferritin - 0.07 ng/ml, soluble transferrin receptor (sTfR) - 0.03 ng/ml, EPO - 0.1 mIU/ml, TNF-α - 0.1 pg/ml, TNF receptor (R) I - 1.58 pg/ml, TNF-RII - 0.21 pg/ml, IFN-γ - 0.04

pg/ml, IL-6 - 1.45 pg/ml, IL-10 - 0.02 pg/ml. Levels of soluble factors were adjusted to account for dilution in anticoagulant at the time of sample collection. For each plasma sample, all analytes were assayed in a single day, thus eliminating freeze/thaw cycles.

Sickle cell variants (HbAA, HbAS and HbSS) were determined by cellulose acetate paper electrophoresis according to the manufacturer's instructions (Helena Laboratories, Beaumont, Texas, USA). Genotyping for α^+-thalassemia and glucose-6-phosphate dehydrogenase (G6PD) variants was performed by polymerase chain reaction (PCR) techniques. DNA was isolated from blood spots on filter paper according to the manufacturer's instructions (Generation® Capture Card Kit, Gentra Inc.). α^+-thalassemia typing was done according to the protocol described by Chong et al. (41).

To type G6PD variants (G6PD B, G6PD A, and G6PD A-), a region spanning the third to fifth exon was amplified by an outer PCR (Forward 5'- GGT GGA TGA TGT ATG TAG-3' and Reverse 5'- GCA ACG CTG CCA CCT TGT G-3'), followed by nested multiplex PCR. Nested primers to detect the residue 202 polymorphism were G6PD-202 F (5'-CCT TCT GCC CGA AAA CAC CTT CA<u>C</u>C-3') and G6PD-202 R (5'- GTC CCC GAA GCT GGC CAT GCT GG -3'); and primers to detect the residue 376 polymorphism were G6PD-376 F (5'- TAC CAG CGC CTC AAC AGC C<u>C</u>C ATG –3') and G6PD-376 R (5'- GGA CTC GTG AAT GTT CTT GGT GAC G-3'). The PCR conditions for the first reaction were as follows: samples were subjected to initial denaturation for 60 seconds at 94°C followed by 30 cycles of 94°C for 60 seconds, 58°C for 45 seconds and 72°C for 60 seconds, followed by 7 minutes at 72°C. The nested multiplex PCR conditions were similar to the above except the annealing temperature was set at 56°C. Mismatches in the primers (at the underlined residues) introduced NcoI digestion sites into the amplified products of the variant alleles, leading to digestion of the G6PD-202 product in G6PD A individuals and digestion of the G6PD-376 product in G6PD A- individuals.

Clinical and Parasitological Definitions

Maternal anemia was defined as maternal venous blood hemoglobin concentration less than 11.0 g/dl. Fetal anemia was defined as cord blood hemoglobin concentration less than 12.5 g/dl (6). Placental malaria status was determined from thick and thin smear of mechanically extracted placental blood, and the presence of placental parasites, inflammation and pigment in PM+ women was characterized by histology as previously described (42). Iron deficiency was defined as ferritin concentration <30 ng/ml when C-reactive protein (CRP) was ≤8.2 µg/ml (iron deficiency in the absence of inflammation), or ferritin concentration <70 ng/ml when CRP was >8.2 µg/ml (iron deficiency in the presence of inflammation) (42).

Statistical Analysis

Analyses were performed using Statview 5.0.1 (SAS Institute, Cary, NC, USA). Differences between proportions were compared by χ^2 test. Normally distributed continuous data were compared by the Student's *t* test and analysis of variance. Data that did not conform to a normal distribution were compared by Mann-Whitney or Kruskal-Wallis tests. Simple and multiple logistic regression models were used to test for associations of maternal and fetal factors to fetal anemia. Two-sided p ≤0.05 was considered to be statistically significant.

In a stepwise approach (see **Supplementary Figure S1**), we searched for maternal and fetal factors related to fetal anemia. We first used a Chi-square test for categorical variables and a Student's t-test for continuous variables to examine their direct relationship to fetal anemia. Because parity was strongly related to fetal anemia risk in that analysis, and is known to impact numerous pregnancy outcomes in malarious areas, we used ANOVA to examine the interactions of parity with other baseline maternal and fetal factors for their relationships to cord hemoglobin level. Secondly, we employed a simple logistic regression analysis to identify fetal soluble factors (iron regulatory proteins, erythropoietin, cytokines and cytokine receptors) related to fetal anemia. We then examined maternal and fetal factors that were seen to be significant in univariate analysis, for their independent association with fetal anemia in multiple logistic regression analysis. Finally, because the interaction term parity*maternal iron deficiency was related to cord hemoglobin level, we stratified the multivariate logistic regression analysis by maternal iron deficiency, and then by parity groups among mothers with iron deficiency.

RESULTS

Fetal Anemia Is Related to Parity but Not to Maternal Anemia

We determined the hemoglobin level in 610 cord blood and 658 maternal blood samples (90 with PM) obtained at delivery. The overall prevalence of fetal anemia defined as cord hemoglobin below 12.5g/dL (6) was 46.2% and increased with successive pregnancies. 95.7% of deliveries were spontaneous vaginal deliveries without any recorded complications of labor. 26/610 (4.3%) were delivered *via* C-section, and 8/26 (30.8%) C-sections had fetal anemia. Mean (SD) cord hemoglobin (g/dL) was 12.5 (2.7), 12.6 (2.3) and 12.1 (3.0) in offspring of primigravidae, secundigravidae and multigravidae, respectively. Fetal anemia was present in 38.9%, 41.3% and 63.3% of first, second and later offspring, respectively (χ^2=9.4, p = 0.008). Cord hemoglobin tended to be inversely correlated with increasing parity although this relationship was not statistically significant (r = - 0.071; p = 0.07).

Most women (356/658 (57.1%)) were anemic at delivery (hemoglobin < 11 g/dL), and this did not differ by parity (54.6%, 56.5% and 58.9% (χ^2 = 0.93, p = 0.62) in primigravidae, secundigravidae and multigravidae respectively). The proportion of infants with fetal anemia did not differ significantly among offspring of mothers with anemia versus offspring of mothers without anemia (50.6% versus 43.6%; χ^2 = 2.7, p = 0.1). This pattern was similar in the different parity groups (primigravid, 46.2% versus 36.6%, χ^2 = 1.4, p = 0.2; secundigravid, 44.7% versus 41.3%, χ^2 = 0.14, p = 0.7; multigravid, 55.6% versus 49.1, χ^2 = 1.1, p = 0.3). When treated as a continuous variable, maternal and fetal hemoglobin were related, but the correlation was weak (Linear correlation coefficient = 0.15; p = 0.04)

Fetal Anemia Is Not Related to Placental Malaria (PM) at Delivery

Fetal anemia was present in 240/520 (46.1%) offspring of PM- versus 49/90 (46.4%) offspring of PM+ mothers (p = 0.9). Although fetal anemia was more frequent in the PM+ than the PM- group in each parity category, none of these differences were statistically significant, using cord hemoglobin of either 12.5 g/dL (**Supplementary Table S1**) or of 10.0 g/dL (**Supplementary Table S2**) to stratify the population. Cord hemoglobin levels did not differ significantly between offspring of PM+ (mean (SD) 12.0 (2.9) g/dL) versus PM- women (mean (SD) 12.3 (2.7) g/dL). Mean (SD) cord hemoglobin levels were 12.3 (2.8) g/dL and 12.2 (2.8) g/dL in offspring of PM+ mothers with inflammation and PM+ mothers without inflammation respectively. The proportions of newborns with fetal anemia did not differ significantly between PM- (46.1%), PM+ without placental inflammation (46.4%), and PM+ with placental inflammation (57.6%), defined histologically as presence of intervillous inflammatory cells (χ^2 = 1.3, p = 0.51). The proportion with fetal anemia did not differ between offspring of mothers with active, past or no placental malaria by histology (p = 0.8).

TABLE 1 | Maternal and newborn characteristics in relation to fetal anemia*.

Characteristic	Fetal Anemia	No Fetal Anemia	P value
	MATERNAL		
Age (Years), Mean (SD)	26.46 (6.3)	25.25 (6.0)	**0.02**
Iron deficiency (n = 461)	211 (45.8%)	250 (54.2%)	0.8
Anemia (n = 314)	159 (50.6%)	155 (49.4%)	0.1
Parity			
Primigravidae (n = 167)	65 (38.9%)	102 (61.1%)	**0.009**
Secundigravidae (n = 146)	61 (41.8%)	85 (58.2%)	
Multigravidae (n = 297)	156 (52.5%)	141 (47.5%)	
PM (Histology) (n=610)			
No infection (n = 498)	227 (45.6%)	271 (54.4%)	0.8
Active infection (n = 78)	38 (48.7%)	40 (51.3%)	
Past infection (n = 34)	17 (50.0%)	17 (50.0%)	
PM (Microscopy)			
PM+ (n = 90)	42/90 (46.7%)	48/90 (53.3%)	0.9
PM– (n = 520)	240/520 (46.2%)	280/520 (53.8%)	
	NEWBORN		
Birth Weight (g), Mean (SD)	3162 (0.41)	3203 (0.43)	0.3
Female/Male (n)	157/171	142/139	0.6
Iron deficiency (n =73)	33 (45.2%)	40 (54.8%)	1.0
Sickle hemoglobin			
AA (n = 488)	232 (84.0%)	256 (80%)	0.4
AS (n = 103)	42 (15.3%)	61 (19.1%)	
SS (n = 5)	2 (0.7%)	3 (0.9%)	
G6PD status			
A (n = 72)	35 (12.65%)	37 (11.7%)	0.2
A- (n = 72)	27 (9.7%)	45 (14.2%)	
A Heterozygous (n =52)	24 (8.6%)	15 (4.7%)	
A- Heterozygous (n = 39)	22 (8.0%)	30 (9.4%)	
B (n = 361)	170 (61.1%)	191 (60.0%)	
Thalassemia			
$\alpha\alpha/\ \alpha\alpha$ (n = 247)	104 (44.9%)	143 (54.2%)	**0.0005**
$-\alpha/\ \alpha\alpha$ (n = 199)	92 (39.6%)	107 (40.5%)	
$-\alpha/\ -\alpha$ (n = 50)	36 (15.5%)	14 (5.3%)	

All variables were analyzed by Chi-square t-test except for maternal age and birth weight (unpaired t-test).
Bold values represent significant differences.

Maternal Iron Status and Parity Interact to Modify Risk of Fetal Anemia

Parity was significantly related to fetal anemia (**Table 1**) and is well-known to impact numerous maternal and fetal outcomes in malarious areas, including its strong effect on placental malaria risk as women acquire protective immunity over successive pregnancies (43). We therefore examined whether the interaction of parity with other maternal and fetal baseline factors was related to cord hemoglobin levels, as an indication whether these interactions might be confounding analyses of fetal anemia risk. Among all interactions examined (**Supplementary Table S3**), only the interaction of parity with maternal iron status was significantly related to cord blood hemoglobin levels (factorial ANOVA, p = 0.03), suggesting that fetal anemia risk factors should be examined after stratification by maternal iron status and parity.

Among mothers with available measurements, 81.6% (618/757) were iron-deficient, and iron deficiency was less common in primigravid (76.6%) than in secundigravid (85.7%) or multigravid women (82.7%; χ^2 = 5.9, p = 0.05). By comparison, only 12.2% (93/726) of newborns had iron deficiency and this did not differ significantly by parity (12.2% in first, 10.2% in second, and 14.3% in third or later offspring; χ^2 = 1.6, P = 0.4). The frequency of maternal or fetal iron deficiency did not differ between newborns with or without fetal anemia, whether defined as hemoglobin below 12.5 g/dL (**Table 1**) or below 10 g/dL (**Supplementary Tables S4** and **S5**).

When mothers were iron-deficient, cord hemoglobin levels decreased (**Figure 1A**, p = 0.01) and the prevalence of fetal anemia increased over successive pregnancies (35.0%, 44.6% and 52.0% of first, second and later offspring, respectively; χ^2 = 8.9, p = 0.001). The opposite pattern was observed when mothers had adequate iron stores: cord hemoglobin levels increased (**Figure 1B**, p = 0.15) and the prevalence of fetal anemia decreased with increasing parity, although this was not statistically significant (51.1%, 31.6% and 42.8% of first, second and later offspring, respectively; χ^2 = 2.1, p = 0.34).

Thalassemia but No Other Red Cell Disorder Is Associated With Fetal Anemia

Samples from 496 newborns were genotyped for α^+-thalassemia, 596 for G6PD deficiency and 596 for sickle cell hemoglobin phenotype. The frequency of neonatal genotypes/phenotypes did not vary by PM or by parity (**Supplementary Table S6**).

α^+-thalassemia but not G6PD deficiency nor sickle hemoglobin increased fetal anemia risk. Overall, thalassemia homozygous ($-\alpha/\ -\alpha$) offspring had the lowest hemoglobin levels (mean (SD) g/dL of 12.5 (2.9), 12.4 (2.7) and 10.9 (2.1) in normal, heterozygous or homozygous offspring; Kruskal Wallis test, p < 0.0001) and the highest frequency of fetal anemia (**Table 1**) compared to heterozygous ($-\alpha/\ \alpha\alpha$) or normal newborns.

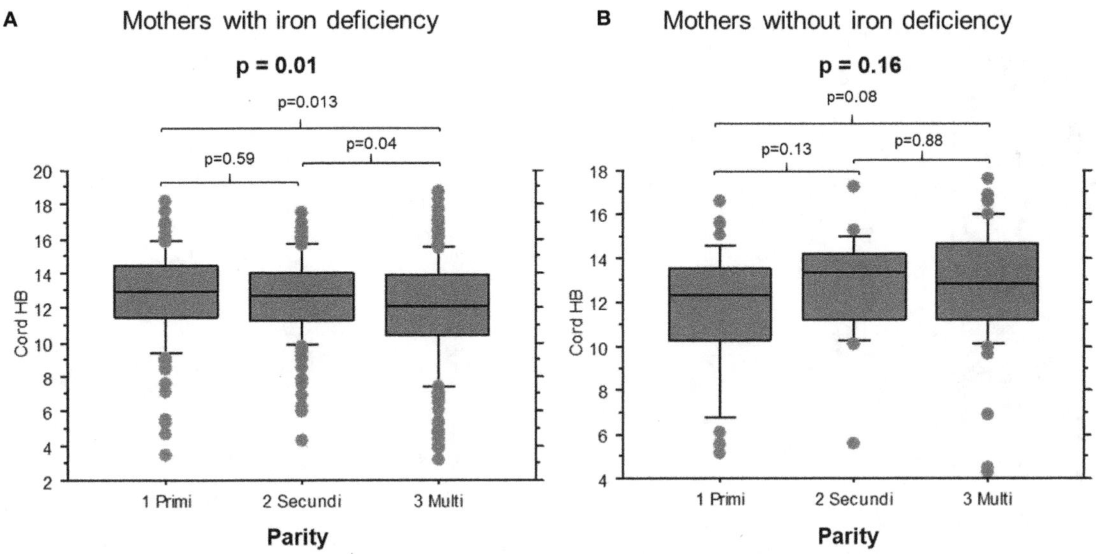

Prevalence of fetal anemia increases with parity of mothers with iron deficiency

Primigravidae = 35.0%,
Secundigravidae = 44.6%
Multigravidae = 52.0%
P = 0.001

Prevalence of fetal anemia does not increase with parity of mothers without iron deficiency

Primigravidae = 51.1%
Secundigravidae = 31.6%
Multigravidae = 48.2%
P = 0.34

FIGURE 1 | Cord blood hemoglobin levels in offspring of mothers with and without iron deficiency, stratified by parity. **(A)** Cord samples from mothers with iron deficiency: 1, primigravidae (n = 53); 2, secundigravidae (n = 72); 3, multigravidae (n = 132). **(B)** Cord samples from mothers with normal iron status: 1, primigravidae (n = 29); 2, secundigravidae (n = 14); 3, multigravidae (n = 31). The box plots indicate the median (horizontal line) and interquartile range (box), and the whiskers represent $10^{th}/90^{th}$ percentiles. The differences between groups were analyzed by the Kruskal-Wallis test. Associated P values are shown.

Thalassemia significantly decreased fetal hemoglobin levels in offspring of multigravidae but not in offspring of primigravidae or secundigravidae. Mean (SD) cord hemoglobin (g/dL) was 12.5 (3.0), 12.4 (2.8) or 10.4 (1.8) in normal, heterozygous or homozygous offspring, respectively, of multigravidae (Kruskal-Wallis test, p = 0.0002), versus 12.4 (2.7), 12.4 (3.0) or 12.4 (2.7) in those of primigravidae (Kruskal-Wallis test, p = 0.86) and 12.7 (2.7), 12.8 (2.0) or 11.4 (2.0) in those of secundigravidae (Kruskal-Wallis test, p = 0.06). Thalassemia increased the frequency of fetal anemia in offspring of multigravidae (χ^2 = 5.64, p = 0.02) but not primigravidae (χ^2 = 0.001, p = 0.9) or secundigravidae (χ^2 = 0.56, p = 0.45).

Cytokine Balance, sTfR and Fetal Thalassemia Are Associated With Fetal Anemia Risk in Univariate and Multivariate Analyses

We performed a simple logistic regression analysis of cord soluble factors and risk of fetal anemia. Higher levels of TNFRII and IL-6 increased the risk of fetal anemia, whereas higher levels of TNF-RI and sTfR decreased the risk (**Table 2**). In an un-stratified multiple logistic regression analysis of these significant factors, –a/–a thalassemia and higher levels of IL-6 and TNF-RII independently increased, whereas higher levels of TNF-RI and sTfR decreased, the risk of fetal anemia (**Table 3**).

TABLE 2 | Simple logistic regression analysis of soluble fetal factors in relation to fetal anemia.

FETAL FACTOR	OR	95% CI	P value
TNF-α (n = 576)	0.80	(0.49 - 1.21)	0.3
TNF-RI (n = 583)	0.46	(0.23 - 0.90)	**0.02**
TNF-RII (n = 583)	2.19	(1.24 - 3.90)	**0.007**
IFN-γ (n = 121)	1.71	(0.82 - 3.56)	0.2
IL-10 (n = 523)	1.08	(0.63 - 1.85)	0.8
IL-6 (n = 476)	1.62	(1.21 - 2.17)	**0.001**
sTfR (n = 583)	0.30	(0.14 - 0.62)	**0.001**
EPO (n = 402)	1.40	(0.78 - 2.52)	0.3

Bold values represent significant differences.

TABLE 3 | Multiple logistic regression analysis of factors in relation to fetal anemia risk (n = 358).

FACTOR	aOR*	95% CI	P value
Secundigravidae	0.41	0.12-1.47	0.2
Multigravidae	0.27	0.02-2.72	0.3
Maternal iron deficiency	0.29	0.07-1.26	0.1
Maternal iron deficiency * Parity	1.63	0.89-3.08	0.1
−α/ αα thalassemia	1.34	0.84-2.15	0.2
−α/ −α thalassemia	4.30	1.78-10.34	**0.001**
TNF-RI	0.26	0.09-0.70	**0.008**
TNF-RII	2.31	1.08-4.94	**0.03**
sTfR	0.24	0.07-0.63	**0.005**
IL-6	2.05	1.38-3.02	**0.0003**

**Adjusted Odds Ratio.*
Bold values represent significant differences.

TABLE 4 | Multivariate logistic regression analysis of risk factors for fetal anemia in offspring of mothers with OR without iron deficiency.

FACTOR	IRON DEFICIENCY (n = 287)			NO IRON DEFICIENCY (n = 71)		
	aOR*	95% CI	P value	aOR	95% CI	P value
Secundigravidae	1.54	0.72-3.28	0.3	0.13	0.03-0.69	**0.02**
Multigravidae	2.12	1.13-4.00	**0.02**	0.57	0.18-1.82	0.3
−α/ αα	1.68	0.97-2.91	0.1	0.58	0.20-1.69	0.3
−α/ −α	7.02	2.62-18.84	**0.0001**	0.22	0.01-4.24	0.3
TNF-RI	0.19	0.06-0.59	**0.005**	1.10	0.10-10.32	1.0
TNF-RII	2.07	0.90-4.79	0.1	5.64	0.55-57.70	0.1
sTfR	0.12	0.03-0.43	**0.001**	1.68	0.15-18.30	0.7
IL-6	2.60	1.60-4.21	**0.0001**	1.47	0.70-3.12	0.3

**Adjusted Odds Ratio.*
Bold values represent significant differences.

TABLE 5 | Multivariate logistic regression analysis of risk factors for fetal anemia in offspring of mothers with iron deficiency in different parity groups.

FACTOR	PRIMIGRAVIDAE (n = 75)			SECUNDIGRAVIDAE (n = 66)			MULTIGRAVIDAE (n = 146)		
	aOR*	95% CI	P value	aOR	95% CI	P value	aOR	95% CI	P value
−α/ αα	1.68	0.50-5.69	0.4	2.21	0.57-8.59	0.3	1.79	0.85-3.75	0.1
−α/ −α	29.92	1.88-475.28	**0.02**	7.92	1.14-55.17	**0.04**	7.87	1.87-33.10	**0.005**
TNF-RI	0.02	0.001-0.33	**0.006**	0.18	0.01-2.49	0.2	0.23	0.05-1.20	0.1
TNF-RII	3.19	0.37-27.84	0.3	0.96	0.15-6.25	1.0	1.83	0.62-5.40	0.3
sTfR	0.006	0.0001-0.24	**0.007**	0.003	0.0004-0.19	**0.006**	0.40	0.08-1.96	0.3
IL-6	1.92	0.68-5.45	0.2	2.50	0.84-7.41	0.1	2.67	1.33-5.47	**0.006**

**Adjusted Odds Ratio.*
Bold values represent significant differences.

Since maternal iron deficiency interacted with parity to modify the levels of cord blood hemoglobin, we stratified the multiple regression analysis by maternal iron status (**Table 4**). All relationships between newborn risk factors and fetal anemia occurred in the maternal iron deficiency group and were absent in the group with normal maternal iron status.

We therefore conducted analyses after stratifying only the maternal iron deficiency group by parity (**Table 5**). Among all parity groups, fetal anemia risk was higher in newborns with thalassemia, higher cord levels of IL-6, and lower cord levels of TNF-RI and sTfR (**Table 5**). Other than −α/ −α thalassemia, these relationships achieved statistical significance in only some parity groups: increased cord TNF-RI and sTfR significantly reduced fetal anemia risk in first pregnancies, increased cord sTfR significantly reduced fetal anemia risk in second pregnancies, and increased cord IL-6 significantly increased fetal anemia risk in third pregnancies. Of note, reduced sample sizes may limit the power of these subgroup analyses to identify significant relationships.

Erythropoietin Levels Are Decreased During Severe Fetal Anemia

Cord EPO levels did not differ significantly between anemic (median (interquartile range), 70.8 mIU/mL (35.2 - 85.3)) and non-anemic newborns (62.3 mIU/mL (37.5 – 95.9); p = 0.1, Mann-Whitney test) indicating that EPO is not responding

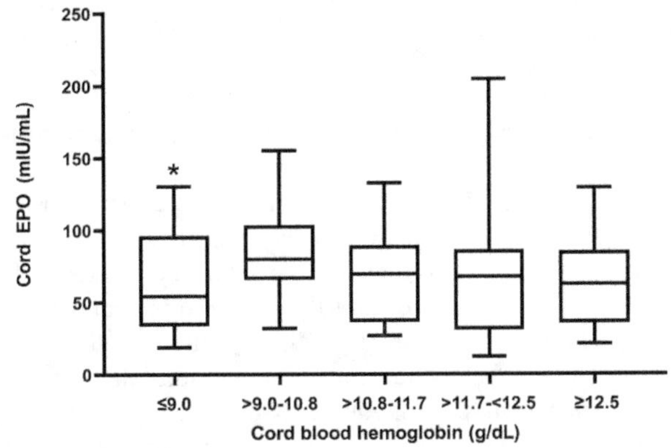

FIGURE 2 | Cord blood EPO levels in relation to degree of fetal anemia. Q1 (Hb ≤ 9 mg/dl); Q2 (Hb > 9 -10.8 mg/dl); Q3 (Hb >10.8-11.7 mg/dl); Q4 (Hb > 11.7-<12.5 mg/dl; and Q5, no fetal anemia (≥12.5). The box plots indicate the median (horizontal line) and interquartile range (box), and the whiskers represent 10th/90th percentiles. The differences between groups were analyzed by the Kruskal-Wallis test; *Q1 was significantly lower than the reference group Q5 (p = 0.03).

appropriately to declining hemoglobin levels. We stratified anemic newborns in quartiles by fetal hemoglobin levels and compared them to normal newborns for their EPO levels (**Figure 2**). Newborns with fetal anemia showed a non-significant trend to increase EPO as cord hemoglobin decreased, except for newborns in the lowest Hb quartile (Hb ≤ 9.0 g/dl) in whom EPO was significantly lower versus normal children.

DISCUSSION

Fetal anemia predisposes to anemia in infancy (4) and is a risk factor for infant mortality (5). Fetal anemia is more frequent in malarious areas (6) but the cause is unclear, so we sought to identify maternal and fetal factors that increase the risk of fetal anemia in Tanzania. We confirmed that fetal anemia is common in an area of intense malaria transmission, but that it is not related to PM at the time of delivery. Instead, inappropriately low EPO levels were associated with the most severe fetal anemia in this population. Further, α^+-thalassemia, sTfR and the cytokine balance (involving TNF-RI, TNF-RII, and IL-6) of the newborn were related to fetal anemia, but these relationships were limited to offspring of iron-deficient mothers in whom all but thalassemia were modified by parity.

We found a high proportion (46.2%) of infants with fetal anemia in our population. The mean cord hemoglobin level of 12.3 g/dl in the present study is lower than levels reported in developing countries without malaria but is comparable to levels from other malarious countries (6). However, placental malaria at delivery was not related to fetal anemia in this study, suggesting that active malaria is not a direct cause. Contradictory findings on the association between malaria in pregnancy and fetal anemia have been reported with some studies showing no association (7–9) but others reporting an association (10–12). Our study suggests that malaria may increase fetal anemia risk through indirect means, such as by causing maternal iron deficiency (44) or by its evolutionary selection of thalassemia (10–12).

Iron is an essential micronutrient for erythropoiesis. The fetus obtains iron from the maternal circulation, and iron deficiency in the mother reduces iron stores in the newborns (45). Recently, animal and human studies have indicated that in the setting of maternal iron deficiency, regulation of placental iron uptake and export to the fetus favors preservation of placental iron sufficiency rather than fetal iron content in order to maintain global function of the healthy placenta (46). We expected that iron deficiency would increase the risk of fetal anemia. However, cord hemoglobin levels did not differ between iron-deficient mothers and mothers with normal iron stores.

Instead, the interaction of maternal iron status and parity was related to cord hemoglobin levels (**Supplementary Table S3**). Fetal anemia prevalence increased significantly with parity when mothers were iron-deficient but tended to decrease when mothers had normal iron stores (**Figure 1**). Maternal iron status modified the relationships of several other factors to fetal anemia. For example, increased levels of cord IL-6 increased the odds and cord TNF-RI decreased the odds of fetal anemia, but only when the mother was iron-deficient. This suggests roles for fetal cytokine balance in the pathogenesis of fetal anemia only during maternal iron deficiency, which suggests that distinct mechanisms converge in the fetus to cause anemia.

Fetal immune activation has been proposed as a mechanism by which placental malaria itself might increase the risk of fetal anemia (6), albeit this and earlier studies (10–12) do not find a direct relationship of placental malaria to fetal anemia. Notably, inflammatory cytokines do not increase in fetal blood during placental malaria (47) and this may explain in part why active placental malaria does not influence the immediate risk of fetal anemia. We cannot rule out that infections prior to delivery may contribute to fetal anemia, as mothers were enrolled in this study at the time of delivery. Future studies should explore whether malaria episodes occurring earlier during pregnancy contribute to the risk of fetal anemia.

The mechanism through which the fetal cytokine milieu may be mediating anemia requires further study. IL-6 is known to induce hypoferremia of infection and inflammation by stimulating the synthesis of hepcidin (48). Hepcidin limits the iron that is available for erythropoiesis by inhibiting its efflux through ferroportin, an iron exporter that is expressed in the small intestine, hepatocytes, macrophages, and placental trophoblast cells (23). Studies to examine IL-6 and hepcidin for their interrelationships to fetal anemia are warranted. Elevated fetal IL-6 was reported in fetal anemia due to maternal Rh alloimmunisation, and presumed to be a marker of fetal systemic inflammatory response syndrome (SIRS) secondary to red blood cell destruction in the reticuloendothelial system (49, 50). Conversely, TNF-RI protects against fetal anemia and might do so by binding and neutralizing TNF-α, an inflammatory cytokine that has been associated with anemia. For this reason, free TNF-α levels in cord blood should be examined in future studies to see whether they have a stronger relationship with fetal anemia than total TNF-α levels.

Maternal iron deficiency and parity also modified the effect of α^+-thalassemia to cause fetal anemia (**Table 4**). α^+-thalassemia is the most common hemoglobinopathy of humans and leads to mild hypochromic microcytic anemia. The prevalence of fetal thalassemia in this population (10.1% $-\alpha/-\alpha$ and 40.1% $-\alpha/\alpha\alpha$) is comparable to that found in other malarious areas of Africa (49). Thalassaemia has been related to hematological status of the fetus in a non-malarious area. In New Zealand, cord levels of hemoglobin, mean corpuscular hemoglobin (MCH) and mean corpuscular volume (MCV) were significantly lower in heterozygous and homozygous thalassemic newborns compared to normal newborns (51, 52).

In the present study, decreased sTfR levels were associated with increased odds of fetal anemia. Erythropoietic activity has been found to be the most important determinant of sTfR levels (51, 53). In conditions such as α-thalassemia which are characterized by stimulated erythropoiesis, sTfR levels are increased; elevated levels of sTfR in older children with thalassemia were previously reported from Vanuatu where malaria is endemic (54). Elevated sTfR may reflect stimulated erythropoiesis in the fetus with thalassemia and anemia.

EPO levels were not significantly increased in newborns with fetal anemia, and this inappropriately blunted response may have contributed to anemia in our study population. EPO is the primary growth factor regulating red blood cell production, and increased cord blood EPO levels are a marker of chronic fetal hypoxia and intrauterine fetal growth retardation (55), as well as Rh isoimmunization (28). EPO does not cross the placenta (56) and therefore must emanate from fetal sources, such as kidneys, liver, and placenta which are known to express the EPO gene (57). We speculate that the degree of fetal anemia observed in Tanzanian newborns may not cause sufficient hypoxia to induce EPO production. Rodent studies suggest that the EPO response to hypoxia is markedly reduced in newborn compared to adult rats (58), possibly because the high oxygen-affinity fetal hemoglobin mitigates tissue hypoxia due to anemia. Alternatively, TNF-α and IL-1 have been shown to inhibit EPO production (59) and therefore the inflammatory environment could suppress EPO production by the fetus during anemia. Indeed, EPO levels were significantly decreased in newborns with the most severe anemia (**Figure 2**), suggesting that a failed EPO response might actively contribute to fetal anemia.

In summary, this study has shown that fetal α-thalassemia, cytokine balance, and sTfR levels, but not PM, are related to fetal anemia risk in an area of high malaria transmission. The relationship of these factors to fetal anemia was only seen when mothers were iron-deficient, suggesting that measures to prevent maternal iron deficiency may reduce fetal anemia risk, albeit maternal iron status was not directly related to fetal anemia. The opposing effects of inflammatory (IL-6) and anti-inflammatory (soluble TNF-RI) factors suggest that conditions that alter fetal cytokine balance may be involved in the pathogenesis of fetal anemia. Future studies are needed to elucidate the causes of altered fetal cytokine balance and their roles in the pathogenesis of fetal anemia. Inadequate EPO may also be a contributor to the most severe cases of anemia in Tanzanian newborns.

AUTHOR CONTRIBUTIONS

PD and MF designed the MOMS Project. JK and EK completed the cytokine assays. GM determined variants of red cell abnormalities. AM performed histological studies. EK and PD analyzed the data and wrote the manuscript with the contribution of all other authors. All authors contributed to the article and approved the submitted version.

ACKNOWLEDGMENTS

The authors are grateful to Muheza Designated District Hospital in Tanzania that hosted the Mother-Offspring Malaria Studies (MOMS) Project in partnership with Seattle Biomedical Research Institute. The authors gratefully acknowledge the participation of the mothers and their infants in the MOMS Project, and the work of the MOMS Project staff, including assistant medical officers, nurses, village health workers, laboratory technicians, microscopists, and data entry personnel. Gretchen Langdon organized the cytokine assays.

REFERENCES

1. Radunovic N, Lockwood CJ, Alvarez M, Plecas D, Chitkara U, Berkowitz RL. The severely anemic and hydropic isoimmune fetus: changes in fetal hematocrit associated with intrauterine death. *Obstet Gynecol* (1992) 79:390–3. doi: 10.1097/00006250-199203000-00013
2. van Kamp IL, Klumper FJ, Bakkum RS, Oepkes D, Meerman RH, Scherjon SA, et al. The severity of immune fetal hydrops is predictive of fetal outcome after intrauterine treatment. *Am J Obstet Gynecol* (2001) 185:668–73. doi: 10.1067/mob.2001.116690
3. Kalanda B, Verhoeff F, le Cessie S, Brabin J. Low birth weight and fetal anaemia as risk factors for infant morbidity in rural Malawi. *Malawi Med J* (2009) 21:69–74. doi: 10.4314/mmj.v21i2.44553
4. le Cessie S, Verhoeff FH, Mengistie G, Kazembe P, Broadhead R, Brabin BJ. Changes in haemoglobin levels in infants in Malawi: effect of low birth weight and fetal anaemia. *Arch Dis Child Fetal Neonatal Ed* (2002) 86:F182–187. doi: 10.1136/fn.86.3.F182
5. van Eijk AM, Ayisi JG, Ter Kuile FO, Slutsker L, Shi YP, Udhayakumar V, et al. HIV, malaria, and infant anemia as risk factors for postneonatal infant mortality among HIV-seropositive women in Kisumu, Kenya. *J Infect Dis* (2007) 196:30–7. doi: 10.1086/518441
6. Brabin B. Fetal anaemia in malarious areas: its causes and significance. *Ann Trop Paediatr* (1992) 12:303–10. doi: 10.1080/02724936.1992.11747589
7. Brabin BJ, Kalanda BF, Verhoeff FH, Chimsuku LH, Broadhead RL. Risk factors for fetal anaemia in a malarious area of Malawi. *Ann Trop Paediatr* (2004) 24:311–21. doi: 10.1179/027249304225019136
8. Laar AK, Grant FE, Addo Y, Soyiri I, Nkansah B, Abugri J, et al. Predictors of fetal anemia and cord blood malaria parasitemia among newborns of HIV-positive mothers. *BMC Res Notes* (2013) 6:350. doi: 10.1186/1756-0500-6-350

9. Rogawski ET, Chaluluka E, Molyneux ME, Feng G, Rogerson SJ, Meshnick SR. The effects of malaria and intermittent preventive treatment during pregnancy on fetal anemia in Malawi. *Clin Infect Dis* (2012) 55:1096–102. doi: 10.1093/cid/cis597
10. Abrams ET, Kwiek JJ, Mwapasa V, Kamwendo DD, Tadesse E, Lema VM, et al. Malaria during pregnancy and foetal haematological status in Blantyre, Malawi. *Malar J* (2005) 4:39. doi: 10.1186/1475-2875-4-39
11. McClure EM, Meshnick SR, Mungai P, Malhotra I, King CL, Goldenberg RL, et al. The association of parasitic infections in pregnancy and maternal and fetal anemia: a cohort study in coastal Kenya. *PloS Negl Trop Dis* (2014) 8: e2724. doi: 10.1371/journal.pntd.0002724
12. Van Santen S, de Mast Q, Luty AJ, Wiegerinck ET, Van der Ven AJ, Swinkels DW. Iron homeostasis in mother and child during placental malaria infection. *Am J Trop Med Hyg* (2011) 84:148–51. doi: 10.4269/ajtmh.2011.10-0250
13. Harrington WE, Mutabingwa TK, Kabyemela E, Fried M, Duffy PE. Intermittent treatment to prevent pregnancy malaria does not confer benefit in an area of widespread drug resistance. *Clin Infect Dis* (2011) 53:224–30. doi: 10.1093/cid/cir376
14. Adachi M, Manji K, Ichimi R, Nishimori H, Shindo K, Matsubayashi N, et al. : Detection of congenital malaria by polymerase-chain-reaction methodology in Dar es Salaam, Tanzania. *Parasitol Res* (2000) 86:615–8. doi: 10.1007/PL00008540
15. Allen DA, Breen C, Yaqoob MM, Macdougall IC. Inhibition of CFU-E colony formation in uremic patients with inflammatory disease: role of IFN-gamma and TNF-alpha. *J Investig Med* (1999) 47:204–11.
16. Clark IA, Chaudhri G. Tumour necrosis factor may contribute to the anaemia of malaria by causing dyserythropoiesis and erythrophagocytosis. *Br J Haematol* (1988) 70:99–103. doi: 10.1111/j.1365-2141.1988.tb02440.x
17. Kurtzhals JA, Adabayeri V, Goka BQ, Akanmori BD, Oliver-Commey JO, Nkrumah FK, et al. Low plasma concentrations of interleukin 10 in severe malarial anaemia compared with cerebral and uncomplicated malaria. *Lancet* (1998) 351:1768–72. doi: 10.1016/S0140-6736(97)09439-7
18. Othoro C, Lal AA, Nahlen B, Koech D, Orago AS, Udhayakumar V. A low interleukin-10 tumor necrosis factor-alpha ratio is associated with malaria anemia in children residing in a holoendemic malaria region in western Kenya. *J Infect Dis* (1999) 179:279–82. doi: 10.1086/314548
19. Fried M, Muga RO, Misore AO, Duffy PE. Malaria elicits type 1 cytokines in the human placenta: IFN-gamma and TNF-alpha associated with pregnancy outcomes. *J Immunol* (1998) 160:2523–30.
20. Bodnar LM, Siega-Riz AM, Arab L, Chantala K, McDonald T. Predictors of pregnancy and postpartum haemoglobin concentrations in low-income women. *Public Health Nutr* (2004) 7:701–11. doi: 10.1079/PHN2004597
21. Massawe SN, Urassa EN, Mmari M, Ronquist G, Lindmark G, Nystrom L. The complexity of pregnancy anemia in Dar-es-Salaam. *Gynecol Obstet Invest* (1999) 47:76–82. doi: 10.1159/000010067
22. Jaime-Perez JC, Herrera-Garza JL, Gomez-Almaguer D. Sub-optimal fetal iron acquisition under a maternal environment. *Arch Med Res* (2005) 36:598–602. doi: 10.1016/j.arcmed.2005.03.023
23. Bastin J, Drakesmith H, Rees M, Sargent I, Townsend A. Localisation of proteins of iron metabolism in the human placenta and liver. *Br J Haematol* (2006) 134:532–43. doi: 10.1111/j.1365-2141.2006.06216.x
24. Donovan A, Brownlie A, Zhou Y, Shepard J, Pratt SJ, Moynihan J, et al. : Positional cloning of zebrafish ferroportin1 identifies a conserved vertebrate iron exporter. *Nature* (2000) 403:776–81. doi: 10.1038/35001596
25. Maier RF, Bohme K, Dudenhausen JW, Obladen M. Cord blood erythropoietin in relation to different markers of fetal hypoxia. *Obstet Gynecol* (1993) 81:575–80.
26. Seikku L, Rahkonen L, Tikkanen M, Hamalainen E, Rahkonen P, Andersson S, et al. Amniotic fluid erythropoietin and neonatal outcome in pregnancies complicated by intrauterine growth restriction before 34 gestational weeks. *Acta Obstet Gynecol Scand* (2015) 94:288–94. doi: 10.1111/aogs.12553
27. Gruslin A, Perkins SL, Manchanda R, Fleming N, Clinch JJ. Maternal smoking and fetal erythropoietin levels. *Obstet Gynecol* (2000) 95:561–4. doi: 10.1097/00006250-200004000-00016
28. Moya FR, Grannum PA, Widness JA, Clemons GK, Copel JA, Hobbins JC. Erythropoietin in human fetuses with immune hemolytic anemia and hydrops fetalis. *Obstet Gynecol* (1993) 82:353–8.
29. Voutilainen PE, Widness JA, Clemons GK, Schwartz R, Teramo KA. Amniotic fluid erythropoietin predicts fetal distress in Rh-immunized pregnancies. *Am J Obstet Gynecol* (1989) 160:429–34. doi: 10.1016/0002-9378(89)90466-3
30. Raj DK, Das Mohapatra A, Jnawali A, Zuromski J, Jha A, Cham-Kpu G, et al. Anti-PfGARP activates programmed cell death of parasites and reduces severe malaria. *Nature* (2020) 582:104–8. doi: 10.1038/s41586-020-2220-1
31. Park S, Nixon CE, Pond-Tor S, Kabyemela ER, Fried M, Duffy PE, et al. Impact of maternally derived antibodies to Plasmodium falciparum Schizont Egress Antigen-1 on the endogenous production of anti-PfSEA-1 in offspring. *Vaccine* (2019) 37:5044–50. doi: 10.1016/j.vaccine.2019.06.084
32. Muehlenbachs A, Fried M, Lachowitzer J, Mutabingwa TK, Duffy PE. Natural selection of FLT1 alleles and their association with malaria resistance in utero. *Proc Natl Acad Sci USA* (2008) 105:14488–91. doi: 10.1073/pnas.0803657105
33. Kurtis JD, Raj DK, Michelow IC, Park S, Nixon CE, McDonald EA, et al. : Maternally-derived Antibodies to Schizont Egress Antigen-1 and Protection of Infants From Severe Malaria. *Clin Infect Dis* (2019) 68:1718–24. doi: 10.1093/cid/ciy728
34. Kabyemela ER, Muehlenbachs A, Fried M, Kurtis JD, Mutabingwa TK, Duffy PE. Maternal peripheral blood level of IL-10 as a marker for inflammatory placental malaria. *Malar J* (2008) 7:26. doi: 10.1186/1475-2875-7-26
35. Kabyemela ER, Fried M, Kurtis JD, Mutabingwa TK, Duffy PE. Decreased susceptibility to Plasmodium falciparum infection in pregnant women with iron deficiency. *J Infect Dis* (2008) 198:163–6. doi: 10.1086/589512
36. Gwamaka M, Fried M, Domingo G, Duffy PE. Early and extensive CD55 loss from red blood cells supports a causal role in malarial anaemia. *Malar J* (2011) 10:386. doi: 10.1186/1475-2875-10-386
37. Goncalves BP, Fried M, Duffy PE. Parasite burden and severity of malaria in Tanzanian children. *N Engl J Med* (2014) 371:482. doi: 10.1056/NEJMc1407114
38. Brickley EB, Kabyemela E, Kurtis JD, Fried M, Wood AM, Duffy PE. Developing a novel risk prediction model for severe malarial anemia. *Glob Health Epidemiol Genom* (2017) 2:e14. doi: 10.1017/gheg.2017.8
39. Leenstra T, Coutinho HM, Acosta LP, Langdon GC, Su L, Olveda RM, et al. Schistosoma japonicum reinfection after praziquantel treatment causes anemia associated with inflammation. *Infect Immun* (2006) 74:6398–407. doi: 10.1128/IAI.00757-06
40. Corchia C, Balata A, Meloni GF, Meloni T. Favism in a female newborn infant whose mother ingested fava beans before delivery. *J Pediatr* (1995) 127:807–8. doi: 10.1016/S0022-3476(95)70178-8
41. Chong SS, Boehm CD, Higgs DR, Cutting GR. Single-tube multiplex-PCR screen for common deletional determinants of alpha-thalassemia. *Blood* (2000) 95:360–2. doi: 10.1182/blood.V95.1.360
42. Muehlenbachs A, Fried M, McGready R, Harrington WE, Mutabingwa TK, Nosten F, et al. A novel histological grading scheme for placental malaria applied in areas of high and low malaria transmission. *J Infect Dis* (2010) 202:1608–16. doi: 10.1086/656723
43. Fried M, Nosten F, Brockman A, Brabin BJ, Duffy PE. Maternal antibodies block malaria. *Nature* (1998) 395:851–2. doi: 10.1038/27570
44. Muriuki JM, Mentzer AJ, Mitchell R, Webb EL, Etyang AO, Kyobutungi C, et al. : Malaria is a cause of iron deficiency in African children. *Nat Med* (2021). doi: 10.1038/s41591-021-01238-4
45. Gambling L, Danzeisen R, Gair S, Lea RG, Charania Z, Solanky N, et al. Effect of iron deficiency on placental transfer of iron and expression of iron transport proteins in vivo and in vitro. *Biochem J* (2001) 356:883–9. doi: 10.1042/bj3560883
46. Sangkhae V, Fisher AL, Wong S, Koenig MD, Tussing-Humphreys L, Chu A, et al. Effects of maternal iron status on placental and fetal iron homeostasis. *J Clin Invest* (2020) 130:625–40. doi: 10.1172/JCI127341
47. Kabyemela ER, Fried M, Kurtis JD, Mutabingwa TK, Duffy PE. Fetal responses during placental malaria modify the risk of low birth weight. *Infect Immun* (2008) 76:1527–34. doi: 10.1128/IAI.00964-07
48. Nemeth E, Rivera S, Gabayan V, Keller C, Taudorf S, Pedersen BK, et al. IL-6 mediates hypoferremia of inflammation by inducing the synthesis of the iron regulatory hormone hepcidin. *J Clin Invest* (2004) 113:1271–6. doi: 10.1172/JCI200420945

49. Mockenhaupt FP, Falusi AG, May J, Ademowo OG, Olumese PE, Meyer CG, et al. The contribution of alpha+-thalassaemia to anaemia in a Nigerian population exposed to intense malaria transmission. *Trop Med Int Health* (1999) 4:302–7. doi: 10.1046/j.1365-3156.1999.00386.x
50. Vaisbuch E, Romero R, Gomez R, Kusanovic JP, Mazaki-Tovi S, Chaiworapongsa T, et al. An elevated fetal interleukin-6 concentration can be observed in fetuses with anemia due to Rh alloimmunization: implications for the understanding of the fetal inflammatory response syndrome. *J Matern Fetal Neonatal Med* (2011) 24:391–6. doi: 10.3109/14767058.2010.507294
51. Kohgo Y, Nishisato T, Kondo H, Tsushima N, Niitsu Y, Urushizaki I. Circulating transferrin receptor in human serum. *Br J Haematol* (1986) 64:277–81. doi: 10.1111/j.1365-2141.1986.tb04120.x
52. Mickleson KN, Dixon MW, Hill PJ, Bluck R, Eales M, Rutherford J, et al. Influence of alpha thalassaemia on haematological parameters in Polynesian patients. *N Z Med J* (1985) 98:1036–8.
53. Beguin Y, Huebers HA, Josephson B, Finch CA. Transferrin receptors in rat plasma. *Proc Natl Acad Sci USA* (1988) 85:637–40. doi: 10.1073/pnas.85.2.637
54. Rees DC, Williams TN, Maitland K, Clegg JB, Weatherall DJ. Alpha thalassaemia is associated with increased soluble transferrin receptor levels. *Br J Haematol* (1998) 103:365–9. doi: 10.1046/j.1365-2141.1998.00971.x
55. Ostlund E, Lindholm H, Hemsen A, Fried G. Fetal erythropoietin and endothelin-1: relation to hypoxia and intrauterine growth retardation. *Acta Obstet Gynecol Scand* (2000) 79:276–82. doi: 10.1080/j.1600-0412.2000.079004276.x
56. Schneider H, Malek A. Lack of permeability of the human placenta for erythropoietin. *J Perinat Med* (1995) 23:71–6. doi: 10.1515/jpme.1995.23.1-2.71
57. Conrad KP, Benyo DF, Westerhausen-Larsen A, Miles TM. Expression of erythropoietin by the human placenta. *FASEB J* (1996) 10:760–8. doi: 10.1096/fasebj.10.7.8635693
58. Caro J, Erslev AJ, Silver R, Miller O, Birgegard G. Erythropoietin production in response to anemia or hypoxia in the newborn rat. *Blood* (1982) 60:984–8. doi: 10.1182/blood.V60.4.984.bloodjournal604984
59. Faquin WC, Schneider TJ, Goldberg MA. Effect of inflammatory cytokines on hypoxia-induced erythropoietin production. *Blood* (1992) 79:1987–94. doi: 10.1182/blood.V79.8.1987.bloodjournal7981987

6

The Potential Contribution of ABO, Lewis and Secretor Histo-Blood Group Carbohydrates in Infection by *Toxoplasma gondii*

Luiz Carlos De Mattos [1*†], *Ana Iara Costa Ferreira* [1†], *Karina Younan de Oliveira* [1], *Fabiana Nakashima* [1†] *and Cinara Cássia Brandão* [1,2†]

[1] *Immunogenetics Laboratory, Molecular Biology Department, Faculty of Medicine – FAMERP, São José do Rio Preto, Brazil,*
[2] *FAMERP Toxoplasma Research Group, Molecular Biology Department, Faculty of Medicine – FAMERP, São José do Rio Preto, Brazil*

Correspondence:
Luiz Carlos De Mattos
luiz.demattos@edu.famerp.br

The glycosyltransferases encoded by genes from the human ABO, Lewis, and Secretor histo-blood group systems synthesize part of the carbohydrate antigens in hematopoietic and non-hematopoietic tissues. The combined action of these glycosyltransferases strongly influences cell, tissue, mucosa, and exocrine secretion carbohydrate phenotypes, including those serving as habitat for mutualistic and pathogenic microorganisms. A set of reports investigated associations between *Toxoplasma gondii* infection and the ABO histo-blood group system, but the results are contradictory. As *T. gondii* uses the gastrointestinal tract as a route for infection, and in this organ, the expression of ABO, Lewis, and Secretor histo-blood group carbohydrates occurs, it is reasonable to suppose some biological relationship between them. This text reviewed association studies published in recent decades focusing on the potential contribution of the ABO, Lewis, and Secretor histo-blood group carbohydrates and infection by *T. gondii*.

Keywords: histo-blood group systems, carbohydrates, secretor, lewis phenotype, secretor phenotype, ABO blood group, *Toxoplasma gondii*

INTRODUCTION

Toxoplasma gondii, the etiologic agent of toxoplasmosis, was first identified in 1908 by Alphonso Splendore, in São Paulo, Brazil, in tissues of a rabbit, and by Nicolle and Manceaux in Tunisia, North Africa, in the tissues of a rodent *Ctenodoactylus gundi* (Ferguson, 2009; Innes, 2010). According to the current taxonomic classification, this parasite belongs to the Phylum Apicomplexa, which contains other pathogens such as *Plasmodium, Theileria, Eimeria, Neospora, Cryptosporidium*, and *Babesia* species (Arisue and Hashimoto, 2015).

T. gondii presents a heteroxenous life cycle, with felines being the definitive hosts. All warm-blooded animals, including humans, are intermediate hosts. The life cycle of *T. gondii* has three different developmental stages. Tachyzoites, the free form found in the peripheral blood during the acute phase of infection, can cross the placenta, reaching the fetus during pregnancy, allowing congenital toxoplasmosis. Bradyzoites, which form tissue cysts and remain in the latent stage, can infect humans by raw or undercooked meat consumption. Oocysts, shed in the feline's feces, constitute the environmentally resistant stage of *T. gondii* and can infect humans by ingesting contaminated water and vegetables (Dubey, 2009).

T. gondii is a cosmopolitan obligatory intracellular parasite that infects all nucleated cells from warm-blooded animals (Furtado et al., 2011; Subauste et al., 2011). It presents tropism for some human organs and tissues such as the brain, choroid, retina, as well as placenta (Dadimoghaddam et al., 2014). Depending on the site of infection, different clinical forms of toxoplasmosis, such as neuro-toxoplasmosis and neurological disorders (McConkey et al., 2013), ocular toxoplasmosis (Ferreira et al., 2014), and congenital toxoplasmosis, arise (Chung et al., 2018). Some other clinical manifestations of this disease have been reported but seem uncommon (Saxena et al., 2018). These clinical entities place *T. gondii* and toxoplasmosis in a prominent position in contemporary medicine (Furtado et al., 2011; Subauste et al., 2011).

The global serological prevalence of infection by *T. gondii* is high, affecting about one-third of the world's population (Pappas et al., 2009; Foroutan-Rad et al., 2016). However, the rates vary according to the region and the habits of the population. South American countries such as Brazil present infection rates above 60% (Dubey et al., 2012), while some Asian countries such as Taiwan have less than 10% (Chiang et al., 2012). Socioeconomic conditions such as illiteracy, low family income, and unemployment influence high infection rates (Meier et al., 2016; Mareze et al., 2019).

Different routes contribute to the transmission of *T. gondii* to humans. Although congenital transmission is an essential route of dissemination to fetuses and newborns, the infection acquired after birth can be due to different factors, including the consumption of raw or undercooked meat, the ingestion of contaminated vegetables and water, as well as contact with soil and cat feces (Furtado et al., 2011; Dubey et al., 2012; Ferreira et al., 2014). Transfusion of blood components and organ and tissue transplantation is also among the potential transmission routes (Foroutan-Rad et al., 2016; Dard et al., 2018).

Laboratory diagnosis of toxoplasmosis is essentially serological, but a set of molecular methods detect *T. gondii* genomic DNA in different biological samples (Liu et al., 2015; Dard et al., 2016). Serology detecting IgM and IgG anti-*T. gondii* antibodies and PCR (conventional PCR, Nested PCR, Real-Time PCR) are standard methods in determining acute and chronic infection (Okay et al., 2009; Saki et al., 2019; Murata et al., 2020).

T. gondii infection and the different clinical forms of toxoplasmosis have gained importance as public health issues. The risks that this parasite present to humans is considerable, especially to HIV-AIDS patients (Laboudi, 2017), cancer patients (Anvari et al., 2019), organ recipients (Robert-Gangneux et al., 2018), pregnant women, fetuses, and neonates (Chung et al., 2018). Therefore, understanding the different aspects of *T. gondii* infection contributes to better understanding the epidemiology of toxoplasmosis.

The susceptibility to *T. gondii* infection is heterogeneous and depends on parasite strains, environmental factors, and genetic traits of the human hosts. A set of human host genetic factors related to the acquisition risk of infection by *T. gondii* in diseased and healthy individuals is available in the literature. Polymorphisms of cell receptors such as Toll-Like Receptors (TLR-2: 2258G>A; TLR-4: 896A>G and 1196C>T, TLR-9: 2848G>A) (Wujcicka et al., 2017) and coreceptors (CCR5: 59029 AA or AG genotypes) (De Faria Junior et al., 2018) were associated with increased susceptibility. Genes and alleles controlling the immune response such as MICA and their HLA ligands (MICA-HLA: MICA*002~HLA-B*35), and KIR (KIR: KIR3DS1-Bw4-80Ile; KIR2DS1^{+}/C2^{++} KIR3DS1^{+}/Bw4-80Ile^{+}) increase the risk of infection (Ayo et al., 2015; Ayo et al., 2016). High levels of the cytokines IL-6, IL-10, IL-12 and TNF-α were associated with increased susceptibility to infection and development of different clinical forms of toxoplasmosis (Maia et al., 2017).

A set of host risk factors are known (Pinto-Ferreira et al., 2019), but others need to be investigated further. This text discusses the potential contribution of histo-blood group carbohydrates from ABO, Lewis, and Secretor systems in infection by *T. gondii*. The carbohydrate profiles of these genetic systems have high diversity in the gastrointestinal tract (Henry, 2001), a site used by *T. gondii* as a route to infect humans (Dubey, 2009). These two independent events occur in the same organ, and it is reasonable to suppose that there is some biological relationship between them.

Human ABO, Lewis and Secretor Histo-Blood Group Carbohydrates

The name human histo-blood systems bring together genetic systems whose genes control the expression of specific glycosyltransferases responsible for the biosynthesis of carbohydrate antigens in cells of the hematopoietic and non-hematopoietic tissues and exocrine secretions. The ABO, Lewis, and Secretor systems express part of the repertoire of carbohydrate antigens in the gastrointestinal tract (Henry, 2001; Nydegger et al., 2005). The glycosyltransferases encoded by FUT2 (Secretor), FUT3 (Lewis), and ABO (GTA, GTB) interact in the biosynthesis of ABO and Lewis carbohydrate antigens by adding specific monosaccharides to precursor oligosaccharides, creating new carbohydrate antigens. Specific polyclonal and monoclonal antibodies and some lectins recognize these carbohydrate antigens allowing the serological characterization of ABO and Lewis phenotypes in red blood cells, tissue phenotypes, and salivary Secretor and Nonsecretor phenotypes (Schenkel-Brunner, 2000; Imberty et al., 2003). The transfusion procedures and tissue and organ transplantation require the correct identification of the four main ABO phenotypes to match recipients and blood donors and recipients and organ donors (Edinur et al., 2015).

The frequencies of ABO, Lewis, and Secretor phenotypes are well established in all human populations, but variations in the rates occur worldwide (Daniels, 2013). The translational applications of these histo-blood group systems are under investigation, offering opportunities to develop new technologies, personalized medicine, and improve public health (Korchagina and Henry, 2015; Dotz and Wuhrer, 2016; Ryzhov et al., 2016). For example, the influence of the histo-blood group carbohydrates in the susceptibility to infection and immunity (Cooling, 2015; Brandão de Mattos and de Mattos, 2017; Stowell and Stowell, 2019a), in thrombosis, cardiovascular diseases, and metabolism (Stowell and Stowell, 2019b) as well as developing enteric virus vaccines (Ramani and Giri, 2019), are of importance in public health.

The histo-blood group carbohydrate antigens synthesized by ABO, Lewis, and Secretor glycosyltransferases are involved in the glycosylation of proteins and lipids in eukaryotic cells (Corfield, 2017; Brandão de Mattos et al., 2019). Six types of monosaccharides constitute the structure of histo-blood carbohydrates: β-D-Glucose (Glc), β-D-N-Acetylglucosamine (GlcNAc), β-D-Galactose (Gal), β-D-N-Acetylgalactosamine (GalNAc), α-Fucose (Fuc) and D-Mannose (Man). Some of them are the immunodominant sugars that define the antigenic epitopes recognized by polyclonal and monoclonal antibodies and lectins in serological phenotyping. GalNAc defines the A antigen, whereas Gal defines the B antigen in the ABO histo-blood group system. The Fuc defines the H, Le^a, and Le^b antigens depending on their position in the precursor oligosaccharide chains (Gilliver and Henry, 2003).

Different precursor oligosaccharides serve as the substrate for the histo-blood group glycosyltransferase. The addition of the above monosaccharides to each precursor oligosaccharide by the ABO, Lewis, and Secretor glycosyltransferases gives rise to different carbohydrate antigens, which may differ in the spatial conformation and affinity to monoclonal antibodies (Imberty et al., 2003; De Mattos, 2016). Data from ABO, Lewis, and Secretor histo-blood group systems are present in **Table 1**. For more details of biochemical and structural characteristics of histo-blood group carbohydrates, readers should refer to Schenkel-Brunner (2000) and De Mattos (2016).

The biosynthesis of histo-blood group carbohydrates in the gastrointestinal tract and exocrine secretions is a complex biological process. Depending on the presence, absence or combination of ABO, Lewis, and Secretor glycosyltransferases, variable levels of histo-blood group carbohydrate will be synthesized at the gastrointestinal tract and in the exocrine secretions. For example, the FUTII glycosyltransferase synthesizes the H carbohydrate antigen, the primary substrate for GTA, GTB, and FUTIII glycosyltransferases synthesize new carbohydrate antigens. Since Secretors carry a functional FUTII glycosyltransferase synthesizing H carbohydrate antigen, they can express high variability of histo-blood group carbohydrates compared to Nonsecretor, which has no functional FUTII glycosyltransferase (Henry et al., 1995; Imberty et al., 2003). **Table 2** shows the relative quantities of histo-blood group carbohydrates expressed in the exocrine secretions and mucosal tissues according to the combination of the ABO, Lewis and Secretor functional glycosyltransferases, as proposed by Perry and colleagues (Perry et al., 2007).

ABO and Lewis red blood cell phenotyping predict part of the carbohydrate profile expressed in the gastrointestinal tract. However, a combination of serological, histological analysis such as immunohistochemistry and molecular methods are required to determine the correct tissue phenotypes and the level of expression of histo-blood group carbohydrates (Henry et al., 1994; Henry, 2001). Determining the correct histo-blood group carbohydrate profile is crucial to establish correct associations with infections and diseases (Henry et al., 1995). These approaches were critical in studies investigating the human gastrointestinal pathogen *Helicobacter pylori*, which is able to bind the histo-blood group carbohydrate Lewis b (Le^b) expressed in the stomach mucosae (Borén et al., 1993; Martins et al., 2006).

Associations Between *T. gondii* Infection and ABO, Lewis, and Secretor Histo-Blood Groups

The histo-blood group carbohydrates and *T. gondii* infection studies mostly focused on of associations enrolling seropositive patients and seronegative controls. Some reported statistically significant differences favoring one or more ABO phenotypes, while others did not find these differences. The majority of the studies examined only the ABO system and neglected the Secretor and Lewis histo-blood groups.

Positive and negative associations have been reported in the literature in the last three decades. A study carried out in Norway enrolling volunteers from different areas found a high proportion of anti-*T. gondii* antibodies in B (28.8%) and AB (18.0%) phenotypes (Midtvedt and Vaage, 1989). These frequencies were higher than those from the general population (9.1% and 3.4%, respectively). These authors proposed that the B histo-blood group carbohydrate, which contains two galactose units in its terminal structure, might be an important receptor for *T. gondii* in the gastrointestinal tract.

Subsequent reports were published confirming the observations from the study from Norway. In one of them, the authors found IgG anti-*T. gondii* antibodies in 75% of Cuban blood donors from AB histo-blood phenotype, a rate elevated compared to the general population (3.6%) (Lópes et al., 1993).

TABLE 1 | ABO, Lewis, and Secretor histo-blood group systems data. Modified from De Mattos (2016).

Systems	HGNC[1]	ISBT[2]	Chromosomes	Glycosyltransferase (Abbreviations)	IUBMB[3] Code	Immunodominant sugar	Antigens
Secretor	*FUT2*	SE	19q13.3	α1,2-Fucosyltransferase (FUTII)	EC 2.4.1.69	Fuc	H type 1
Lewis	*FUT3*	LE	19p13.3	α1,3/4-Fucosyltransferase (FUTIII)	EC 2.4.1.65	Fuc, GalNAc, Gal	Le^a, Le^b, ALe^b, BLe^b
ABO	*ABO*	ABO	9q.34.1	α1,3-N-Acetylgalactosaminyltransferase (GTA)	EC 2.4.1.40	GalNAc	A type 1, A type 2
				α1,3-N-Galactosyltransferase (GTB)	EC 2.4.1.37	Gal	B type 1, B type 2

[1]HGNC, Human Genome Nomenclature Committee; [2]ISBT, International Society for Blood Transfusion; [3]International Union of Biochemistry and Molecular Biology.

TABLE 2 | The relative level of histo-blood group carbohydrates expressed in tissues and exocrine secretions according to the combination of histo-blood group glycosyltransferases. Modified from Perry et al., 2007.

Systems	Glycosyltransferases	OP type 1	H	Le^a	Le^b	A type 1	B type 1	ALe^b	BLe^b	RBC phenotypes
ABO, Lewis, Secretor	FUTII + FUTIII + GTA	(+)	(+)	+	+++	+++	0	++++	0	A Le(a-b+)
ABO, Lewis, Secretor	FUTII + FUTIII + GTB	(+)	(+)	+	+++	+++	++	0	++++	B Le(a-b+)
ABO, Lewis, Secretor	FUTII + FUTIII + GTA + GTB	(+)	(+)	+	+++	+++	++	++++	++++	AB Le(a-b+)
ABO, Lewis, Secretor	FUTII + FUTIII	(+)	(+)	+	+++++					O Le(a-b+)
ABO, Lewis, Secretor	FUTII + GTA	+	++			+++++				A Le(a-b-)
ABO, Lewis, Secretor	FUTII + GTB	+	++				+++++			B Le(a-b-)
ABO, Lewis, Secretor	FUTII + GTA + GTB	+	++			+++++	+++++			AB Le(a-b-)
ABO, Lewis, Secretor	FUTII	+	+++++							O Le(a-b-)
ABO, Lewis, Non-Secretor	FUTIII + GTA	+		+++++						A Le(a+b-)
ABO, Lewis, Non-Secretor	FUTIII + GTB	+		+++++						B Le(a+b-)
ABO, Lewis, Non-Secretor	FUTIII + GTA + GTB	+		+++++						AB Le(a+b-)
ABO, Lewis, Non-Secretor	FUTIII	+		+++++						O Le(a+b-)

OP, Oligosaccharide precursor; RBC, Red blood cell; (+): Very low expression; +, ++: Low expression; +++, ++++ Moderate expression; +++++: High expression.

Another study from Russia reported that 54% of the blood donors having anti-*T. gondii* antibodies were from the AB histo-blood group phenotype, and 27% were from the O histo-blood group phenotype (Zhiburt et al., 1997). Two other studies in the Czech Republic enrolling military personnel and in the Philippines enrolling individuals from urban and suburban areas also found an association between IgG anti-*T. gondii* antibodies with B and AB histo-blood group phenotypes (Kolbekova et al., 2007; Salibay et al., 2008). The data from these studies align with experimental observations showing galactose as an important monosaccharide in the interactions between humans and *T. gondii*. Galactose is a common component of many oligosaccharides involved in the glycosylation of proteins and lipids, but its presence is not exclusive to the B histo-blood group carbohydrate structure (Coelho et al., 2015).

Reports of no association between infection by *T. gondii* and ABO histo-blood group system are found in the literature. In Tanzania, Africa, statistically significant differences were not found in ABO phenotypes frequencies and anti-*T. gondii* antibodies in blood donors (Gill, 1985). Another study enrolling 4,000 pregnant French women found no differences in the frequencies of the ABO phenotypes in those seropositive and seronegative (Lécolier et al., 1990).

Our group carried out studies in northwestern São Paulo State, Brazil, a region with high infection rates by *T. gondii* (Gonçalves et al., 2010; Ferreira et al., 2014). In one of them, investigating only the ABO histo-blood group phenotypes, no statistically significant differences were observed in the proportions of seropositive and seronegative pregnant women (Rodrigues et al., 2011). No associations were observed in a second study, combining the ABO and Secretor histo-blood group phenotypes (Brandão de Mattos et al., 2008). This study considered that the expression of ABO histo-blood group carbohydrates in the gastrointestinal tract is under control of the FUT2 gene. In another one, we investigated the profile of histo-blood group carbohydrates resulting from the integrated action of the glycosyltransferases encoded by *FUT2*, *FUT3*, and *ABO* genes (Nakashima et al., 2019). This study showed that the Leb carbohydrate confers some protection against infection by *T. gondii*. We recently investigated only the ABO histo-blood group phenotypes in a series of 1,730 blood donors, and no evidence of an association between seropositivity and the ABO phenotypes was found (Unpublished). In the light of these observations, the biological role of ABO, Lewis, and Secretor histo-blood group carbohydrates in the infection by *T. gondii* remains unsolved and requires new strategies for investigations. **Table 3** shows the data of positive and negative associations between ABO, Lewis, and Secretor histo-blood group carbohydrates and infection by *T. gondii*.

Experimental Demonstrations That *Toxoplasma gondii* Binds Carbohydrates

The investigation of potential biological relationships between the infection by *T. gondii* and the ABO, H, Lewis, and Secretor histo-blood group carbohydrates is attractive. A set of experiments carried out *in vitro* demonstrated that these histo-blood group carbohydrates act as receptors favoring the attachment of microorganisms at the gastrointestinal mucosae such as *Helicobacter pylori* (Borén et al., 1993), *Candida albicans* (Cameron and Douglas, 1996), Rotavirus (Sun et al., 2018), and Norovirus (Esseili et al., 2019). These microorganisms bind histo-blood group carbohydrates in a specific manner, increasing the susceptibility of individuals who express some of these oligosaccharide structures. However, *in vivo* experiments demonstrating the attachment of *T. gondii* to ABO, H, Lewis, and Secretor histo-blood group carbohydrates are scarce.

Some studies demonstrated that carbohydrates are involved in one or more steps of the cell invasion process exploited by *T. gondii*. One of them investigated the ultrastructural localization of carbohydrate residues and sugar-binding sites in the rhoptries from *T. gondii* tachyzoites (De Carvalho et al., 1991). Their results suggested that these sugar-binding sites play an essential role during the process of *T. gondii*-host cell interaction. Another one demonstrated that *T. gondii* micronemal protein MIC1, one of the first proteins released in the cell invasion process, is a critical lactose-binding lectin (Lourenço et al., 2001). *T. gondii* induces conformational changes in the microneme complex TgMIC4. This complex can bind various galactose-containing carbohydrates (Marchant et al., 2012; Santos et al., 2015). Chinese hamster ovary

TABLE 3 | Studies of the association between ABO, H, Lewis, and Secretor histo-blood group carbohydrates and infection by *Toxoplasma gondii* and toxoplasmosis.

Place/ Positive	Source	N	Seropositivity		Methods	HBG systems	Association	Phenotypes	Effects	References
			n	%						
Tanzania	Blood donors	208	79	38.0	IHA*	ABO	No	–	–	Gill, 1985
Norway	Volunteers	1,788	395	22.1	TcT€	ABO	Yes	B and AB	Susceptibility	Midtvedt & Vaage, 1989
France	Pregnant (MR)	4,000	3,127	78.0	NR#	ABO	No	–	–	Lécolier et al., 1990
Russia	Patients	38	15	39.5	NR#	ABO	Yes	A	Susceptibility	Teplinskaia & Kaliberdina, 1992
Cuba	Blood donors	1,036	684	66.0	IgG ELISA	ABO	Yes	AB	Susceptibility	López et al., 1993
Russia	Blood donors	323	NR	NR	NR	ABO	Yes	B and AB	Susceptibility	Zhiburt et al., 1997
Czech Republic	Military	3,250	748	23.0	IgM, IgG ELISA CFT&	ABO	Yes	B and AB	Susceptibility	Kolbekova et al., 2007
Philippines	Urban, suburban residents	140	38	27.1	LAT¥	ABO	Yes	B	Susceptibility	Salibay et al., 2008
Brazil	Pregnant women	367	182	49.6	IHA*	ABO, Secretor	No	–	–	Brandão de Mattos et al., 2008
Egypt	Blood donors	260	155	59.6	IgG ELISA	ABO	Yes	O	Susceptibility	Elsheikha et al., 2009
Brazil	Pregnant women (MR)	1006	645	64.1	IgM, IgG ELISA	ABO	No	–	–	Rodrigues et al., 2011
Taiwan	Blood donors	1,783	166	9.3	IgM, IgG ELISA	ABO	No	–	–	Chiang et al., 2012
Czech Republic	Military	491	154	31.4	IgM, IgG ELISA	ABO	No	–	–	Flegr et al., 2013
Iraq	Blood donors	400	131	32.7	IgM, IgG ELISA	ABO	Yes	AB	Susceptibility	Mahmood et al., 2013
			136	34.0	LAT					
Iran	Blood donors	1,480	286	19.3	IgM, IgG ELISA	ABO	No	–	–	Sarkari et al., 2014
Iran	Blood products	250	59	23.6	IgM, IgG ELISA	ABO	Yes	B, AB	Susceptibility	Shaddel et al., 2014
Iran	Blood donors	375	94	25.0	IgM, IgG ELISA	ABO	No	–	–	Modrek et al., 2014
Iran	Blood donors	500	160	32.0	IgM, IgG ELISA	ABO	Yes	B	Susceptibility	Mahmoudvand et al., 2015
Côte d'Ivoire	Blood donors	106	68	64.1	IgM, IgG ELISA	ABO	No	–	–	Siransy et al., 2016
Iran	Blood donors	491	200	40.7	IgM, IgG ELISA	ABO	No	–	–	Sadooghian et al., 2017
Iran	Blood donors	285	48	16.8	IgM, IgG ELISA	ABO	No	–	–	Moshfe et al., 2018
Iraq	Miscarriage	200	67	33.5	IgM LAT, ELISA	ABO	No	–	–	Smael et al., 2018
Egypt	Blood donors	276	150	54.3	IgM, IgG ELISA	ABO	No	–	–	Abd El Wahab et al., 2018
Brazil	Pregnant women	244	158	64.7	IgM, IgG ELISA	ABO, Lewis, Secretor	Yes	Le(a-b+)	Resistance	Nakashima et al., 2019
Brazil	Blood donors	1,730	835	48.3	IgM, IgG ELISA	ABO	No	–	–	Nakashima et al. (Unpublished data)

**IHA, Indirect Hemagglutination; €TcT, Toxoplasmin Cutaneous Test; &CFT, Complement Fixation Test; ¥LAT, Latex Agglutination Test; #Non Referred; MD, Data from Medical Records.*

cells deficient in sialic acid, a widely distributed monosaccharide on the cell surface of all vertebrates, are resistant to infection by *T. gondii* (Monteiro et al., 1998). These authors proposed that sialic acid is a critical monosaccharide for cell attachment and invasion of *T. gondii.* A recent paper supports their data that *T. gondii* uses the sialic acid-binding protein-1 localized on its outer membrane to bind sialic acid for host cell attachment and invasion (Xing et al., 2020). These reports reinforce the potential role of the host's oligosaccharides in the host-*T. gondii* interactions.

Oligosaccharide chains containing galactose in the inner structure and the terminal monosaccharide are the precursors for ABO, Lewis, and Secretor histo-blood group carbohydrates expressed in the gastrointestinal tract (De Mattos, 2016). The combined action of the glycosyltransferases encoded by the *ABO*, *FUT1*, *FUT2*, and *FUT3* genes in the gastrointestinal tract create a carbohydrate repertoire that acts as receptors containing galactose that modify the susceptibility or resistance to pathogens (Henry, 2001). It is reasonable to speculate the potential contribution of the repertoire of histo-blood group carbohydrates as a host's risk factors for infection by *T. gondii.* However, experiments demonstrating that *T. gondii* tachyzoites or oocysts bind specific histo-blood group carbohydrates are required.

The Significance of Positive and Negative Associations Between ABO, Lewis and Secretor Histo-Blood Group Systems and *T. gondii* Infection

In the general context, studying associations between biomarkers and infectious diseases is a good starting point to understand the epidemiology and pathophysiology of a disease. Carrying out experimental demonstrations resolving the contribution of a genetic trait in the susceptibility or resistance to disease reinforces the importance of association studies, providing a background concerning the contributions of biomarkers in disease screening, diagnosis, prognosis, and therapy (Timpson et al., 2018). The reported associations between ABO, Lewis, and Secretor histo-blood group systems and susceptibility to infection by pathogenic microorganisms are crucial to initiate experimental investigations aiming to demonstrate the contribution of the histo-blood group carbohydrates as receptors for pathogens (Cooling, 2015; Stowell and Stowell, 2019a).

In this scenario, experimental demonstrations that histo-blood group carbohydrates can act as receptors or coreceptors for *T. gondii* in the gastrointestinal tract would allow translational applications in areas with a high prevalence of this parasite. Maybe these carbohydrates could be helpful to estimate the risk for the different clinical forms, disease progression, and personalized treatment, and prevention of toxoplasmosis, especially in contemporary personalized medicine.

Without experimental demonstrations, the associations between the ABO, Lewis, and Secretor histo-blood group systems and infection by *T. gondii* weaken. The studies investigating only the ABO red blood cell phenotypes require at least two considerations. Firstly, *T. gondii* does not use erythrocytes as a host cell but infects nucleated cells. Secondly, the ABO tissue phenotypes result from the action of FUTI, FUTII, FUTIII, GTA and GTB glycosyltransferases (Henry and Samuelsson, 2000). The presence, absence, or combination of these glycosyltransferases affects the tissue carbohydrate profiles, varying according to ethnicity (Henry, 2001). Genetic events such as single nucleotide polymorphisms, deletions, insertions, and recombinations might affect the efficiency of the encoded glycosyltransferases, adding complexities to the carbohydrate profiles (De Mattos, 2016). This set of events can misinterpret the associations between the infection by *T. gondii* and ABO, Lewis and Secretor histo-blood group systems.

The contradictory data that emerged from the studies enlisted in **Table 3** might be due to different reasons. Individuals such as pregnant women, volunteers, military personnel, urban and suburban area residents, and blood donors were enrolled. The number of individuals in each study varies from a few tens to thousands, and the inclusion and exclusion criteria are not clear. Furthermore, the detection of anti-*T. gondii* antibodies did not follow standard laboratory tests. This heterogeneity creates contradictory results and weakens the comparisons among them.

From 25 studies in **Table 3**, eighteen used the ELISA method to identify IgM and IgG anti-*T. gondii* antibodies. ELISA is an excellent method to detect antigens and antibodies in infectious diseases due to its excellent sensitivity and specificity. Besides being cheaper, it indicates the serological immune status of the infected and noninfected individual at low costs (Shah and Maghsoudlou, 2016). However, limitations of serological tests such as ELISA to detect anti-*T. gondii* antibodies may also be related to different antigens (native versus recombinant) present in the commercial kits (Zhang et al., 2017). Some studies have shown that some commercial kits failed to detect low levels of IgG anti-*T. gondii* (Douet et al., 2019).

Considering that *T. gondii* has high genetic variability from one region to another, recombinant antigens present in commercial kits can vary among manufacturers affecting their sensitivity and specificity. Commercial kits manufactured with different recombinant antigens may fail to detect some *T. gondii* strains, especially in South American countries, due to the diversity of strains (Arranz-Solís et al., 2019). These differences might produce false-positive or false-negative results and fail to identify individuals with a reagent and non-reagent serology (Wilson et al., 1997). These characteristics might contribute to the contradictory data reported by studies associating histo-blood group carbohydrates and infection by *T. gondii*.

The amount of histo-blood group carbohydrates linked to proteins and lipids varies in exocrine secretions and the blood plasma depending on epistatic interactions between histo-blood group FUTI, FUTII, FUTIII, GTA and GTB glycosyltransferases (Henry et al., 1997; Achermann et al., 2005; Cooling, 2015). A previous study reported quantities of ALe^b carbohydrate three times higher than A type 1, representing almost 3% of the neutral glycosphingolipids in the blood plasma (Lindstrom et al., 1992). One can speculate that these quantitative differences impact the susceptibility or resistance to infections by pathogens such as *T. gondii*.

Old reports showed that some human pathogens such as the juvenile forms of *Schistosoma mansoni* (Goldring et al., 1976), *Fasciola hepática* (Ben-Ismail et al., 1982) and *Toxocara canis* (Smith et al., 1983) could synthesize histo-blood group carbohydrates or adsorb them to their surface from human blood and exocrine secretions. These authors propose that adsorbing histo-blood group carbohydrates could represent a strategy of evasion from innate and adaptive immune responses giving parasites an advantage for survival in the host. Without experimental evidence showing that *T. gondii* explores these strategies in humans, the proposition made by the Norwegian group that B histo-blood group carbohydrate facilitates the infection by this parasite remains speculative.

An alternative explanation to the associations shown in **Table 3** could be related to the presence of α-Gal epitopes in *T. gondii* tachyzoites and oocysts. The α-Gal epitope (Galα1→3Galβ1→4GlcNAc-R) is an oligosaccharide synthesized by the α-1,3-Galactoyltransferase whose gene α1,3GT, was lost by humans and anthropoid primates during evolution (Galili, 1997). The α-Gal epitope is structurally related to B histo-blood group carbohydrate (Galα1→3[Fucα1→2]Galβ1→4GlcNAc-R) (Cabezas-Cruz et al., 2017). The absence of this epitope in humans coincides with their ability to produce a natural anti-α-Gal antibody such as IgG, IgM and IgA isotypes, possibly due to the stimulus given by the α-Gal epitope present in gut microorganisms (Huai et al., 2016). The production of an anti-α-Gal antibody by humans is independent of ABO, Lewis and Secretor histo-blood group systems. However, its plasma level is low in individuals from B blood group, making them more prone to infectious diseases such as malaria and tuberculosis (Cabezas-Cruz et al., 2017). This observation does not align with the infection by *T. gondii* due to the lack of α-Gal epitope in tachyzoites (Hodžić et al., 2020). Considering that the infection by *T. gondii* after birth occurs essentially by the gastrointestinal tract, studies aiming to demonstrate α-Gal epitope in this parasite would help clarify the associations with B and AB blood groups.

EXPLORING ANIMAL MODELS

Experimental animal models help understand many aspects of the pathophysiology of infectious and parasitic diseases. Although many experimental studies focus on the strategies used by *T. gondii* to invade nucleated cells (Subauste, 2012; Dunay et al., 2018), this approach exploring relationships between this parasite and histo-blood group carbohydrates are scant. These models could help understand how *T. gondii* explores histo-blood group carbohydrates as potential receptors or coreceptors and favors new strategies for managing infection, disease treatment, and prevention.

Using Rhesus monkeys as an animal model, it was possible to understand some aspects of *H. pylori* and histo-blood group carbohydrates (Lindén et al., 2008). This human pathogen uses the gastrointestinal tract as a route of infection. Primates such as Rhesus monkeys express ABO, Lewis and Secretor histo-blood group carbohydrates in the gastrointestinal tract and exocrine secretions besides red blood cells (Blancher and Socha, 1997 Therefore, they could be helpful as an animal model to experimentally verify if any particular histo-blood group carbohydrate facilitates the infection by *T. gondii* through the gastrointestinal tract. These studies could also evaluate if the predisposition to infection by *T. gondii* linked to a particular histo-blood group carbohydrate depends on age, gender, ways of transmission, and virulent and nonvirulent strains. Data arising from these animal models could offer insights for translational applications in prevention, diagnosis, and outcome of disease and treatment.

CONCLUDING REMARKS

Studies comparing the ABO, Lewis, and Secretor histo-blood group systems and infection by *T. gondii* reported contradictory results. Experimental demonstrations that galactose is involved in the cell invasion by this parasite could, per se, explain these associations. However, this monosaccharide is widespread in many human cells, tissues, and exocrine secretions as part of the glycosylation process, and it is not present only in the B histo-blood group carbohydrate. Galactose is a unit of sugar composing many of the precursor oligosaccharide substrates for the histo-blood group glycosyltransferases. Therefore, the biological role of histo-blood group carbohydrates as receptors or coreceptors to *T. gondii* remains unexplained and requires further investigations.

The histo-blood group glycosyltransferases have evolved to synthesize and diversify a portion of oligosaccharides expressed in the gastrointestinal tract. This strategy represents a crucial biological process for changing potential receptors for pathogenic microorganisms (Henry, 2001). The FUTII glycosyltransferase diversifies the carbohydrate structures and reduces the extension of histo-blood group carbohydrate chains in secretors compared to nonsecretors (Angstrom et al., 2004). Units of galactose are present in the terminal structure and inner core of histo-blood group carbohydrate antigens. Better understanding these characteristics of histo-blood group carbohydrates may improve understanding of how ABO, Lewis, and Secretor contribute to infection by *T. gondii*.

Future studies focusing on the binomial histo-blood group carbohydrates and *T. gondii* infection should address questions regarding the role of these carbohydrates in the infection and the different clinical forms of toxoplasmosis. Also, experimental tests must determine if *T. gondii* virulent and nonvirulent strains bind histo-blood carbohydrates in a specific manner. Answering these questions could offer some translational applications for susceptibility, treatment, and prevention. The investigation of these factors offers an attractive field for research to understand the contribution of histo-blood group carbohydrates in the infection by *T. gondii*.

AUTHOR CONTRIBUTIONS

LM and CB design the study and wrote the manuscript. AF, KY, and FN collected the data from the literature and drew the tables in the manuscript. All authors contributed to the article and approved the submitted version.

ACKNOWLEDGMENTS

Jim Hesson copyedited the manuscript (https://www.academicenglishsolutions.com/editing-service).

REFERENCES

1. Abd El Wahab, W. M., Shaapan, R. M., El Hafiz Hassanain, M. E. D. A., Elfadaly, H. A., and Hamdy, D. A. (2018). *Toxoplasma gondii* Infection and Associated Sociodemographic and Behavioral Risk Factors Among Blood Donors. *Asian J. Epidemiol.* 11 (2), 52–58. doi: 10.3923/aje.2018.52.58
2. Achermann, F. J., Julmy, F., Gilliver, L. G., Carrel, T. P., and Nydegger, U. E. (2005). Soluble Type A Substance in Fresh-Frozen Plasma as a Function of ABO and Secretor Genotypes and Lewis Phenotype. *Transfus. Apher. Sci.* 32, 255–262. doi: 10.1016/j.transci.2004.05.007
3. Angstrom, J., Larsson, T., Hansson, G. C., Karlsson, K., and Henry, S. (2004). Default Biosynthesis Pathway for Blood Group-Related Glycolipids in Human Small Intestine as Defined by Structural Identification of Linear and Branched Glycosilceramides in a Group O Le(a–B–) Nonsecretor. *Glycobiology* 14, 1–12. doi: 10.1093/glycob/cwh003
4. Anvari, D., Sharif, M., Sarvi, S., Aghayan, S. A., Gholami, S., Pagheh, A. S., et al. (2019). Seroprevalence of *Toxoplasma gondii* Infection in Cancer Patients: A Systematic Review and Meta-Analysis. *Microb. Pathog.* 129, 30–42. doi: 10.1016/j.micpath.2019.01.040
5. Arisue, N., and Hashimoto, T. (2015). Phylogeny and Evolution of Apicoplasts and Apicomplexan Parasites. *Parasitol. Int.* 64 (3), 254–259. doi: 10.1016/ j.parint.2014.10.005
6. Arranz-Solıs, D., Cordeiro, C., Young, L. H., Darde, M. L., Commodaro, A. G., Grigg, M. E., et al. (2019). Serotyping of *Toxoplasma gondii* Infection Using Peptide Membrane Arrays. *Front. Cell. Infect. Microbiol.* 9, 408. doi: 10.3389/ fcimb.2019.00408
7. Ayo, C. M., Camargo, A. V., Frederico, F. B., Siqueira, R. C., Previato, M., Murata, F. H., et al. (2015). MHC Class I Chain-Related Gene A Polymorphisms and Linkage Disequilibrium With HLA-B and HLA-C Alleles in Ocular Toxoplasmosis. *PloS One* 10 (12), e0144534. doi: 10.1371/journal.pone.0144534
8. Ayo, C. M., Frederico, F. B., Siqueira, R. C., Brandão de Mattos, C. C., Previato, M., Barbosa, A. P., et al. (2016). Ocular Toxoplasmosis: Susceptibility in Respect to the Genes Encoding the KIR Receptors and Their HLA Class I Ligands. *Sci. Rep.* 6, 36632. doi: 10.1038/srep36632
9. Ben-Ismail, R., Mulet-Clamagirand, C., Carme, B., and Gentilini, M. (1982). Biosynthesis of A, H, and Lewis Blood Group Determinants in Fasciola Hepatica. *J. Parasitol.* 68, 402–407. doi: 10.2307/3280949
10. Blancher, A., and Socha, W. W. (1997). "The ABO, Hh and Lewis Blood Group in Humans and Nonhuman Primates", in *Molecular Biology and Evolution of Blood Group and MHC Antigens in Primates*. Eds. A. Blancher, J. Klein and W. W. Socha (Berlin: Spring Verlag), p. 30–92. doi: 10.1007/978-3-642-59086-3_3
11. Boren, T., Falk, P., Roth, K. A., Larson, G., and Normark, S. (1993). Attachment of *Helicobacter pylori* to Human Gastric Epithelium Mediated by Blood Group Antigens. *Science* 262 (5141), 1892–1895. doi: 10.1126/science.8018146
12. Brandão de Mattos, C. C., and de Mattos, L. C. (2017). Histo-Blood Group Carbohydrates as Facilitators for Infection by *Helicobacter pylori*. *Infect. Genet. Evol.* 53, 167–174. doi: 10.1016/j.meegid.2017.05.025
13. Brandão de Mattos, C. C., Cintra, J. R., Ferreira, A. I., Spegiorin, L. C., Galisteu, K. J., Machado, R. L., et al. (2008). Lack of Association Between ABO Histo-Blood Groups, Secretor and Nonsecretor Phenotypes, and Anti-*Toxoplasma gondii* Antibodies Among Pregnant Women From the Northwestern Region of São Paulo State, Brazil. *Arch. Med. Sci.* 4 (3), 254–258.
14. Brandão de Mattos, C. C., Miola, M. P., and De Mattos, L. C. (2019). Abo, H, Lewis and Secretor Histo-Blood Group-Like Carbohydrates in Pathogenic and Non- Pathogenic Invertebrates. *Clin. Microbiol. Res.* 1 (1), 2–6. doi: 10.31487/ j.CMR.2018.01.08
15. Cabezas-Cruz, A., Mateos-Hernandez, L., Alberdi, P., Villar, M., Riveau, G., Hermann, E., et al. (2017). Effect of Blood Type on Anti-Alpha-Gal Immunity and the Incidence of Infectious Diseases. *Exp. Mol. Med.* 49 (3), e301. doi: 10.1038/emm.2016.164
16. Cameron, B. J., and Douglas, L. J. (1996). Blood Group Glycolipids as Epithelial Cell Receptors for *Candida albicans*. *Infect. Immun.* 64 (3), 891–896. doi: 10.1128/iai.64.3.891-896
17. Chiang, T. Y., Hsieh, H. H., Kuo, M. C., Chiu, K. T., Lin, W. C., Fan, C. K., et al. (2012). Seroepidemiology of *Toxoplasma gondii* Infection Among Healthy Blood Donors in Taiwan. *PloS One* 7 (10), e48139. doi: 10.1371/journal.pone.0048139
18. Chung, M. H., Shin, C. O., and Lee, J. (2018). TORCH (Toxoplasmosis, Rubella, Cytomegalovirus, and Herpes Simplex Virus) Screening of Small for Gestational Age and Intrauterine Growth Restricted Neonates: Efficacy Study in a Single Institute in Korea. *Korean J. Pediatr.* 61 (4), 114–120. doi: 10.3345/kjp.2018.61.4.114
19. Coelho, A. I., Berry, G. T., and Rubio-Gozalbo, M. E. (2015). Galactose Metabolism and Health. *Curr. Opin. Clin. Nutr. Metab. Care* 18 (4), 422–427. doi: 10.1097/MCO.000000
20. Cooling, L. (2015). Blood Groups in Infection and Host Susceptibility. *Clin. Microbiol. Rev.* 28, 801–870. doi: 10.1128/CMR.00109-14
21. Corfield, A. (2017). Eukaryotic Protein Glycosylation: A Primer for Histochemists and Cell Biologists. *Histochem. Cell Biol.* 147 (2), 119–147. doi: 10.1007/ s00418-016-1526-4
22. Dadimoghaddam, Y., Daryani, A., Sharif, M., Ahmadpour, E., and Hossienikhah, Z. (2014). Tissue Tropism and Parasite Burden of *Toxoplasma gondii* RH Strain in Experimentally Infected Mice. *Asian Pac. J. Trop. Med.* 7 (7), 521–524. doi: 10.1016/S1995-7645(14)60087-0
23. Daniels, G. (2013). *Human Blood Groups: Introduction. 3rd* (Oxford, UK: Wiley- Blackwell). doi: 10.1002/9781118493595
24. Dard, C., Fricker-Hidalgo, H., Brenier-Pinchart, M. P., and Pelloux, H. (2016). Relevance of and New Developments in Serology for Toxoplasmosis. *Trends Parasitol.* 32 (6), 492–506. doi: 10.1016/j.pt.2016.04.001
25. Dard, C., Marty, P., Brenier-Pinchart, M. P., Garnaud, C., Fricker-Hidalgo, H., Pelloux, H., et al. (2018). Management of Toxoplasmosis in Transplant Recipients: An Update. *Expert Rev. Anti Infect. Ther.* 16 (6), 447–460. doi: 10.1080/14787210.2018.1483721
26. De Carvalho, L., Souto-Padron, T., and de Souza, W. (1991). Localization of Lectin-Binding Sites and Sugar-Binding Proteins in Tachyzoites of *Toxoplasma gondii*. *J. Parasitol.* 77 (1), 156–161. doi: 10.2307/3282574
27. De Faria Junior, G. M., Ayo, C. M., de Oliveira, A. P., Lopes, A. G., Frederico, F. B., Silveira-Carvalho, A. P., et al. (2018). CCR5 Chemokine Receptor Gene Polymorphisms in Ocular Toxoplasmosis. *Acta Trop.* 178, 276–280. doi: 10.1016/j.actatropica.2017.12.012
28. De Mattos, L. C. (2016). Structural Diversity and Biological Importance of ABO, H, Lewis and Secretor Histo-Blood Group Carbohydrates. *Rev. Bras. Hematol. Hemoter.* 38 (4), 331–340. doi: 10.1016/j.bjhh.2016.07.005
29. Dotz, V., and Wuhrer, M. (2016). Histo-Blood Group Glycans in the Context of Personalized Medicine. *Biochim. Biophys. Acta* 1860 (8), 1596–1607. doi: 10.1016/j.bbagen.2015.12.026
30. Douet, T., Armengol, C., Charpentier, E., Chauvin, P., Cassaing, S., Iriart, X., et al. (2019). Performance of Seven Commercial Automated Assays for the Detection of Low Levels of Anti-Toxoplasma IgG in French Immunocompromised Patients. *Parasite* 26, 51. doi: 10.1051/parasite/2019052
31. Dubey, J. P. (2009). History of the Discovery of the Life Cycle of *Toxoplasma gondii*. *Int. J. Parasitol.* 39 (8), 877–882. doi: 10.1016/j.ijpara.2009.01.005
32. Dubey, J. P., Lago, E. G., Gennari, S. M., Su, C., and Jones, J. L. (2012). Toxoplasmosis in Humans and Animals in Brazil: High Prevalence, High Burden of Disease, and Epidemiology. *Parasitology* 139 (11), 1375–1424. doi: 10.1017/S0031182012000765
33. Dunay, I. R., Gajurel, K., Dhakal, R., Liesenfeld, O., and Montoya, J. G. (2018). Treatment of Toxoplasmosis: Historical Perspective, Animal Models, and Current Clinical Practice. *Clin. Microbiol. Rev.* 31 (4), e00057–e00017. doi: 10.1128/CMR.00057-17
34. Edinur, H. A., Chambers, G. K., and Dunn, P. P. (2015). Recent Developments in Transplantation and Transfusion Medicine. *Ann. Transplant.* 20, 424–429. doi: 10.12659/AOT.894003
35. Elsheikha, H. M., Azab, M. S., Abousamra, N. K., Rahbar, M. H., Elghannam, D. M., and Raafat, D. (2009). Seroprevalence of and Risk Factors for *Toxoplasma gondii* Antibodies Among Asymptomatic Blood Donors in Egypt. *Parasitol. Res.* 104 (6), 1471–1476. doi: 10.1007/s00436-009-1350-z
36. Esseili, M. A., Gao, X., Boley, P., Hou, Y., Saif, L. J., Brewer-Jensen, P., et al. (2019). Human Norovirus Histo-Blood Group Antigen (HBGA) Binding Sites Mediate the Virus Specific Interactions With Lettuce Carbohydrates. *Viruses* 11 (9), pii: E833. doi: 10.3390/v11090833
37. Ferguson, D. J. (2009). *Toxoplasma gondii*: 1908-2008, Homage to Nicolle, Manceaux and Splendore. *Mem. Inst. Oswaldo Cruz* 104 (2), 133–148. doi: 10.1590/S0074-02762009000200003
38. Ferreira, A. I. C., De Mattos, C. B., Frederico, F. B., Meira, C. S., Almeida, G. C., Nakashima, F., et al. (2014). Risk Factors for Ocular Toxoplasmosis in Brazil. *Epidemiol. Infect.* 142 (1), 142–148. doi: 10.1017/S0950268813000526
39. Flegr, J., Preiss, M., and Klose, J. (2013). Toxoplasmosis-Associated Difference in Intelligence and Personality in Men Depends on Their Rhesus Blood Group But Not ABO Blood Group. *PloS One* 8 (4), e61272. doi: 10.1371/ journal.pone.0061272
40. Foroutan-Rad, M., Majidiani, H., Dalvand, S., Daryani, A., Kooti, W., Saki, J., et al. (2016). Toxoplasmosis in Blood Donors: A Systematic Review and Meta-Analysis. *Transfus. Med. Rev.* 30 (3), 116–122. doi: 10.1016/j.tmrv.2016.03.002
41. Furtado, J. M., Smith, J. R., Belfort, R. Jr, Gattey, D., and Winthrop, K. L. (2011). Toxoplasmosis: A Global Threat. *J. Glob. Infect. Dis.* 3 (3), 281–284. doi: 10.4103/0974-777X.83536
42. Galili, U. (1997). "The *a*-Galactoyl Epitope (Gala1!3 Galb1!4glcNAc-R)

and the Natural anti-Gal Antibody", in *Molecular Biology and Evolution of Blood Group and MHC Antigens in Primates.* Eds. A. Blancher, J. Klein and W. W. Socha (Berlin: Spring Verlag), 236–253. doi: 10.1007/978-3-642-59086-3_8

43. Gill, H. S. (1985). Occurrence of *Toxoplasma gondii* Antibodies in Tanzanian Blood Donors. *East. Afr. Med. J.* 62 (8), 585–588.
44. Gilliver, L. G., and Henry, S. M. (2003). Biochemistry of Carbohydrate Blood Group Antigens. *Immunohematology* 19 (2), 33–42. doi: 10.21307/ immunohematology-2019-472
45. Goldring, O. L., Clegg, J. A., Smithers, S. R., and Terry, R. J. (1976). Acquisition of Human Blood Group Antigens by *Schistosoma mansoni. Clin. Exp. Immunol.* 26, 181–187.
46. Gonçalves, M. A. S., de Matos, C. C. B., Spegiorin, L. C. J. F., Oliani, D. C. M. V., Oliani, A. H., and de Mattos, L. C. (2010). Seropositivity Rates for Toxoplasmosis, Rubella, Syphilis, Cytomegalovirus, Hepatitis and HIV Among Pregnant Women Receiving Care at a Public Health Service, São Paulo State, Brazil. *Braz. J. Infect. Dis.* 14 (6), 601–605. doi: 10.1590/S1413-86702010000600009
47. Henry, S. M. (2001). Molecular Diversity in the Biosynthesis of GI Tract Glycoconjugates. A Blood-Group-Related Chart of Microorganism Receptors. *Transfus. Clin. Biol.* 8 (3), 226–230. doi: 10.1016/s1246-7820(01)00112-4
48. Henry, S., Jovall, P. A., Ghardashkhani, S., Elmgren, A., Martinsson, T., Larson, G., et al. (1997). Structural and Immunochemical Identification of Le(a), Le(B), H Type 1, and Related Glycolipids in Small Intestinal Mucosa of a Group O Le(a- B-) Nonsecretor. *Glycoconj. J.* 14 (2), 209–223. doi: 10.1023/a:1018541821819
49. Henry, S., Oriol, R., and Samuelsson, B. (1995). Lewis Histo-Blood Group System and Associated Secretory Phenotypes. *Vox Sang* 69 (3), 166–182. doi: 10.1111/ j.1423-0410.1995.tb02591.x
50. Henry, S. M., and Samuelsson, B. (2000). "ABO Polymorphisms and Their Putative Biological Relationships With Disease", in *Human Blood Cells. Consequences of Genetic Polymorphisms and Variations.* Ed. M.-J. King (London, UK: Imperial College Press) 15–03. doi: 10.1142/97818481 60309_0002
51. Henry, S. M., Samuelsson, B. E., and Oriol, R. (1994). Immunochemical and Immunohistological Expression of Lewis Histo-Blood Group Antigens in Small Intestine Including Individuals of the Le(a+b+) and Le(a-b-) Nonsecretor Phenotypes. *Glycoconj. J.* 11 (6), 600–607. doi: 10.1007/ BF00731312
52. Hodzic, A., Mateos-Hernandez, L., Frealle, E., Roman-Carrasco, P., Alberdi, P., Pichavant, M., et al. (2020). Infection With *Toxocara canis* Inhibits the Production of IgE Antibodies to Alpha-Gal in Humans: Towards a Conceptual Framework of the Hygiene Hypothesis? *Vaccines (Basel)* 8 (2), 167. doi: 10.3390/vaccines8020167
53. Huai, G., Qi, P., Yang, H., and Wang, Y. (2016). Characteristics of Alpha-Gal Epitope, Anti-Gal Antibody, Alpha1,3 Galactosyltransferase and Its Clinical Exploitation (Review). *Int. J. Mol. Med.* 37 (1), 11–20. doi: 10.3892/ ijmm.2015.2397
54. Imberty, A., Breton, C., Oriol, R., Mollicone, R., and Perez, S. (2003). Biosynthesis, Structure and Conformation of Blood Group Carbohydrate Antigens. *Adv. Macromol. Carbohydr. Res. Elsevier*, 2, 67–130.
55. Innes, E. A. (2010). A Brief History and Overview of *Toxoplasma gondii. Zoonoses Public Health* 57 (1), 1–7. doi: 10.1111/j.1863-2378.2009.01276.x
56. Kolbekova, P., Kourbatova, E., Novotna, M., Kodym, P., and Flegr, J. (2007). New and Old Risk-Factors for *Toxoplasma gondii* Infection: Prospective Cross- Sectional Study Among Military Personnel in the Czech Republic. *Clin. Microbiol. Infect.* 13 (10), 1012–1017. doi: 10.1111/j.1469-0691.2007.01771.x
57. Korchagina, E. Y., and Henry, S. M. (2015). Synthetic Glycolipid-Like Constructs as Tools for Glycobiology Research, Diagnostics, and as Potential Therapeutics. *Biochem. (Mosc.)* 80 (7), 857–871. doi: 10.1134/ S0006297915070068
58. Laboudi, M. (2017). Review of Toxoplasmosis in Morocco: Seroprevalence and Risk Factors for Toxoplasma Infection Among Pregnant Women and HIV-Infected Patients. *Pan. Afr. Med. J.* 27, 269. doi: 10.11604/ pamj.2017.27.269.11822
59. Lecolier, B., Grynberg, H., and Freund, M. (1990). Absence of Relationship Between *Toxoplasma gondii* Antibodies and Blood Group in Pregnant Women in France. *Eur. J. Clin. Microbiol. Infect. Dis.* 9 (2), 152–153. doi: 10.1007/BF01963648
60. Linden, S., Mahdavi, J., Semino-Mora, C., Olsen, C., Carlstedt, I., Boren, T., et al. (2008). Role of ABO Secretor Status in Mucosal Innate Immunity and *H. pylori* Infection. *PloS Pathog.* 4 (1), e2. doi: 10.1371/journal.ppat.0040002
61. Lindstrom, K., Breimer, M. E., Jovall, P.-E., Lanne, B., Pimlott, W., and Samuelsson, B. E. (1992). Non-Acid Glycosphingolipid Expression in Plasma of an A1 Le(a-B+) Secretor Human Individual: Identification of an ALeb Heptaglycosylceramide as Major Blood Group Component. *J. Biochem.* 111, 337–345. doi: 10.1093/oxfordjournals.jbchem.a123759
62. Liu, Q., Wang, Z. D., Huang, S. Y., and Zhu, X. Q. (2015). Diagnosis of Toxoplasmosis and Typing of *Toxoplasma gondii*. *Parasit. Vectors* 8, 292. doi: 10.1186/s13071-015-0902-6
63. Lopez, R., Fano, R., Contreras, R., and Font, L. (1993). Igg Antibodies Against *Toxoplasma gondii* in Cuban Blood Donors. *Rev. Latinoam Microbiol.* 35 (2), 207–210. Lourenço, E. V., Pereira, S. R., Faca, V. M., Coelho-Castelo, A. A., Mineo, J. R., Roque- Barreira, M. C., et al. (2001). *Toxoplasma gondii* Micronemal Protein MIC1 Is a Lactose-Binding Lectin. *Glycobiology* 11 (7), 541–547. doi: 10.1093/glycob/11.7.541 Mahmood, S. H., AL-Qadhi, B. N., and Zghair, K. H. (2013). Prevalence of Toxoplasmosis of Males Blood Donors in Baghdad. *Iraqi J. Sci.* 54 (4), 832–841.
64. Mahmoudvand, H., Saedi Dezaki, E., Soleimani, S., Baneshi, M. R., Kheirandish, F., Ezatpour, B., et al. (2015). Seroprevalence and Risk Factors of *Toxoplasma gondii* Infection Among Healthy Blood Donors in South-East of Iran. *Parasit. Immunol.* 37 (7), 362–367. doi: 10.1111/pim.12198
65. Maia, M. M., Meira-Strejevitch, C. S., Pereira-Chioccola, V. L., de Hippolito, D. D. C., Silva, V. O., Brandão de Mattos, C. C., et al. (2017). Evaluation of Gene Expression Levels for Cytokines in Ocular Toxoplasmosis. *Parasit. Immunol.* 39, e12462. doi: 10.1111/pim.12462
66. Marchant, J., Cowper, B., Liu, Y., Lai, L., Pinzan, C., Marq, J. B., et al. (2012). Galactose Recognition by the Apicomplexan Parasite *Toxoplasma gondii*. *J. Biol. Chem.* 287 (20), 16720–16733. doi: 10.1074/jbc.M111.325928
67. Mareze, M., Benitez, A. D. N., Brandão, A. P. D., Pinto-Ferreira, F., Miura, A. C., Martins, F. D. C., et al. (2019). Socioeconomic Vulnerability Associated to *Toxoplasma gondii* Exposure in Southern Brazil. *PloS One* 14 (2), e0212375. doi: 10.1371/journal.pone.0212375
68. Martins, L. C., de Oliveira Corvelo, T. C., Oti, H. T., do Socorro Pompeu Loiola, R., Aguiar, D. C., dos Santos Barile, K. A., et al. (2006). ABH and Lewis Antigen Distributions in Blood, Saliva and Gastric Mucosa and *H. pylori* Infection in Gastric Ulcer Patients. *World J. Gastroenterol.* 12 (7), 1120–1124. doi: 10.3748/ wjg.v12.i7.1120
69. McConkey, G. A., Martin, H. L., Bristow, G. C., and Webster, J. P. (2013). *Toxoplasma gondii* Infection and Behaviour - Location, Location, Location? *J. Exp. Biol.* 216 (Pt 1), 113–119. doi: 10.1242/jeb.074153
70. Meier, H. C. S., Haan, M. N., Mendes de Leon, C. F., Simanek, A. M., Dowd, J. B., and Aiello, A. E. (2016). Early Life Socioeconomic Position and Immune Response to Persistent Infections Among Elderly Latinos. *Soc. Sci. Med.* 166, 77–85. doi: 10.1016/j.socscimed.2016.07.004
71. Midtvedt, T., and Vaage, L. (1989). Relationship Between *Toxoplasma gondii* Antibodies and Blood Group. *Eur. J. Clin. Microbiol. Infect. Dis.* 8 (6), 575–576. doi: 10.1007/BF01967490
72. Modrek, M. J., Mousavi, M., and Saravani, R. (2014). *Toxoplasma gondii* Seroprevalence Among Blood Donors in Zahedan, Southeastern Iran. *Int. J. Infect.* 1 (2), e21111. doi: 10.17795/iji-21111
73. Monteiro, V. G., Soares, C. P., and de Souza, W. (1998). Host Cell Surface Sialic Acid Residues Are Involved on the Process of Penetration of *Toxoplasma gondii* Into Mammalian Cells. *FEMS Microbiol. Lett.* 164, 323–327. doi: 10.1111/j.1574-6968.1998.tb13105.x
74. Moshfe, A., Arefkhah, N., Sarkari, B., Kazemi, S., and Mardani, A. (2018). *Toxoplasma gondii* in Blood Donors: A Study in Boyer-Ahmad County, Southwest Iran. *Interdiscip. Perspect. Infect. Dis.* 2018, 3813612. doi: 10.1155/2018/3813612
75. Murata, F. H. A., Previato, M., Frederico, F. B., Barbosa, A. P., Nakashima, F., de Faria, G. M. Jr, et al. (2020). Evaluation of Serological and Molecular Tests Used for the Identification of *Toxoplasma gondii* Infection in Patients Treated in an Ophthalmology Clinic of a Public Health Service in São Paulo State, Brazil. *Front. Cell. Infect. Microbiol.* 9, 472. doi: 10.3389/ fcimb.2019.00472
76. Nakashima, F., Brandãode Mattos, C. C., Ferreira, A. I. C., Spergiorin, L. C. J. F., Meira- Strejevitch, C. S., Oliani, A. H., et al. (2019). FUT3 and FUT2 Genotyping and Glycoconjugate Profile Lewis[b] as a Protective Factor to *Toxoplasma gondii* Infection. *Acta Trop.* 193, 92–98. doi: 10.1016/j. actatropica.2019.02.031
77. Nydegger, U. E., Tevaearai, H., Berdat, P., Rieben, R., Carrel, T., Mohacsi, P., et al. (2005). Histo-Blood Group Antigens as Allo- and Autoantigens. *Ann. N. Y. Acad. Sci.* 1050, 40–51. doi: 10.1196/annals.1313.006
78. Okay, T. S., Yamamoto, L., Oliveira, L. C., Manuli, E. R., Andrade Junior,

H. F., and Del Negro, G. M. (2009). Significant Performance Variation Among PCR Systems in Diagnosing Congenital Toxoplasmosis in São Paulo, Brazil: Analysis of 467 Amniotic Fluid Samples. *Clinics (Sao Paulo)* 64 (3), 171–176. doi: 10.1590/s1807-59322009000300004

79. Pappas, G., Roussos, N., and Falagas, M. E. (2009). Toxoplasmosis Snapshots: Global Status of *Toxoplasma gondii* Seroprevalence and Implications for Pregnancy and Congenital Toxoplasmosis. *Int. J. Parasitol.* 39, 1385–1394. doi: 10.1016/j.ijpara.2009.04.003
80. Perry, H. E., Franklin, R. A., Bray, S. J., Lo, M. K., Svensson, L. A., and Henry, S. M. (2007). A Novel Study of Association Between *Neisseria gonorrhoeae* and the Human Carbohydrate Blood Groups. *Immunohematology* 23 (3), 100–104. doi: 10.21307/immunohematology-2019-327
81. Pinto-Ferreira, F., Caldart, E. T., Pasquali, A. K. S., Mitsuka-Bregano, R., Freire, R. L., and Navarro, I. T. (2019). Patterns of Transmission and Sources of Infection in Outbreaks of Human Toxoplasmosis. *Emerg. Infect. Dis.* 25 (12), 2177–2182. doi: 10.3201/eid2512.181565
82. Ramani, S., and Giri, S. (2019). Influence of Histo Blood Group Antigen Expression on Susceptibility to Enteric Viruses and Vaccines. *Curr. Opin. Infect. Dis.* 32 (5), 445–452. doi: 10.1097/QCO.0000000000000571
83. Robert-Gangneux, F., Meroni, V., Dupont, D., Botterel, F., Garcia, J. M. A., Brenier-Pinchart, M. P., et al. (2018). Toxoplasmosis in Transplant Recipients, Europe 2010-2014. *Emerg. Infect. Dis.* 24 (8), 1497–1504. doi: 10.3201/eid2408.180045
84. Rodrigues, A. C. F., Uezato, S., Vono, M. B., Pandossio, T., Spegiorin, L. C. J. F., Oliani, A. H., et al. (2011). Non-Association Between Anti-*Toxoplasma gondii* Antibodies and ABO Blood Group System. *J. Venom. Anim. Toxins incl. Trop. Dis.* 17 (2), 184–189. doi: 10.1590/S1678-91992011000200009
85. Ryzhov, I. M., Korchagina, E. Y., Tuzikov, A. B., Popova, I. S., Tyrtysh, T. V., and Pazynina, G. V. (2016). Function-Spacer-Lipid Constructs of Lewis and Chimeric Lewis/ABH Glycans. Synthesis and Use in Serological Studies. *Carbohydr. Res.* 435, 83–96. doi: 10.1016/j.carres.2016.09.016
86. Sadooghian, S., Mahmoudvand, H., Mohammadi, M. A., Sarcheshmeh, N. N., Kareshk, A. T., Kamiabi, H., et al. (2017). Prevalence of *Toxoplasma gondii* Infection Among Healthy Blood Donors in Northeast of Iran. *Iran J. Parasitol.* 12 (4), 554–562.
87. Saki, J., Foroutan, M., Khodkar, I., Khodadadi, A., and Nazari, L. (2019). Seroprevalence and Molecular Detection of *Toxoplasma gondii* in Healthy Blood Donors in Southwest Iran. *Transfus. Apher. Sci.* 58 (1), 79–82. doi: 10.1016/j.transci.2018.12.003
88. Salibay, C. C., Dungca, J. Z., and Claveria, F. G. (2008). Serological Survey of *Toxoplasma gondii* Infection Among Urban (Manila) and Suburban (Dasmariñas, Cavite) Residents, Philippines. *J. Protozool. Res.* 18, 26–33. doi: 10.32268/jprotozoolres.18.1_26
89. Santos, A., Carvalho, F. C., Roque-Barreira, M. C., Zorzetto-Fernandes, A. L., Gimenez- Romero, D., Monzo, I., et al. (2015). Evidence for Conformational Mechanism on the Binding of TgMIC4 With *b*-Galactose-Containing Carbohydrate Ligand. *Langmuir* 31 (44), 12111–12119. doi: 10.1021/acs.langmuir.5b03141
90. Sarkari, B., Shafiei, R., Zare, M., Sohrabpour, S., and Kasraian, L. (2014). Seroprevalence and Molecular Diagnosis of *Toxoplasma gondii* Infection Among Blood Donors in Southern Iran. *J. Infect. Dev. Ctries.* 8 (4), 543–547. doi: 10.3855/jidc.3831
91. Saxena, S., Kumar, S., and Kharbanda, J. (2018). Toxoplasmosis Submandibular Lymphadenitis: Report of an Unusual Case With a Brief Review. *J. Oral. Maxillofac. Pathol.* 22 (1), 116–120. doi: 10.4103/jomfp.JOMFP_268_17
92. Schenkel-Brunner, H. (2000). *Human Blood Groups: Chemical and Biochemical Basis of Antigen Specificity. 2nd* (New York: Springer Wien), 54–248. doi: 10.1007/978-3-7091-6294-1
93. Shaddel, M., Mirzaii-Dizgah, I., and Hoshangi, M. (2014). Anti-*Toxoplasma gondii* Antibody Levels in Blood Supply of Shiraz Blood Transfusion Institute, Iran. *Iran J. Parasitol.* 9 (1), 120–124.
94. Shah, K., and Maghsoudlou, P. (2016). Enzyme-Linked Immunosorbent Assay (ELISA): The Basics. *Br. J. Hosp. Med. (Lond.)* 77 (7), C98–101. doi: 10.12968/ hmed.2016.77.7.C98
95. Siransy, L., Dasse, S. R., Gonat, S. P., Legbedji, A., N'guessan, K., Kouacou, P. A., et al. (2016). Immunity Status of Blood Donors Regarding *Toxoplasma gondii* Infection in a Low-Income District of Abidjan, Cote d'ivoire, West Africa. *J. Immunol. Res.* 2016, 6830895. doi: 10.1155/2016/6830895
96. Smael, B. S., Palpitany, A. S., and Hamarahim, K. H. (2018). Association of Rhesus Blood Group (RhD) and Toxoplasmosis in Women With Miscarriage in Erbil. *Erbil. J. Nurs. Midwifery* 1 (2), 94–100. doi: 10.15218/ejnm.2018.12
97. Smith, H. V., Kusel, J. R., and Girdwood, R. W. (1983). The Production of Human A and B Blood Group Like Substances by *In Vitro* Maintained Second Stage *Toxocara canis* Larvae: Their Presence on the Outer Larval Surfaces and in Their Excretions/Secretions. *Clin. Exp. Immunol.* 54, 625–633.
98. Stowell, C. P., and Stowell, S. R. (2019a). Biologic Roles of the ABH and Lewis Histo-Blood Group Antigens Part I: Infection and Immunity. *Vox Sang* 114 (5), 426–442. doi: 10.1111/vox.12787.a
99. Stowell, S. R., and Stowell, C. P. (2019b). Biologic Roles of the ABH and Lewis Histo-Blood Group Antigens Part II: Thrombosis, Cardiovascular Disease and Metabolism. *Vox Sang* 114 (6), 535–552. doi: 10.1111/vox.12786.b
100. Subauste, C. (2012). Animal Models for *Toxoplasma gondii* Infection. *Curr. Protoc. Immunol.* Chapter 19, Unit 19.3.1–23. doi: 10.1002/0471142735.im1903s96
101. Subauste, C. S., Ajzenberg, D., and Kijlstra, A. (2011). Review of the Series "Disease of the Year 2011: Toxoplasmosis" Pathophysiology of Toxoplasmosis. *Ocul. Immunol. Inflamm.* 19, 297–306. doi: 10.3109/09273948.2010.605198
102. Sun, X., Wang, L., Qi, J., Li, D., Wang, M., Cong, X., et al. (2018). Human Group C Rotavirus VP8*s Recognize Type A Histo-Blood Group Antigens as Ligands. *J. Virol.* 92 (11), e00442–e00418. doi: 10.1128/JVI.00442-18
103. Teplinskaia, L. E., and Kaliberdina, A. F. (1992). The Immunological Factors Characterizing Neurochorioretinitis. *Vestn. Oftalmol.* 108 (4-6), 26–29.
104. Timpson, N. J., Greenwood, C. M. T., Soranzo, N., Lawson, D. J., and Richards, J. B. (2018). Genetic Architecture: The Shape of the Genetic Contribution to Human Traits and Disease. *Nat. Rev. Genet.* 19 (2), 110–124. doi: 10.1038/nrg.2017.101
105. Wilson, M., Remington, J. S., Clavet, C., Varney, G., Press, C., and Ware, D. (1997). Evaluation of Six Commercial Kits for Detection of Human Immunoglobulin M Antibodies to *Toxoplasma gondii*. The FDA Toxoplasmosis Ad Hoc Working Group. *J. Clin. Microbiol.* 35 (12), 3112–3115. doi: 10.1128/JCM.35.12.3112-3115.1997
106. Wujcicka, W., Wilczynski, J., and Nowakowska, D. (2017). Genetic Alterations Within TLR Genes in Development of *Toxoplasma gondii* Infection Among Polish Pregnant Women. *Adv. Med. Sci.* 62 (2), 216–222. doi: 10.1016/j.advms.2017.02.002
107. Xing, M., Yang, N., Jiang, N., Wang, D., Sang, X., Feng, Y., et al. (2020). A Sialic Acid-Binding Protein SABP1 of *Toxoplasma gondii* Mediates Host Cell Attachment and Invasion. *J. Infect. Dis.* 222 (1), 126–135. doi: 10.1093/infdis/jiaa072
108. Zhang, K., Lin, G., Han, Y., and Li, J. (2017). The Standardization of 5 Immunoassays for anti-Toxoplasma Immunoglobulin G(IgG). *Clin. Chim. Acta* 472, 20–25. doi: 10.1016/j.cca.2017.07.007
109. Zhiburt, E. B., Ionova, A. I., Danil'chenko, V. V., Serebrianaia, N. B., Bel'gesov, N. V., and Trofimenko, E. V. (1997). The Spread of Antibodies to Cytomegalovirus and Toxoplasma Among Donors of Blood Components. *Zh. Mikrobiol. Epidemiol. Immunobiol.* 1, 59–61.

7

Myeloperoxidase and Other Markers of Neutrophil Activation Associate with Malaria and Malaria/HIV Coinfection in the Human Placenta

Demba Sarr[1], Lilian J. Oliveira[2,3], Brittany N. Russ[3], Simon O. Owino[3,4,5,6], Joab D. Middii[4,5,7], Stephen Mwalimu[4,5,8], Linda Ambasa[4,5,9], Faris Almutairi[1,10], John Vulule[4†], Balázs Rada[1] and Julie M. Moore[3,4,5]*

[1] Department of Infectious Diseases, College of Veterinary Medicine, University of Georgia, Athens, GA, United States, [2] Department of Pathology, College of Veterinary Medicine, University of Georgia, Athens, Georgia, United States, [3] Department of Infectious Diseases and Immunology, College of Veterinary Medicine, University of Florida, Gainesville, FL, United States, [4] Vector Biology and Control Research Centre, Kenya Medical Research Institute, Kisian, Kenya, [5] University of Georgia/Kenya Medical Research Institute Placental Malaria Study, Siaya District Hospital, Siaya, Kenya, [6] Faculty of Science, Department of Zoology, Maseno University, Maseno, Kenya, [7] Kisumu Specialists Hospital Laboratory, Kisumu, Kenya, [8] Animal and Human Health Program, International Livestock Research Institute, Nairobi, Kenya, [9] #1 Heartsaved Adult Family Care, Marysville, WA, United States, [10] Department of Pharmaceutical and Biomedical Sciences, College of Pharmacy, University of Georgia, Athens, GA, United States

***Correspondence:**
Julie M. Moore
juliemoore@ufl.edu

†This manuscript is dedicated to the memory of our dear friend and colleague

Introduction: Placental malaria (PM) is characterized by accumulation of inflammatory leukocytes in the placenta, leading to poor pregnancy outcomes. Understanding of the underlying mechanisms remains incomplete. Neutrophils respond to malaria parasites by phagocytosis, generation of oxidants, and externalization of Neutrophil Extracellular Traps (NETs). NETs drive inflammation in malaria but evidence of NETosis in PM has not been reported. Neutrophil activity in the placenta has not been directly investigated in the context of PM and PM/HIV-co-infection.

Methods: Using peripheral and placental plasma samples and placental tissue collected from Kenyan women at risk for malaria and HIV infections, we assessed granulocyte levels across all gravidities and markers of neutrophil activation, including NET formation, in primi- and secundigravid women, by ELISA, western blot, immunohistochemistry and immunofluorescence.

Results: Reduced peripheral blood granulocyte numbers are observed with PM and PM/HIV co-infection in association with increasing parasite density and placental leukocyte hemozoin accumulation. In contrast, placental granulocyte levels are unchanged across infection groups, resulting in enhanced placental: peripheral count ratios with PM. Within individuals, PM- women have reduced granulocyte counts in placental relative to peripheral blood; in contrast, PM stabilizes these relative counts, with HIV coinfection tending to elevate placental counts relative to the periphery. In placental blood, indicators of neutrophil activation, myeloperoxidase (MPO) and proteinase 3 (PRTN3), are significantly elevated with PM and, more profoundly, with PM/HIV co-infection, in association with placental parasite density and hemozoin-bearing leukocyte accumulation. Another neutrophil marker, matrix metalloproteinase (MMP9), together with MPO and PRTN3, is elevated with self-reported fever. None of these factors, including the neutrophil chemoattractant, CXCL8, differs in relation to infant birth weight or gestational age. CXCL8 and MPO levels in the peripheral blood do not differ with infection status nor associate with birth outcomes. Indicators of NETosis in the placental plasma do not vary with infection, and while structures consistent with NETs are observed in placental tissue, the results do not support an association with PM.

Conclusions: Granulocyte levels are differentially regulated in the peripheral and placental blood in the presence and absence of PM. PM, both with and without pre-existing HIV infection, enhances neutrophil activation in the placenta. The impact of local neutrophil activation on placental function and maternal and fetal health remains unclear. Additional investigations exploring how neutrophil activation and NETosis participate in the pathogenesis of malaria in pregnant women are needed.

Keywords: neutrophils, pregnancy, NETs (neutrophil extracellular traps), placental malaria, myeloperoxidase, *Plasmodium falciparum*

INTRODUCTION

Malaria infection during pregnancy is a significant public health problem with substantial effects on the mother, her fetus, and the newborn child [reviewed by (1)]. Accumulation of parasites in the placenta is a common feature of *Plasmodium falciparum* infection in pregnant women, mediated by VAR2CSA, a parasite protein exported to the surface of infected red blood cells, which binds to chondroitin sulfate A on proteoglycans, including syndecan-1 (2), in the placenta. Paucigravid women (in the first or second pregnancy) are especially vulnerable and are more likely than multigravidae (three or more pregnancies) and nonpregnant women to develop severe malaria (1). The interplay between parasites and the placenta is associated with inflammation characterized by the recruitment, retention, and activation of innate immune cells including polymorphonuclear leukocytes (neutrophils) (3) and is known as placental malaria (PM) (4). PM is associated with adverse pregnancy outcomes such as maternal anemia, stillbirth, and low birth weight (LBW) due to intrauterine growth restriction, and is most severe in the first pregnancy (5). How neutrophils in particular may affect placental pathology and fetal growth in the context of malaria remains a mystery.

Previous studies addressing potential interactions between PM and HIV infection suggest that the latter impairs immunity against malaria (6). HIV-infected pregnant women have more frequent and higher density parasitemia than HIV-negative pregnant women (7–11). Importantly, malaria accelerates HIV disease progression and higher viral load among pregnant women. Fetal complications in PM and association between maternal HIV status and fetal outcome have also been addressed (11–17). A definitive role for neutrophils in pathogenesis of PM alone and co-infections with HIV has been rarely studied. In one study, the number of circulating pigmented (Hz-bearing) neutrophils negatively correlated with birth weight, suggesting that these cells may have a pathogenic role in PM and thus may serve as prognostic markers for malaria-associated low birth weight (18). Another study reported that circulating neutrophils were reduced in pregnant women with *P. falciparum* malaria compared to negative controls (3). Others have found elevated neutrophil levels in placental relative to peripheral blood in malaria-infected women (19). Limited studies that performed direct measures have noted increased neutrophil levels by placental histopathology (20, 21). Consistent with this, cytokines and chemokines that can attract neutrophils, namely MIF, CXCL8/IL-8, and CCL3, are elevated in human PM (22–27).

Neutrophils are essential effector cells of the innate immune system. In humans, neutrophils are the most abundant type of white blood cell, accounting for 70% of all leukocytes in the blood of healthy adults (28). During pregnancy, the neutrophil count begins to increase in the second month and plateaus in the second or third trimester, a time at which the total number of white blood cells ranges from 9,000 to 15,000 X10^6/L (29). These cells are classically considered to be short-lived and act as the first line of defense in innate immunity, ensuring tissue restitution following resolution of infection (30–32). Neutrophils can rapidly be recruited to sites of infection and tissue injury (33), where they generate reactive oxygen species (ROS) through the activity of NADPH oxidase, thereby initiating antibacterial/antiparasitic defense (34). Neutrophils clear infections by phagocytosis, generation of ROS, release of potent bactericidal enzymes by degranulation, and formation of neutrophil extracellular traps (NETs) (35).

As evidenced in malaria, however, neutrophils represent a double-edged sword. These cells are activated and are capable of clearing malaria parasites by a variety of mechanisms (reviewed by (36), yet they are implicated in pathogenic mechanisms as well (37). Mice developing malaria-associated acute lung injury/acute respiratory distress syndrome (ALI/ARDS) had greater neutrophil accumulation in the lungs compared to mice that did not develop pulmonary complications (38). In these mice, targeting of neutrophils decreased the development of malaria-associated ALI/ARDS and significantly increased mouse survival (38), suggesting that neutrophils play a significant role in the pathogenesis of ALI/ARDS during experimental severe malaria and could be targeted to improve disease outcome.

Oxidative damage to tissues is also a key attribute of malaria pathogenesis that may be in part attributable to neutrophils.

Retinopathy-positive cerebral malaria is associated with accumulation of neutrophils (39). Likewise, previous work with *P. chabaudi* and *P. berghei* ANKA infection in mice indicated that neutrophils were responsible for liver damage, cerebral complications, and ALI/ARDS (38, 40, 41). Uptake of hemozoin (Hz)-containing digestive vacuoles by neutrophils drives a rapid oxidative burst but suppresses subsequent neutrophil activity (42). Oxidative damage in PM has been reported in humans and in mouse models, but key drivers remain unclear (43–46).

NETs are generated by the extrusion of DNA strands into the extracellular milieu, where they can entrap invasive pathogens (47, 48). The most common method for NET detection *in vitro* is microscopic observation (49), with immunodetection of neutrophil-derived proteins such as myeloperoxidase (MPO) and proteinase 3 (PRTN3) (50, 51) colocalized with DNA (49). NETs in tissue samples have similarly been shown as extracellular DNA colocalized with neutrophil-derived proteins (49). NET remnants such as DNA and neutrophil-derived protein complexes (MPO-DNA; neutrophil elastase (NE)-DNA) and citrullinated histones can be determined by ELISA in fluid samples (50, 51) or detected by flow cytometry (52, 53) as indicators of NETosis.

A role for NETosis in both protection and pathogenesis in malaria is emerging. *P. falciparum*-infected red blood cells reportedly stimulate human neutrophils to release NETs *in vitro* (38). The latest mechanistic investigations of NETs in malaria show that they are released by neutrophils exposed to malaria parasites and impede parasite spread thereby controlling infection (54). Furthermore, these studies provide evidence that NET release in malaria is independent of cell-cell contact and is mediated by macrophage migration inhibitory factor and peptidylarginine deiminase 4 (PAD4)-dependent histone citrullination (54). Interestingly, malaria parasite species have been shown to produce DNase that degrades NETs and the deficiency of this enzyme resulted in lower parasitemia in mice (55). Importantly, NETosis has been linked to severe malaria in human infection and in mouse models (38, 56–58). Using human samples and a mouse model for malaria, Knackstedt et al. demonstrated that heme-induced NETs are essential for malaria pathogenesis, with granulopoiesis and endothelial cell activation as two mechanisms of NET-mediated inflammation of the vasculature (58).

The present study investigates granulocyte levels and neutrophil activity in the peripheral and placental blood and tissue of parturient Kenyan women exposed to malaria and HIV. Neutrophils and associated markers appear to be influenced by these infections and preliminary evidence of NETosis in the placenta blood is offered. These data show a potential implication of neutrophils in the pathogenesis of PM but further studies are required to characterize the mechanisms by which this occurs.

MATERIAL AND METHODS

Ethics Statement

The study supporting collection of samples used in this report was approved by the Kenya Medical Research Institute, the Centers for Disease Control and Prevention, and the University of Georgia Institutional Review Boards. All study participants provided written informed consent before enrollment and procedures and instruments involving human subjects, sample collection and data analysis, processing, and testing were approved throughout the conduct of patient recruitment. All samples and data are anonymized.

Study Participants and Sample Collection

Participant recruitment and sample collection have been previously described (11, 59) (Matthias et al., manuscript in preparation). Briefly, the recruitment of 222 participants was performed at New Nyanza Provincial General Hospital, a public referral hospital, in Kisumu from November, 2002 to May, 2004. Subsequently, 825 participants were recruited at Siaya District Hospital, a public secondary health facility in Siaya until September, 2008. Women of all gravidities and uncomplicated vaginal deliveries were randomly recruited from patients admitted to the Delivery Ward of these hospitals. Only women with no health issues aside from malaria or HIV were eligible for full participation in the study. Maternal demographic and clinical information was collected and summarized, including whether or not participants self-reported fever within the two weeks prior to delivery. Infant gestational age was estimated using the modified Dubowitz score, and birth weight in grams was measured within eight hours after delivery. Maternal placental (intervillous) blood (IVB) was collected by the prick method within five minutes of placental expulsion (60). Peripheral blood was collected by venipuncture of the cubital vein within 12 hours post-partum. Platelet-free plasma was prepared as described (59) and stored continuously at -80°C, avoiding multiple cycles of freeze-thaw. Complete blood count (CBC) of both peripheral blood and IVB to estimate total white blood cell (WBC) and granulocyte counts was performed simultaneously with a Beckman Coulter AcT diff2 (Beckman Coulter Corporation, Miami, FL) within eight hours of blood collection. Although the majority of granulocytes detected by CBC are expected to be neutrophils, differential analysis for granulocytes was not available; thus, granulocyte levels are reported for this study. Full thickness placental tissue sections were collected from three unique regions of the placental disk, and fixed in Streck Tissue Fixative (Streck Inc., Omaha, NE). Five-micron sections were stained with hematoxylin and eosin for histopathological examination or left unstained for immunohistochemical analysis. From the same placental regions, 125 mm^3 sections of villus tissue underlying the placental basal plate were collected and flash frozen in liquid nitrogen for future molecular analysis and with Tissue-Tek OCT compound (Sakura Finetek USA, Inc., Torrance, CA) for immunofluorescence assessments and stored continuously at ≤-80°C until use.

Parasitemia was assessed on thick and thin smears of peripheral and placental blood and estimation of thick smear parasite density assumed 8,000 WBCs per μL of blood for both peripheral and placental blood. Percentage of leukocytes in the maternal placental vascular space bearing Hz was calculated from these thick smears. HIV serostatus was determined by rapid tests as previously described (11, 59).

Study Designs

Among the 1047 women recruited into the study, samples and data from a subset of 379 women are included in the work described here. Sample selection and use are summarized in **Figure 1** and **Supplemental Figure 1**, and patient characteristics are summarized in **Table 1**. All malaria infections are attributable to *P. falciparum;* a single participant was diagnosed with a *P. falciparum/P. malariae* mixed infection. Paired peripheral and placental data from Complete Blood Count were available from 224 women (79 primigravidae, 54 secundigravidae and 91 multigravidae, representing four infection groups (uninfected, malaria only (PM+HIV-), HIV only (PM-HIV +), and co-infected (PM+HIV+)). Gravidity differs significantly across the infection groups providing CBC data (*P*=0.0093 by Kruskal-Wallis test with post-hoc group-wise comparisons by Dunn's multiple comparisons test; median, interquartile range (IQR): PM-HIV-, 2, 1 – 3; PM+HIV-, 1, 1 - 2; PM-HIV+, 3, 2 – 4; PM+HIV+, 2, 1 – 3). Subsequent analyses focused on primigravid and secundigravid (paucigravid) women who experience the most significant outcomes with malaria and HIV infections in this setting (10, 61) (Matthias et al., manuscript in preparation).

Pilot data to detect markers of neutrophil activation and NETosis (cell-free DNA, DNA-human neutrophil elastase (NE) complexes, histones) in placental plasma were generated using HIV seronegative primigravid placental plasma (**Figure 1**), selected on the basis of placental histopathological status (uninfected, and infected: acute, chronic, chronic inflammatory). Acute infection is defined as the presence of infected red blood cells (iRBC), white blood cell (WBC) count by CBC <13,000/uL, and hemozoin scores [as described in (Avery et al., 2012)] ≤1 in WBCs and in fibrin. Chronic infection is defined as presence of iRBC, WBC count <13,000/uL, and hemozoin scores ≥2 in WBCs and in fibrin. Chronic inflammatory infection is defined as presence of iRBC, WBC count >13,000/uL, and hemozoin scores ≥2 in WBCs and in fibrin. Uninfected samples were confirmed parasite PCR negative and lacked iRBCs in histological sections. Subsequent ELISA data were generated from paucigravid women (**Figure 1**), representing malaria and HIV positive and negative women, with balanced selection of primigravid and secundigravid women within each infection group (PM-HIV-, PM+HIV-, PM-HIV+, PM+HIV+), and with matched selection across groups of infant birth weights, in both cases to the extent that sample availability allowed. Frozen placental tissues for immunofluorescence were selected to represent each infection group from among samples with MPO data, based on sample availability (**Figure 1**). Immunohistochemistry and western blot experiments utilized paucigravid samples (**Figure 1**), representing the four infection groups, with matched selection for granulocyte count (by CBC) ranges across each group.

ELISA

Levels of myeloperoxidase (MPO), proteinase 3 (PRTN3), matrix metalloproteinase (MMP9), and CXCL8 were quantified in peripheral and placental blood using a commercial ELISA kit

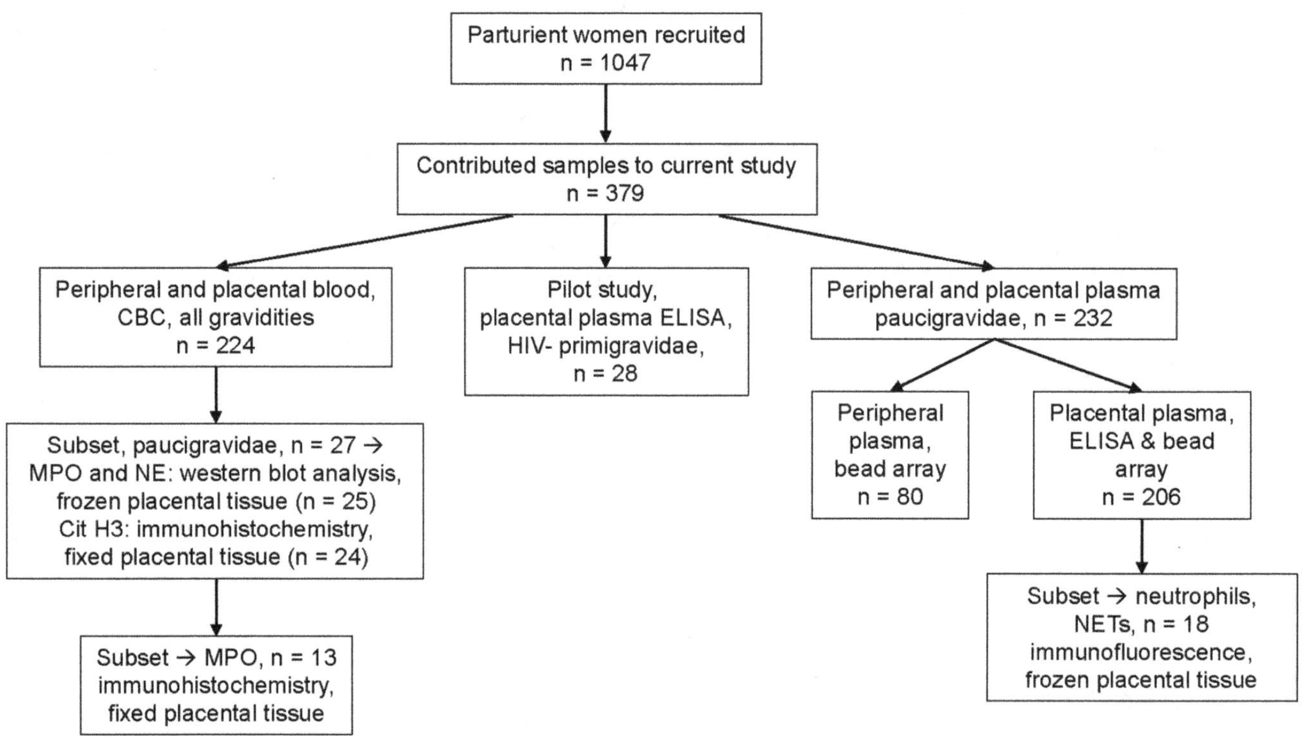

FIGURE 1 | Diagram of sample collection and testing. Shown are the number of patients recruited in a large cohort of parturient women in western Kenya, and samples contributed and tested in this study. Details of sample selection criteria are described in Materials and methods. Overlap of sample assessment on a per patient basis is depicted in **Supplemental Figure 1**.

TABLE 1 | Descriptive characteristics of study population stratified by gravidity.

Characteristics	All Women (n = 379)	Paucigravid (n = 288)	Multigravid[a] (n = 91)	*P*-value[b]
Maternal Sociodemographic				
Gravidity	1 (1-11)	1 (1-2)	4 (3-11)	-
Primigravid (%)	192 (50.6)	192 (66.7)	-	-
Age (years)	21 (13-39)	19 (13-32)	26 (20-39)	<0.0001
Married (%)	258 (68.1)	171 (59.4)	87 (95.6)	<0.0001
Luo ethnicity (%)	348 (91.8) (n=377)	259 (90.5) (n=286)	89 (97.8)	0.0230
Siaya[c] residence (%)	342 (90.2)	251 (87.1)	91 (100)	<0.0001
Laboratory				
Fever[d] at admission (%)	4 (3.3) (n=123)	3 (3.1) (n=97)	1 (3.8) (n=26)	1
HIV[e] seropositive* (%)	103 (27.2)	75 (26)	28 (30.8)	0.4177
Malaria smear positive* (%)	131 (34.6)	113 (39.2)	18 (19.8)	0.0006
Parasite density/μL[f] (range; interquartile range)	4,976 (40-226,208; 618-25,345) (n=131)	5,208 (40-226,208; 958-31,188) (n=113)	2,433 (83-119,107; 479-7,521) (n=18)	0.0752
Peripheral hemoglobin[g] (g/dL)	11.3 (5.30-20.4) (n=319)	11.3 (5.30-20.2) (n=228)	11.4 (5.80-20.4) (n=91)	0.5433
Placental hemozoin load[h]	3.5 (0.3-82) (n=127)	3.7 (0.3-82) (n=108)	1.6 (0.6-54) (n=19)	0.1820
Newborn				
Birth weight (g)	3,200 (2,000-4,500)	3,000 (2,000-4,400)	3,400 (2,600-4,500)	<0.0001
Low birth weight (≤ 2500 g) (%)	61 (16.1)	61 (21.2)	0 (0)	<0.0001
Gestational age (weeks)	38 (34-42) (n=376)	38 (34-40) (n=285)	38 (35-42)	0.0116
Preterm birth (<37 weeks) (%)	56 (14.9) (n=376)	49 (17.2) (n=285)	7 (7.7)	0.0277
Male infant (%)	193 (50.9)	150 (52.1)	43 (47.2)	0.4709
Self-reported history				
Fever, past two weeks[i] (%)	77 (20.3)	63 (21.9)	14 (15.4)	0.2315

Data are shown as number (percent) or median (range) unless otherwise noted. Sample sizes are shown where missing data reduce group numbers for specific parameters or only a subset of the group have values >0.
[a]Multigravidae contribute complete blood count data only;
[b]Comparison of paucigravidae with multigravidae by two-tailed Fisher's exact test (proportions), Mann Whitney test (continuous data) or Welch's t test (log transformed continuous data).
[c]remainder were recruited in Kisumu;
[d]defined as >37.6°C.
[e]HIV, human immunodeficiency virus;
[f]parasitemia measured in placental blood, analysis done on log-transformed data;
[g]by complete blood count.
[h]percent white blood cells observed on placental blood thick smear with engulfed hemozoin;
[i]self-reported fever or malaria in the last two weeks;
**factors used to guide sample selection.*

(R&D Systems, DuoSet, Minneapolis, MN) or bead arrays (R&D Systems) following manufacturer instructions and as previously described (62, 63). The experimental lower limits of detection for MPO were 125 pg/ml (ELISA) and 130 pg/mL (bead array), 125 pg/mL for MMP9, 10 pg/mL for PRTN3 and 3.9 pg/mL for CXCL8. Citrullinated histone H3 was measured using a kit from Cayman Chemical (Ann Arbor, MI), with a lower limit of detection at 0.1 ng/mL. Levels of NE-DNA complexes were assessed using an in-house protocol established to detect NET formation (64). In this assay, rabbit anti-NE (1:2,000, Calbiochem, San Diego, CA) was used as capture antibody and horseradish peroxidase-conjugated anti-DNA antibody (1:500, Roche, Indianapolis, IN) as detection antibody. Cell-free double stranded DNA was detected using the Quant-iT™ PicoGreen™ dsDNA Assay Kit (ThermoFisher Scientific, Grand Island, NY, USA) according to the manufacturer's instructions. DNA concentrations were quantitated using a known DNA standard with a lower limit of detection of 5 ng/mL as previously described (65). Total histone H3 levels were detected using a commercial kit (Active Motif, Carlsbad, CA) according to manufacturer instructions; the lower limit of detection was 150 ng/mL.

Immunohistochemistry and Immunofluorescence

Unstained 5 μm placental tissue sections were dewaxed for 15 minutes at 65°C followed by two incubations in xylene (2x5 minutes). Sections were then rehydrated in alcohol and antigen-retrieved with Sodium Citrate Buffer as previously described (66). Sections were then brought to room temperature and exposed to endogenous peroxidase activity block (DAKO, Cat#S2023) for 15 minutes. After washing with 1X TBST, sections were incubated with 10% Goat Serum for 10 minutes and incubated with the primary antibody (1/500 for MPO or 1/500 for citH3 in 1% Goat Serum) overnight at 4°C. The next day, samples were washed with 1X TBST (3x5 minutes) and incubated with polymer HRP anti-rabbit IgG for 30 minutes at RT. After three washes in 1X TBST, sections were exposed to DAB for 5 minutes, washed with distilled water, counterstained with hematoxylin (Cat#H3401-500, Vector Laboratories), dehydrated, and mounted with acrytol mounting medium (Cat#13518, Electron Microscopy Sciences, Hatfield, USA).

Immunofluorescent analysis was performed on 5 µm cryosections of OCT-preserved placental tissue. The sections were fixed in ice-cold acetone for 10 minutes and air dried for 1 hour. Following a rehydration step with 0.05 mM Tris-buffered saline (TBS; pH 7.5), sections were incubated with Protein Block, Serum-Free solution from Agilent DAKO (X0909, Santa Clara, CA, USA) for 1 hour. Rabbit anti-human MPO was purchased from Agilent DAKO (A039829-2, Santa Clara, CA, USA) and rabbit -anti-NE was purchased from Millipore-Sigma (481001, Burlington, MA, USA). Antibodies were pre-labeled using the Zenon Alexa Fluor 488 rabbit IgG1 labeling kit for anti-human MPO and Zenon Alexa Fluor 594 rabbit IgG1 labeling kit for anti-NE from Thermo Fisher Scientific (Waltham, MA USA). The labeled antibodies were diluted in Antibody Diluent reagent from Agilent DAKO (X0909, Santa Clara, CA, USA) at 1:100 and the sections incubated overnight a 4° C. Negative controls were labelled with an irrelevant prelabeled isotype control at the same concentration and same labeling as the primary antibody. The sections were then washed three times in TBS and labeled with Hoescht 33342 reagent (2.3 µg/ml) for 15 minutes. The slides were washed again, and cover slips were mounted using Prolong Antifade mounting medium (Thermo Fisher Scientific, Waltham, MA USA).

Slides were examined using a Leica DM2500 LED microscope with filters 02 (DAPI filter), 03 (FITC filter) and 15 (rhodamine filter) at 20 X magnification. Digital images were acquired using Leica LASX software and a high-resolution Leica DMC6200 digital camera. Five random fields within each villi section were captured for morphometric analysis within a 197.7 mm^2 field of view (FOV). A total cell number was generated and analyzed for each sample based on the sum of the average number of cells per FOV in each sample.

For image analysis of immunohistochemistry samples, several random FOV were acquired in RBG format and exported as tag image format (*tif) with the respective metadata. Using QuPath v0.2.3-m4 software (67), the digital images were preprocessed using the built-in visual stain editor to estimate and adjust stain vectors to improve staining quality. The round cells in the intervillous spaces were manually annotated based on hematoxylin filter to warrant the selection of all nucleated cells in the analyzed FOV. The intensity of MPO staining was measured as optical density (OD) and classified by the module "positive cell detection" using adjusted pixel size (0.1465 µM) to match the image resolution and automatic thresholds. The cell detection measurements were compiled. The number of positive cells and the intensity of DAB staining (per mm^2) were used in the statistical analysis. All analyzed images were blindly evaluated by an observer for quality control purposes prior to data export. Due to the variability of preservation of intervillous blood among the samples, the minimum for evaluation was three FOV or at least 100 intervillous round cells.

Analysis of immunofluorescence samples was also performed using QuPath v0.2.3-m4 software (67). Images of three fluorescence channels (green, red and blue) were overlaid. The positive cells for either MPO or NE or dually positive cells were manually annotated. The annotated cells were always associated with blue stained nuclei (DNA material). The fluorescence intensity of MPO staining was measured in the green channel and intensity of NE staining was measured in the red channel using the "Analysis" and "Calculate features" with automatic thresholds. Additional overlays of negative controls were exported, and random areas were analyzed to set a threshold of nonspecific fluorescence by average of intensity of fluorescence in these areas in the green and red channels. An annotated cell was considered positive when the fluorescence intensity was higher than the average fluorescence intensity in either or both of the green and red channels in the negative controls. NETs were identified as dual positive for MPO and NE, associated with DNA staining, and with a size higher than 102 μM^2 as reported (68). All analyzed images were blindly evaluated by an observer for quality control purposes prior to data export.

Western Blotting

Placental villous tissue (30 mg frozen weight) was homogenized in RIPA buffer supplemented with proteinase inhibitor cocktail. Samples were homogenized with Tissue Lyser (Qiagen, Valencia, USA) and centrifuged at 10,000g for 15 minutes. Protein concentrations were determined by bicinchoninic acid (BCA) method (Thermo Scientific, Rockford, USA) with bovine serum albumin (BSA) as a standard. Equal individual protein samples were prepared and stored at -80°C until use. Proteins (30 µg/sample) were separated by SDS-PAGE, blotted onto nitrocellulose membranes (Biorad, Hercules, USA) and probed with monoclonal or polyclonal rabbit antibodies specific for MPO (Agilent Technology, Santa Clara, USA), NE (Abcam, Cambridge, USA), citrullinated histone H3 (Abcam), and Hsp 90 (Cell Signaling Technologies) (as a loading control). Overnight incubation with primary antibody at 4°C was followed by one-hour incubation with anti-rabbit horseradish peroxidase secondary conjugates (Vector Laboratories). Proteins were detected using an enhanced chemiluminescence reagent (Pierce, Rockford, IL, USA). ChemiDoc Touch Imaging System with Image Lab Touch Software (BioRad) was used for image acquisition and densitometry analysis. Densitometry data are presented as ratio of target protein to Hsp90.

Statistical Analysis

Graph Pad Prism 9.1 software was used for all graphical data presentation and statistical analysis. Data are presented as scatter plot (correlation analysis and categorical analysis, with median line). Details for statistical analysis are indicated in the text or in figure legends as appropriate. Parasite density and percent Hz-bearing WBCs were log transformed prior to analyses. Binary analysis of non-normally distributed data of matched samples utilized the Wilcoxon matched-pairs signed rank test; unpaired analyses utilized the Mann-Whitney test. Correlation analysis was performed using the Spearman's correlation test. Multiple group comparisons were performed with Kruskal-Wallis test with post-hoc group-wise comparisons by Dunn's multiple comparisons test. Two-tailed Fisher's exact test was used to compare proportions. Statistical significance was set at $P < 0.05$.

RESULTS

Granulocyte Counts Are Differentially Impacted by Malaria and HIV Infection in the Peripheral and Placental Blood

To determine the extent to which granulocyte levels are influenced by PM, and how pre-existing HIV infection may modify this response, granulocyte counts derived from CBC analysis of peripheral and placental blood from women of all gravidities were assessed. Counts do not vary with gravidity in peripheral (median, IQR: paucigravid, 10.0 (6.90 – 13.7) $x10^3/\mu L$; multigravid, 9.10 (7.30 – 11.5) $x10^3/\mu L$; $P = 0.6543$, Mann Whitney test) or placental blood (paucigravid, 7.80 (5.70 – 11.9) $x10^3/\mu L$; multigravid, 7.80 (5.70 – 10.4); $P = 0.4889$). Compared with control PM-HIV- women, peripheral granulocyte counts are reduced in PM+HIV- and PM+HIV+ women (**Figure 2A**). The lower levels in the latter are strongly attributable to HIV infection, as levels between the two HIV+ groups are not significantly different ($P = 0.5044$). In contrast to peripheral blood, no differences in neutrophil counts in the placenta are evident (**Figure 2B**). Interestingly, the ratio of placental to peripheral blood granulocyte counts is enhanced by PM in both HIV- and HIV+ women (**Figure 2C**). Pairwise comparison of peripheral to placental granulocyte counts among individuals within the infection groups shows that while placental granulocyte levels are reduced relative to the periphery in uninfected and HIV seronegative women, this difference is lost with PM, with a tendency toward a reversed pattern in co-infected women (**Figure 2D** and **Supplemental Table 1**). Additionally, with the exception of PM+HIV+ women, in whom total WBC counts are strongly elevated in placental relative to peripheral blood, relative patterns of granulocyte levels between the peripheral and placental blood vary independently of total WBC counts (**Supplemental Table 1** and **Supplemental Figure 2A**). In terms of proportion of total WBCs, granulocytes are universally substantially reduced in the placenta relative to the peripheral blood (**Supplemental Figure 2B** and **Supplemental Table 1**). However, whereas granulocyte percentages in the peripheral blood (**Supplemental Figure 2C**) follow the same trends observed with granulocyte counts (**Figure 2A**), placental granulocyte percentages reveal a distinct pattern of reduction in HIV+PM+ women (**Supplemental Figure 2D**) that is not observed in placental granulocyte counts (**Figure 2B**).

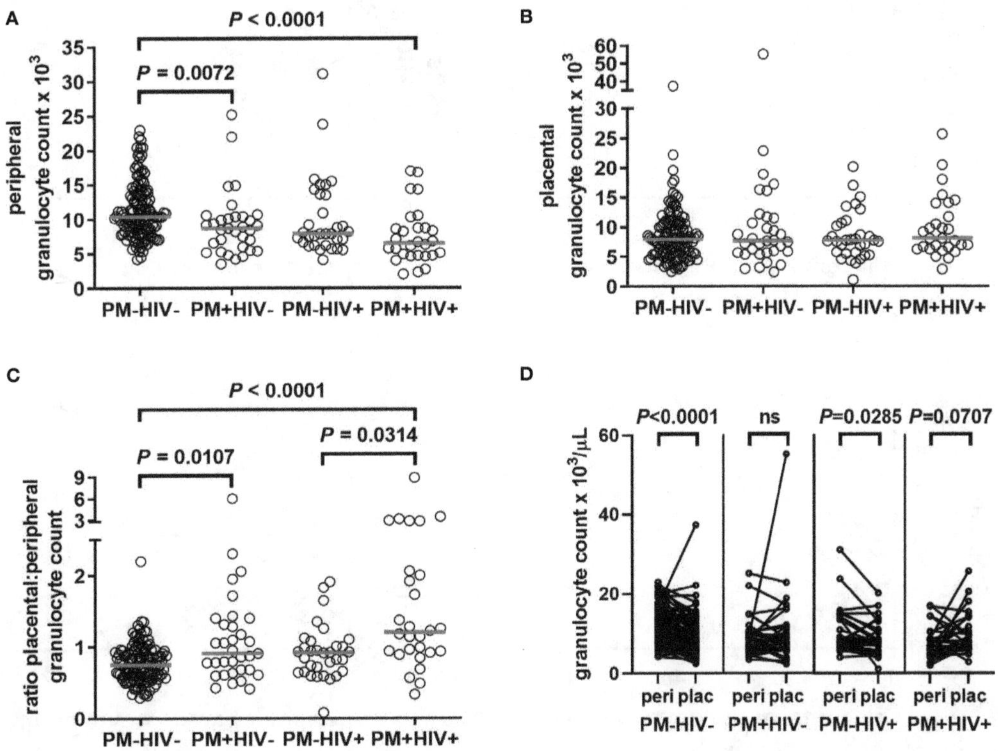

FIGURE 2 | Placental malaria and HIV infections differentially alter granulocyte levels in peripheral and placental blood. Peripheral and placental blood were subjected to complete blood count. Granulocyte numbers in **(A)** peripheral and **(B)** placental blood are shown. **(C)** Depicts the ratio of placental to peripheral blood granulocyte numbers, HIV-/PM-, n = 131; HIV-/PM+, n = 33; HIV+/PM-, n = 32; HIV+/PM+, n = 28. **(A–C)** Statistics by Kruskal-Wallis test with post-hoc group-wise comparisons by Dunn's multiple comparisons test. **(D)**, pairwise comparisons by Wilcoxon matched-pairs signed rank test. PM-=placental malaria negative; PM+=placental malaria positive; HIV-=human immunodeficiency virus seronegative; HIV+=human immunodeficiency virus seropositive.

Granulocyte Counts Correlate With Indicators of PM Severity but Not Birth Outcomes

PM often manifests as a chronic maternal inflammatory response dominated by accumulation of monocytes (5, 20, 26, 69). To assess the extent to which granulocyte counts might be influenced by severity of PM, correlation analysis of counts among PM+ women (combined HIV- and HIV+) were performed with parasite density and the percentage of WBCs bearing Hz in the placental blood space, which is taken as an indicator of chronicity of placental infection. The placental granulocyte count is unrelated to placental parasite density (**Figure 3A**) but positively correlates with Hz-bearing WBCs (**Figure 3C**). In contrast, the peripheral granulocyte count is inversely related to peripheral parasite density (**Figure 3B**) and Hz-bearing WBCs in the placenta (**Figure 3D**).

While granulocyte levels appear to be influenced by the intensity of the PM infection, no relationship with infant birth weight or gestational age is evident (**Supplemental Table 2**) nor do counts vary as a function of maternal self-reported fever (data not shown).

Placental Blood MPO Increases With Placental Inflammation

Based upon parameters including presence of parasites, inflammatory cell infiltration, and presence of Hz, PM has been variously categorized in histopathological examination in attempts to summarize severity and longevity of PM and associated birth outcomes (70–73). As a first step toward probing functional attributes of neutrophils in PM, a pilot study was conducted to measure levels of MPO in placental plasma from HIV-seronegative primigravidae whose placentae were histologically categorized into four groups (uninfected, acute, chronic, and chronic, inflammatory infection). MPO is released upon activation of neutrophils in the blood and tissues into both the phagolysosomal compartment and the extracellular environment, as well as in NETs (74, 75). Relative to uninfected samples, placental plasma from tissues with evidence of chronic, inflammatory infection shows significantly elevated MPO levels (**Figure 4A**). Correspondingly, this group tends toward lower infant birth weights relative to uninfected women (**Figure 4B**). Placental MPO levels correlate positively with percent of Hz-bearing WBCs in the placenta (**Figure 4C**). MPO levels are

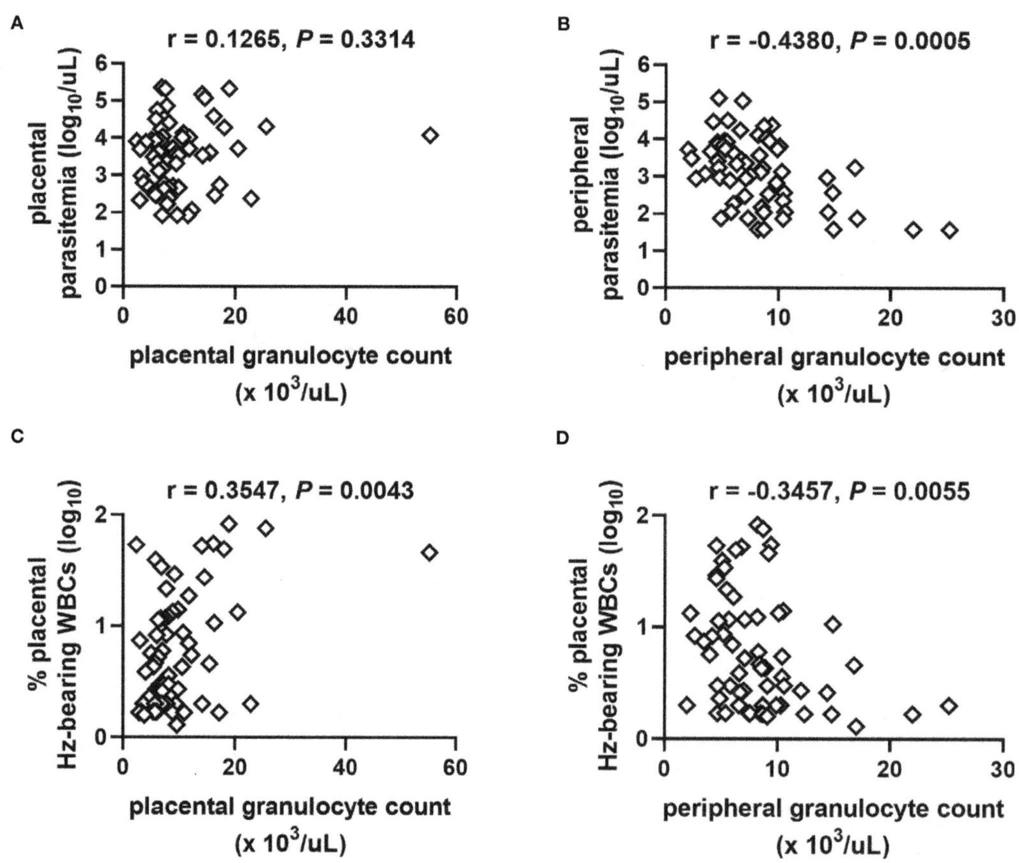

FIGURE 3 | Relationships of granulocyte numbers with measures of placental malaria vary as a function of blood source. Placental granulocyte counts measured by complete blood count in women with PM are unrelated to **(A)** placental parasite density but positively correlate with **(C)** the level of Hz-bearing WBCs in the placental intervillous space. Peripheral granulocyte counts negatively correlate with **(B)** peripheral parasite density and **(D)** level of Hz-bearing WBCs in the placental intervillous space. Both infection measures are log transformed. Results of Spearman's correlation analysis are shown. **(A, B)** n = 61; **(C, D)** n = 63.

elevated with self-reported fever in these women and tend toward higher levels in those delivering low birth weight infants (**Figure 4D**). Overall, these data indicate that high MPO concentrations are associated with PM, especially chronic, inflammatory infection, and relevant clinical outcomes.

Malaria and HIV Infection Impact Placental but Not Peripheral Levels of Soluble Markers of Neutrophil Activation

Building upon these initial observations, a larger analysis was undertaken to identify the extent to which malaria and PM/HIV co-infections in pregnant women impact indicators of neutrophil function. In addition to MPO, key markers of activated neutrophils, MMP9, and PRTN3, and a key neutrophil chemoattractant, CXCL8, were measured in peripheral and placental plasma of paucigravid women. In peripheral blood, MPO and CXCL8 levels are not impacted by PM, regardless of HIV infection status (**Figures 5A, B**). Additionally, peripheral MPO and CXCL8 levels are unrelated to infant birth weight and gestational age at birth (**Supplemental Figures 3E, F**). In contrast, placental blood levels of MPO are significantly elevated with PM and PM/HIV co-infection relative to uninfected and HIV+ women, respectively (**Figure 6A**), and in mothers who reported recent fever (**Figure 6B**). CXCL8 levels in PM+HIV+ women are elevated relative to levels in uninfected women (**Figure 6C**), and tend toward a weak enhancement with reported fever (**Figure 6D**). While MMP9 levels remain unchanged with infection (**Figure 6E**), levels are enhanced with reported fever (**Figure 6F**). Finally, like MPO, PRTN3 levels are enhanced by PM in both HIV- and HIV+ women (**Figure 6G**), and are increased with recent fever (**Figure 6H**). Despite associations with PM, none of the measured markers differ as a function of birth weight or gestational age (**Supplemental Figure 3**). Placental levels of all of these factors significantly positively correlate with each other (**Table 2**), and with the exception of CXCL8, all positively correlate with placental parasite density (**Figures 7A–D**), and percent Hz-bearing WBCs in the placenta (**Figures 7E–H**). However, contrary to expectation, none of these factors correlate with granulocyte counts or percentages (data not shown).

Placental MPO Detection by Immunohistochemistry and Western Blot

To further characterize MPO expression in the placenta, tissue sections from a subgroup of patients were probed using

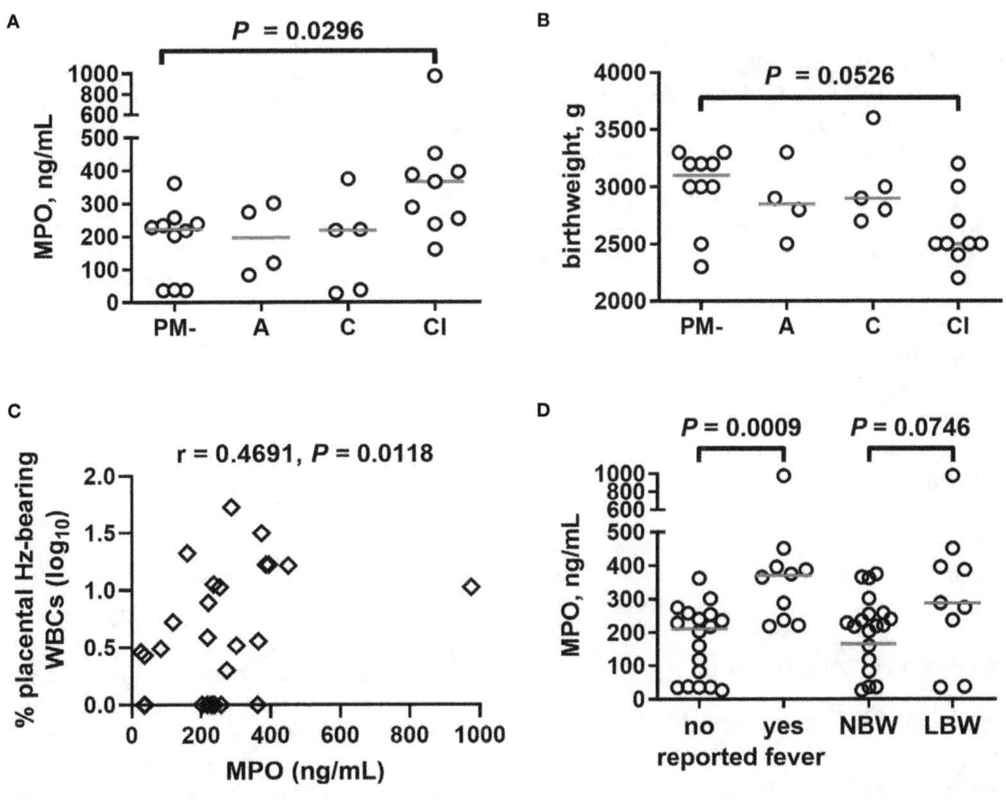

FIGURE 4 | Placental blood MPO levels increase in chronic, inflammatory placental malaria, together with reduced birth weight. **(A)** MPO measured in placental plasma by ELISA from primigravid women with and without PM stratified by placental histopathological status (see Methods). **(B)** Infant birth weight from the same women is similarly stratified. **(C)** MPO levels collectively analyzed by Spearman's correlation test with percent placental leukocytes (WBCs) bearing engulfed hemozoin. **(D)** Placental MPO levels measured by ELISA assessed for relationships with self-reported fever and infant birth weight. Statistics by Kruskal-Wallis test with post-hoc group-wise comparisons by Dunn's multiple comparisons test. PM- = placental malaria negative (n = 10); A = acute infection (n = 4); C = chronic infection (n = 5); CI = chronic inflammatory infection (n = 9); NBW= normal birth weight (n = 19); LBW = low birth weight (n = 9); no self-reported fever (n = 18), reported fever (n = 10).

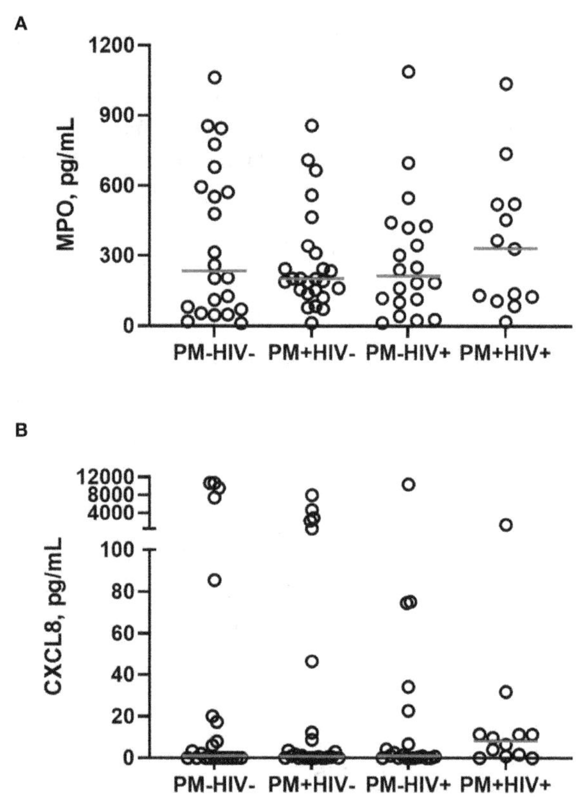

FIGURE 5 | Peripheral blood MPO and CXCL8 levels do not change as a function of placental malaria and HIV seropositivity. Peripheral plasma samples from paucigravid women were analyzed for **(A)** MPO and **(B)** CXCL8 levels by bead array. No statistically significant differences among the groups are evident (Kruskal-Wallis test with post-hoc group-wise comparisons by Dunn's multiple comparisons test). HIV-/PM-, n = 22; HIV-/PM+, n = 25; HIV+/PM-, n = 20; HIV +/PM+, n = 14 (MPO), n = 13 (CXCL8.) Groups as defined in **Figure 2**.

immunohistochemistry. MPO+ cells are frequently observed in these placentae, even in the absence of PM (**Figures 8A–D**). Frequency (**Figure 8E**) and intensity of MPO expression (**Figure 8F**), however, tend to be enhanced in PM+HIV- but not PM+HIV+ tissues. Probing for MPO by western blot of proteins derived from whole placental tissue may serve as a proxy for intensity of MPO expression, but preliminary analysis thereto does not reveal compelling evidence for influence of protein levels by infection status (**Supplemental Figures 4A, C**). Similarly, NE protein levels in whole placental tissue extracts are independent of infection status (**Supplemental Figure 4B, D**).

Plasma Markers of NETosis Are Not Affected by PM

Although NETosis has been linked to severe malaria in nonpregnant patients (38, 56, 57), this mechanism has not to our knowledge been explored in PM. Using detection of nonspecific (cell-free DNA; **Supplemental Figure 5A**) and known markers of NET formation (NE-DNA, **Supplemental Figure 5B;** cell-free histones, **Supplemental Figure 5C**), no evidence of significant PM-induced NETosis in placental plasma is observed in HIV- primigravidae (as in **Figure 4**), regardless of placental histopathological status. Similarly, citrullinated histone H3 (citH3), an additional marker of NET formation, does not differ in paucigravid placental plasma as a function of PM regardless of HIV infection (**Supplemental Figure 6A**), although elevated levels are evident in two PM+ women. Nonetheless, citrullinated histone H3 levels tend to positively correlate with placental granulocyte count (**Supplemental Figure 6B**).

In Situ Evidence for Netosis in Placental Tissue

As an alternate indicator of NETosis, fixed placental tissue was probed by immunohistochemistry for citH3. Some weakly positive cells are evident in the intervillous space, and, surprisingly, occasional stronger staining is seen in syncytiotrophoblast (**Supplemental Figure 7A, B**). Extracellular evidence of citH3, structures that would be consistent with NETosis, however, is rarely observed (**Supplemental Figure 4B**).

Although attempts to identify soluble components of NETosis in placental plasma and *in situ* in fixed, paraffin-embedded placental tissue does not provide compelling evidence of PM with or without HIV co-infection as a driver of placental NETosis, it is not possible to conclude that this process does not occur in PM, since sample collection, processing and storage, for example, could impede such detection. As an alternate approach, placental tissues flash-frozen in OCT were assessed by immunofluorescence staining for MPO, NE and DNA. In most samples, regardless of infection status, structures that are suggestive of NETs are evident (**Figure 9; Supplemental Figure 8**). The presumptive NETs are highly pleomorphic. Some structures are composed of single cells in the intervillous space that have streaky, comet-like nuclei and cytoplasm containing blue fluorescence (DNA) that colocalizes with green fluorescence (MPO) and red fluorescence (NE) (**Figures 9M–P, R–T**). Most frequently, the NETs are characterized by small to large aggregates of two or more pleomorphic cells with indistinct cell limits and pleomorphic nuclei encroached in a large MPO+/NE+ cytoplasm (**Figures 9M–O, Q–S**). Frequently, the cytoplasmic projections colocalize with MPO, NE and DNA material (**Figures 9M–O, Q–S**). These presumptive NETs are observed in maternal intervillous blood spaces, within the villus stroma, and occasionally inside the fetal vasculature (**Figures 9S, T**).

The small sample size of this experiment impacts statistical power; however, counts of singly stained MPO+, NE+ and MPO +/NE+ double stained cells do not vary with PM, including with stratification by HIV serostatus (**Supplemental Figures 8A–C**). Small, non-NETosing neutrophils (double MPO+/NE+, <102 μm^2) tend to be more numerous with PM (median, IQR, PM-: 12, 4.5 - 60; PM+: 22, 18 - 41; P = 0.0928) whereas larger putatively NETosing MPO+/NE+ cells are unchanged (median, IQR, PM-: 9.0, 2.0 - 35; PM+: 19, 15 - 34; P = 0.3735). Further stratification by HIV infection status yields no significant differences between the groups for small and large cells, including assessment of large NETosing cells as a percent of all MPO+/NE+ cells (**Supplemental Figures 8D–F**). Counts of MPO+/NE+ cells, including those classified as large, positively correlate with placental levels of CXCL8 (**Figures 10A, B**), with a similar tendency for small MPO+/NE+ neutrophils

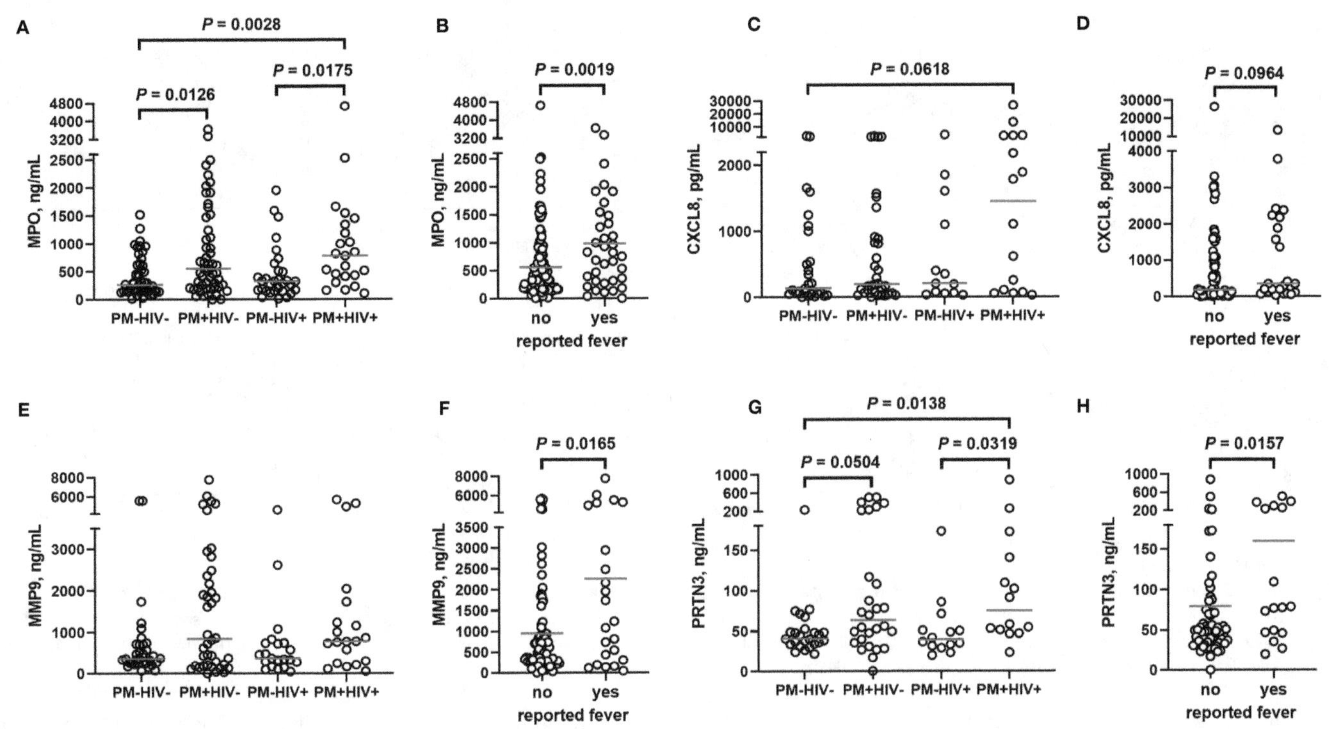

FIGURE 6 | Markers of neutrophil activation are variably altered by placental malaria and HIV seropositivity. Placental plasma from paucigravid women was analyzed for **(A, B)** myeloperoxidase (MPO), **(C, D)** CXCL8, **(E, F)** matrix metalloproteinase 9 (MMP9), and **(G, H)** proteinase 3 (PRTN3) levels by bead array and ELISA and stratified by **(A, C, E, G)** infection status and **(B, D, F, H)** self-reported fever (independent of infection status). **(A, C, E, G)** Statistics by Kruskal-Wallis test with post-hoc group-wise comparisons by Dunn's multiple comparisons test and **(B, D, F, H)** by Mann-Whitney U test. MPO: HIV-/PM-, n = 50; HIV-/PM+, n = 53; HIV+/PM-, n = 31; HIV+/PM+, n = 24. CXCL8, HIV-/PM-, n = 27; HIV-/PM+, n = 33; HIV+/PM-, n = 13; HIV+/PM+, n = 16. MMP9, HIV-/PM-, n = 35; HIV-/PM+, n = 40; HIV+/PM-, n = 21; HIV+/PM+, n = 21. PRTN3, HIV-/PM-, n = 25; HIV-/PM+, n = 28; HIV+/PM-, n = 14; HIV+/PM+, n = 15. Groups as defined in **Figure 2**.

(**Figure 10C**). Likewise, weak positive correlations are observed between MMP9 and MPO+/NE+ cells as well as small neutrophils (**Figures 10D, F**) but not between MMP9 and large cell count (**Figure 10E**). Placental levels of MPO are unrelated to these cell counts (**Supplemental Figure 9**).

DISCUSSION

In this study, we analyzed maternal peripheral and placental granulocyte levels as well as markers of neutrophil activation, including NET-specific markers and structures, in women with and without PM and HIV infection at the time of delivery. The results show that maternal peripheral granulocyte counts decrease with PM in the presence and absence of pre-existing HIV infection. Although a differential to discern neutrophil counts among the granulocytes was not performed, these findings are consistent with previous work that reported reduced neutrophil counts in malaria-infected pregnant compared to uninfected women (3, 76). A study in rhesus monkeys (*Macaca mulatta*) infected with *P. coatneyi* also showed a significant decrease in neutrophil levels starting at gestation week 9 (77). This contrasts with the observation that neutrophil counts are enhanced with HIV infection in pregnant women (78). Our results suggest that PM overcomes this apparent HIV-driven neutrophilia, since HIV seropositive women with PM

TABLE 2 | Correlation matrix of placental markers of neutrophil activation.

	MPO		MMP9		PRTN3		CXCL8	
	r, IQR*	P	r, IQR	P	r, IQR	P	r, IQR	P
MPO	1	-	0.7287, 0.6273 - 0.8058	<0.0001	0.9179, 0.8737 - 0.9471	<0.0001	0.4485, 0.2002 - 0.6426	0.0006
MMP9	0.7287, 0.6273 - 0.8058	<0.0001	1	-	0.7626, 0.6500 - 0.8424	<0.0001	0.3797, 0.0804 - 0.6161	0.0120
PRTN3	0.9179, 0.8737 - 0.9471	<0.0001	0.7626, 0.6500 - 0.8424	<0.0001	1	-	0.4106, 0.0615 - 0.6701	0.0196
CXCL8	0.4485, 0.2002 - 0.6426	0.0006	0.3796, 0.0804 - 0.6161	0.0120	0.4106, 0.0615 - 0.6701	0.0196	1	-

**Data represent results of Spearman's test with IQR, interquartile range.*

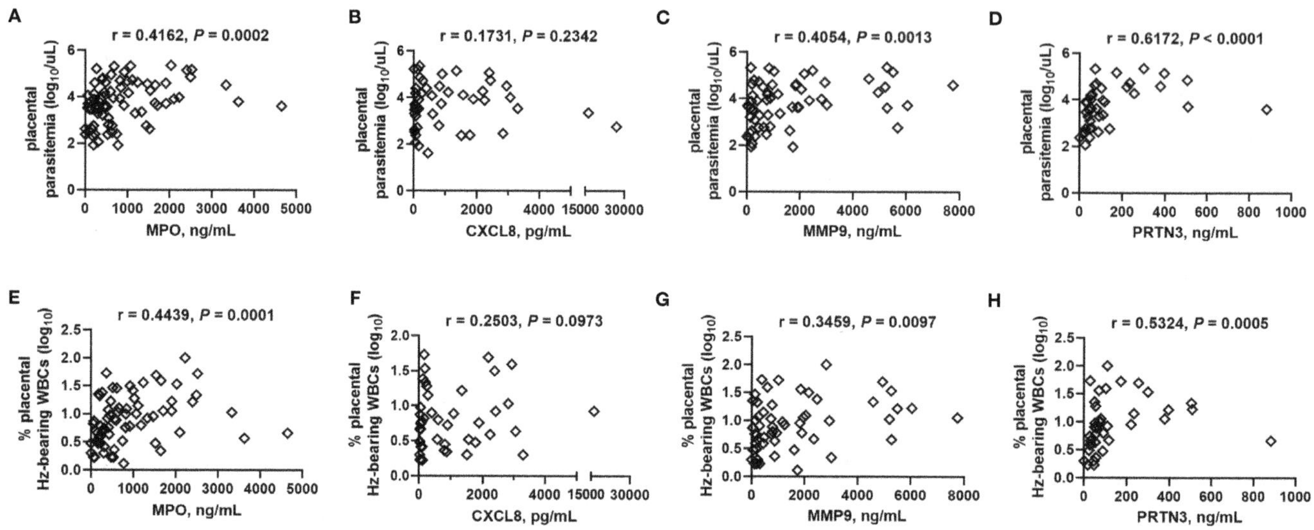

FIGURE 7 | Placental blood MPO, MMP9, and PRTN3 levels positively correlate with placental parasite density and hemozoin-bearing white blood cells. **(A, E)** MPO, **(B, F)** CXCL8, **(C, G)** MMP9, and **(D, H)** PRTN3 levels measured by bead array in plasma are collectively analyzed by Spearman's correlation test with **(A–D)** thick smear placental parasite density (log transformed) and **(E–H)** percent placental WBCs bearing engulfed hemozoin (log transformed). **(A)**, n = 77; **(B)**, n = 49; **(C)**, n = 61; **(D)**, n = 43; **(E)**, n = 73; **(F)**, n = 47; **(G)**, n = 57; **(H)**, n = 40.

have significantly suppressed granulocyte counts in the peripheral blood.

Contrary to expectation, no differences in granulocyte counts in the placenta are evident in this cohort of women. However, the enhanced ratios of placental to peripheral blood granulocyte numbers at the population level support the conclusion that during PM and PM/HIV co-infection, granulocytes accumulate in the placenta at the expense of the periphery, or, at minimum, are relatively more stable in the placenta. The physiological control of this phenomenon is worthy of further investigation, particularly given our observation that overall, granulocytes make up a lower proportion of total leukocytes in the placenta than in the peripheral blood and thus may be differentially regulated in these two blood spaces. Neutrophils are a key component of the normal process of labor, with accumulation of these cells in the uterine wall; the reductions observed here may be indicative of an exodus of neutrophils from the intervillous space to the myometrium [reviewed in (79)]. Despite the tendency toward lower granulocyte percentages and counts in placental relative to peripheral blood in the absence of infection, pairwise comparison at the individual patient level shows an overall tendency for granulocyte counts in placenta to increase uniquely with PM/HIV co-infection. However, granulocytes as a percent of total WBCs in the placenta are significantly reduced with co-infection. This may indicate that the massive overall increase in placental WBCs seen in this group (**Supplemental Table 1**) is heavily attributable to other cell subsets, likely monocytes (20).

Other researchers have reported significant accumulation of neutrophils in the placenta with PM (19, 20). What may be driving accumulation or preservation of these cells in the maternal placental blood, and why the current study shows placental granulocyte count stability but not accumulation with PM is unclear. Aside from the obvious differences in methodology and cell identification, placental granulocyte levels as measured here appear to be influenced by infection intensity, as counts positively correlate with the percent of placental WBCs bearing phagocytosed Hz. Thus, differences across studies could also be due to differences in infection intensity or chronicity. In general, local production of chemokines, including CXCL8, a factor that promotes neutrophil chemotaxis (80), may be an important determining factor in granulocyte/neutrophil presence in the intervillous blood, as is the case for recruitment to the uterus at parturition [reviewed in (79)]. Importantly, CXCL8 is elevated in PM+HIV+ placentae. The source of CXCL8 in the placenta that might participate in this response is not clear but could be maternal monocytes (22, 26), fetal syncytiotrophoblast (3, 22, 81, 82), or uterine/decidual stromal cells (83).

Previous studies have indicated that neutrophils may play a pathogenic role in PM and could serve as prognostic markers for malaria-associated low birth weight (18). We report that in this population of parturient women, granulocyte counts do not associate with infant birth outcomes. This may be due to inadequate sample size, lack of differential analysis to directly count neutrophils, or may be related to the overall patient recruitment strategy, which excluded complicated pregnancies and deliveries and health issues other than malaria and HIV infections. Because an interesting relationship between neutrophils and malaria parasites is emerging [reviewed in (36)] and neutrophils are key cells at multiple stages of normal and abnormal pregnancy [reviewed in (79)], it is imperative for future studies to definitively identify neutrophils in the granulocyte population, and to further consider neutrophil

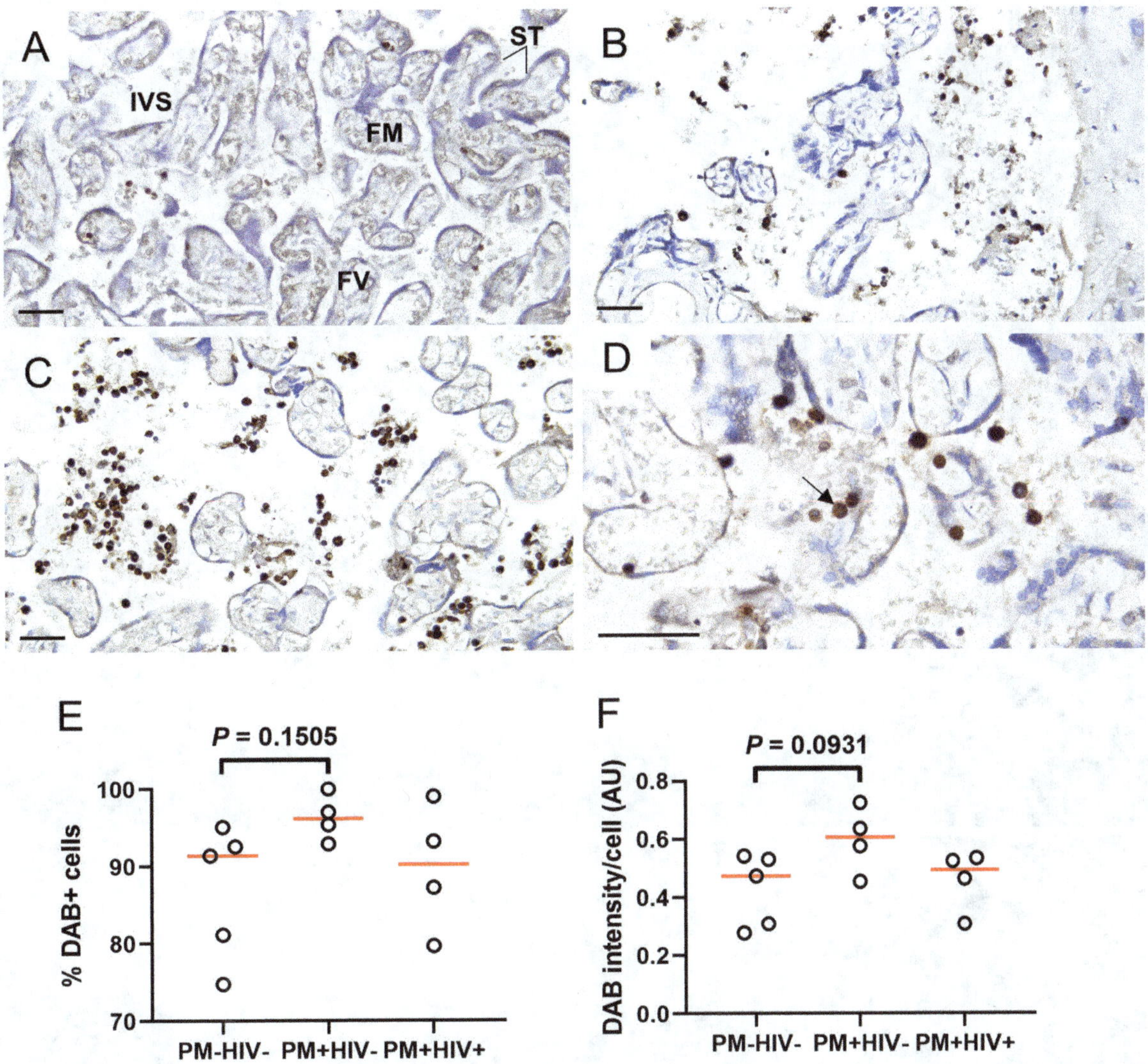

FIGURE 8 | Placental WBCs from PM+HIV- women show more robust MPO expression by immunohistochemistry relative to uninfected and co-infected women. Frequency and intensity of MPO staining is lower in **(A)** uninfected placenta and **(B)** PM+HIV+ placenta relative to **(C)** PM+HIV- placenta. **(D)** Segmented nucleus clearly delineates MPO staining in a neutrophil (arrow). ST, syncytiotrophoblast; FM, fetal mesenchyme; FV, fetal vessel; IVS, intervillous space. Scale bars represent 50 μm. **(E)** Percent cells expressing MPO weakly tends to be higher in PM+HIV- relative to uninfected women. **(F)** MPO staining intensity tends to be higher in PM+ HIV- relative to uninfected women. Statistics by Kruskal-Wallis test with post-hoc group-wise comparisons by Dunn's multiple comparisons test. PM-/HIV-, n = 5; PM+/HIV-, n = 4; PM+/HIV+, n = 4. Groups as defined in **Figure 2**.

subsets and functional parameters to discern potential relationships with pathogenic outcomes of PM.

One of the many consequences of neutrophil activation is the secretion of granules containing MPO, MMP9, NE, and PRTN3. Neutrophils produce massive amounts of these proteins, in the case of MPO, representing 5% of the total cellular protein (84). Our data show for the first time that placental blood MPO and PRTN3 levels are elevated with PM in both HIV- and HIV+ paucigravid women relative to PM-HIV- women. It was unexpected to find that none of these markers correlates with placental granulocyte counts, emphasizing the need for further work to definitively identify the source of these factors in placental plasma and fully characterize neutrophil function in PM. Importantly, observations of MPO in fixed placental tissue sections suggest that this factor may be produced by both intervillous neutrophils and monocytes, yet most MPO-expressing cells observed by immunofluorescence are co-stained for NE, identifying them as neutrophils.

Placental levels of MPO, MMP9, and PRTN3 all positively correlate with placental parasitemia as well as placental hemozoin bearing WBCs, suggesting that production is enhanced by chronic infection. Since MPO attenuates pathogen clearance during *P. yoelii* nonlethal infection (85), it is tempting to speculate that this enzyme may inhibit parasite clearance in PM as well. In an initial pilot study, we found placental blood MPO levels to be increased significantly with

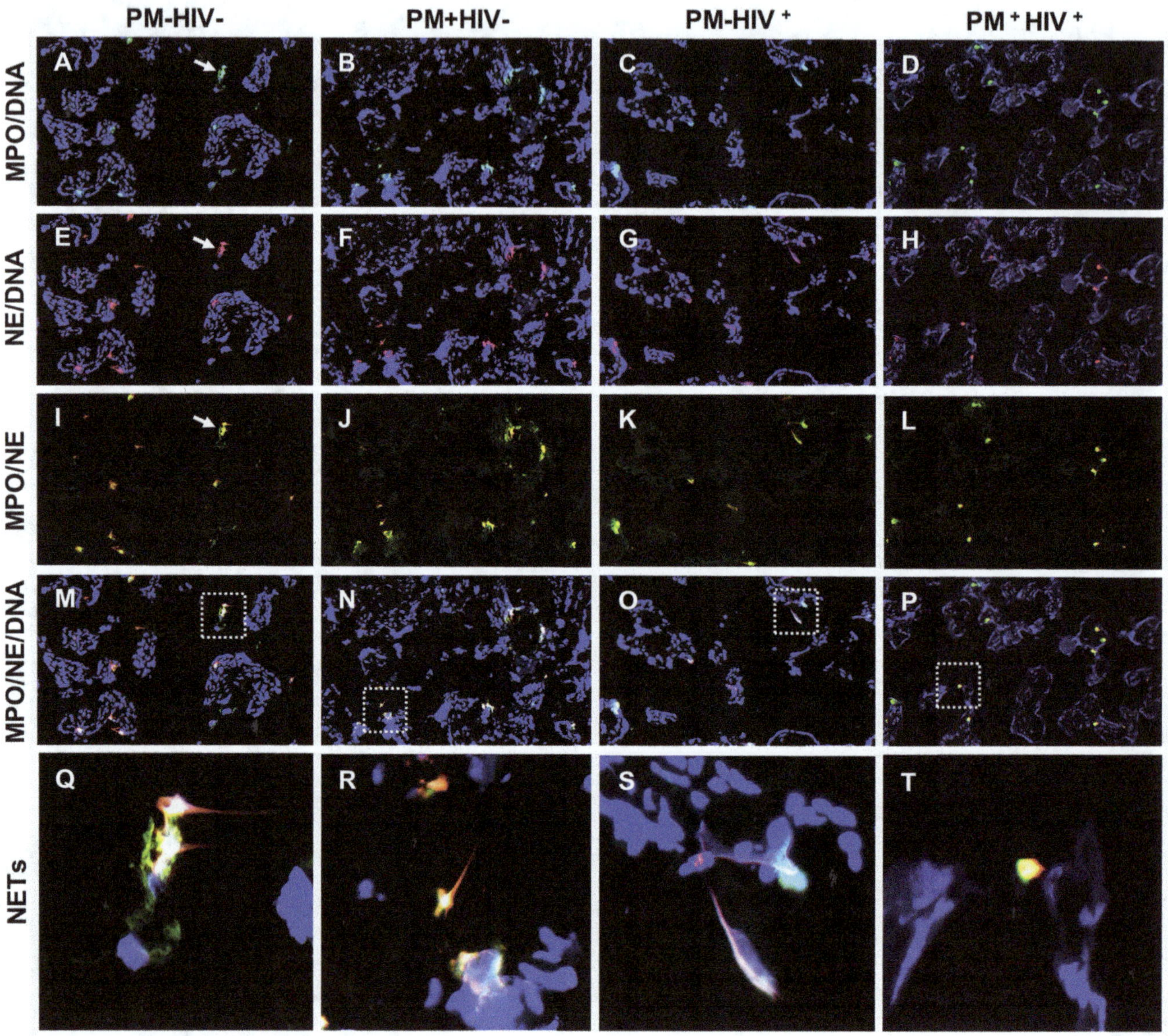

FIGURE 9 | Detection of NETs by immunfluorescence in placental tissue. Immunolocalization of MPO (green), NE (red) in term placenta. The DNA was labeled with Hoescht 33342 (blue). **(A, E, I, M, Q)** uninfected placenta; **(B, F, J, N, R)** PM+HIV- placenta; **(C, G, K, O, S)** PM-HIV+ placenta; and **(D, H, L, P, T)** PM+HIV+ placenta. The first row **(A–D)** shows the colocalization of MPO with DNA, the second row **(E–H)**, colocalization of NE and DNA, the third row **(I–L)**, colocalization of MPO and NE and the fourth row **(M–P)**, colocalization of MPO, NE and DNA. The last row shows in higher magnification the dotted areas in panels **(M–P)** that contain putative NET-like structures **(Q–T)**. Arrows in panels **(A, E, I)** indicate NET-like structures. Groups are as defined in **Figure 2**.

chronic, inflammatory PM in primigravidae. MPO is associated with vascular dysfunction (86) and underlies the pathophysiology of numerous vascular inflammatory diseases including arteriosclerosis and coronary artery disease (87, 88). Inflammation and endothelial dysfunction are characteristics of preeclampsia, and increased MPO levels in placental and peripheral circulation in preeclamptic women have been described (89, 90). The extent to which PM and PM/HIV coinfection may contribute to preeclampsia *via* MPO production or modification of other neutrophil functions remains to be determined. This may be an exciting avenue to pursue given increasing evidence that malaria predisposes women to this hypertensive disorder (91, 92).

Elevated neutrophil activation, as evidenced by higher plasma concentrations not only of MPO but also of PRTN3 and NE, is associated with severe pediatric malaria (39). Likewise, MMP9, an endopeptidase released by neutrophils and monocytes, is implicated in the pathogenesis of severe malaria (93–95). An MMP9 polymorphism protects against PM, further implicating an important role for this enzyme in *P. falciparum* infection (96). Importantly, MPO, MMP9 and PRTN3 levels in the placenta associate with self-reported fever in this cohort of parturient

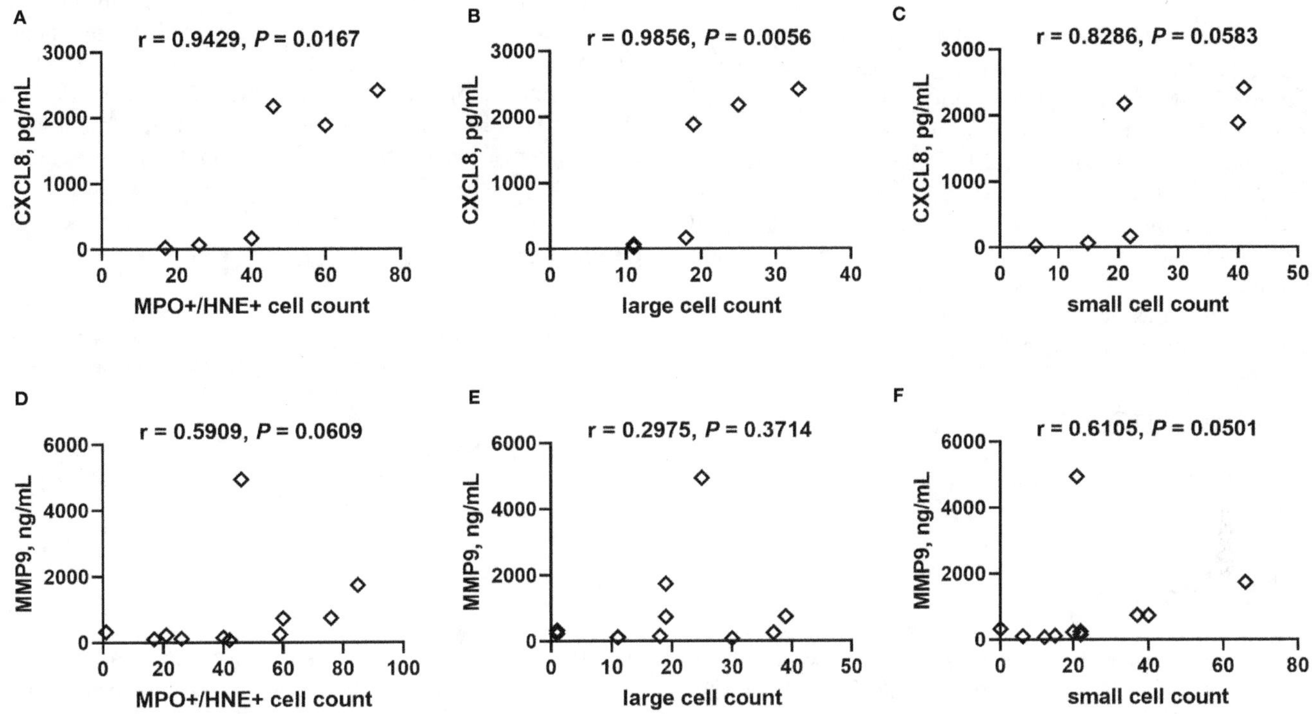

FIGURE 10 | Correlation analysis of CXCL8 and MMP9 with neutrophils in placental tissue. Counts of neutrophils detected in frozen cryosections as **(A, D)** MPO+/NE+, and MPO+/NE+ cells stratified by size as **(B, E)** large: >102 μm^2, and **(C, F)** small: <102 μm^2 collectively correlated with placental plasma levels of **(A–C)** CXCL8 and **(D–F)** MMP9. Cell counts determined by analysis of immunofluorescence of tissues. Statistics by Spearman's correlation test. PM-/HIV-, n = 5; PM+/HIV-, n = 5; PM-/HIV+, n = 4; PM+/HIV+, n = 4. Groups as defined in **Figure 2**.

women. However, while pilot data in HIV seronegative primigravidae suggest a tendency for placental MPO to be higher in women with low birth weight infants, in a larger cohort of paucigravid malaria-exposed women that also considered HIV infection, no relationship with birth weight or gestational age emerges for any of these markers. This is unexpected given that the factors do correlate with parameters (placental parasite density and Hz-bearing WBCs) that are typically associated with poor outcomes in PM. Indeed, Hz-bearing neutrophils in the peripheral blood of pregnant women predict low birth weight (18). While additional work will be required to resolve this discrepancy, these results suggest that the mechanism by which neutrophils mediate poor birth outcomes may not be directly related to the release of neutrophil granules in the placental blood space. One potential alternate mechanism may be downstream effects of these factors, which were not measured here. High concentrations of neutrophil-derived antimicrobial compounds can make these cells detrimental to the host (97–99). For example, activated neutrophils exacerbate preeclampsia by releasing ROS (100–105). Of note, MPO catalyzes the formation of aggressive reactive oxygen intermediates, including hypochlorous, hypobromous, and hypothiocyanous acids, respectively (106, 107), which contribute to oxidative killing (108). Oxidative stress is a feature of PM (43, 44), but the extent to which neutrophils contribute to it remains to be established.

Contrary to expectation, this study finds no evidence of a relationship between PM and levels of soluble markers of NETosis in the placenta. Similarly, while structures consistent with NETs (MPO, NE, and DNA co-localization) are observed in the intervillous space, a relationship with PM is not evident. Alternatively, non-activated, resting, "small" neutrophils tend to be elevated with PM in this study. Because NETs have been observed in the placental intervillous space in pregnancies complicated by preeclampsia (103, 105), and given parallels between PM and preeclampsia, it was our expectation that NETosis would be enhanced in placentae of infected women. While further research designed specifically to address this question is warranted, it is tempting to speculate that NETosis may be subject to unique and as yet poorly understood control mechanisms in the placenta that are not specifically activated or perturbed by PM. The overall reduction of granulocyte counts in the placenta relative to the peripheral blood hints at this possibility.

In conclusion, the present study demonstrates that PM and PM/HIV co-infection perturb granulocyte levels, and soluble signatures of neutrophil activation associate with indicators of PM infection and associated symptoms. The findings do not authoritatively distinguish between a protective or pathogenic role for neutrophils or products of their activation, nor is an association of PM with NETosis established. Further exploration of neutrophil function in the context of malaria and HIV in pregnant women, particularly direct assessment of activity, is required to fill remaining gaps in knowledge.

AUTHOR CONTRIBUTIONS

JMM, LJO, BR, and DS conceived and designed the experiments. LA, JDM, JMM, SM, and SO coordinated sample and clinical data collection. FA, JMM, LJO, SO, BR, BNR, and DS performed the experiments. LJO performed the Qupath analysis and prepared micrographs. JMM, LJO, BNR, and DS prepared the figures and tables. JMM performed descriptive statistical analyses. JMM, LJO, and DS wrote the manuscript. JV provided logistical and infrastructural support for sample collection, processing, storage and shipment, and facilitated local ethical reviews in Kenya. All authors (with the exception of JV, deceased) contributed to the article and approved the submitted version.

ACKNOWLEDGMENTS

We thank the parturient women and Labour Ward staff at New Nyanza Provincial General Hospital, Kisumu and Siaya District Hospital, Siaya, Kenya, and the Kenya-based UGA/KEMRI team, including Meshak Auma, Mary Kibatha, Jackline Midoro, Brisson Muia, Philip Naluande, Benson Odhiambo, Fenner Odhiambo, Dorothy Odidi, Milka Okwach, Dickens Olang, Francis Omwalo, Elkana Ondere, Godfrey Owenga, Rose Oyucho, Moses Sichangi, and Benson Vibhakar, without whose participation, active support and dedication this study would not have been possible.

SUPPLEMENTARY MATERIAL

Supplementary Table 1 | Pairwise comparison of peripheral and placental white blood cell (WBC) and granulocyte counts. PM = placental malaria; HIV = human immunodeficiency virus. Data are shown in graphical form in **Supplemental Figure 2A**, and **Supplemental Figure 2B**

Supplementary Table 2 | Granulocyte numbers as a function of infant birth weight and gestational age at birth. NBW, normal birth weight, LBW, low birth weight; TB, term birth; PTB, preterm birth.

REFERENCES

1. Bauserman M, Conroy AL, North K, Patterson J, Bose C, Meshnick S. An Overview of Malaria in Pregnancy. *Semin Perinatol* (2019) 43(5):282–90. doi: 10.1053/j.semperi.2019.03.018
2. Ayres Pereira M, Mandel Clausen T, Pehrson C, Mao Y, Resende M, Daugaard M, et al. Placental Sequestration of Plasmodium Falciparum Malaria Parasites Is Mediated by the Interaction Between VAR2CSA and Chondroitin Sulfate A on Syndecan-1. *PloS Pathogens* (2016) 12(8): e1005831. doi: 10.1371/journal.ppat.1005831
3. Bostrom S, Schmiegelow C, Abu Abed U, Minja DTR, Lusingu J, Brinkmann V, et al. Neutrophil Alterations in Pregnancy-Associated Malaria and Induction of Neutrophil Chemotaxis by Plasmodium Falciparum. *Parasite Immunol* (2017) 39(6):1–6. doi: 10.1111/pim.12433
4. Rogerson SJ, Mwapasa V, Meshnick SR. Malaria in Pregnancy: Linking Immunity and Pathogenesis to Prevention. *Am J Trop Med Hygiene* (2007) 77(6 Suppl):14–22. doi: 10.4269/ajtmh.77.6.suppl.14
5. Rogerson SJ, Pollina E, Getachew A, Tadesse E, Lema VM, Molyneux ME. Placental Monocyte Infiltrates in Response to Plasmodium Falciparum Malaria Infection and Their Association With Adverse Pregnancy Outcomes. *Am J Trop Med Hygiene* (2003) 68(1):115–9. doi: 10.4269/ajtmh.2003.68.1.0680115
6. Serghides L, Finney CA, Ayi K, Loutfy M, Kain KC. Chronic HIV Infection Impairs Nonopsonic Phagocytosis of Malaria Parasites. *J Acquir Immune Defic Syndr* (2015) 68(2):128–32. doi: 10.1097/QAI.0000000000000427
7. Steketee RW, Wirima JJ, Bloland PB, Chilima B, Mermin JH, Chitsulo L, et al. Impairment of a Pregnant Woman's Acquired Ability to Limit Plasmodium Falciparum by Infection With Human Immunodeficiency Virus Type-1. *Am J Trop Med Hygiene* (1996) 55(1 Suppl):42–9. doi: 10.4269/ajtmh.1996.55.42
8. Parise ME, Ayisi JG, Nahlen BL, Schultz LJ, Roberts JM, Misore A, et al. Efficacy of Sulfadoxine-Pyrimethamine for Prevention of Placental Malaria in an Area of Kenya With a High Prevalence of Malaria and Human Immunodeficiency Virus Infection. *Am J Trop Med Hygiene* (1998) 59 (5):813–22. doi: 10.4269/ajtmh.1998.59.813
9. Verhoeff FH, Brabin BJ, Hart CA, Chimsuku L, Kazembe P, Broadhead RL. Increased Prevalence of Malaria in HIV-Infected Pregnant Women and its Implications for Malaria Control. *Trop Med Int Health* (1999) 4(1):5–12. doi: 10.1046/j.1365-3156.1999.00349.x
10. van Eijk AM, Ayisi JG, ter Kuile FO, Misore A, Otieno JA, Kolczak MS, et al. Human Immunodeficiency Virus Seropositivity and Malaria as Risk Factors for Third-Trimester Anemia in Asymptomatic Pregnant Women in Western Kenya. *Am J Trop Med Hygiene* (2001) 65(5):623–30. doi: 10.4269/ajtmh.2001.65.623
11. Perrault SD, Hajek J, Zhong K, Owino SO, Sichangi M, Smith G, et al. Human Immunodeficiency Virus Co-Infection Increases Placental Parasite Density and Transplacental Malaria Transmission in Western Kenya. *Am J Trop Med Hygiene* (2009) 80(1):119–25. doi: 10.4269/ajtmh.2009.80.119
12. Bloland PB, Wirima JJ, Steketee RW, Chilima B, Hightower A, Breman JG. Maternal HIV Infection and Infant Mortality in Malawi: Evidence for Increased Mortality Due to Placental Malaria Infection. *AIDS* (1995) 9 (7):721–6. doi: 10.1097/00002030-199507000-00009
13. Mwapasa V, Rogerson SJ, Molyneux ME, Abrams ET, Kamwendo DD, Lema VM, et al. The Effect of Plasmodium Falciparum Malaria on Peripheral and Placental HIV-1 RNA Concentrations in Pregnant Malawian Women. *AIDS* (2004) 18(7):1051–9. doi: 10.1097/00002030-200404300-00014
14. Briand V, Badaut C, Cot M. Placental Malaria, Maternal HIV Infection and Infant Morbidity. *Ann Trop Paediatr* (2009) 29(2):71–83. doi: 10.1179/146532809X440699
15. Mockenhaupt FP, Bedu-Addo G, von Gaertner C, Boye R, Fricke K, Hannibal I, et al. Detection and Clinical Manifestation of Placental Malaria in Southern Ghana. *Malaria J* (2006) 5:119. doi: 10.1186/1475-2875-5-119
16. Naseem S, Anwar S, Ihsanullah M. Outcome and Complications of Malaria in Pregnancy. *Gomal J Med Sci* (2004) 6:98–101.
17. Nielson KS, Melo M, Vanella I. Primary HIV Infection During Pregnancy: High Rate of HIV-1 MTCT in a Cohort of Patients in South Brazil. *Retrovirology* (2008) 5(1). doi: 10.1186/1742-4690-5-S1-O1
18. Chua CL, Robinson LJ, Baiwog F, Stanisic DI, Hamilton JA, Brown GV, et al. High Numbers of Circulating Pigmented Polymorphonuclear Neutrophils as a Prognostic Marker for Decreased Birth Weight During Malaria in Pregnancy. *Int J Parasitol* (2015) 45(2-3):107–11. doi: 10.1016/j.ijpara.2014.12.002
19. Okamgba OC, Ifeanyichukwu MO, Ilesanmi AO, Chigbu LN. Variations in the Leukocyte and Cytokine Profiles Between Placental and Maternal Circulation in Pregnancy-Associated Malaria. *Res Rep Trop Med* (2018) 9:1–8. doi: 10.2147/RRTM.S137829
20. Ordi J, Menendez C, Ismail MR, Ventura PJ, Palacin A, Kahigwa E, et al. Placental Malaria Is Associated With Cell-Mediated Inflammatory Responses With Selective Absence of Natural Killer Cells. *J Infect Dis* (2001) 183(7):1100–7. doi: 10.1086/319295
21. Ordi J, Ismail MR, Ventura PJ, Kahigwa E, Hirt R, Cardesa A, et al. Massive Chronic Intervillositis of the Placenta Associated With Malaria Infection. *Am J Surg Pathol* (1998) 22(8):1006–11. doi: 10.1097/00000478-199808000-00011
22. Moormann AM, Sullivan AD, Rochford RA, Chensue SW, Bock PJ, Nyirenda T, et al. Malaria and Pregnancy: Placental Cytokine Expression

and Its Relationship to Intrauterine Growth Retardation. *J Infect Dis* (1999) 180(6):1987–93. doi: 10.1086/315135

23. Chaisavaneeyakorn S, Moore JM, Othoro C, Otieno J, Chaiyaroj SC, Shi YP, et al. Immunity to Placental Malaria. IV. Placental Malaria Is Associated With Up-Regulation of Macrophage Migration Inhibitory Factor in Intervillous Blood. *J Infect Dis* (2002) 186(9):1371–5.
24. Chaisavaneeyakorn S, Moore JM, Mirel L, Othoro C, Otieno J, Chaiyaroj SC, et al. Levels of Macrophage Inflammatory Protein 1 Alpha (MIP-1 Alpha) and MIP-1 Beta in Intervillous Blood Plasma Samples From Women With Placental Malaria and Human Immunodeficiency Virus Infection. *Clin Diagn Lab Immunol* (2003) 10(4):631–6. doi: 10.1128/cdli.10.4.631-636.2003
25. Chaisavaneeyakorn S, Lucchi N, Abramowsky C, Othoro C, Chaiyaroj SC, Shi YP, et al. Immunohistological Characterization of Macrophage Migration Inhibitory Factor Expression in Plasmodium Falciparum-Infected Placentas. *Infect Immun* (2005) 73(6):3287–93. doi: 10.1128/IAI.73.6.3287-3293.2005
26. Abrams ET, Brown H, Chensue SW, Turner GD, Tadesse E, Lema VM, et al. Host Response to Malaria During Pregnancy: Placental Monocyte Recruitment Is Associated With Elevated Beta Chemokine Expression. *J Immunol* (2003) 170(5):2759–64. doi: 10.4049/jimmunol.170.5.2759
27. Suguitan AL Jr, Leke RG, Fouda G, Zhou A, Thuita L, Metenou S, et al. Changes in the Levels of Chemokines and Cytokines in the Placentas of Women With Plasmodium Falciparum Malaria. *J Infect Dis* (2003) 188 (7):1074–82. doi: 10.1086/378500
28. Ambayya A, Su AT, Osman NH, Nik-Samsudin NR, Khalid K, Chang KM, et al. Haematological Reference Intervals in a Multiethnic Population. *PloS One* (2014) 9(3):e91968. doi: 10.1371/journal.pone.0091968
29. Sato R, Ikuma M, Takagi K, Yamagishi Y, Asano J, Matsunaga Y, et al. Exposure of Drugs for Hypertension, Diabetes, and Autoimmune Disease During Pregnancy and Perinatal Outcomes: An Investigation of the Regulator in Japan. *Med (Baltimore)* (2015) 94(1):e386. doi: 10.1097/MD.0000000000000386
30. Mayadas TN, Cullere X, Lowell CA. The Multifaceted Functions of Neutrophils. *Annu Rev Pathol* (2014) 9:181–218. doi: 10.1146/annurev-pathol-020712-164023
31. Schauer C, Janko C, Munoz LE, Zhao Y, Kienhofer D, Frey B, et al. Aggregated Neutrophil Extracellular Traps Limit Inflammation by Degrading Cytokines and Chemokines. *Nat Med* (2014) 20(5):511–7. doi: 10.1038/nm.3547
32. Fullerton JN, Gilroy DW. Resolution of Inflammation: A New Therapeutic Frontier. *Nat Rev Drug Discov* (2016) 15(8):551–67. doi: 10.1038/nrd.2016.39
33. Kolaczkowska E, Kubes P. Neutrophil Recruitment and Function in Health and Inflammation. *Nat Rev Immunol* (2013) 13(3):159–75. doi: 10.1038/nri3399
34. Choi JW, Im MW, Pai SH. Nitric Oxide Production Increases During Normal Pregnancy and Decreases in Preeclampsia. *Ann Clin Lab Sci* (2002) 32(3):257–63.
35. Liew PX, Kubes P. The Neutrophil's Role During Health and Disease. *Physiol Rev* (2019) 99(2):1223–48. doi: 10.1152/physrev.00012.2018
36. Aitken EH, Alemu A, Rogerson SJ. Neutrophils and Malaria. *Front Immunol* (2018) 9:3005. doi: 10.3389/fimmu.2018.03005
37. Amulic B, Moxon CA, Cunnington AJ. A More Granular View of Neutrophils in Malaria. *Trends Parasitol* (2020) 36(6):501–3. doi: 10.1016/j.pt.2020.03.003
38. Sercundes MK, Ortolan LS, Debone D, Soeiro-Pereira PV, Gomes E, Aitken EH, et al. Targeting Neutrophils to Prevent Malaria-Associated Acute Lung Injury/Acute Respiratory Distress Syndrome in Mice. *PloS Pathogens* (2016) 12(12):e1006054. doi: 10.1371/journal.ppat.1006054
39. Feintuch CM, Saidi A, Seydel K, Chen G, Goldman-Yassen A, Mita-Mendoza NK, et al. Activated Neutrophils Are Associated With Pediatric Cerebral Malaria Vasculopathy in Malawian Children. *mBio* (2016) 167(1): e01300–15. doi: 10.1128/mBio.01300-15
40. Porcherie A, Mathieu C, Peronet R, Schneider E, Claver J, Commere PH, et al. Critical Role of the Neutrophil-Associated High-Affinity Receptor for IgE in the Pathogenesis of Experimental Cerebral Malaria. *J Exp Med* (2011) 208(11):2225–36. doi: 10.1084/jem.20110845
41. Rocha BC, Marques PE, Leoratti FMS, Junqueira C, Pereira DB, Antonelli L, et al. Type I Interferon Transcriptional Signature in Neutrophils and Low-Density Granulocytes Are Associated With Tissue Damage in Malaria. *Cell Rep* (2015) 13(12):2829–41. doi: 10.1016/j.celrep.2015.11.055
42. Dasari P, Reiss K, Lingelbach K, Baumeister S, Lucius R, Udomsangpetch R, et al. Digestive Vacuoles of Plasmodium Falciparum Are Selectively Phagocytosed by and Impair Killing Function of Polymorphonuclear Leukocytes. *Blood* (2011) 118(18):4946–56. doi: 10.1182/blood-2011-05-353920
43. Sarr D, Cooper CA, Bracken TC, Martinez-Uribe O, Nagy T, Moore JM. Oxidative Stress: A Potential Therapeutic Target in Placental Malaria. *ImmunoHorizons* (2017) 1(4):29–41. doi: 10.4049/immunohorizons.1700002
44. Megnekou R, Djontu JC, Bigoga JD, Medou FM, Tenou S, Lissom A. Impact of Placental Plasmodium Falciparum Malaria on the Profile of Some Oxidative Stress Biomarkers in Women Living in Yaounde, Cameroon. *PloS One* (2015) 10(8):e0134633. doi: 10.1371/journal.pone.0134633
45. Sharma L, Kaur J, Shukla G. Role of Oxidative Stress and Apoptosis in the Placental Pathology of Plasmodium Berghei Infected Mice. *PloS One* (2012) 7(3):e32694. doi: 10.1371/journal.pone.0032694
46. Sharma L, Kaur J, Rishi P, Shukla G. Plasmodium Berghei: Influence of Infection on the Oxidant and Antioxidants Levels in Pregnant BALB/c Mice. *Exp Parasitol* (2012) 131(2):215–22. doi: 10.1016/j.exppara.2012.04.005
47. Brinkmann V, Zychlinsky A. Beneficial Suicide: Why Neutrophils Die to Make NETs. *Nat Rev Microbiol* (2007) 5(8):577–82. doi: 10.1038/nrmicro1710
48. Brinkmann V, Reichard U, Goosmann C, Fauler B, Uhlemann Y, Weiss DS, et al. Neutrophil Extracellular Traps Kill Bacteria. *Science* (2004) 303 (5663):1532–5. doi: 10.1126/science.1092385
49. Masuda S, Nakazawa D, Shida H, Miyoshi A, Kusunoki Y, Tomaru U, et al. NETosis Markers: Quest for Specific, Objective, and Quantitative Markers. *Clinica Chimica Acta; Int J Clin Chem* (2016) 459:89–93. doi: 10.1016/j.cca.2016.05.029
50. Kessenbrock K, Krumbholz M, Schonermarck U, Back W, Gross WL, Werb Z, et al. Netting Neutrophils in Autoimmune Small-Vessel Vasculitis. *Nat Med* (2009) 15(6):623–5. doi: 10.1038/nm.1959
51. Nakazawa D, Tomaru U, Suzuki A, Masuda S, Hasegawa R, Kobayashi T, et al. Abnormal Conformation and Impaired Degradation of Propylthiouracil-Induced Neutrophil Extracellular Traps: Implications of Disordered Neutrophil Extracellular Traps in a Rat Model of Myeloperoxidase Antineutrophil Cytoplasmic Antibody-Associated Vasculitis. *Arthritis Rheumatol* (2012) 64(11):3779–87. doi: 10.1002/art.34619.Citedin:Pubmed
52. Gavillet M, Martinod K, Renella R, Harris C, Shapiro NI, Wagner DD, et al. Flow Cytometric Assay for Direct Quantification of Neutrophil Extracellular Traps in Blood Samples. *Am J Hematol* (2015) 90(12):1155–8. doi: 10.1002/ajh.24185
53. Tucker SL, Sarr D, Rada B. Neutrophil Extracellular Traps Are Present in the Airways of ENaC-Overexpressing Mice With Cystic Fibrosis-Like Lung Disease. *BMC Immunol* (2021) 22(1):7. doi: 10.1186/s12865-021-00397-w
54. Rodrigues DAS, Prestes EB, Gama AMS, Silva LS, Pinheiro AAS, Ribeiro JMC, et al. CXCR4 and MIF Are Required for Neutrophil Extracellular Trap Release Triggered by Plasmodium-Infected Erythrocytes. *PloS Pathogens* (2020) 16(8):e1008230. doi: 10.1371/journal.ppat.1008230
55. Chang Z, Jiang N, Zhang Y, Lu H, Yin J, Wahlgren M, et al. TatD-Like DNase of Plasmodium Is a Virulence Factor and a Potential Malaria Vaccine Candidate. *Nat Commun* (2016) 7:11537. doi: 10.1038/ncomms11537
56. Baker VS, Imade GE, Molta NB, Tawde P, Pam SD, Obadofin MO, et al. Cytokine-Associated Neutrophil Extracellular Traps and Antinuclear Antibodies in Plasmodium Falciparum Infected Children Under Six Years of Age. *Malaria J* (2008) 7:41. doi: 10.1186/1475-2875-7-41
57. Kho S, Minigo G, Andries B, Leonardo L, Prayoga P, Poespoprodjo JR, et al. Circulating Neutrophil Extracellular Traps and Neutrophil Activation Are Increased in Proportion to Disease Severity in Human Malaria. *J Infect Dis* (2019) 219(12):1994–2004. doi: 10.1093/infdis/jiy661
58. Knackstedt SL, Georgiadou A, Apel F, Abu-Abed U, Moxon CA, Cunnington AJ, et al. Neutrophil Extracellular Traps Drive Inflammatory Pathogenesis in Malaria. *Sci Immunol* (2019) 4(40):1–9. doi: 10.1126/sciimmunol.aaw0336

59. Avery JW, Smith GM, Owino SO, Sarr D, Nagy T, Mwalimu S, et al. Maternal Malaria Induces a Procoagulant and Antifibrinolytic State That Is Embryotoxic But Responsive to Anticoagulant Therapy. *PloS One* (2012) 7 (2):e31090. doi: 10.1371/journal.pone.0031090
60. Othoro C, Moore JM, Wannemuehler K, Nahlen BL, Otieno J, Slutsker L, et al. Evaluation of Various Methods of Maternal Placental Blood Collection for Immunology Studies. *Clin Vaccine Immunol* (2006) 13(5):568–74. doi: 10.1128/CVI.13.5.568-574.2006
61. Ayisi JG, van Eijk AM, ter Kuile FO, Kolczak MS, Otieno JA, Misore AO, et al. The Effect of Dual Infection With HIV and Malaria on Pregnancy Outcome in Western Kenya. *AIDS* (2003) 17(4):585–94. doi: 10.1097/00002030-200303070-00014
62. Yoo DG, Winn M, Pang L, Moskowitz SM, Malech HL, Leto TL, et al. Release of Cystic Fibrosis Airway Inflammatory Markers From Pseudomonas Aeruginosa-Stimulated Human Neutrophils Involves NADPH Oxidase-Dependent Extracellular DNA Trap Formation. *J Immunol* (2014) 192(10):4728–38. doi: 10.4049/jimmunol.1301589
63. Floyd M, Winn M, Cullen C, Sil P, Chassaing B, Yoo DG, et al. Swimming Motility Mediates the Formation of Neutrophil Extracellular Traps Induced by Flagellated Pseudomonas Aeruginosa. *PloS Pathogens* (2016) 12(11): e1005987. doi: 10.1371/journal.ppat.1005987
64. Yadav R, Yoo DG, Kahlenberg JM, Bridges SL Jr, Oni O, Huang H, et al. Systemic Levels of Anti-PAD4 Autoantibodies Correlate With Airway Obstruction in Cystic Fibrosis. *J Cyst Fibros* (2019) 18(5):636–45. doi: 10.1016/j.jcf.2018.12.010
65. Yadav R, Linnemann RW, Kahlenberg JM, Bridges LS Jr, Stecenko AA, Rada B. IgA Autoantibodies Directed Against Self DNA Are Elevated in Cystic Fibrosis and Associated With More Severe Lung Dysfunction. *Autoimmunity* (2020) 53(8):476–84. doi: 10.1080/08916934.2020.1839890
66. Sarr D, Bracken TC, Owino SO, Cooper CA, Smith GM, Nagy T, et al. Differential Roles of Inflammation and Apoptosis in Initiation of Mid-Gestational Abortion in Malaria-Infected C57BL/6 and a/J Mice. *Placenta* (2015) 36(7):738–49. doi: 10.1016/j.placenta.2015.04.007
67. Bankhead P, Loughrey MB, Fernandez JA, Dombrowski Y, McArt DG, Dunne PD, et al. QuPath: Open Source Software for Digital Pathology Image Analysis. *Sci Rep* (2017) 7(1):16878. doi: 10.1038/s41598-017-17204-5
68. Ginley BG, Emmons T, Lutnick B, Urban CF, Segal BH, Sarder P. Computational Detection and Quantification of Human and Mouse Neutrophil Extracellular Traps in Flow Cytometry and Confocal Microscopy. *Sci Rep* (2017) 7(1):17755. doi: 10.1038/s41598-017-18099-y
69. Menendez C, Ordi J, Ismail MR, Ventura PJ, Aponte JJ, Kahigwa E, et al. The Impact of Placental Malaria on Gestational Age and Birth Weight. *J Infect Dis* (2000) 181(5):1740–5. doi: 10.1086/315449
70. Bulmer JN, Rasheed FN, Francis N, Morrison L, Greenwood BM. Placental Malaria. I. Pathological classification. *Histopathology* (1993) 22(3):211–8. doi: 10.1111/j.1365-2559.1993.tb00110.x
71. Ismail MR, Ordi J, Menendez C, Ventura PJ, Aponte JJ, Kahigwa E, et al. Placental Pathology in Malaria: A Histological, Immunohistochemical, and Quantitative Study. *Hum Pathol* (2000) 31(1):85–93. doi: 10.1016/S0046-8177(00)80203-8
72. Rogerson SJ, Hviid L, Duffy PE, Leke RF, Taylor DW. Malaria in Pregnancy: Pathogenesis and Immunity. *Lancet Infect Dis* (2007) 7(2):105–17. doi: 10.1016/S1473-3099(07)70022-1
73. Muehlenbachs A, Fried M, McGready R, Harrington WE, Mutabingwa TK, Nosten F, et al. A Novel Histological Grading Scheme for Placental Malaria Applied in Areas of High and Low Malaria Transmission. *J Infect Dis* (2010) 202(10):1608–16. doi: 10.1086/656723
74. Urban CF, Ermert D, Schmid M, Abu-Abed U, Goosmann C, Nacken W, et al. Neutrophil Extracellular Traps Contain Calprotectin, a Cytosolic Protein Complex Involved in Host Defense Against Candida Albicans. *PloS Pathogens* (2009) 5(10):e1000639. doi: 10.1371/journal.ppat.1000639
75. Papayannopoulos V, Metzler KD, Hakkim A, Zychlinsky A. Neutrophil Elastase and Myeloperoxidase Regulate the Formation of Neutrophil Extracellular Traps. *J Cell Biol* (2010) 191(3):677–91. doi: 10.1083/jcb.201006052
76. Sarr D, Marrama L, Gaye A, Dangou JM, Niang M, Mercereau-Puijalon O, et al. High Prevalence of Placental Malaria and Low Birth Weight in Sahelian Periurban Area. *Am J Trop Med Hygiene* (2006) 75(1):171–7. doi: 10.4269/ajtmh.2006.75.171
77. Davison BB, Kaack MB, Rogers LB, Rasmussen KK, Rasmussen T, Henson EW, et al. Alterations in the Profile of Blood Cell Types During Malaria in Previously Unexposed Primigravid Monkeys. *J Infect Dis* (2005) 191 (11):1940–52. doi: 10.1086/430004
78. Mandala WL, Gondwe EN, Molyneux ME, MacLennan JM, MacLennan CA. Leukocyte Counts and Lymphocyte Subsets in Relation to Pregnancy and HIV Infection in Malawian Women. *Am J Reprod Immunol* (2017) 78(3):1–7. doi: 10.1111/aji.12678
79. Giaglis S, Stoikou M, Grimolizzi F, Subramanian BY, van Breda SV, Hoesli I, et al. Neutrophil Migration Into the Placenta: Good, Bad or Deadly? *Cell Adh Migr* (2016) 10(1-2):208–25. doi: 10.1080/19336918.2016.1148866
80. Knall C, Worthen GS, Johnson GL. Interleukin 8-Stimulated Phosphatidylinositol-3-Kinase Activity Regulates the Migration of Human Neutrophils Independent of Extracellular Signal-Regulated Kinase and P38 Mitogen-Activated Protein Kinases. *Proc Natl Acad Sci USA* (1997) 94 (7):3052–7. doi: 10.1073/pnas.94.7.3052
81. Lucchi NW, Sarr D, Owino SO, Mwalimu SM, Peterson DS, Moore JM. Natural Hemozoin Stimulates Syncytiotrophoblast to Secrete Chemokines and Recruit Peripheral Blood Mononuclear Cells. *Placenta* (2011) 32 (8):579–85. doi: 10.1016/j.placenta.2011.05.003
82. Vasquez AM, Segura C, Blair S. Induction of Pro-Inflammatory Response of the Placental Trophoblast by Plasmodium Falciparum Infected Erythrocytes and TNF. *Malaria J* (2013) 12:421. doi: 10.1186/1475-2875-12-421
83. Stockfelt M, Larsson G, Engstrom H, Puttonen H, Zetterberg H, Blennow K, et al. Activated Low-Density Granulocytes in Peripheral and Intervillous Blood and Neutrophil Inflammation in Placentas From SLE Pregnancies. *Lupus Sci Med* (2021) 8(1):1–12. doi: 10.1136/lupus-2020-000463
84. Pullar JM, Vissers MC, Winterbourn CC. Living With a Killer: The Effects of Hypochlorous Acid on Mammalian Cells. *IUBMB Life* (2000) 50(4-5):259–66. doi: 10.1080/713803731
85. Theess W, Sellau J, Steeg C, Klinke A, Baldus S, Cramer JP, et al. Myeloperoxidase Attenuates Pathogen Clearance During Plasmodium Yoelii Nonlethal Infection. *Infect Immun* (2017) 85(1):1–10. doi: 10.1128/IAI.00475-16
86. Vita JA, Brennan ML, Gokce N, Mann SA, Goormastic M, Shishehbor MH, et al. Serum Myeloperoxidase Levels Independently Predict Endothelial Dysfunction in Humans. *Circulation* (2004) 110(9):1134–9. doi: 10.1161/01.CIR.0000140262.20831.8F
87. Sugiyama S, Okada Y, Sukhova GK, Virmani R, Heinecke JW, Libby P. Macrophage Myeloperoxidase Regulation by Granulocyte Macrophage Colony-Stimulating Factor in Human Atherosclerosis and Implications in Acute Coronary Syndromes. *Am J Pathol* (2001) 158(3):879–91. doi: 10.1016/S0002-9440(10)64036-9
88. Klebanoff SJ. Myeloperoxidase: Friend and Foe. *J Leukoc Biol* (2005) 77 (5):598–625. doi: 10.1189/jlb.1204697
89. Gandley RE, Rohland J, Zhou Y, Shibata E, Harger GF, Rajakumar A, et al. Increased Myeloperoxidase in the Placenta and Circulation of Women With Preeclampsia. *Hypertension* (2008) 52(2):387–93. doi: 10.1161/HYPERTENSIONAHA.107.107532
90. Hung TH, Chen SF, Lo LM, Li MJ, Yeh YL, Hsieh TT. Myeloperoxidase in the Plasma and Placenta of Normal Pregnant Women and Women With Pregnancies Complicated by Preeclampsia and Intrauterine Growth Restriction. *Placenta* (2012) 33(4):294–303. doi: 10.1016/j.placenta.2012.01.004
91. Mruma HA, McQuillan R, Norrie J. The Association of Malaria Infection and Gestational Hypertension in Africa: Systematic Review and Meta-Analysis. *J Glob Health* (2020) 10(2):20417. doi: 10.7189/jogh.10.020417
92. Obiri D, Erskine IJ, Oduro D, Kusi KA, Amponsah J, Gyan BA, et al. Histopathological Lesions and Exposure to Plasmodium Falciparum Infections in the Placenta Increases the Risk of Preeclampsia Among Pregnant Women. *Sci Rep* (2020) 10(1):8280. doi: 10.1038/s41598-020-64736-4
93. Prato M, Giribaldi G, Polimeni M, Gallo V, Arese P. Phagocytosis of Hemozoin Enhances Matrix Metalloproteinase-9 Activity and TNF-Alpha Production in Human Monocytes: Role of Matrix Metalloproteinases in the Pathogenesis of Falciparum Malaria. *J Immunol* (2005) 175(10):6436–42 doi: 10.4049/jimmunol.175.10.6436
94. Prato M, Gallo V, Giribaldi G, Arese P. Phagocytosis of Haemozoin (Malarial Pigment) Enhances Metalloproteinase-9 Activity in Human Adherent Monocytes: Role of IL-1beta and 15-HETE. *Malaria J* (2008) 7:157. doi: 10.1186/1475-2875-7-157
95. Prato M, Giribaldi G. Matrix Metalloproteinase-9 and Haemozoin: Wedding

Rings for Human Host and Plasmodium Falciparum Parasite in Complicated Malaria. *J Trop Med* (2011) 2011:628435. doi: 10.1155/2011/628435

96. Apoorv TS, Babu PP, Meese S, Gai PP, Bedu-Addo G, Mockenhaupt FP. Matrix Metalloproteinase-9 Polymorphism 1562 C > T (Rs3918242) Associated With Protection Against Placental Malaria. *Am J Trop Med Hygiene* (2015) 93(1):186–8. doi: 10.4269/ajtmh.14-0816
97. Porto BN, Stein RT. Neutrophil Extracellular Traps in Pulmonary Diseases: Too Much of a Good Thing? *Front Immunol* (2016) 7:311. doi: 10.3389/fimmu.2016.00311
98. Rada B. Neutrophil Extracellular Traps. *Methods Mol Biol* (2019) 1982:517–28. doi: 10.1007/978-1-4939-9424-3_31
99. Rada B. Interactions Between Neutrophils and Pseudomonas Aeruginosa in Cystic Fibrosis. *Pathogens* (2017) 6(1):1–24. doi: 10.3390/pathogens6010010
100. Tsukimori K, Nakano H, Wake N. Difference in Neutrophil Superoxide Generation During Pregnancy Between Preeclampsia and Essential Hypertension. *Hypertension* (2007) 49(6):1436–41. doi: 10.1161/HYPERTENSIONAHA.106.086751
101. Agarwal A, Aponte-Mellado A, Premkumar BJ, Shaman A, Gupta S. The Effects of Oxidative Stress on Female Reproduction: A Review. *Reprod Biol Endocrinol* (2012) 10:49. doi: 10.1186/1477-7827-10-49
102. Aly AS, Khandelwal M, Zhao J, Mehmet AH, Sammel MD, Parry S. Neutrophils Are Stimulated by Syncytiotrophoblast Microvillous Membranes to Generate Superoxide Radicals in Women With Preeclampsia. *Am J Obstetrics Gynecol* (2004) 190(1):252–8. doi: 10.1016/j.ajog.2003.07.003
103. Gupta AK, Hasler P, Holzgreve W, Hahn S. Neutrophil NETs: A Novel Contributor to Preeclampsia-Associated Placental Hypoxia? *Semin Immunopathol* (2007) 29(2):163–7. doi: 10.1007/s00281-007-0073-4
104. Hahn S, Giaglis S, Hoesli I, Hasler P. Neutrophil NETs in Reproduction: From Infertility to Preeclampsia and the Possibility of Fetal Loss. *Front Immunol* (2012) 3:362. doi: 10.3389/fimmu.2012.00362
105. Marder W, Knight JS, Kaplan MJ, Somers EC, Zhang X, O'Dell AA, et al. Placental Histology and Neutrophil Extracellular Traps in Lupus and Pre-Eclampsia Pregnancies. *Lupus Sci Med* (2016) 3(1):e000134. doi: 10.1136/lupus-2015-000134
106. Pattison DI, Davies MJ, Hawkins CL. Reactions and Reactivity of Myeloperoxidase-Derived Oxidants: Differential Biological Effects of Hypochlorous and Hypothiocyanous Acids. *Free Radic Res* (2012) 46 (8):975–95. doi: 10.3109/10715762.2012.667566
107. Rayner BS, Love DT, Hawkins CL. Comparative Reactivity of Myeloperoxidase-Derived Oxidants With Mammalian Cells. *Free Radical Biol Med* (2014) 71:240–55. doi: 10.1016/j.freeradbiomed.2014.03.004
108. Winterbourn CC, Kettle AJ. Redox Reactions and Microbial Killing in the Neutrophil Phagosome. *Antioxid Redox Signal* (2013) 18(6):642–60. doi: 10.1089/ars.2012.4827

8

Do Antibodies to Malaria Surface Antigens Play a Role in Protecting Mothers from Maternal Anemia?

Madeleine C. Wiebe[1] *and Stephanie K. Yanow*[1,2*]

[1] Department of Medical Microbiology and Immunology, University of Alberta, Edmonton, AB, Canada, [2] School of Public Health, University of Alberta, Edmonton, AB, Canada

***Correspondence:**
Stephanie K. Yanow
yanow@ualberta.ca*

Pregnancy-associated malaria (PAM) caused by *Plasmodium falciparum* can result in detrimental outcomes for both mother and infant, including low infant birth weight, preterm birth, maternal anemia, spontaneous abortion, and maternal and/or infant mortality. Maternal anemia is a particularly complex outcome, as the body must both maintain erythropoiesis and tolerance of the growing fetus, while directing a Th1 response against the parasite. Underlying the pathogenesis of PAM is the expression of variant surface antigens (VSA_{PAM}) on the surface of infected red blood cells (iRBC) that mediate sequestration of the iRBC in the placenta. Naturally acquired antibodies to VSA_{PAM} can block sequestration and activate opsonic phagocytosis, both associated with improved pregnancy outcomes. In this review, we ask whether VSA_{PAM} antibodies can also protect mothers against malarial anemia. Studies were identified where VSA_{PAM} antibody titres and/or function were associated with higher maternal hemoglobin levels, thus supporting additional protective mechanisms for these antibodies against PAM. Yet these associations were not widely observed, and many studies reported no association between protection from maternal anemia and VSA_{PAM} antibodies. We discuss the epidemiological, biological and technical factors that may explain some of the variability among these studies. We appraise the current evidence of these complex interactions between PAM-specific immunity and maternal anemia, propose potential mechanisms, and discuss knowledge gaps.

Keywords: pregnancy-associated malaria, anemia, inflammation, placenta, VAR2CSA antibodies, VSA_{PAM} antibodies

INTRODUCTION

Pregnant women are especially vulnerable to malaria compared to non-pregnant adults in Africa (1) and 11 million pregnancies are at risk for complications from pregnancy-associated malaria (PAM) on this continent (2) in addition to those in lower transmission regions elsewhere (3). PAM is attributed to poor fetal outcomes including stillbirths (4), low birth weight infants (2) and premature births (5). PAM also significantly contributes to severe maternal anemia (6).

During a *Plasmodium falciparum* infection in high transmission settings, primigravid women have an especially high risk of poor pregnancy outcomes, and this risk decreases with gravidity [reviewed in (7)]. Pregnancy outcomes can affect both mother (maternal anemia, maternal morbidity and mortality) and child (low infant birth weight, pre-term birth, and spontaneous abortion). After several instances of PAM, protection may be conferred by acquired immunity (8). Specifically, antibodies to pregnancy-specific variant surface antigens (VSA_{PAM}) expressed on the surface of the infected red blood cell (iRBC) are known to disrupt the adherence of iRBCs to chondroitin sulfate A (CSA) in the placenta and prevent parasite sequestration here (9, 10). One of the key targets of these maternal antibodies is VAR2CSA, a VSA expressed on the iRBC surface that directly binds to CSA (11). VAR2CSA antibodies are associated with improved pregnancy outcomes (12) and as a result, are the focus of vaccines to prevent PAM (13, 14).

While antibody-mediated immune mechanisms are associated with improved birth outcomes, particularly increased infant birth weight, we do not know whether these humoral mechanisms could protect women from developing anemia. By preventing sequestration of iRBCs in the placenta or opsonizing VSAs on the surface of iRBCs, VSA_{PAM} antibodies may promote iRBC phagocytosis in the intervillous spaces (IVS) of the placenta or parasite killing in the spleen, lowering parasitemia and reducing the risk of maternal anemia. However, the development of anemia in PAM and its connection to humoral immunity is not well defined and potential underlying mechanisms of protection warrant investigation (15). Here, we first consider the causes of maternal anemia in PAM, and then examine the studies that investigated associations between anemia and VSA_{PAM} antibodies.

MECHANISMS OF ANEMIA IN THE CONTEXT OF PAM

Maternal anemia is a common, but particularly complex consequence of PAM, typically defined as a hemoglobin level less than 11 g/dL, with mild and severe anemia for pregnant women defined at 10–10.9 g/dL and less than 7 g/dL, respectively (16). In a healthy pregnancy, the maternal vasculature must vasodilate approximately 5 weeks into pregnancy, with total blood volume and red cell mass significantly increased (17). An increase in plasma volume compared to red cell production results in physiological anemia during pregnancy that usually resolves by the third trimester (reviewed in (18, 19)). However, anemia is exacerbated by poor nutrition, iron deficiency, and maternal hypertension (reviewed in (20)).

If anemia develops due to malaria infection, this can result in maternal morbidity and mortality as the red cell population is compromised. Some mechanisms of anemia are shared between uncomplicated malaria and PAM, such as obligate hemolysis as the schizont ruptures, which triggers a pro-inflammatory response. In uncomplicated malaria, a profound loss of nRBCs contributes to anemia (21), as red cell deformability is reduced, which has been correlated with a lower hemoglobin concentration (22, 23) but whether this also occurs in the placenta is not known. This loss of non-infected RBCs (nRBCs) is yet to be observed in the PAM setting. Dysregulated erythropoiesis is also reported in uncomplicated malaria, often due to production of pro-inflammatory mediators including cytokines, nitric oxide, and lipoperoxides that can lead to bone marrow dysfunction [reviewed in (24, 25)].

In pregnancy, tolerance to the fetus must be maintained primarily with a T helper (Th) 2 response, through secretions of TGF-β, IL-4, and IL-6 (26–28). However, a *P. falciparum* infection triggers a Th1 response, increasing pro-inflammatory cytokine secretions including IL-1β, TNFα, and IFNγ. Moore et al. observed that intervillous blood mononuclear cells from multigravid women negative for placental malaria had the highest secretions of IFNγ, while cells from primigravid and secundigravid women positive for placental malaria had low IFNγ secretions (29). Thus, an increased production of IFNγ may help control a placental infection. However, pro-inflammatory mediators have also been associated with detrimental placental inflammation. Increased TNFα in primigravid women was associated with placental lesions, while increased IL-1β was associated with congenital malaria (30). This pro-inflammatory response was associated with severe maternal anemia (27). The increase in pro-inflammatory cytokines may also inhibit erythropoiesis in the bone marrow, leading to bone marrow dysfunction and contributing to overall maternal anemia (reviewed in (31), though this has not been shown specifically for PAM. In response to the pro-inflammatory state in the placenta, IL-10 is frequently elevated along with pro-inflammatory mediators in PAM (32, 33) in attempts to maintain a healthy pregnancy (reviewed in (34). Thus, IL-10 can be considered a marker for dangerous placental inflammation (29, 32, 35, 36) and levels of IL-10 correlated with maternal anemia (32, 33).

A source of these cytokines in the placenta are monocytes and macrophages (34, 37, 38), which often accumulate in the IVS during infection. Antibodies may fine-tune this response by directly targeting the parasite, blocking iRBC sequestration in the placenta and/or increasing opsonic phagocytosis by targeting iRBCs for engulfment. These potential mechanisms, as illustrated in **Figure 1**, may lower parasitemia in the placenta so that a prolonged inflammatory response is not required.

Further investigation is required to elucidate the mechanisms of anemia in PAM compared with uncomplicated malaria. Far less is published on anemia in PAM, and yet there may be significant differences due to changes in immune regulation that occur in pregnancy. For example, a Th1 response to combat a malaria infection could pose a greater risk in pregnancy compared to uncomplicated malaria as maintenance of a Th2 response is important for the health of the fetus. The investigation of the role of VSA_{PAM} antibodies is further complicated by the multifactorial causes of anemia during PAM, which may alter the relationship between antibody titre/function and maternal anemia. Thus, a connection between VSA_{PAM} antibodies and maternal anemia may be difficult to elucidate.

STUDIES OF VSA_{PAM} ANTIBODIES AND MATERNAL ANEMIA

Women without prior exposure to PAM lack antibodies to the unique pregnancy-specific VSA that mediate sequestration of iRBCs to the placenta. Pregnant women can eventually acquire antibodies against these VSA and the levels of these antibodies increase with gravidity (8, 39). There is evidence for an

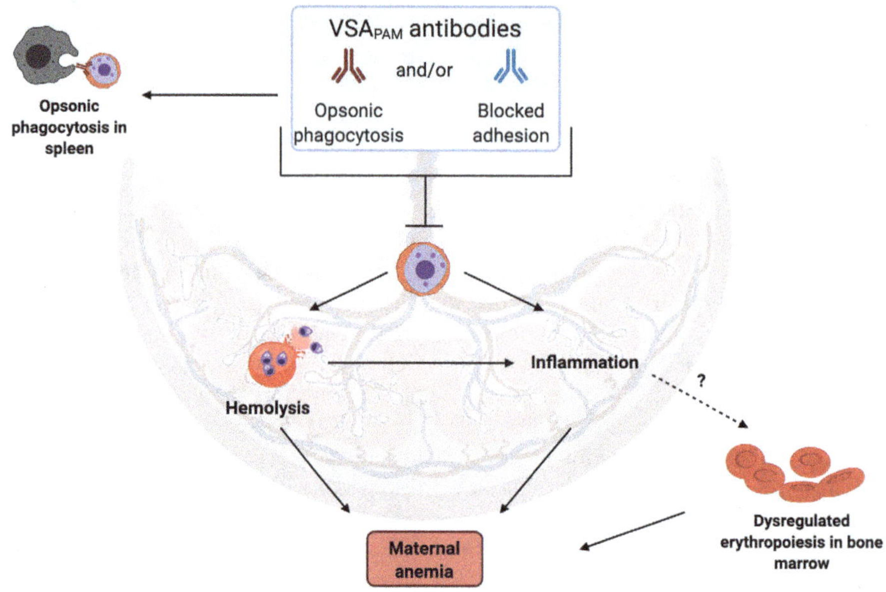

FIGURE 1 | Mechanisms by which VSA$_{PAM}$ antibodies could protect against anemia in PAM. VSA$_{PAM}$ antibodies that bind to the surface of iRBCs can promote iRBC clearance from the placenta by preventing sequestration and/or promoting opsonic phagocytosis in the IVS of the placenta or in the spleen. Both of these mechanisms would reduce placental parasitemia and could prevent several of the downstream mechanisms that lead to maternal anemia; one of these is iRBC hemolysis, where parasite material is released and detected by toll-like receptors present on cells in the IVS, activating a pro-inflammatory response. Reduced inflammation may in turn prevent dysregulated erythropoiesis in the bone marrow, further protecting against maternal anemia. (Created with BioRender.com).

association between VSA$_{PAM}$ antibodies and improved birth weight (40), but less is known whether these antibodies can also protect women from maternal anemia. Here, we discuss the limited studies on VSA$_{PAM}$ antibodies and anemia (**Table 1**).

Studies With No Correlation Between VSA$_{PAM}$ Antibodies and Maternal Anemia

In the first study to relate measures of VSA$_{PAM}$ antibodies to birth outcomes, plasma from Kenyan pregnant mothers was tested in the inhibition of binding assay (IBA) with placental isolates and correlated to infant birth weight, gestational age, and maternal hemoglobin at delivery (40). Plasma that blocked >35% of parasite binding to CSA was considered positive for blocking antibodies. Such antibodies were only observed in 1 of 47 primigravid women, while in secondigravid women, anti-adhesion activity was greater and associated with both increased infant birth weight and gestational age. However, there was no relationship between anti-adhesion antibodies and maternal hemoglobin levels (40).

This association was also observed in a study in Benin, where antibody titres were measured against the recombinant proteins DBL1-DBL2X, DBL5ϵ, and DBL6ϵ by ELISA, and functional activity was assessed by IBA (41). Increased anti-adhesion activity was associated with a decreased risk of placental infection at delivery and low birth weight, but there was no association between antibody titres or anti-adhesion activity and maternal anemia at delivery (41).

Opsonic phagocytosis of iRBCs is an important measure of antibody function. In primigravid women from Malawi, serum samples were collected in the late third trimester and tested for reactivity to CS2 parasites by flow cytometry and opsonic phagocytosis (42). No association was observed with maternal anemia or infant birth weight and VSA$_{PAM}$ antibodies. The study was continued with third trimester samples from secundigravid women (43). Again, no association was observed between maternal anemia and VSA$_{PAM}$ IgG or opsonic activity, but a positive correlation between opsonic phagocytosis and infant birth weight was observed.

Other studies compared hemoglobin measurements to IgG titres but not to antibody function. In Mozambique, serum samples collected at delivery were tested by ELISA for reactivity against a number of malarial antigens expressed in uncomplicated malaria and during PAM, including DBL5ϵ and DBL6ϵ, along with reactivity to two placental isolates (44). VSA$_{PAM}$ IgG against one isolate was associated with increased birth weight and gestational age of infants, but no association was found with maternal anemia. In Senegal, IgG was measured against the VAR2CSA subdomains DBL1X, DBL5ϵ, and DBL6ϵ by ELISA and compared with maternal anemia at enrollment and delivery in samples from primigravid, secondigravid, and multigravid women (45). IgG levels against DBL5ϵ and DBL6ϵ at enrollment and delivery were parity-dependent, and high IgG titres correlated with past malaria infection rather than acute PAM. In this study, there was no association between the levels of antibodies against these VAR2CSA domains and maternal anemia or birth weight at any measured time point. Similarly, in a study from Mozambique, the levels of antibody that stained the native VSA on CS2 parasites in flow cytometry did not associate with maternal anemia at delivery (46). Surprisingly, these

TABLE 1 | Summary of studies on VSA_{PAM} antibodies and maternal anemia.

Citation	Setting	Assays used	Time of serum/ plasma collection	Anemia-related outcomes
No association between VSA_{PAM} antibodies and maternal anemia				
Duffy and Fried (40)	Kenya	IBA	Delivery	VSA_{PAM} blocking antibodies were not associated with maternal hemoglobin at delivery
Ndam et al. (41)	Benin	ELISA, IBA	Delivery	VSA_{PAM} blocking antibodies were not associated with maternal anemia at delivery
Ataide et al. (42)	Malawi	Flow, opsonic phagocytosis	Late third trimester	VSA_{PAM} antibodies from primigravid women were not associated with maternal hemoglobin
Ataide et al. (43)	Malawi	Flow, opsonic phagocytosis	Late third trimester	VSA_{PAM} antibodies from secundigravid women were not associated with maternal hemoglobin
Mayor et al. (44)	Mozambique	ELISA, Flow	Delivery	VSA_{PAM} antibodies were not associated with maternal anemia
Ndam et al., 2006 (45)	Senegal	ELISA	First to second trimester and delivery	Seroreactive antibodies against VAR2CSA subdomains were not associated with maternal anemia
Serra-Casas et al. (46)	Mozambique	Flow	Delivery	VSA_{PAM} antibodies were not associated with maternal anemia
Aitken et al. (47)	Malawi	Flow	28–34 weeks gestation	VSA_{PAM} antibodies were not associated with maternal hemoglobin
Fried et al. (48)	Mali	Multiplex	Second trimester	Seroreactive antibodies against VAR2CSA subdomains were not correlated with a reduced risk of maternal anemia
Mixed association between VSA_{PAM} antibodies and maternal anemia				
Lloyd et al. (49)	Cameroon	Multiplex	Delivery	Seroreactive antibodies against VAR2CSA were associated with lower hematocrit levels and increased prevalence of anemia in women negative for placental infection
Staalsoe et al. (50)	Kenya	Flow	Delivery	Levels of VSA_{PAM} antibodies correlated with hemoglobin in women with chronic placental infection but not acute or past infection
Association between VSA_{PAM} antibodies and maternal anemia				
Feng et al., (51)	Malawi	Opsonic phagocytosis	14–20 weeks gestation	Two-fold increase in opsonic phagocytosis index was associated with reduced odds of maternal anemia
Jaworowski et al. (52)	Malawi	Opsonic phagocytosis	Third trimester	VSA_{PAM} antibodies from anemic women displayed significantly lower opsonizing activity compared to non-anemic women
Chandrasiri et al. (53)	Malawi	Flow, opsonic phagocytosis	Before 20 weeks gestation	10% increase in opsonic phagocytosis index was associated with maternal hemoglobin increase of 0.4 g/L at 36 weeks gestation
Sander et al. (54)	Cameroon	Detection of *var2csa* copy number	First, second, and third trimester	In Ngali II, increasing *var2csa* copy number, which correlated with antibodies against DBL4ϵ, was associated with higher maternal hemoglobin
Chandrasiri et al. (55)	Sudan	Flow, opsonic phagocytosis, cytokine profiles	Second and third trimester	DBL5ϵ antibodies and maternal hemoglobin were negatively correlated with pro-inflammatory cytokines; opsonizing antibodies were positively associated with hemoglobin
Gavina et al. (56)	Colombia	ELISA, IBA	First and second trimester	VSA_{PAM} blocking antibodies were positively associated with maternal hemoglobin

antibodies did not correlate with other birth outcomes either, including preterm birth or low birth weight.

Two longitudinal studies reported VSA_{PAM} antibody and hemoglobin levels throughout pregnancy, and both failed to identify a correlation between antibody levels at enrollment and pregnancy outcomes. The first study reported IgG titres in pregnant Malawi women from serum collected at various points in pregnancy including study enrollment, 28–34 gestational weeks, and 1–6 months postpartum (47). There was a non-significant downward trend in antibody levels against VSA-expressing parasites CS2 and HCS3-VSA from enrollment to one month postpartum, but IgG remained detectable 6 months after delivery in 72% of women. Despite the persistence of the VSA_{PAM} antibodies, they were not associated with an increase in maternal hemoglobin levels. Fried et al. published findings from Mali with plasma samples collected at enrollment, 30–32 gestational weeks, and at delivery (48). A multiplex bead assay was used to determine seropositivity to a large number of VAR2CSA subdomains, including DBL2X, DBL4ϵ, and ID1-ID2a, but notably not the full-length protein. Increased antibody titres against either of the DBL domains were not significantly associated with any type of protection.

Mixed Association Between VSA_{PAM} Antibodies and Maternal Anemia

In Cameroon, two groups of women, one positive and one negative for placental malaria, both had overall low antibody levels to full-length VAR2CSA at delivery (49). Among women positive for placental malaria, higher seropositivity against VAR2CSA was associated with a reduced risk of placental parasitemia and low birth weight infants, but not maternal anemia at delivery. Interestingly, in women negative for placental malaria, the presence of VAR2CSA antibodies was associated with lower hematocrit at delivery and increased prevalence of maternal anemia. This is hypothesized to be the product of a malaria infection that was cleared early in pregnancy, with the presence of antibodies marking this past infection. But, the maternal hematocrit and prevalence of anemia are only slightly different between women with and without VAR2CSA antibodies, thus this effect may not be biologically relevant.

With samples from a large cohort of pregnant women from Kilifi, VSA_{PAM} IgG levels were measured by flow cytometry against various *P. falciparum* placental isolates and compared to hemoglobin levels (57). Increased severity of maternal anemia was correlated with low IgG levels in chronic cases of PAM (placentas infected with parasites and hemozoin pigment present) and the level of VSA_{PAM} antibodies in these women was a strong predictor of maternal hemoglobin levels. However, no correlation was observed in women with acute or past placental infection.

Studies That Inversely Correlate VSA_{PAM} Antibodies to Maternal Anemia

The findings from six studies suggest that VSA_{PAM} antibodies can reduce the severity of maternal anemia. In Malawi, two studies investigated the function of VSA_{PAM} antibodies by testing for opsonic phagocytosis. The first study revealed that a two-fold increase in the phagocytosis index was associated with a significant, 70% reduction in the odds of developing maternal anemia at delivery (51). Another study investigated third trimester serum samples and found that VSA_{PAM} IgG reactivity in flow correlated with activity in the opsonic phagocytosis assay ($r = 0.60$), but serum from anemic women displayed significantly lower opsonic activity (52). Notably, coinfection with HIV reduced opsonic activity, but did not affect inhibition of binding levels or total IgG against VSA_{PAM} (52).

In a later study from Malawi, antibody titres and function correlated to maternal hemoglobin at 36 weeks gestation, infant birth weight, gestational age, infant length, and placental histology at delivery (53). There was a significant positive association between IgG reactivity against CS2 parasites and maternal hemoglobin levels; a 10% increase in reactivity in flow corresponded to a hemoglobin increase of 0.5 g/L. Similarly, a 10% increase in the phagocytosis index corresponded to a hemoglobin increase of 0.4 g/L. Collectively, these studies support the hypothesis that opsonic phagocytosis could be an important effector mechanism of protection from maternal anemia.

VSA_{PAM} antibody-mediated protection from anemia may relate to the number of *var2csa* genes per *P. falciparum* genome in the parasites that infect pregnant women (54). Parasites with more than one *var2csa* gene are more common in PAM, compared to the non-pregnant population, and may provide a selective advantage over parasites with only one *var2csa* gene. In the Cameroonian village of Ngali II, increasing *var2csa* copy numbers in the parasites infecting pregnant women were associated with higher hemoglobin levels at delivery, but not with birth weight. However, in another region, Yaoundé, this relationship was reversed, with a negative correlation observed between *var2csa* copy number and birth weight. In Ngali II, IgG against DBL4ϵ, but not the full-length VAR2CSA, correlated positively with gene copy number. The authors hypothesized that parasites with multiple copies of *var2csa* may elicit immunity to specific DBL domains of VAR2CSA, and the protection observed might be due to a strong immune response that develops in women infected with these parasites.

Along with titre and functional assays, Chandrasiri et al. examined cytokine profiles of pregnant women from Sudan (55). Cytokine profiles were measured with a multiplex bead array that detected IL-1β, IL-6, IL-8, IL-10, IL-12, and TNFα. IFNγ was also measured by ELISA. Distinct cytokine profiles were observed in women with severe PAM compared to uninfected controls, with IFNγ, IL-6, and IL-10 significantly elevated. Parasite density was positively associated with levels of pro-inflammatory cytokines IL-6 and IL-8. Women with severe cases had low levels of IgG against VSA_{PAM} tested in flow, compared to uninfected controls. However, antibodies against DBL5ϵ were significantly greater than controls and negatively correlated with IL-1β, IL-6, and IL-8. Hemoglobin levels in these women were also negatively associated with IL-1β, IL-6, IL-8, and TNFα. Consistent with the studies from Malawi, opsonizing activity was positively associated with maternal hemoglobin at study enrollment. This study revealed associations between cytokine levels and VSA_{PAM} antibodies. An influx of pro-inflammatory cytokines could increase the risk of maternal anemia, but the presence of antibodies may have an effect on cytokine profiles.

Only one study from outside Africa identified a positive correlation between VSA_{PAM} antibodies and hemoglobin levels. This study was based in Colombia and examined a cohort of women with submicroscopic PAM (56). While VAR2CSA-specific antibody levels did not correlate with hemoglobin levels, the activity of these sera in the IBA was significantly associated with higher maternal hemoglobin levels at delivery. Interestingly, an association between antibody titre or function was not seen with birth weight, which is more commonly observed than associations with maternal anemia.

TRENDS AND CAVEATS

The results summarized above are divided on whether VSA_{PAM} antibodies contribute to protection from maternal anemia induced by PAM. These conclusions are consistent with a recent meta-analysis that examined associations between VSA_{PAM} antibodies and poor pregnancy outcomes, and included many of the same studies (58). Overall, the meta-analysis suggested that VSA_{PAM} antibodies are more likely to be markers of infection, instead of a source of protection against adverse outcomes, including anemia (58). However, additional analyses of the primary data provided by the authors revealed heterogeneous associations of VSA_{PAM} antibodies with anemia depending on a number of variables, such as gravidity, study design and the type of assay used to characterize antibodies. Considering these data and the results from the studies described previously, we identified various factors that may explain the discrepancies between these study findings.

Study Setting

The level of malaria transmission in the study region influences the frequency of exposure to parasites and the diversity of strains.

In turn, this could impact the magnitude and breadth of antibodies to VSA. Lloyd et al. collected samples from Yaoundé, a low transmission area with an entomological inoculation rate of approximately one infectious bite per person per month (49). In this study, just over half of women with a placental infection had antibodies to VAR2CSA, and this frequency was only 26.9% among multigravid women. Without sufficient exposure during pregnancy, a correlation between antibodies and pregnancy outcomes may not be detected. However, the study site of Fried et al. had intense seasonal transmission but there was no association between VSA_{PAM} antibodies and anemia, despite a positive correlation between infection history and antibody titres against several VAR2CSA subdomains (48). In this setting submicroscopic infections (SMI) were common, with a frequency between 19.8% and 25.4% in women who were blood smear negative at enrollment, and these infections were associated with an increase in VSA_{PAM} antibody levels, particularly in multigravid women. SMI may boost antibody responses without contributing to poor pregnancy outcomes, thus an association between VSA_{PAM} antibody titres and outcomes may not be observed. A similar finding was observed in Colombia, a low transmission setting, where history of SMI did not correlate directly with maternal hemoglobin measurements (56). Based on these few studies, it is unclear how transmission intensity impacts associations between VSA_{PAM} antibodies and anemia.

In certain settings, the fraction of anemia attributable to malaria may be low, masking a protective effect of VSA_{PAM} antibodies. In one of the cohorts from Malawi, 62% of women were anemic and the mean hemoglobin level was 10.6 g/dL, likely reflecting non-malarial causes of anemia (43). In Kenya, Staalsoe et al. also reported overall low hemoglobin values, with 15.6% of women having hemoglobin concentrations under 7 g/dL (57). Ndam et al. reported 62% of women were anemic at enrollment and 45% at delivery in a cohort from Benin, with only 16% and 12% of women testing positive for malaria infection at enrollment and delivery, respectively (41). Several factors besides malaria could influence maternal anemia, including micronutrient deficiency, coinfections, and quality of prenatal care [reviewed in (24, 25)]. Interestingly, in the cohort investigated by Chandrasiri et al. where there was a protective association between VSA_{PAM} antibodies and maternal anemia, women were given supplements (including iron) and the median hemoglobin was 11 g/dL (53). Perhaps this supplementation controlled for malaria-independent causes of anemia, revealing an association between the VSA_{PAM} antibodies and malaria-attributable anemia.

Study Design

Depending on the study design, samples are collected at various times during pregnancy and/or at delivery and this could affect the interpretation of study findings. For example, VSA_{PAM} antibodies detected early in pregnancy may indicate a prior exposure to VSA_{PAM} in a previous pregnancy; thus, a pregnant woman may begin pregnancy with some immunity that may be boosted during subsequent pregnancies. Staalsoe et al. found that by six months postpartum, titres of VSA_{PAM} IgG decreased, but levels were boosted in women by the second trimester of their next pregnancy (59). Modeling studies estimate that VAR2CSA antibodies can persist over many years (60). Of those studies that reported an association between VSA_{PAM} antibodies and maternal hemoglobin levels, 4 out of 6 assessed antibody titre and/or function measured at first to second trimester (51, 53, 55, 56). In contrast, most of the studies that did not find a protective association with maternal anemia collected samples late in pregnancy, in the third trimester and at delivery (40, 41, 44, 46, 49, 45). If these VSA_{PAM} antibodies developed as a result of infection late in pregnancy, increased antibody levels may reflect recent boosting from infection and obscure a relationship between antibody and protection from anemia. Thus, VSA_{PAM} antibodies detected later in pregnancy may be markers of infection, rather than a source of protection, as noted by Cutts et al. (58), and others.

The gravidity of women included in the study can also greatly impact the titre, persistence and quality of antibodies investigated. Antibodies against VSA expressed in PAM develop with each successive infection in pregnancy; in high transmission settings, multigravid women are more likely to have antibodies that correlate with better pregnancy outcomes than primigravid women, supporting that these antibodies are maintained into the next pregnancy. Fried et al. reported that VSA_{PAM} antibodies from primigravid women are short-lived, compared to those from secundigravid and multigravid women (48). In the 2010 Ataide et al. study, only primigravid women were included and samples were collected in the late third trimester, with no protective association between VSA_{PAM} antibodies and anemia observed (42). The same cohort was followed into the second pregnancy, and again there was no association between maternal hemoglobin and VSA_{PAM} IgG or opsonic phagocytosis activity (43). Thus, protective qualities of VSA_{PAM} antibodies might not fully develop until infections in multiple pregnancies have occurred. In Malawi, recognition of iRBCs by VSA_{PAM} antibodies from secundigravid and multigravid women, but not primigravid women, was associated with a reduced odds of anemia (47, 58). In contrast to the related studies discussed above, this association was observed in samples collected in the third trimester of pregnancy.

Another important consideration is treatment history. IPTp with 1500/75 mg of sulphadoxine and pyrimethamine (SP) during antenatal care visits is recommended by WHO in most areas in sub-Saharan Africa to reduce placental malaria (61). This treatment has the potential to affect the acquisition of VSA_{PAM} antibodies, as parasitemia is prevented or cleared to the point that plasma cells will not produce antibodies against VSA_{PAM} targets. In Ndam et al. where no association was observed between VSA_{PAM} antibodies and maternal anemia at delivery, women received two doses of SP during pregnancy (41). Aitken et al. reported lower levels of VSA_{PAM} antibodies associated with IPTp treatment (47). Similar observations were made in other studies from Kenya (50) and Ghana (62), where reductions in antibody titres were associated with IPTp treatment (though pregnancy outcomes were not reported). In contrast, Serra-Casas et al. failed to observe an effect of IPTp on VSA_{PAM} antibody levels (46). Therefore, the effects of IPTp on VSA_{PAM} antibodies in relation to anemia are unclear. But, it is unlikely that IPTp treatment contributes to the severity of maternal anemia itself, as a controlled or lowered parasitemia should benefit the health of the mother.

Finally, HIV is known to affect the humoral response in PAM, which was observed by a number of studies examined in this review (42–44, 46, 52). In the two studies by Ataide et al. VSA_{PAM} phagocytic antibodies were reduced in HIV positive women compared to women who were HIV negative but this was only observed when antibody activity was measured using a functional assay; there was no change in the antibody reactivity to iRBCs by flow cytometry (42, 43). The presence of HIV in a cohort may therefore reduce VSA_{PAM} antibody levels and/or function to a level too low to improve outcomes, particularly in lower transmission settings (49) or when women are treated with IPTp (46).

Assay Selection

It is necessary to assess antibody titre and particularly function to make comparisons with pregnancy outcomes. From the group of studies that did not find an association with maternal anemia, IBA was the primary functional assay used, with only two studies in this group that measured opsonic phagocytosis activity (42 43). Inhibition of adhesion by VSA_{PAM} antibodies is more commonly associated with higher infant birth weight due to *P. falciparum* infections during pregnancy (40). In only one study, from Colombia, adhesion-blocking activity was associated with increased maternal hemoglobin at delivery (56). Several of the studies point to opsonic phagocytic activity as a particularly important correlate of protection against maternal anemia. Chandrasiri et al. showed that only antibodies with opsonic phagocytic activity were associated with reduced odds of severe malaria, rather than antibody titre measured by ELISA (55). Similarly, Feng et al. observed a correlation between a reduced odds ratio of maternal anemia and VSA_{PAM} antibody activity both by flow cytometry and opsonic phagocytosis, but the relationship between phagocytic activity was stronger than VSA_{PAM} seroreactivity in flow (51). Interestingly, in one study, VSA_{PAM} IgG measured by flow correlated more strongly with opsonic activity than anti-adhesion activity in the IBA (52).

Functional assays can also focus on specific IgG subclasses, rather than measuring total IgG by flow cytometry or ELISA. IgG1 and IgG3 are cytophilic subclasses that interact with Fc receptors on other immune cells, including monocytes and macrophages, and promote opsonic phagocytosis (63). These are the dominant subclasses in PAM, while IgG2 and IgG4 levels do not significantly change (64). Opsonic phagocytosis assays specifically measure these cytophilic subclasses, whereas testing for total IgG may not reveal a relationship with pregnancy outcomes. Future studies should characterize antibody populations using functional assays, along with assessments of titre and subclass, to test for associations with anemia.

Overall, there are many factors that can affect the relationship between maternal anemia and VSA_{PAM} antibodies. Based on our interpretation of the studies described above, the discordance between the study findings may be attributed in part to the timing of sample collection and assay selection.

Potential Mechanisms of Antibody-Mediated Protection from Maternal Anemia in PAM

Though evidence for a specific role for VSA_{PAM} antibodies in protection against maternal anemia is currently inconclusive, we can speculate on putative mechanisms of protection to help inform future research (**Figure 1**). We hypothesize that protective antibodies could directly target the iRBCs in the placental environment, either through opsonization or by physically blocking adhesion to CSA. Based on the group of studies that found an association with improved outcomes, VSA_{PAM} antibodies that mediate opsonic phagocytosis of iRBCs may be more likely to be protective against maternal anemia than antibodies that inhibit parasite binding to the placenta, suggesting these antibodies may have distinct effector mechanisms. Antibodies with dual functions may also exist.

Antibody binding to iRBCs can lead to different downstream effects. Clearing the iRBC from the placenta either by preventing sequestration and/or recruiting immune cells would prevent the hemolysis associated with anemia and the associated inflammatory response. Erythropoiesis is also susceptible to a dysregulated pro-inflammatory response, a common cause of anemia in uncomplicated malaria and PAM [reviewed in (24)]. VSA_{PAM} antibodies can potentially contribute to these responses by reducing cytokine dysregulation and targeting immune cells to iRBCs. As observed by Chandrasiri et al. pro-inflammatory cytokines IL-1β, IL-6, and IL-8 negatively correlated with antibody titres against DBL5ϵ in pregnant women with severe malaria (55). In this study, opsonizing antibody activity and cytokine profiles were not compared directly, but maternal hemoglobin levels increased with increasing levels of opsonizing antibodies (53). In another study, cytokine secretions were measured after opsonic phagocytosis of CS2 parasites had occurred, using serum from Malawian pregnant women. These results were compared to antibody-independent phagocytosis and a shift in the cytokine profile was observed, with an increase in production of IL-1β and TNFα when antibodies were present (65). Opsonized iRBCs activated the inflammasome and production of IL-1β by macrophages, but this was also observed with unopsonized iRBCs. Thus, the secretion of pro-inflammatory mediators likely occurs in the placenta with and without sufficient titres of VSA_{PAM} antibodies. Perhaps the labeling of iRBCs with VSA_{PAM} antibodies leads to Th1-like immune responses to appropriately respond to the parasite without leading to dysregulated inflammation and inhibition of erythropoiesis.

FUTURE DIRECTIONS

As the pathways leading to anemia in PAM are complicated and multifactorial, further research is critical to better understand any potential underlying immune mechanisms in response to malaria infection that contribute to or protect women from anemia. Longitudinal studies should be continued in and outside of Africa to increase the body of knowledge available on infection, VSA_{PAM} antibody levels, and pregnancy outcomes. Studies should be conducted in many diverse settings to reveal context-specific effects on the acquisition of PAM immunity and the prevalence of maternal anemia. Treatment practices and circulation of other pathogens in a particular area can also affect humoral immunity.

In those studies where VSA_{PAM} antibodies are associated with higher hemoglobin levels in mothers, it will be exciting to unravel the underlying mechanisms of protection. We propose a basic model for how these antibodies that target placental iRBCs could block downstream pathogenic effects that lead to anemia, yet the mechanisms that directly contribute to this process need to be delineated. While the data support a role for these antibodies in blocking sequestration in the placenta and promoting opsonic phagocytosis, emerging evidence linking the innate and adaptive immune systems merit exploration. For example, data is emerging on the role of the complement system in uncomplicated malaria. The antibody-mediated activation of the classical complement pathway was observed in samples from children and was an indicator of protective immunity (66). In addition, NK cells may participate in the response to PAM. Long et al. showed that antibodies from VAR2CSA-immunized rabbits induced iRBC lysis *in vitro* (67). Further, human IgG pooled from plasma of multigravid women and incubated with parasites and NK cells inhibited parasite growth by approximately 50%. No connection to anemia was examined, but this is an interesting component of the PAM response that should be further investigated with respect to pregnancy outcomes.

This review highlights the complexity of the body's response to PAM and the large gaps in the current knowledge on immune mechanisms underlying protection. Pregnant women and young children remain at great risk of morbidity and mortality from malaria. Continued research in this area will add to our understanding of PAM and potentially reveal novel therapy and vaccine strategies to combat this disease.

AUTHOR CONTRIBUTIONS

MCW conducted the literature review. MCW and SKY jointly wrote the manuscript. All authors contributed to the article and approved the submitted version.

ACKNOWLEDGEMENT

We thank Michael Good and Sedami Gnidehou for their valuable feedback during the preparation of this review.

REFERENCES

1. McGregor IA. Epidemiology, malaria and pregnancy. *Am J Trop Med Hyg* (1984) 33(4):517–25. doi: 10.4269/ajtmh.1984.33.517
2. WHO. *World malaria report 2019.* Geneva: World Health Organization (2019). p. 2019.
3. Dellicour S, Tatem AJ, Guerra CA, Snow RW, ter Kuile FO. Quantifying the number of pregnancies at risk of malaria in 2007: a demographic study. *PLoS Med* (2010) 7(1):e1000221. doi: 10.1371/journal.pmed.1000221
4. Moore KA, Simpson JA, Scoullar MJL, McGready R, Fowkes FJI. Quantification of the association between malaria in pregnancy and stillbirth: a systematic review and meta-analysis. *Lancet Glob Health* (2017) 5(11):e1101–e12. doi: 10.1016/S2214-109X(17)30340-6
5. Laelago T, Yohannes T, Tsige G. Determinants of preterm birth among mothers who gave birth in East Africa: systematic review and meta-analysis. *Ital J Pediatr* (2020) 46(1):10. doi: 10.1186/s13052-020-0772-1
6. Brabin B, Rogerson S. The epidemiology and outcomes of maternal malaria. In: E Patrick, MF Duffy, editors. *Malaria in Pregnancy: Deadly Parasite, Susceptible Host.* London: CRC Press (2001). p. 28–55.
7. Ataide R, Mayor A, Rogerson SJ. Malaria, primigravidae, and antibodies: knowledge gained and future perspectives. *Trends Parasitol* (2014) 30(2):85–94. doi: 10.1016/j.pt.2013.12.007
8. Fried M, Nosten F, Brockman A, Brabin BJ, Duffy PE. Maternal antibodies block malaria. *Nature* (1998) 395(6705):851–2. doi: 10.1038/27570
9. Fried M, Duffy PE. Adherence of Plasmodium falciparum to chondroitin sulfate A in the human placenta. *Science* (1996) 272(5267):1502–4. doi: 10.1126/science.272.5267.1502
10. Ricke CH, Staalsoe T, Koram K, Akanmori BD, Riley EM, Theander TG, et al. Plasma antibodies from malaria-exposed pregnant women recognize variant surface antigens on Plasmodium falciparum-infected erythrocytes in a parity-dependent manner and block parasite adhesion to chondroitin sulfate A. *J Immunol* (2000) 165(6):3309–16. doi: 10.4049/jimmunol.165.6.3309
11. Salanti A, Staalsoe T, Lavstsen T, Jensen AT, Sowa MP, Arnot DE, et al. Selective upregulation of a single distinctly structured var gene in chondroitin sulphate A-adhering Plasmodium falciparum involved in pregnancy-associated malaria. *Mol Microbiol* (2003) 49(1):179–91. doi: 10.1046/j.1365-2958.2003.03570.x
12. Salanti A, Dahlback M, Turner L, Nielsen MA, Barfod L, Magistrado P, et al. Evidence for the involvement of VAR2CSA in pregnancy-associated malaria. *J Exp Med* (2004) 200(9):1197–203. doi: 10.1084/jem.20041579
13. Sirima SB, Richert L, Chene A, Konate AT, Campion C, Dechavanne S, et al. PRIMVAC vaccine adjuvanted with Alhydrogel or GLA-SE to prevent placental malaria: a first-in-human, randomised, double-blind, placebo-controlled study. *Lancet Infect Dis* (2020) 20(5):585–97. doi: 10.1016/S1473-3099(19)30739-X
14. Mordmuller B, Sulyok M, Egger-Adam D, Resende M, de Jongh WA, Jensen MH, et al. First-in-human, Randomized, Double-blind Clinical Trial of Differentially Adjuvanted PAMVAC, A Vaccine Candidate to Prevent Pregnancy-associated Malaria. *Clin Infect Dis* (2019) 69(9):1509–16. doi: 10.1093/cid/ciy1140
15. Rogerson SJ, Mwapasa V, Meshnick SR. Malaria in pregnancy: linking immunity and pathogenesis to prevention. *Am J Trop Med Hyg* (2007) 77(6 Suppl):14–22.
16. WHO. *Haemoglobin concentrations for the diagnosis of anaemia and assesment of severity.* Geneva: World Health Organizaiton (2011). Available at: http://www.who.int/vmnis/indicators/haemoglobin.
17. Chapman AB, Abraham WT, Zamudio S, Coffin C, Merouani A, Young D, et al. Temporal relationships between hormonal and hemodynamic changes in early human pregnancy. *Kidney Int* (1998) 54(6):2056–63. doi: 10.1046/j.1523-1755.1998.00217.x

18. Sanghavi M, Rutherford JD. Cardiovascular physiology of pregnancy. *Circulation* (2014) 130(12):1003–8. doi: 10.1161/CIRCULATIONAHA.114.009029
19. Vricella LK. Emerging understanding and measurement of plasma volume expansion in pregnancy. *Am J Clin Nutr* (2017) 106(Suppl 6):1620S–5S. doi: 10.3945/ajcn.117.155903
20. Cao C, O'Brien KO. Pregnancy and iron homeostasis: an update. *Nutr Rev* (2013) 71(1):35–51. doi: 10.1111/j.1753-4887.2012.00550.x
21. Jakeman GN, Saul A, Hogarth WL, Collins WE. Anaemia of acute malaria infections in non-immune patients primarily results from destruction of uninfected erythrocytes. *Parasitology* (1999) 119(Pt 2):127–33. doi: 10.1017/s0031182099004564
22. Dondorp AM, Angus BJ, Chotivanich K, Silamut K, Ruangveerayuth R, Hardeman MR, et al. Red blood cell deformability as a predictor of anemia in severe falciparum malaria. *Am J Trop Med Hyg* (1999) 60(5):733–7. doi: 10.4269/ajtmh.1999.60.733
23. Looareesuwan S, Davis TM, Pukrittayakamee S, Supanaranond W, Desakorn V, Silamut K, et al. Erythrocyte survival in severe falciparum malaria. *Acta Trop* (1991) 48(4):263–70. doi: 10.1016/0001-706x(91)90014-b
24. Ghosh K, Ghosh K. Pathogenesis of anemia in malaria: a concise review. *Parasitol Res* (2007) 101(6):1463–9. doi: 10.1007/s00436-007-0742-1
25. White NJ. Anaemia and malaria. *Malar J* (2018) 17(1):371. doi: 10.1186/s12936-018-2509-9
26. de Moraes-Pinto MI, Vince GS, Flanagan BF, Hart CA, Johnson PM. Localization of IL-4 and IL-4 receptors in the human term placenta, decidua and amniochorionic membranes. *Immunology* (1997) 90(1):87–94. doi: 10.1046/j.1365-2567.1997.00139.x
27. Fried M, Muga RO, Misore AO, Duffy PE. Malaria elicits type 1 cytokines in the human placenta: IFN-gamma and TNF-alpha associated with pregnancy outcomes. *J Immunol* (1998) 160(5):2523–30.
28. Achidi EA, Apinjoh TO, Titanji VP. Malaria parasitemia and systemic cytokine bias in pregnancy. *Int J Gynaecol Obstet* (2007) 97(1):15–20. doi: 10.1016/j.ijgo.2006.12.015
29. Moore JM, Nahlen BL, Misore A, Lal AA, Udhayakumar V. Immunity to placental malaria. I. Elevated production of interferon-gamma by placental blood mononuclear cells is associated with protection in an area with high transmission of malaria. *J Infect Dis* (1999) 179(5):1218–25. doi: 10.1086/314737
30. Dobano C, Berthoud T, Manaca MN, Nhabomba A, Guinovart C, Aguilar R, et al. High production of pro-inflammatory cytokines by maternal blood mononuclear cells is associated with reduced maternal malaria but increased cord blood infection. *Malar J* (2018) 17(1):177. doi: 10.1186/s12936-018-2317-2
31. Perkins DJ, Were T, Davenport GC, Kempaiah P, Hittner JB, Ong'echa JM. Severe malarial anemia: innate immunity and pathogenesis. *Int J Biol Sci* (2011) 7(9):1427–42. doi: 10.7150/ijbs.7.1427
32. Kabyemela ER, Muehlenbachs A, Fried M, Kurtis JD, Mutabingwa TK, Duffy PE. Maternal peripheral blood level of IL-10 as a marker for inflammatory placental malaria. *Malar J* (2008) 7:26. doi: 10.1186/1475-2875-7-26
33. Hountohotegbe T, Gbedande K, Agbota G, Ibitokou S, Massougbodji A, Deloron P, et al. Circulating Cytokines Associated with Poor Pregnancy Outcomes in Beninese Exposed to Infection with Plasmodium falciparum. *Infect Immun* (2020) 88(8). doi: 10.1128/IAI.00042-20
34. Thaxton JE, Sharma S. Interleukin-10: a multi-faceted agent of pregnancy. *Am J Reprod Immunol* (2010) 63(6):482–91. doi: 10.1111/j.1600-0897.2010.00810.x
35. Suguitan ALJr., Leke RG, Fouda G, Zhou A, Thuita L, Metenou S, et al. Changes in the levels of chemokines and cytokines in the placentas of women with Plasmodium falciparum malaria. *J Infect Dis* (2003) 188(7):1074–82. doi: 10.1086/378500
36. Suguitan ALJr., Cadigan TJ, Nguyen TA, Zhou A, Leke RJ, Metenou S, et al. Malaria-associated cytokine changes in the placenta of women with pre-term deliveries in Yaounde, Cameroon. *Am J Trop Med Hyg* (2003) 69(6):574–81. doi: 10.4269/ajtmh.2003.69.574
37. Walter PR, Garin Y, Blot P. Placental pathologic changes in malaria. A histologic and ultrastructural study. *Am J Pathol* (1982) 109(3):330–42.
38. Ismail MR, Ordi J, Menendez C, Ventura PJ, Aponte JJ, Kahigwa E, et al. Placental pathology in malaria: a histological, immunohistochemical, and quantitative study. *Hum Pathol* (2000) 31(1):85–93. doi: 10.1016/s0046-8177(00)80203-8
39. O'Neil-Dunne I, Achur RN, Agbor-Enoh ST, Valiyaveettil M, Naik RS, Ockenhouse CF, et al. Gravidity-dependent production of antibodies that inhibit binding of Plasmodium falciparum-infected erythrocytes to placental chondroitin sulfate proteoglycan during pregnancy. *Infect Immun* (2001) 69(12):7487–92. doi: 10.1128/IAI.69.12.7487-7492.2001
40. Duffy PE, Fried M. Antibodies that inhibit Plasmodium falciparum adhesion to chondroitin sulfate A are associated with increased birth weight and the gestational age of newborns. *Infect Immun* (2003) 71(11):6620–3. doi: 10.1128/IAI.71.11.6620-6623.2003
41. Ndam NT, Denoeud-Ndam L, Doritchamou J, Viwami F, Salanti A, Nielsen MA, et al. Protective Antibodies against Placental Malaria and Poor Outcomes during Pregnancy, Benin. *Emerg Infect Dis* (2015) 21(5):813–23. doi: 10.3201/eid2105.141626
42. Ataide R, Hasang W, Wilson DW, Beeson JG, Mwapasa V, Molyneux ME, et al. Using an improved phagocytosis assay to evaluate the effect of HIV on specific antibodies to pregnancy-associated malaria. *PLoS One* (2010) 5(5): e10807. doi: 10.1371/journal.pone.0010807
43. Ataide R, Mwapasa V, Molyneux ME, Meshnick SR, Rogerson SJ. Antibodies that induce phagocytosis of malaria infected erythrocytes: effect of HIV infection and correlation with clinical outcomes. *PLoS One* (2011) 6(7): e22491. doi: 10.1371/journal.pone.0022491
44. Mayor A, Kumar U, Bardaji A, Gupta P, Jimenez A, Hamad A, et al. Improved pregnancy outcomes in women exposed to malaria with high antibody levels against Plasmodium falciparum. *J Infect Dis* (2013) 207(11):1664–74. doi: 10.1093/infdis/jit083
45. Tuikue Ndam NG, Salanti A, Le-Hesran JY, Cottrell G, Fievet N, Turner L, et al. Dynamics of anti-VAR2CSA immunoglobulin G response in a cohort of senegalese pregnant women. *J Infect Dis* (2006) 193(5):713–20. doi: 10.1086/500146
46. Serra-Casas E, Menendez C, Bardaji A, Quinto L, Dobano C, Sigauque B, et al. The effect of intermittent preventive treatment during pregnancy on malarial antibodies depends on HIV status and is not associated with poor delivery outcomes. *J Infect Dis* (2010) 201(1):123–31. doi: 10.1086/648595
47. Aitken EH, Mbewe B, Luntamo M, Maleta K, Kulmala T, Friso MJ, et al. Antibodies to chondroitin sulfate A-binding infected erythrocytes: dynamics and protection during pregnancy in women receiving intermittent preventive treatment. *J Infect Dis* (2010) 201(9):1316–25. doi: 10.1086/651578
48. Fried M, Kurtis JD, Swihart B, Morrison R, Pond-Tor S, Barry A, et al. Antibody levels to recombinant VAR2CSA domains vary with Plasmodium falciparum parasitaemia, gestational age, and gravidity, but do not predict pregnancy outcomes. *Malar J* (2018) 17(1):106. doi: 10.1186/s12936-018-2258-9
49. Lloyd YM, Fang R, Bobbili N, Vanda K, Ngati E, Sanchez-Quintero MJ, et al. Association of Antibodies to VAR2CSA and Merozoite Antigens with Pregnancy Outcomes in Women Living in Yaounde, Cameroon. *Infect Immun* (2018) 86(9):e00166-18. doi: 10.1128/IAI.00166-18
50. Staalsoe T, Shulman CE, Dorman EK, Kawuondo K, Marsh K, Hviid L. Intermittent preventive sulfadoxine-pyrimethamine treatment of primigravidae reduces levels of plasma immunoglobulin G, which protects against pregnancy-associated Plasmodium falciparum malaria. *Infect Immun* (2004) 72(9):5027–30. doi: 10.1128/IAI.72.9.5027-5030.2004
51. Feng G, Aitken E, Yosaatmadja F, Kalilani L, Meshnick SR, Jaworowski A, et al. Antibodies to variant surface antigens of Plasmodium falciparum-infected erythrocytes are associated with protection from treatment failure and the development of anemia in pregnancy. *J Infect Dis* (2009) 200(2):299–306. doi: 10.1086/599841
52. Jaworowski A, Fernandes LA, Yosaatmadja F, Feng G, Mwapasa V, Molyneux ME, et al. Relationship between human immunodeficiency virus type 1 coinfection, anemia, and levels and function of antibodies to variant surface antigens in pregnancy-associated malaria. *Clin Vaccine Immunol* (2009) 16(3):312–9. doi: 10.1128/CVI.00356-08
53. Chandrasiri UP, Fowkes FJ, Beeson JG, Richards JS, Kamiza S, Maleta K, et al. Association between malaria immunity and pregnancy outcomes among Malawian pregnant women receiving nutrient supplementation. *Malar J* (2016) 15(1):547. doi: 10.1186/s12936-016-1597-7

54. Sander AF, Salanti A, Lavstsen T, Nielsen MA, Theander TG, Leke RG, et al. Positive selection of Plasmodium falciparum parasites with multiple var2csa-type PfEMP1 genes during the course of infection in pregnant women. *J Infect Dis* (2011) 203(11):1679–85. doi: 10.1093/infdis/jir168
55. Chandrasiri UP, Randall LM, Saad AA, Bashir AM, Rogerson SJ, Adam I. Low antibody levels to pregnancy-specific malaria antigens and heightened cytokine responses associated with severe malaria in pregnancy. *J Infect Dis* (2014) 209(9):1408–17. doi: 10.1093/infdis/jit646
56. Gavina K, Gnidehou S, Arango E, Hamel-Martineau C, Mitran C, Agudelo O, et al. Clinical Outcomes of Submicroscopic Infections and Correlates of Protection of VAR2CSA Antibodies in a Longitudinal Study of Pregnant Women in Colombia. *Infect Immun* (2018) 86(4):e00797-17. doi: 10.1128/IAI.00797-17
57. Staalsoe T, Shulman CE, Bulmer JN, Kawuondo K, Marsh K, Hviid L. Variant surface antigen-specific IgG and protection against clinical consequences of pregnancy-associated Plasmodium falciparum malaria. *Lancet* (2004) 363 (9405):283–9. doi: 10.1016/S0140-6736(03)15386-X
58. Cutts JC, Agius PA, Zaw L, Powell R, Moore K, Draper B, et al. Pregnancy-specific malarial immunity and risk of malaria in pregnancy and adverse birth outcomes: a systematic review. *BMC Med* (2020) 18(1):14. doi: 10.1186/s12916-019-1467-6
59. Staalsoe T, Megnekou R, Fievet N, Ricke CH, Zornig HD, Leke R, et al. Acquisition and decay of antibodies to pregnancy-associated variant antigens on the surface of Plasmodium falciparum-infected erythrocytes that protect against placental parasitemia. *J Infect Dis* (2001) 184(5):618–26. doi: 10.1086/322809
60. Fowkes FJ, McGready R, Cross NJ, Hommel M, Simpson JA, Elliott SR, et al. New insights into acquisition, boosting, and longevity of immunity to malaria in pregnant women. *J Infect Dis* (2012) 206(10):1612–21. doi: 10.1093/infdis/jis566
61. WHO. *A Strategic Framework for Malaaria Prevention and Control During Pregnancy in the African Region*. Brazzaville: WHO Regional Office for Africa (2004). Contract No.: AFR/MAL/04/01.
62. Stephens JK, Kyei-Baafour E, Dickson EK, Ofori JK, Ofori MF, Wilson ML, et al. Effect of IPTp on Plasmodium falciparum antibody levels among pregnant women and their babies in a sub-urban coastal area in Ghana. *Malar J* (2017) 16(1):224. doi: 10.1186/s12936-017-1857-1
63. Tebo AE, Kremsner PG, Luty AJ. Fcgamma receptor-mediated phagocytosis of Plasmodium falciparum-infected erythrocytes in vitro. *Clin Exp Immunol* (2002) 130(2):300–6. doi: 10.1046/j.1365-2249.2002.01972.x
64. Elliott SR, Brennan AK, Beeson JG, Tadesse E, Molyneux ME, Brown GV, et al. Placental malaria induces variant-specific antibodies of the cytophilic subtypes immunoglobulin G1 (IgG1) and IgG3 that correlate with adhesion inhibitory activity. *Infect Immun* (2005) 73(9):5903–7. doi: 10.1128/IAI.73.9.5903-5907.2005
65. Zhou J, Ludlow LE, Hasang W, Rogerson SJ, Jaworowski A. Opsonization of malaria-infected erythrocytes activates the inflammasome and enhances inflammatory cytokine secretion by human macrophages. *Malar J* (2012) 11:343. doi: 10.1186/1475-2875-11-343
66. Reiling L, Boyle MJ, White MT, Wilson DW, Feng G, Weaver R, et al. Targets of complement-fixing antibodies in protective immunity against malaria in children. *Nat Commun* (2019) 10(1):610. doi: 10.1038/s41467-019-08528-z
67. Arora G, Hart GT, Manzella-Lapeira J, Doritchamou JY, Narum DL, Thomas LM, et al. NK cells inhibit Plasmodium falciparum growth in red blood cells via antibody-dependent cellular cytotoxicity. *Elife* (2018) 7. doi: 10.7554/eLife.36806

9

Safety of a Novel *Listeria monocytogenes*-Based Vaccine Vector Expressing NcSAG1 (*Neospora caninum* Surface Antigen 1)

William Robert Pownall[1†], Dennis Imhof[2†], Nerea Fernandez Trigo[3], Stephanie C. Ganal-Vonarburg[3], Philippe Plattet[4], Camille Monney[4], Franck Forterre[1], Andrew Hemphill[2] and Anna Oevermann[4*]

[1] Division of Small Animal Surgery, Department of Clinical Veterinary Sciences, Vetsuisse Faculty, University of Bern, Bern, Switzerland, [2] Institute of Parasitology, DIP, Vetsuisse Faculty, University of Bern, Bern, Switzerland, [3] Department for BioMedical Research (DBMR), Universitätsklinik für Viszerale Chirurgie und Medizin, Inselspital, Bern University Hospital, University of Bern, Bern, Switzerland, [4] Division of Neurological Sciences, DCR-VPH, Vetsuisse Faculty, University of Bern, Bern, Switzerland

***Correspondence:**
Anna Oevermann
anna.oevermann@vetsuisse.unibe.ch

[†]These authors have contributed equally to this work

Listeria monocytogenes (LM) has been proposed as vaccine vector in various cancers and infectious diseases since LM induces a strong immune response. In this study, we developed a novel and safe LM-based vaccine vector platform, by engineering a triple attenuated mutant (Lm3Dx) (ΔactA, ΔinlA, ΔinlB) of the wild-type LM strain JF5203 (CC 1, phylogenetic lineage I). We demonstrated the strong attenuation of Lm3Dx while maintaining its capacity to selectively infect antigen-presenting cells (APCs) *in vitro*. Furthermore, as proof of concept, we introduced the immunodominant *Neospora caninum* (Nc) surface antigen NcSAG1 into Lm3Dx. The NcSAG1 protein was expressed by Lm3Dx_SAG1 during cellular infection. To demonstrate safety of Lm3Dx_SAG1 *in vivo*, we vaccinated BALB/C mice by intramuscular injection. Following vaccination, mice did not suffer any adverse effects and only sporadically shed bacteria at very low levels in the feces (<100 CFU/g). Additionally, bacterial load in internal organs was very low to absent at day 1.5 and 4 following the 1st vaccination and at 2 and 4 weeks after the second boost, independently of the physiological status of the mice. Additionally, vaccination of mice prior and during pregnancy did not interfere with pregnancy outcome. However, Lm3Dx_SAG1 was shed into the milk when inoculated during lactation, although it did not cause any clinical adverse effects in either dams or pups. Also, we have indications that the vector persists more days in the injected muscle of lactating mice. Therefore, impact of physiological status on vector dynamics in the host and mechanisms of milk shedding requires further investigation. In conclusion, we provide strong evidence that Lm3Dx is a safe vaccine vector in non-lactating animals. Additionally, we provide first indications that mice vaccinated with Lm3Dx_SAG1 develop a strong and Th1-biased immune response against the Lm3Dx-expressed neospora antigen. These results encourage to further investigate the efficiency of Lm3Dx_SAG1 to prevent and treat clinical neosporosis.

Keywords: microbial vaccine, *Listeria monocytogenes*, neosporosis, *Neospora caninum*, immune response, *in vitro* safety, *in vivo* safety

INTRODUCTION

In both human and veterinary medicine, the implementation of vaccines revealed to be one of the most effective strategies to prevent morbidity and mortality from infectious diseases. Case in points include small-pox (Meyer et al., 2020), rabies (Fischer and Schnell, 2018), polio, mumps, measles, rubella, varicella (Di Pietrantonj et al., 2020), meningococcal infections, Ebola (Henao-Restrepo et al., 2017), myxomatosis, canine distemper, parvovirosis, herpesvirus infections, and leptospirosis (Davis-Wurzler, 2014; Afghah et al., 2017; Jiang et al., 2019). Currently, many marketed vaccines rely on live-attenuated or killed/inactivated pathogens. For improved safety and immunogenicity, significant efforts have been made to develop alternative approaches using subunit-, DNA-, mRNA- or vector-based vaccines, even more so in the past months in the light of the COVID-19 pandemic (Griot et al., 2004; Nielsen et al., 2012; Fukuhara et al., 2016; Sharma et al., 2020).

Although to this day quantification of induced antibodies is used to evaluate immunogenicity of vaccines, it is increasingly recognized that T-cell responses are instrumental for a protective and sustained immunity against numerous infectious diseases (Gilbert, 2011; Gray et al., 2018; Jameson and Masopust, 2018; Peng et al., 2020; Sharma et al., 2020). Indeed, humoral responses proved insufficient in the control of certain pathogens (Fischer and Schnell, 2018; Vetter et al., 2018) and there is still an unmet need for vaccines against diseases such as tuberculosis, HIV (Gray et al., 2018) or protozoan parasites such as *Toxoplasma gondii* and the closely related *Neospora caninum* (Nc) (Leong et al., 2009; Wang et al., 2014).

Nc is an obligatory intracellular protozoan parasite belonging to the phylum apicomplexa and a major infectious cause of abortion and reproductive failure in cattle and small ruminants due to transplacental passage of rapidly proliferating tachyzoites and subsequent infection of the fetus (Schares et al., 1998; Moreno et al., 2012). Economic losses in the global cattle industry due to Nc-associated abortion and premature culling are estimated to amount up to 1.3 billion US $ yearly (Reichel et al., 2013). Models predict vaccination to be the most cost-effective approach to reduce abortions and reproductive failure in cattle herds with high Nc prevalence (Liu et al., 2020). Additionally, vaccines might prevent severe neuromuscular disease (Anvari et al., 2020) and fecal oocyst shedding in infected dogs, which are a major source of exogenous transmission to cattle (McAllister et al., 1998; Monney et al., 2011). However, despite strong efforts of the researcher community, no commercial vaccine is currently available.

Most vaccine trials provided evidence that a Th1-biased or a balanced Th1/Th2 immune response offer protection against horizontal and vertical transmission because they simulate the immune response during Nc infection that is associated with a robust development of specific $CD4^+$ and $CD8^+$ T-cells targeting the intracellular stage of the parasite (Hemphill et al., 2006; Aguado-Martínez et al., 2019). In contrast, vaccines triggering only a humoral immune response proved to be insufficient in preventing the disease because antibodies act only against the extracellular stage (Monney et al., 2011; Hemphill et al., 2016).

Over the last decades, *Listeria monocytogenes* (Lm), a gram-positive and facultatively intracellular bacterium, has evolved to a paradigmatic pathogen for immunology research (Cossart and Lebreton, 2014). Lm infection generates strong innate and adaptive immune responses and, thus, Lm has been increasingly recognized as a vaccine vector for the prevention and therapy of tumors and infectious diseases showing promising results in clinical trials (Liu, 2006; Singh and Wallecha, 2011; Wood and Paterson, 2014; Flickinger et al., 2018; Wendel Naumann and Leath, 2020).

Lm is an opportunistic pathogen that may cause serious disease including gastroenteritis, septicemia, abortions and neurolisteriosis in humans and animals (Schlech, 2019; Matle et al., 2020). Virulence of Lm is essentially governed by a defined set of crucial virulence factors regulating cellular invasion and intercellular spread. Invasion of most cells is mediated by the bacterial surface proteins InlA and InlB that bind cellular receptors present on a wide range of host cells and induce bacterial endocytosis (Lecuit et al., 1997). However, phagocytosis of Lm by professional phagocytes including antigen-presenting cells (APCs) is independent of theses receptors. Once internalized, Lm is either processed by the phagolysosome, or escapes the phagosome prior to phagolysosomal fusion and enters the cytosol, a process dependent of proteins encoded by *hly*, *plcA* and *plcB* (Radoshevich and Cossart, 2018). Once in the cytosol, Lm relies on an actin-assembly inducing protein encoded by the *actA* gene, to highjack the cellular actin machinery enabling Lm to spread from cell to cell (Radoshevich and Cossart, 2018).

During infection, Lm triggers potent innate and adaptive immune responses when phagocytosed by APCs (Flickinger et al., 2018; D'Orazio, 2019). Importantly, proteins from bacteria that reach the cytosol of infected APCs are processed and loaded on major histocompatibility complex (MHC) class I molecules for presentation to $CD8^+$ cytotoxic T-cells (Ikonomidis et al., 1994; Pamer, 2004; Flickinger et al., 2018; Chávez Arroyo and Portnoy, 2020; Zeng et al., 2020), while bacterial proteins that are degraded within phagolysosomes of APCs are delivered to MHC class II associated epitope presentation for $CD4^+$ T-cell priming (D'Orazio, 2019).

By deleting one or more crucial virulence genes, Lm virulence is easily and significantly attenuated preventing systemic infection of the host, while immunogenicity is maintained (Brockstedt et al., 2004). Thus, attenuated Lm is a promising vaccine vector to be used against diseases including neosporosis, for which a Th1-mediated immune response is required to confer protection (Ikonomidis et al., 1994; Brockstedt et al., 2004; Johnson et al., 2011; Wood and Paterson, 2014; Flickinger et al., 2018; D'Orazio, 2019; Chávez Arroyo and Portnoy, 2020). Additionally, the Lm vector has the advantage over other microbial vectors to overcome pre-existent or vector-induced immunity in the host allowing homologous prime-boost vaccination schemes without compromising its efficacy in T-cell priming (Leong et al., 2009).

The aim of our study was to develop an attenuated Lm vaccine vector (Lm3Dx) platform that is safe and expresses foreign antigen. To demonstrate proof of concept for triggering of a Th1 immune response we selected the NcSAG1 as antigen, which is a highly immunogenic protein, expressed on the surface of Nc tachyzoites and implicated to have a functional role in host cell invasion (Hemphill et al., 1997).

MATERIAL AND METHODS

Experimental Setup

Additionally to the crucial virulence genes *actA*, *inlA*, *inlB*, the fosfomycin resistance gene (*fosX*) was deleted from the parental JF5203 strain (ST1, CC1) (Aguilar-Bultet et al., 2018). *FosX* encodes a protein involved in inherent fosfomycin resistance of Lm outside the host (Scortti et al., 2018), and deletion renders the vaccine vector highly sensitive to this antibiotic and selectable without introducing exogenous antibiotic resistance genes while cloning. The resulting Lm vector Lm3Dx was first tested for genetic stability upon serial passaging and for infection dynamics in canine cell lines as surrogates for epithelial cells and APCs. The gene coding for the major Nc surface antigen NcSAG1 (*sag1*) was fused to the first 300 nucleotides of *actA* containing the signal peptide and PEST sequences to enhance antigen processing (Sewell et al., 2008) and was inserted into Lm3Dx *via* homologous recombination to avoid the introduction of exogenous antibiotic resistance genes. Homologous recombination, as opposed to plasmid integration methods used for other Lm-based vaccine vectors, does not require growth of the engineered vector on selective media containing antibiotics (Sacco et al., 2016) to ensure retention of the antigen encoding genes, thereby conferring high safety and stability to our vaccine strain. Bacterial NcSAG1 expression by the engineered Lm3Dx-NcSAG1 was confirmed by real-time PCR (RT-PCR) and Western Blot (WB) before performing *in vivo* safety and immunogenicity testing. For the latter, female pregnant and non-pregnant BALB/c mice were vaccinated intramuscularly (i.m.) with Lm3Dx expressing NcSAG1 using a homologous prime-boost vaccination scheme. In mice, bacterial spread to organs and to newborn pups, fecal and milk shedding (**Table 1**), genetic stability of isolated Lm3Dx_NcSAG1 and indicators of humoral and cellular immune response to NcSAG1 were evaluated.

Generation and Quality Control of the Vaccine Vector

Bacterial Strains, Plasmids, and Primers

Bacterial strains and plasmids used in this study are listed in **Supplementary Files S2, S3** and primers in **Supplementary File S4**, respectively.

The pMADΔactA plasmid used to remove *actA* was previously described (Henke et al., 2015). To generate the pHOSSΔinlAB plasmid, flanking regions of the *inlAB* region including the first 12 N-terminal nucleotides of *inlA* and the last 36 C-terminal nucleotides of *inlB* were amplified with GoTaq®DNA polymerase (Promega Corporation, Madison, USA) using the primer pairs ΔinlA_n_fw_1_SalI/ΔinlAB_2_rv (617pb) and ΔinlAB_3_F/ΔinlB_R_XmaI, respectively. The two resulting fragments were then ligated using T4 DNA ligase (Thermo Fisher Scientific Inc., Waltham, USA) following digestion of pHOSS1 (Abdelhamed et al., 2015) with XmaI (New England Labs Inc., Ipswich, MA, USA) and SalI (New England Labs Inc.) according to the manufacturer's instruction.

The pMADΔfosX plasmid for deletion of *fosX* was generated by removing the *fosX* sequence from a pMADfosX plasmid containing *fosX* with its flanking regions. The fosX fragment was generated by amplification from JF5203 with Hifi cloning (Takarabio Inc.) and purification with the NucleoSpin® Gel and PCR Clean-up Kit (Macherey-Nagel, Düren, Germany) after gel electrophoresis. Both insertion of the resulting fragment into pMADfosX and subsequent deletion of the *fosX* sequence from pMADfosX to generate pMADΔfosX were performed with the In-fusion® HD Cloning Plus (TakaraBio Inc.) technology according to the manufacturer recommendations. For In-fusion® cloning, the amplification primer pairs pMADfosX3_F/pMADfosX4_R, pMADfosX1_F/pMADfosX2_R and pMADΔfosX1_F/pMADΔfosX2_R were used to generate pMADfosX and pMADΔfosX, respectively. pMADfosX and pMADΔfosX plasmids were Sanger sequenced (3730 DNA Analyzer, Thermo Fisher Scientific Inc., Waltham, USA) using the BigDye® Terminator v3.1 Cycle Sequencing Kit (Thermo Fisher Scientific Inc., Waltham, USA). The primers used for sequencing (fosX_F, fosX_R, pMAD_F, pMAD_R, fosX_ex_F, fosX_ex_R) are listed in **Supplementary File S4**.

For generation of the pMAD_NactA100AA_SAG1_HIS plasmid, NactA100AA_SAG1_HIS was created *in-silico* using the Geneious 8.1 software (Biomatters Inc.) and synthesized and inserted into pMAD by Twist Bioscience (San Francisco, USA). Briefly, the *sag1* sequence NCLIV_033230 was codon-optimized for *L. monocytogenes* using a publicly available web-based software (http://www.jcat.de/). At the *sag1* 5' end, the first 300 nucleotides of *actA* were added and the 3' end was fused with a HIS tag followed by 2 stop codons. In order to ensure insertion of *sag1* into the *actA* locus, this sequence was inserted between the two *actA* flanking regions of the pMAD*ΔactA* plasmid resulting in pMAD_NactA100AA_SAG1_HIS. For deletion of the HIS-tag to generate pMAD_NactA100AA_SAG1 (Map in **Suplementary File S1**) the fragment without HIS tag was amplified with the Hifi cloning system and integrated into pMAD with the In-fusion® HD Cloning Plus using the primer pair SAG1HISdel_F/SAG1HISdel_R (**Supplementary File S4**).

TABLE 1 | Scheme of the vaccination and sampling protocol performed for each mouse experiment.

Day	-3	-2	-1	0	1	2	3	4	5	6	7	8	9	10	11	12	13	14	15	16	17	18	19	20	21	22	23	24	25	26	27	28	29	30	31	32	33	34	35	36	37	38	39	40	41	42	43	44	45	46	47	48	49	50	51	52	53-73	74
***In-vivo* safety**																																																											
Lm3Dx																																																											
Immunization				X														X														X																											
Fecal sampling			X	X	X	X		X	X	X	X			X			X	X	X	X	X	X	X	X	X			X			X	X	X	X	X	X	X	X	X	X			X			X												
Serum sampling			X															X														X														X												
Euthanasia and						X																																								X												
organ sampling																																																											
Splenocyte stimulation																																														X												
WT																																																											
Inoculation				X																																																							
Fecal sampling			X	X	X	X																																																					
Euthanasia and organ sampling						X																																																				
Milk excretion																																																											
Immunization				X																																																							
Milk sampling					X	X	X	X																																																		
Euthanasia, organ sampling								X																																																		
Birth Interference																																																											
Immunization				X														X														X																											
Fecal sampling	X				X	X		X			X								X	X		X			X								X	X		X			X				X			X												
Mating																													X	X	X																											
Pups birth																																																					X	X	X	X		
Serum sampling	X																																																									X
Euthanasia, organ sampling,																																																										X
splenocyte stimulation																																																											

Engineering of Lm-3Dx and Lm-3Dx_SAG1

In order to prevent permanent insertion of antibiotic resistance genes into the vector, all mutant strains were generated from *L. monocytogenes* strain JF5203 (NCBI Reference Sequence: NZ_LT985474.1; https://www.ncbi.nlm.nih.gov/nuccore/NZ_LT985474.1; lineage I, CC 1, ST 1, serotype 4b) by homologous recombination with either pMAD or pHOSS1 plasmid derivates (**Supplementary File S3**). The JF5203Δ*actA* mutant generated in a previous study (Henke et al., 2015) was used as parental mutant to engineer the vaccine vector. The JF5203Δ*actA/inlA/inlB/fosX* vector (Lm3Dx) was generated by sequential in-frame deletion of *inlA/inlB* and *fosX* genes from the JF5203Δ*actA* mutant by homologous recombination with the respective pMAD (Arnaud et al., 2004) and pHOSS1 (Abdelhamed et al., 2015) plasmid derivates described above. Gene deletions were confirmed by DNA sequencing of the intermediate mutants and by full genome sequencing of the final vaccine vector strain (see below).

Finally, Lm3Dx was transformed with the plasmid pMAD_NactA100AA_SAG1 (**Supplementary File S1**) to create Lm3Dx_SAG1 expressing *sag1* fused to the 300 first nucleotides of *actA* under the control of the *actA* promotor.

Quality Control

Fosfomycin minimal inhibitory concentrations (MICs) were determined in Lm WT and Lm3Dx using the fosfomycin E-test strip (Biomérieux SA, France) after 24h incubation at 37°C as previously described (Scortti et al., 2006). Genetic stability of Δ*actA* mutant and Lm3Dx was determined in comparison to the WT by serial passaging under non-selective conditions. Strains were cultured in 10mL of Bacto Brain Heart Infusion broth (BHI, Sigma-Aldrich, Buchs, Switzerland) and sub-cultured every 12 h at a 1/10'000 dilution into fresh BHI broth. Every 10 passages, 10μL of the medium was plated on BHI-Agar plate (Sigma-Aldrich, Buchs, Switzerland) and cultured 24h at 37°C before further passaging was done. Every ten passages until passage number 100, a colony of the plating performed on BHI-Agar was grown in 10mL of BHI broth and DNA was extracted using the DNA extraction kit (Invitrogen, PureLink™ Microbiome, DNA purification Kit). PCR of extracted DNA was performed to ensure stability of the deletion of each virulence gene (primers used are listed in **Supplementary File S4**). Insertion of the *sag1* sequence into Lm3Dx was confirmed by colony PCR using the *actA* flanking region primer pairs (**Supplementary File S4**), resulting in Lm3Dx_SAG1. Furthermore, both Lm3Dx and Lm3Dx_SAG1 were sequenced by INVIEW Resequencing (Eurofins Genomics, Constance, Germany) after the first and 100th passage in BHI broth to analyze for single nucleotide point mutations (SNPs) (https://www.ebi.ac.uk/ena/browser/view/PRJEB43038).

For confirmation of NcSAG1 expression at the RNA level, Lm3Dx_SAG1 was cultured in BHI broth overnight at 37°C. The next day, RNA was extracted with the RNA extraction kit (RiboPure™ Bacteria, Invitrogen, Thermo Fisher Inc., Waltham, USA) and contaminating genomic DNA was eliminated with RQ1 RNaseFree DNase (Promega Corporation, Madison, USA). Purified RNA was then reverse transcribed into cDNA with GoScript™ Reverse Transcriptase (Promega Corporation, Madison, USA) following the instruction of the manufacturer. PCR for NcSAG1 was performed using NcSAG1_F/NcSAG1_R primers (**Supplementary File S4**). NcSAG1 protein expression in Lm3Dx_SAG1 during infection was confirmed by WB of proteins extracted from infected canine histiocytic DH82 cells. Briefly, DH82 cells were cultured to confluency in Corning® Cell culture T150 flasks (Fisher scientific Inc., Waltham, USA) and infected at a multiplicity of infection (MOI) of 40. Six hours post-infection, infected cells were detached by Trypsin-EDTA (Sigma-Aldrich, Buchs, Switzerland), centrifuged and the pellet was frozen at -80°C. After thawing, cells were lysed by sonication (3 cycles of 2 minutes at 40% duty) (Sonifier 450, Branson, Danbury, CT, USA) and proteins were separated from the cell lysate by centrifugation (15.000 x g, 15 minutes at 4°C). Fifteen μg each of the unpurified protein extract, of Nc protein extract as positive control and of the empty Lm3Dx vector as a negative control, were separated by SDS-Page and electrophoretically transferred to a nitrocellulose membrane. The membrane was blocked in PBS/0.1% Tween-20/2% milk powder for 1 h at RT, and the monoclonal mouse anti-*Nc*SAG1 antibody (kindly provided by Prof. Dr. Camilla Björkman, University of Uppsala, Sweden) (Björkman and Hemphill, 1998) was applied at a dilution of 1:1000 overnight at 4°C. Membranes were washed four times with PBS supplemented with 0.1% Tween-20, and were incubated with the goat anti-mouse IgG coupled to alkaline phosphatase (AP) (Promega, Madison, USA), diluted 1:2000 in PBS-Tween-20. Following four more washes in PBS, bound antibodies were visualized by developing the AP reaction using 0.3% NBT/BCIP stock solution (Roche, Basel, Switzerland) in 0.1 M sodium chloride, 5 mM magnesium chloride, and 0.1 M Tris (pH 9.5). The enzymatic reaction was stopped by immersing the membrane in distilled water.

In Vitro Safety

In Vitro Infection Assays

To check whether virulence gene deletion attenuates cellular infection of the vaccine vector Lm3Dx and whether attenuation is cell-type specific, canine cell lines representing epithelial cells (Madin-Darby Canine Kidney, MDCK) and macrophages (DH82) were infected. The day prior to infection, both cell lines were seeded in 24-well plates at densities of 0.8 x 10^5 (MDCK) or 2.5 x 10^5 cells (DH82) per well, respectively, and were grown in DMEM medium supplemented with 10% FCS and 50 μg/mL Penicillin/Streptomycin at 37°C with 5% CO_2. One hour prior to infection, cells were starved in FCS- and antibiotic-free medium. Cells were then infected with Lm WT, Lm Δ*actA*, Lm3Dx and *Listeria innocua* at a MOI of 1.25. The concentration of the inoculum was determined by OD_{600} measurement on a Biospectrometer® basic (Vaudaux-Eppendorf AG, Schönenbuch/Basel, Switzerland) and confirmed by plating of the inoculum on brain heart infusion (BHI) plates (Sigma-Aldrich). After 1h, cells were washed once with PBS and DMEM medium supplemented with FCS (2% for long-term infection assay or 10% for short-term infection assay) and 50 μg/mL gentamicin (Sigma-Aldrich) was added to prevent extracellular replication.

Colony-forming units (CFU) evaluation for the short-term infection assays was performed as previously reported (Rupp et al., 2015). Briefly, infected cells were washed once with PBS and then harvested in 100 µl of 0.5% Triton X-100 (Sigma–Aldrich) in distilled water (dH2O) 2, 4, 6, 24, 48 and 72 h post-infection (pi). Ten-fold serial dilutions of the lysates were plated on BHI-agar plates, and CFUs per well were calculated. At least three independent experiments were performed in triplicate.

For long-term infection assays, cells were infected as described above, but had to be sub-cultured due to cellular proliferation. At determined timepoints (2, 5, 7, 9 and 12 days pi) cells were washed once with PBS and then detached using 100 µL of Trypsin-EDTA solution (Sigma-Aldrich). Half of the cell suspension was transferred in a new 24-well plate with fresh DMEM medium supplemented with 2% FCS and 50µg/mL gentamicin for sub-culturing. The other half was incubated with 2% Triton X-100 (Sigma-Aldrich) in dH_2O for 10 min and then plated in serial dilutions as described above. At the final timepoint (14 days pi) cells were harvested in 100 µL of 2% Triton X-100 and further processed as described above. At least three independent experiments were performed in triplicate.

Immunofluorescence Analysis of *In Vitro* Infection Assays

Coverslips with infected cells (DH82 or MDCK) were collected at 2, 6, 24, 48 and 72 hours pi and were fixed in 4% paraformaldehyde (PFA, Sigma–Aldrich) at 37°C for 15 min. Immunofluorescence was performed as previously reported (Rupp et al., 2015). Coverslips were incubated with *Listeria* O antiserum (BD Difco, 1:1000 in PBS-T) and phalloidin DyLight 633 (Fisher Scientific, Waltham, MA, USA, 1:500) in PBS-T with 10% normal goat serum (NGS, Agilent Technologies, CA, USA). After 1 h, coverslips were washed three times with PBS-T, followed by a 45 min incubation with Alexa Fluor 488 goat anti-rabbit IgG (Life Technologies, 1:500) and DAPI (1:10,000) in PBS-T supplemented with 10% NGS. Coverslips were washed twice with PBS and finally rinsed with dH_2O and mounted using glycergel (Dako). Specimens were imaged using a FV3000 confocal laser scanning microscope (Olympus, Hamburg, Germany) and were analyzed using FIJI (Schindelin et al., 2012).

In Vivo Safety and Immunogenicity

Mouse Vaccination

All mouse experiments were conducted in compliance with the Swiss and European Union (Directive no. 2010/63/EU) legislation for the use of animals for scientific purposes, and animal protocols were approved by the Bernese Animal Welfare Committee (licenses BE113/19 and BE103/20). For the experiments, 6-week-old female and male BALB/c as well as synchronized pregnant mice were obtained from Charles River Laboratories (Sulzfeld, Germany). All mice were maintained under conventional day/night cycle in a temperature-controlled room excepted for the mice used in the milk excretion experiment, where the cages were kept under a sterile hood after vaccination, with water and food *ad libitum*. Two weeks upon arrival at the facility, mice were randomly distributed into groups and individually marked. One additional week of acclimatization was then given to the mice prior to start of the experiment.

For each experiment inoculation doses of Lm3Dx_SAG1 or WT strain were prepared by culturing a colony overnight in 10 mL BHI broth at 37°C. Bacteria were washed 3x with sterile PBS (Sigma-Aldrich) to remove BHI-broth. Prior to injection, they were resuspended to an OD_{600} of 0.8 and sequentially diluted to the desired concentration in each experiment (1×10^6, 5×10^6 and/or 1×10^7 CFU/50 µL). Concentration was confirmed by plating of the inoculum on BHI-Agar plates (Sigma-Aldrich) and CFU counting 24 h after incubation at 37°C. Euthanasia was performed in a euthanasia chamber using isoflurane and CO_2 or cervical dislocation for pups younger than 3 weeks old.

Experiment 1: Biosafety evaluation of Lm3Dx_SAG1 in non-pregnant BALB/c female mice.

Mice were randomly allocated into experimental groups of 5 to 6 mice each, with an additional mouse per group used as sentinel. Three groups were injected i.m. with 50 µL sterile PBS containing the Lm3Dx_SAG1 vaccine strain at different dosages (1×10^6, 5×10^6, 1×10^7 CFU), one group with the WT strain (1×10^7 CFU) and the negative control group with 50 µL sterile PBS. Sentinel mice were used to evaluate Lm transmission between mice in the same experimental cage. Mice were immunized i.m. in the thigh. Lm3Dx_SAG1 groups received a primovaccination and two booster injections, both two weeks apart, and were euthanized 2 weeks following the last immunization (**Table 1**). Because the group receiving WT (1×10^7 CFU) had to be euthanized 1.5d after the first immunization due to severity of clinical signs, 5 additional mice were inoculated i.m. with 50 µl PBS containing 1×10^7 Lm3Dx_SAG1 and euthanized 1.5d after inoculation to assess the attenuation of our Lm3Dx_SAG1 vaccine strain during the acute phase. At euthanasia, liver, spleen, kidney, uterus, brain, thigh musculature and GIT of the Lm3Dx_SAG1 vaccinated mice were retrieved for further evaluation.

Experiment 2: Biosafety evaluation of Lm3Dx_SAG1 in lactating BALB/c dams and suckling pups.

To assess Lm3Dx_SAG1 excretion in milk and the safety of its use in lactating dams, we randomly allocated 14 dams with their respective pups (2-8 days old) into two groups (7 per group). Based on the results of the first experiment, the Lm3Dx_SAG1 group was injected once with 1×10^7 CFU of Lm3Dx_SAG1 and the other group with PBS in the thigh musculature. From day 1 to day 4 after inoculation, dams were separated from their pups 1 hour prior to milking once a day (**Table 1**). Mice were anesthetized with isoflurane and 1 IU of oxytocin (Sigma) was injected intraperitoneally. Ten minutes later, milk collection was started using a custom-made vacuum pump-based milk collection system. Upon milking, dams were returned to their pups in a cage under a sterile hood until the following day. Dams and pups were euthanized at day 4 pi. The liver, spleen, thigh musculature and GIT of the Lm3Dx_SAG1 vaccinated dams and their pups were retrieved for further evaluation.

Experiment 3: Assessment of potential effects of Lm3Dx_SAG1 on pregnancy outcome in BALB/c mice.

The experiment included three experimental groups of 6 mice each. Two groups were inoculated three times at two-week intervals with 50 μl PBS containing the Lm3Dx_SAG1 vaccine strain at $1x10^6$ and $1x10^7$ CFU respectively, while the control group was inoculated with 50 μL sterile PBS at each vaccination (**Table 1**). The first vaccination was done at day 0 and the first booster on day 14. On day 22, mice were estrus-synchronized using the Whitten effect (Whitten, 1957) and were mated from day 25 to 27 by housing two females and one male in the same cage. Subsequently, males were removed from the cage and the third immunization was performed at day 28 (early pregnancy). Data on fertility (number of female mice that became pregnant), litter size (number of delivered pups per dam), stillborn mice and neonatal mortality (number of dead pups from birth until day 2 postpartum (p.p.)); postnatal mortality (number of dead pups from day 3 p.p. to the end of the experiment) and clinical signs that occurred during the observation phase were recorded. Dams and surviving pups were monitored at least 21 days after birth to rule out possible adverse effects due to treatments. At euthanasia, liver, spleen, injected thigh musculature and GIT of the Lm3Dx_SAG1 vaccinated dams and PBS control group were retrieved for further evaluation.

Microbiological Assessments

Mice in experiments 1 and 3 were monitored for fecal shedding as follows. In experiment 1, fecal sampling (100 mg/mouse) and analysis was performed daily from the day prior to the first vaccine administration until day 7 pi and at day 10 pi. Then, the same sampling scheme was repeated for the two booster injections (**Table 1**). In experiment 3, fecal samples of every mice were retrieved 1, 2, 4 and 7 days after each vaccine dose administration and at day 11 and 14 after the third vaccine administration.

Fecal samples were homogenized in Half-Fraser broth (Fisher Scientific) at a 1:10 dilution using 5 mm glass beads (Sigma-Aldrich) in a TissueLyser II (Quiagen, MD, USA). Ten-fold serial dilutions were plated on ALOA Agar plates (Biomérieux, France) and incubated 2 days at 37°C prior to quantification of CFUs. Additionally, bacteria were enriched by culturing fecal homogenates for 24 h at 37°C in Half-Fraser broth followed by plating on ALOA Agar Plates for qualitative evaluation. Ten-fold serial dilution of milk probes were also plated on ALOA Agar plates and enriched in Half-Fraser broth as described for fecal samples. Bacterial isolates were confirmed by phenotype on ALOA Agar plates (round, blue-green colony with an opaque halo) and colony PCR amplification with the primer pairs hly_F/hly_R, actA_F/actA_R, inlA_F/inlA_R, inlB_F/inlB_R, fosX_F/fosX_R and *Nc*SAG1_F/*Nc*SAG1_R (**Supplementary File S4**). CFU sensitivity was set at 10^3 CFU/gram feces or milk for the quantitative assay without prior enrichment and at 10^2 CFU/gram feces or milk for the qualitative assay after enrichment in Half-Fraser broth followed by plating on ALOA Agar plates.

For assessment of bacterial intra-host spread, organs of female mice (experiments 1-3) and pups (experiment 2) were collected under sterile conditions immediately after euthanasia to evaluate the presence of Lm in organs. Organs were divided for immersion-fixation in 4% formaldehyde (for subsequent histological and immunohistological analysis) and for homogenization and enrichment in Half-Fraser Broth (1:10) as described previously for fecal analysis. Additionally, in experiment 3, pups which died in the postnatal phase (before endpoint analysis), were weighted and homogenized in whole in Half-Fraser broth (1:10) using an ULTRA-TURRAX® Tube Drive (Faust AG, Schaffhausen, Switzerland) and serial dilutions were plated on ALOA plates with and without prior enrichment in Half-Fraser broth as described above for qualitative and quantitative evaluation. At endpoint analysis, three weeks after birth, spleen, part of the liver and the gastrointestinal tract (GIT) of every surviving pup were pooled, weighted and homogenized 1:10 in Half-Fraser broth for quantitative and qualitative CFU evaluation as described above.

Histopathological Analysis

To screen for organ lesions caused by Lm WT and Lm3Dx_SAG1, formalin fixed and paraffin embedded muscle, liver, spleen, brain, kidney and uterus of adult mice used in all three experiments were stained with hematoxylin and eosin (H&E) and microscopically analyzed. In experiment 2, histopathology of spleen, liver and GIT of pups was performed. Additionally, most sections were screened for persistence of the vaccine vector by using an immunohistochemical protocol for detection of *Listeria*. Immunohistochemistry was performed as previously described (Oevermann et al., 2010) with a polyclonal rabbit antibody against Listeria (1:200, Difco Laboratories, Detroit MI, USA).

Assessment of the Immune Response Against NcSAG1

To investigate the cellular immune response against Lm3Dx_SAG1, spleens of female mice from the PBS and the different Lm3Dx_SAG1 groups of experiments 1 and 3 were used for splenocyte re-stimulation assays. Following euthanasia, spleen samples were immersed in 5 mL of complete RPMI medium (RPMI 1640 medium containing 1% antibiotic: 100 U of penicillin, 100 μl of streptomycin, 2 mM L-glutamine, 10% FCS and 55 μM β-mercaptoethanol). Splenocyte isolation was performed as previously described (Aguado-Martínez et al., 2016a). Following lysis of red blood cells and two washing steps with complete RPMI medium, cell suspensions containing the splenic lymphocytes were seeded in a 24-well plate at a density of 2×10^6 cells/well.

Ex vivo stimulation of the seeded splenic lymphocytes was performed with concanavalin A (ConA; 5 μg/mL; Sigma-Aldrich) as positive control, with *N. caninum* antigen lysate (20 μg/mL) or recombinant NcSAG1 (20 μg/mL), respectively. Unstimulated splenocytes were used as negative control. Following culture at 37°C/5% CO_2 during 72 h, medium supernatants of stimulated and unstimulated splenocytes were collected and levels of IFN-γ and IL-5 were measured in the supernatants using the BD OptEIA™ mouse ELISA kits (BD Biosciences, CA, USA) according to manufacturer's instructions (Aguado-Martínez et al., 2016a). A Luminex instrument (Bio-PlexTM 200 system) was used to run the microtiter filter plates.

The expression and purification of recombinant NcSAG1 used for stimulation in our experiments was performed as follows. Firstly, the coding sequence of NcSAG1 was cloned in the pET151 TOPO® expression construct (ThermoFisher Scientific, MA, USA). *Nc*SAG1 was expressed in BL21 Star™ (DE3) One Shot® *Escherichia coli* strain and purified afterwards by Ni^{2+} affinity chromatography. For the purification of NcSAG1 Protino® Ni-IDA 1000 packed columns (Macherey-Nagel, Düren, Germany) were used, and proteins were purified under denaturing conditions according to manufacturer's instructions. Purity of NcSAG1 was confirmed by SDS-PAGE and the protein concentration was measured with a BCA Protein Assay Kit (Pierce™).

To determine the humoral response against NcSAG1 in experiment 1 blood samples were collected from the tail vein one day before each immunization and by cardiac puncture 14 days after the 2nd booster, immediately after euthanasia. Blood of the WT group was sampled only prior to the first inoculation and immediately after euthanasia (**Table 1**). In experiment 3, to avoid stress of pregnant dams, blood was sampled only two days prior to the first vaccine application and following euthanasia, 42 days after the second booster. Blood of surviving pups was also collected by cardiac puncture. Anti-NcSAG1 IgG levels were determined by ELISA according to Debache et al. (Debache et al., 2008). In brief, 96-well plates were coated with recombinant NcSAG1 (100 ng/well) and incubated overnight at 4°C. The following day, plates were washed three times with washing buffer (0.05% PBS-Tween-20) before antigens were blocked with 1% bovine serum albumin (BSA) in 0.05% PBS-Tween-20 for 2h at RT. Subsequently, sera of individual mice at a dilution of 1:50 and two-fold sequential dilution up to 1:400 were added to individual wells. Following three washes, secondary antibody (goat anti-mouse IgG conjugated to AP (Promega)) was applied at a dilution of 1:2000. Development was performed with AP substrate buffer (1mg/mL). Absorbance was measured as optical density (OD) at 405 nm in a microplate reader (EnSpire™ 2300 Multilabel Reader, Switzerland). For evaluation, OD values were converted into relative index per cent (RIPC) values using the following formula [RIPC = (OD_{405nm} sample − OD_{405nm} negative control)/(OD_{405nm} positive control − OD_{405nm} negative control)*100 (Aguado-Martínez et al., 2016b). Serum of Nc infected mice was used as positive control.

Statistical Analysis

Differences in arithmetic means of CFU between mutants and JF5203 were evaluated with the parametric student t-test and of the humoral and cellular immune responses between mice groups were compared with the non-parametric Mann-Whitney-U test. For the temporal analysis of the IgG response a one-way ANOVA repeated measure was used to compare each timepoint within each given group. 95% confidence intervals (95%CI) were determined and statistical significance was assigned as follows: P ≤.032 *, P ≤.0021 **, P ≤.0002 ***, P <.0001****. For IFN-γ and IL-5 concentrations, graphs are presented as column charts.

Pup mortality was analyzed with the Kaplan–Meier survival method. Pup survival curves were then compared by the Log-rank (Mantel–Cox) test, and differences in pup's mortality rates between groups were assessed by the $\chi 2$ or Fisher's exact test.

All statistical analysis were performed using the commercially available software Prism 9 (Graphpad Prism version 9.0.2 for MacOSX, GraphPad Software, La Jolla, CA, USA, www.graphpad.com).

RESULTS

Lm3Dx Is Strongly Attenuated in MDCK Cells, but Behaves Similar to WT in Early Stages of DH82 Cell Infection

The parental Lm JF5203 strain (lineage I, CC1, ST1) that was isolated from a bovine rhombencephilitis case induces a strong T-cell and B-cell response (Oevermann et al., 2010). It has been extensively studied in our laboratory, and the complete genome has been published and annotated (Aguilar-Bultet et al., 2018). To evaluate the attenuation of the Lm3Dx strain and its tropism to phagocytic cells, MDCK and DH82 were used as surrogates for canine epithelial cells and APCs, respectively, and were infected with Lm3Dx in comparison to WT JF5203, *ΔactA*, and the related apathogenic bacterium *Listeria innocua* (Li) (**Figure 1**). In MDCK cells, the vaccine strain behaved similarly to the apathogenic Li and was significantly attenuated in cellular invasion compared to WT and *ΔactA* Lm as indicated by 2.5 orders of magnitude lower CFUs at 2h pi (**Figure 1A**). Confirming the CFU data, immunofluorescence microscopy detected clearly lower number of intracellular bacteria and infection foci in Lm3Dx than in WT and *ΔactA* (**Supplementary File S7**) at 2h pi. Interestingly, Lm3Dx exhibited, similar to Li, a lag phase compared to *ΔactA* and WT before the numbers of CFU raised exponentially. Additionally, Lm3Dx reached its plateau phase at a CFU count that was slightly higher than observed for Li but approximately 2 and 4 orders of magnitude lower than CFUs of *ΔactA* and WT, respectively (**Figure 1A**). The lower CFU plateaus indicated deficient intercellular spread of Lm3Dx and *ΔactA*. This was further supported by the small size of their infection foci and lower number of intracellular bacteria compared to the WT at 24h pi when analyzed with immunofluorescence microscopy (**Figure 1B**). Also, no actin polymerization was observed in Lm3Dx, *ΔactA* and Li, proving their inefficiency move intracellularly as opposed to WT and to spread from cell-to-cell (**Figure 1B** and **Supplementary File S7**). During long-term infections, the Lm3Dx vaccine strain continued to follow the infection kinetics of the apathogenic Li and was rapidly cleared in MDCK cells. CFU of Lm3Dx were detected until 2 days pi, while CFU of *ΔactA* and WT were retrieved in MDCK cells up to 7 days and 14 days pi, respectively (**Figure 1C**).

In contrast to the infection in MDCK, infection dynamics of Lm3Dx in DH82 cells were similar to the *ΔactA* mutant rather than Li. This indicates (i) the insignificance of *inlA* and *inlB* for Lm infection of phagocytic cells, and (ii) a stronger intracellular survival of Lm3Dx in phagocytes compared to Li. CFU data at 2h pi indicated that all strains entered DH82 cells with similar efficiency (**Figure 1D**) which was supported by similar numbers of intracellular bacteria and infection foci as visualized by immunofluorescence microscopy at 2h (**Supplementary File S8**). CFU numbers of Li remained constant for the first 6h and then continuously dropped (**Figure 1D**). In contrast, CFU counts of Lm3Dx increased until 6 h pi similar to WT and *ΔactA* reaching a peak of 1 x 10^6 CFU/well (**Figure 1D**). Later, CFU of Lm3Dx and *ΔactA* dropped by approximately one order of magnitude and fewer intracellular bacteria were observed compared to the WT at 24 h (**Figures 1D, E**). Within the following 48 h, the numbers of CFUs

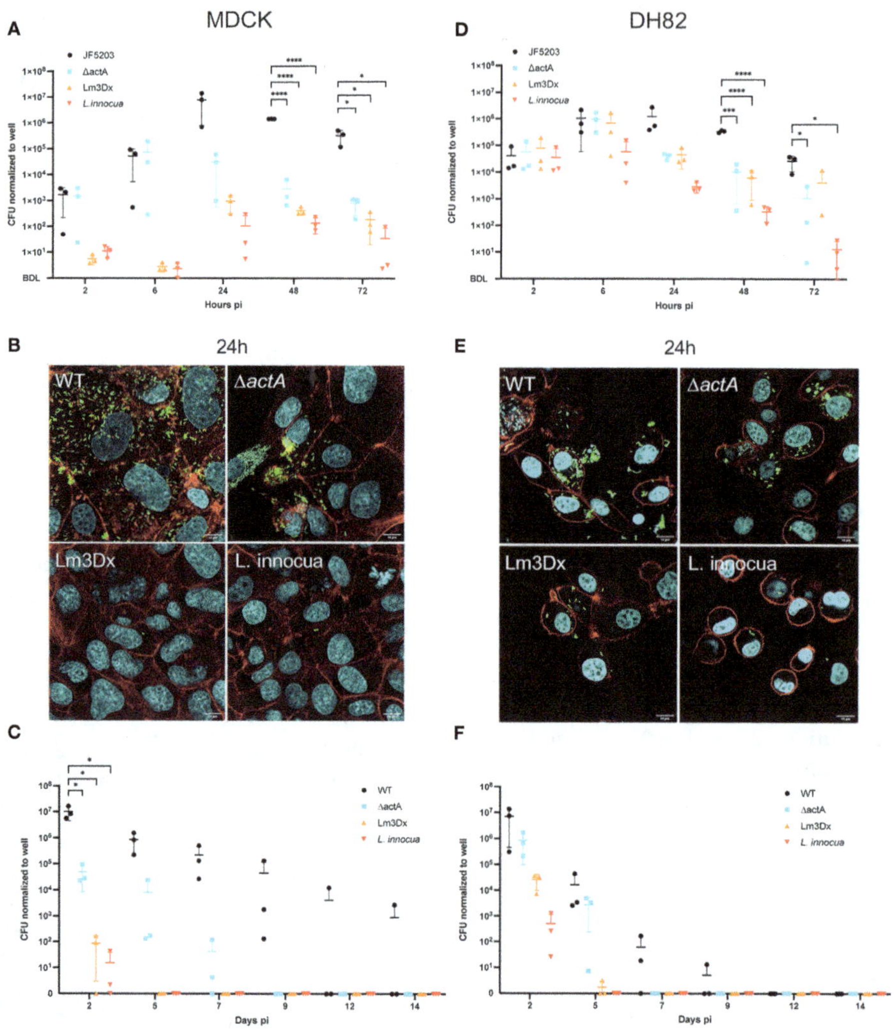

FIGURE 1 | Gentamicin protection assay with the wildtype (WT) parental strain JF5203 (black circles), ΔactA (blue square), Lm3Dx (orange triangle) and *L. innocua* (red triangle) in an epithelial **(A–C)** and macrophage-like cell line **(D–F)**. For the short-term assay until 72h, canine epithelial cells (MDCK) **(A)** and canine macrophage-like cells (DH82) **(D)** were infected for 1h at a multiplicity of infection of 1.25:1. CFU were enumerated at the indicated time points. Immunofluorescence microscopy images of MDCK **(B)** and DH82 **(E)** at 24h post infection with the parental strain, mutants and *L. innocua*. Bacteria are shown in green (Listeria-Antibody), cellular actin is stained with fluorescent phalloidin (red) and cellular and bacterial nuclei with DAPI. At 24h the number of intracellular bacteria is strongly reduced in Lm3Dx-infected MDCK compared to WT-infected and ΔactA-infected MDCK, and rather similar to *L. innocua*-infected MDCK **(B)**. Additionally, Lm3Dx lacks actin polymerization, which is prominent in the WT infected cells (red comet tails). The number of intracellular bacteria is higher in Lm3Dx-infected DH82 cells **(D)** and the reduction compared to WT is less evident than in MDCK. For the long-term assay until 14d, MDCK **(C)** and DH82 **(F)** cells were infected for 1h at a multiplicity of infection of 1.25:1. At the indicated timepoints, cells were detached by trypsin and 50% of cells were transferred to a new well. The remaining cells were lysed and serial dilutions were plated for CFU counting on BHI-Agar. Lm3Dx is cleared more rapidly than the WT from both epithelial and macrophage-like cells. Datapoints in the graphs are from 3 independent experiments performed in triplicate wells and are presented with ± 95% confidence interval; $^*P<0.05$, $^{***}P<0.001$, $^{****}P<0.0001$ (student t test). Because the y-axes of the graphs are in log scale, below detection level (BDL) was added manually to show all values where no CFU were recovered.

of Lm3Dx and *ΔactA* further continued to drop, while the reduction of CFUs in the WT started only at 48 h pi (**Figure 1D**). Immunofluorescence microscopy revealed that Lm3Dx and *ΔactA* had similar number and size of infection foci confirming CFU data (data not shown). Infection foci were smaller than those in WT infected DH82 and larger than those of Li. Lm3Dx had no visible actin tails, indicating that it has lost the spreading ability (**Figure 1E** and **Supplementary File S8**). The clearance of Lm3Dx in DH82 was similar to that of the *ΔactA* mutant. While both Lm3Dx and *ΔactA* persisted in DH82 until 5 days pi, the WT was detected until 9 days pi (**Figure 1F**). Additionally, cell infection assays were performed with the intermediate mutants *ΔactA/fosX* and *ΔactA/ΔinlB/ΔfosX* (up to 72 h pi) and these mutants behaved as the *ΔactA* mutant in DH82 and MDCK cells leading to the conclusion that cell invasion of MDCK was attenuated by deletion of *inlA* but not *inlB* *(data not shown).*

In summary, *in vitro* results showed strong attenuation of Lm3Dx in epithelial cells due to significantly reduced cellular invasion and intercellular spread, while the same strain behaved identical to the WT within phagocytic cells during the early stage of infection as further supported by the number of generations between 2-6h (**Supplementary File S5**).

The Genome of Lm3Dx Remains Stable for 100 Passages After Deletions

Stability of *actA, inlA, inlB and fosX* deletions was confirmed by PCR every 10th passage in BHI (data not shown) up to passage number 100 (**Figure 2**). Additionally, analysis of entire genomic sequences of Lm3Dx at passages 1 and 100 revealed that the genome was stable except the appearance of one SNP identified in the *nifJ* gene, resulting in an isoleucine substituting a methionine (G2752A) in the encoded oxidoreductase. No difference was detected in the infection phenotype of passage 100 in the tested cell lines compared to the initial Lm3Dx mutant, and likewise fosfomycin sensitivity with a MIC of 6 µg/mL compared to ≥1024 µg/mL in the WT was maintained after 100 passages (**Supplementary File S6**).

Lm3Dx Expresses NcSAG1 at the RNA and Protein Level

Based on the *in vitro* results, we anticipated that Lm3Dx would not be able to cause systemic infection of epithelial organs *in vivo*, but that the early infection dynamics of Lm3Dx in phagocytes would be sufficient to trigger an efficient immune response. Therefore, as a proof of concept we created Lm3Dx_SAG1 by inserting the *Neospora caninum* sag1 sequence fused to the first 300 nucleotides of *actA* into the *actA* locus of Lm3Dx, and confirmed NcSAG1 expression in Lm3Dx_SAG1 on RNA (**Figure 3A**) and protein level (**Figure 3B**).

In Vivo Safety Assessment and Immunological Characterization of the Lm3DX Vaccine Strain Expressing the Major *N. caninum* Surface Antigen NcSAG1

None of the Lm3Dx_SAG1 vaccinated mice developed adverse events or clinical signs of listeriosis after vaccination in any of the mouse experiments. In experiment 1, fecal shedding of Lm3Dx_SAG1 was detected only following enrichment in 3/6 mice from the 5 x 10^6 CFU dose group and 1/6 mice from the 1 x 10^7 CFU dose group at day 1 pi. Furthermore, in the 1 x 10^7 CFU/mice group, Lm3Dx_SAG1 was recovered following enrichment at day 3 and day 7 after the first booster injection in one mouse each. In contrast to the Lm3Dx_SAG1 groups, mice injected with the parental WT strain exhibited clinical signs early on. Initial signs appeared 12 h pi and were characterized by mildly reduced general condition and slightly mat fur, while behavior remained normal. However, at 36 h pi, all mice inoculated with the Lm WT strain exhibited strongly impaired health status (isolation, lethargy, hunched posture, ruffled fur, ataxia, paralysis of the injected hindlimb) and had to be humanely euthanized. Feces of WT infected mice were positive only after enrichment in 2/6 mice one day pi, while at day 2, feces of 5/6 mice contained high numbers of bacteria (mean 4.95 x 10^6 CFU/gram feces ± 4.76 x 10^6 (SD)). The feces of one mouse were not recovered at day 2 pi. Feces of sentinel mice in all Lm3Dx groups and the WT group remained negative for Lm throughout the experiment.

After euthanasia of WT injected mice at 36h after injection, CFU count revealed high bacterial loads in most organs (**Figure 4A**). The highest bacterial loads were found in the spleen (mean 2.0 x 10^{10} CFU/gram) and liver (mean 1.62 x 10^7 CFU/gram), while in kidney (mean 4.34 x 10^4 CFU/gram), uterus (mean 5.72 x 10^4 CFU/gram) and brain (mean 2.64 x 10^4 CFU/gram) bacterial numbers were lower (**Figure 4A**). In contrast, at the same timepoint post inoculation, Lm3Dx_SAG1 was recovered only from the spleen of 3/5 mice at a mean 8 x 10^3 CFU/gram organ, 7 orders of magnitude lower than the WT (**Figure 4A**). No Lm3Dx_SAG1 was detected in any other organ 36h after injection, not even following overnight enrichment in broth (**Figure 4A**).

In experiment 2, Lm3Dx_SAG1 excretion into milk of lactating mice was followed up to day 4 post vaccination (**Figure 4B**). Bacterial numbers reached 2.96 x 10^6 CFU/ml of milk at day 2 and remained high until day 4 (**Figure 4B**). Additionally, Lm3Dx_SAG1 was isolated in relatively high numbers from the GIT of pups at day 4 (mean 1,81 x 10^4 CFU/gram) indicating that bacteria were taken up orally with the

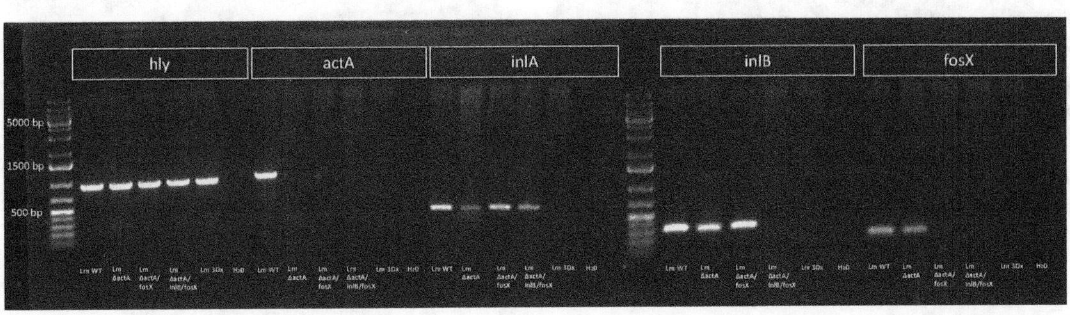

FIGURE 2 | PCR for *hly, actA, inlA, inlB* and *fosX* of WT, Lm3Dx and intermediate mutants at passage 100. All strains harbor the *hly* gene encoding for Listeriolysin O that was used as species control for *Listeria monocytogenes*. Deletions of *actA, inlA, inlB* and *fosX* are stable across 100 passages.

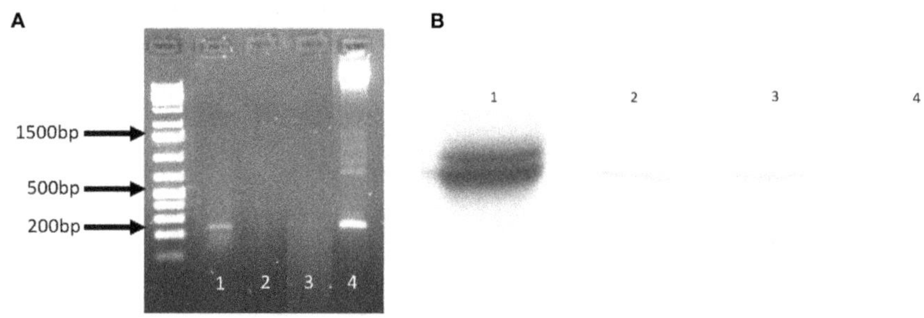

FIGURE 3 | NcSAG1 expression by Lm3Dx_SAG1. **(A)** NcSAG1 mRNA expression. The 200 bp band of NcSAG1 is visible in Lm3Dx_SAG1 (1), but not in the empty vector Lm3Dx (3). H_2O was used as negative control (2) and pMAD_NactA100AA_SAG1 plasmid DNA as positive control (4). **(B)** Bacterial NcSAG1 protein expression in infected cells. WB evidences a specific band of NcSAG1 protein expression at 35kDa in DH82 cells infected with Lm3Dx_SAG1HIS (2) and Lm3Dx_SAG1 (3), but not in DH82 cells infected with the empty vector Lm3Dx (4). Nc crude extract was used as positive control (1).

milk (**Figure 4C**). However, even though Lm3Dx_SAG1 was transmitted with the dam's milk to the pups, none of the pups showed clinical signs of listeriosis. Furthermore, Lm3Dx_SAG1 generally remained restricted to the GI tract of the pups and did not cross the gastrointestinal barrier as indicated by the low incidence of bacteria in internal organs: Lm3Dx_SAG1 was found only following enrichment in the spleen and liver of only 1 and 4/43 pups, respectively (**Figure 4C**). In line with clinical and CFU data, no histopathological lesions were observed in the GIT and internal organs of pups (data not shown). Interestingly, IHC revealed only very few bacteria in the GIT lumen of 5/43 pups, which is in line with the low number of recovered CFU from the GIT. Also in lactating dams, Lm3Dx_SAG1 was isolated from single animals and at low numbers from GIT, spleen and liver at 4d post inoculation (**Figure 4D**). Importantly, at two weeks after the third inoculation (experiment 1) no Lm3Dx_SAG1 was isolated from any organ indicating that the vector is cleared during this time interval (**Figure 4E**).

The differences in bacterial load of the *Listeria monocytogenes* target organs liver, spleen, brain and uterus were reflected in the variation of pathology between WT and Lm3Dx_SAG1. All mice of the WT group suffered severe hepatitis and splenitis with necrosuppurative lesions containing large number of Listeria at 36h, while no significant lesions were present in the liver and spleen of Lm3Dx_SAG1 vaccinated adult mice at this time point (**Figures 5, 6**). Similarly, at later time points (4 days, 2 and 6 weeks post inoculation), no lesions were observed in the target organs, independently of the physiological status of mice (lactation or pregnancy at vaccination). Immunohistochemistry revealed multifocal positivity in few scattered inflammatory cells within the spleen (**Figures 6G, H**), but not in the liver (**Figure 5**), of 4/5 and 4/7 mice at day 1.5 (experiment 1) and 4 (experiment 2), respectively. However, clear bacterial structures were only rarely present (**Figure 6H**). At later time points, no signal was observed anymore. At the site of i.m. injection, all WT inoculated mice showed at 36h large and severe necrosuppurative foci in the muscle, containing myriads of bacteria within phagocytes and myofibers (**Figures 7A, F**). In contrast, Lm3Dx_SAG1-injected mice exhibited a prominent inflammation in the thigh, which was mainly restricted to the subcutaneous and intermuscular fat tissue and occasionally extended between muscle fibers (**Figure 7B**). Myofiber necrosis, which was a prominent feature in the WT group (**Figure 7A**), was rarely observed in the Lm3Dx_SAG1 group. The cellulitis and interstitial myositis was self-limiting in the Lm3Dx_SAG1 group. At day 4 following injection (experiment 2, **Figure 7C**), all lactating mice vaccinated with 1 x 10^7 CFU Lm3Dx_SAG1 had myositis at the site of inoculation in the thigh muscle characterized by focal to multifocal interstitial infiltrations with moderate numbers of neutrophils and fewer macrophages. At two weeks following the third injection (experiment 1, **Figure 7D**), severity of myositis was decreased consisting of mild focal interstitial lymphohistiocytic inflammatory infiltrates in 5/6, 6/6 and 6/6 mice of the 1 x 10^6 CFU, 5 x 10^6 and 1 x 10^7 CFU group, respectively. By 6 weeks following the third injection (experiment 3, **Figure 7E**), the thigh muscle was free of inflammation at the injection site. Interestingly, using immunohistochemistry no bacteria were observed in the interstitial infiltrate of adult mice at 1.5d following vaccination with 1 x 10^7 CFU Lm3Dx_SAG1 (**Figure 7G**). Only in 1/5 mouse, a positive signal was detected in a few cells of the popliteal lymph node (**Figure 7G** insert). However, when mice were vaccinated during early lactation with 1 x 10^7 CFU Lm3Dx_SAG1, moderate numbers of bacteria were multifocally observed in the interstitial infiltrate (**Figure 7H**). At two weeks following the third injection, immunohistochemistry for *Listeria* revealed few bacteria and/or fragments in inflammatory cells of 4/6, 5/6 and 3/6 mice in the 1 x 10^6 CFU, 5 x 10^6 and 1 x 10^7 CFU group, respectively (**Figure 7I**). At 6 weeks following the third injection, no bacteria were detected neither with immunohistochemistry (**Figure 7J**) nor with bacteriology.

The potential effect of vaccination on fertility and pregnancy outcome was evaluated and is summarized in **Table 2**. Vaccination of pregnant mice had no negative impact on the fertility or the number of viable pups. While in the PBS control group one out of 21 pups born died in the neonatal phase, 1/28

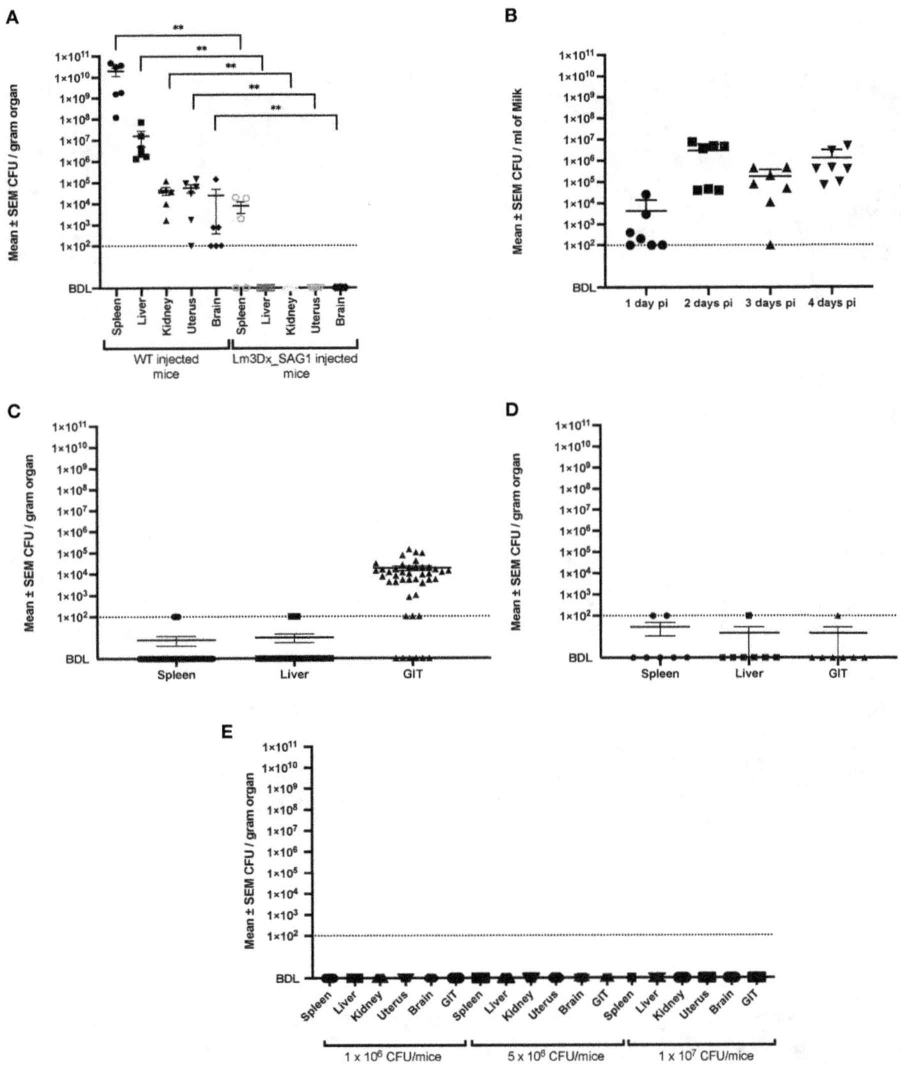

FIGURE 4 | Recovery of WT and Lm3Dx_SAG1 *L. monocytogenes* from internal organs and milk. **(A)** Mean ± SEM CFU/gram organ in adult non-pregnant mice 36h following i.m. inoculation with 1 x 10^7 WT or Lm3Dx_SAG1. Asterisks indicate significant differences to the WT group: $^{**}P \leq 0.0021$ (Mann Whitney-U test). **(B)** Excretion of Lm3Dx_SAG in milk during 4 days following i.m. vaccination of lactating dams, given as mean ± SEM CFU/ml (experiment 2). **(C)** Mean ± SEM CFU/gram organ of pups feeding milk from Lm3Dx_SAG1 dams (experiment 2). **(D)** Mean ± SEM CFU/gram organ in lactating dams 4 days following vaccination with 1 x 10^7 Lm3Dx_SAG1 (experiment 2). **(E)** No CFU were recovered from internal organs of adult mice two weeks following the third vaccination with Lm3Dx_SAG1 (experiment 1). The data points represent individual mouse values. The detection limit for all experiments was set to 10^2 CFU/gram organ or milk following enrichment (dashed line). BDL, Below detection limit.

and 3/21 pups died during the neonatal phase in the 1 x 10^6 CFU and 1 x 10^7 CFU group, respectively ($P > 0.05$) (**Table 2**). Furthermore, vaccination of mice during pregnancy did not negatively impact the development of pups in any of the immunized groups.

Lm3Dx_ SAG1 Triggers a Th1-Biased Immune Response in Both the Non-Pregnant and Pregnant Mouse Model

Vaccination of non-pregnant mice with Lm3Dx_ SAG1 induced a strong Th1 biased immune response when compared to the PBS control group. Comparison to the WT group was not possible, because all WT mice had to be euthanized within 36 h after the first inoculation. We found higher IFN-γ production in splenocytes isolated from spleens of the 1 x 10^6 and 5 x 10^6 CFU of Lm3Dx_ SAG1 vaccinated group compared to the group inoculated with PBS (**Figure 8A**). The IFN-γ response was negatively correlated with the inoculation dose, being strongest in the low-dose group (1 x 10^6 CFU) and lowest in mice vaccinated with 1 x 10^7 CFU. In the latter group, the IFN-γ response was not significantly different to the PBS control group (**Figure 8A**). IFN-γ production was variable between individuals of each group with responses ranging from 5 x 10^3 to 1.5 x 10^4 pg/mL. The Th2-cytokine IL-5 was produced at

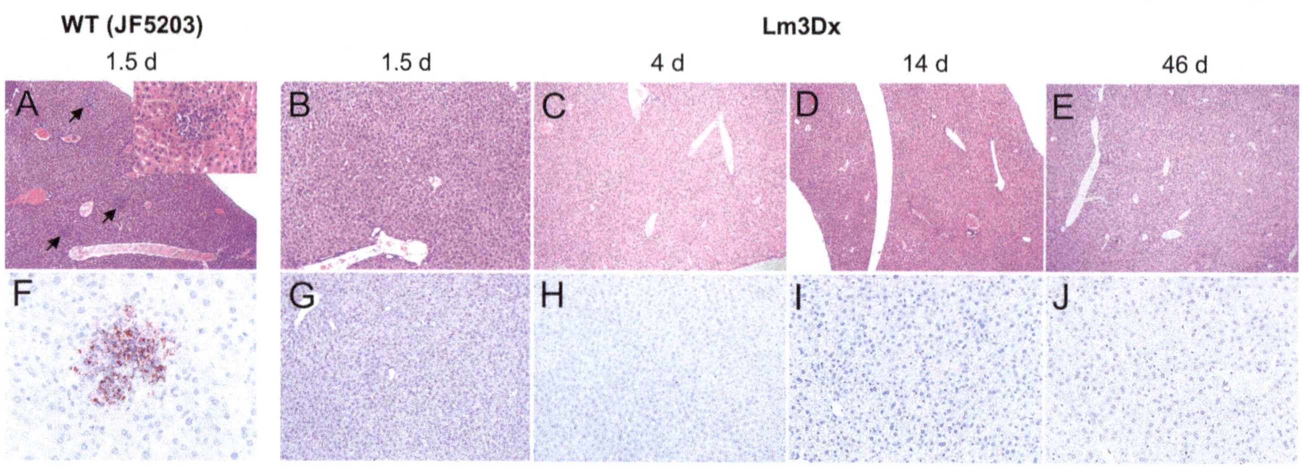

FIGURE 5 | Representative HE **(A–E)** and immunohistochemically (antibody against Lm) **(F–J)** stained liver tissue of WT- and Lm3Dx_SAG1- injected mice. **(A)** Multifocal necrosuppurative hepatitis (arrows) in mice at 36h following injection with WT Lm (40x magnification). Inset: 400x magnification of a small hepatic abscess with aggregations of neutrophils obliterating hepatic cords. **(B–E)** Livers of mice injected with 1 x 10^7 Lm3Dx_SAG1 are normal, without lesions of necrosuppurative hepatitis at all time points: **(B)** 1.5d (100x magnification) and **(C)** 4d (40x magnification) following inoculation, **(D)** 14d (40x magnification) and **(E)** 46d (40x magnification) following the second boost injection. **(F)** Necrosuppurative foci contain myriads of bacteria at 1.5d following inoculation with WT Lm (400x magnification). **(G–J)** Livers of mice injected with 1 x 10^7 Lm3Dx_SAG1 do not contain any bacteria throughout the experiment: **(B)** 1.5d (100x magnification) and **(C)** 4d (100x magnification) following inoculation, **(D)** 14d (200x magnification) and **(E)** 46d (200x magnification) following the second boost injection.

lower levels than IFN-γ, but levels of the 1 x 10^6 CFU/mice group were significantly higher than the PBS group (**Figure 8B**).

In the pregnancy outcome model (experiment 3), stimulated splenocytes isolated from spleens of both, dams and non-pregnant mice, produced increased IFN-γ. No difference in IFN-γ response was observed between pregnant and non-pregnant animals (**Figure 8C**). Similarly to experiment 1, IL-5 levels were increased in Lm3Dx_ SAG1 vaccinated mice compared to the PBS group, albeit at much lower amounts than IFN-γ (**Figure 8D**). For unknown reasons, cytokine

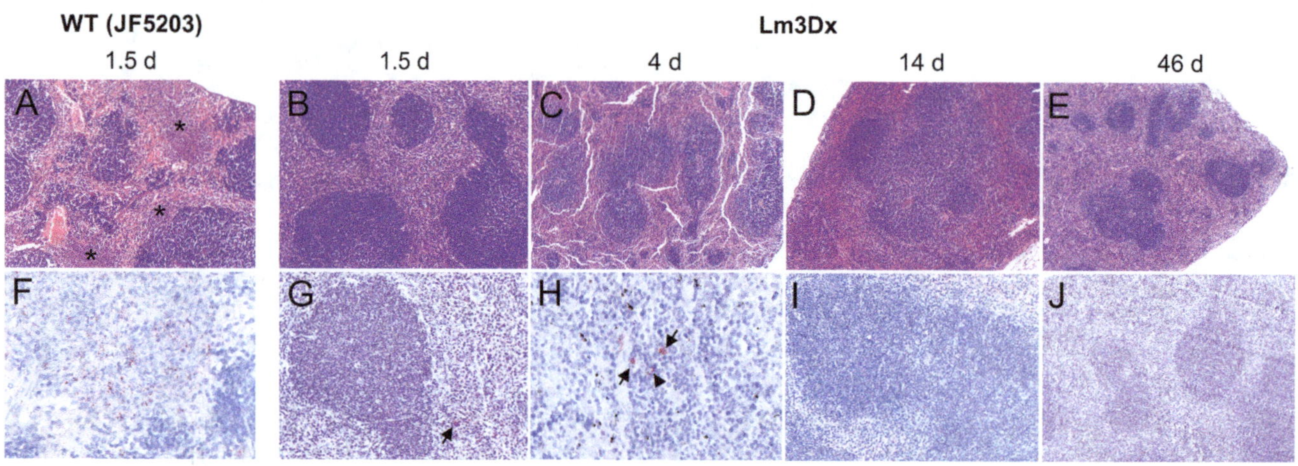

FIGURE 6 | Representative HE **(A–E)** and immunohistochemically (antibody against Lm) **(F–J)** stained spleen tissue of WT- and Lm3Dx_SAG1- injected mice. **(A)** Coalescing necrosuppurative foci in the red pulp of the spleen (asterisks) in mice at 36h following injection with WT Lm (100x magnification). **(B–E)** Spleens of mice injected with 1 x 10^7 Lm3Dx_SAG1 are normal, without lesions of necrosuppurative splenitis at all time points: **(B)** 1.5d (100x magnification) and **(C)** 4d (40x magnification) following inoculation, **(D)** 14d (40x magnification) and **(E)** 46d (40x magnification) following the second boost injection. **(F)** Necrosuppurative foci contain numerous bacteria at 1.5d following inoculation with WT Lm (400x magnification). **(G)** At 1.5d following Lm3Dx_SAG1 injection, 4/5 mice contained multifocal inflammatory cells of the splenic red pulp with a positive Lm signal (arrow), but no clear bacterial structures were observed (200x magnification). **(H)** At 4d following Lm3Dx_SAG1 injection, 4/7 lactating mice contained multifocal inflammatory cells of the splenic red pulp with a positive Lm signal (arrows), and additionally elongated positive structures compatible with bacteria (400x magnification). **(I)** At 14d (200x magnification) and **(E)** 46d (100x magnification) following the second boost injection, no positive signal was observed in Lm3Dx_SAG1 injected mice.

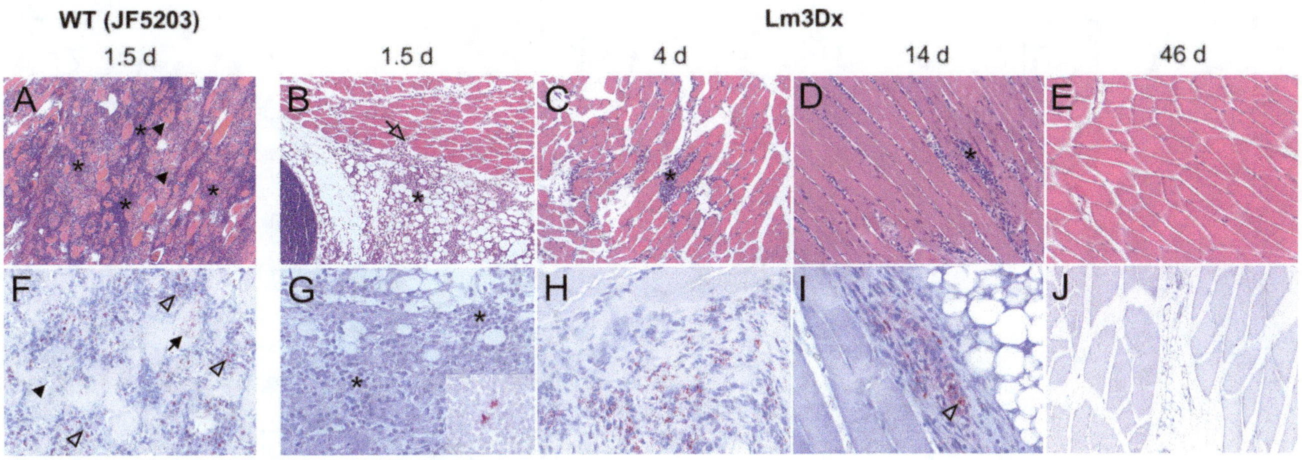

FIGURE 7 | Representative HE **(A–E)** and immunohistochemically (with antibody against Lm) **(F–J)** stained muscle tissue of representative WT- and Lm3Dx_SAG1-injected mice. **(A)** Severe necrosuppurative myositis with marked neutrophilic infiltration (asterisks) and multifocal severe myofiber necrosis (arrowheads) is present in the thigh musculature of WT injected mice at 1.5d after inoculation (100x magnification). **(B)** Focal-extensive and prominent infiltration of the intermuscular fat tissue with neutrophils and macrophages (asterisk) that extends into the muscular interstitium (open arrow) in a mice at 1.5d following injection with 1 x 10^7 Lm3Dx_SAG1 (100x). No myofiber necrosis is present. **(C)** Focal infiltrate with moderate numbers of neutrophils and macrophages (asterisk) that is restricted to the interstitial space between muscle fibers of the thigh musculature in a lactating mouse at 4d following inoculation with Lm3Dx_SAG1 (100x magnification). No myofiber necrosis is present. **(D)** Mild lymphohistiocytic infiltrates (asterisk) are present between muscle fibers of the thigh musculature of mice at 14d following the last boost with Lm3Dx_SAG1 (200x magnification). No myofiber necrosis is present. **(E)** At 46 days following the second boost with Lm3Dx_SAG1, the thigh muscle is free of inflammatory infiltrates (200x magnification). **(F)** Myriads of bacteria are observed in myofibers (arrow) and within neutrophils (open arrowheads) at 1.5d following inoculation with WT (200x magnification). Arrowhead indicates necrotic myofiber. **(G)** At day 1.5 following inoculation of adult mice, no bacteria are observed in the interstitial infiltrate (asterisks, 400x magnification). One/5 mice had a positive signal in the popliteal lymph node (inset, 400x magnification). **(H)** At day 4 following inoculation of lactating mice with Lm3Dx_SAG1, interstitial infiltrates contain moderate numbers of bacteria (400x magnification). Neighboring myofibers are normal. **(I)** Few inflammatory cells within the interstitial infiltrates contain bacteria (open arrowhead) or bacterial fragments at 14 days following the second boost with Lm3Dx_SAG1 (400x magnification). **(J)** No bacteria are present in the thigh muscle of LM3Dx_SAG1 injected mice at 46 days following the second boost (200x magnification).

concentrations were higher than in the first experiment. Factors that may have contributed to the variation might include 1) sample freezing and thawing in experiment 1, which may have led to protein degradation; 2) time point differences: blood samples in experiment 3 were collected three weeks later than in the first experiment, and in this time window the cellular immune response may have further matured; 3) inter-experimental variation.

Lm3Dx_ SAG1 Elicits a Low-Titer Nc Specific IgG Response in Both Non-Pregnant and Pregnant Mice

Lm3Dx_SAG1 triggered only low titers of NcSAG1 specific IgG. In experiment 1, when compared to the baseline titers of animals before vaccination, a significant increase of IgG titers was only observed following the second booster in the 1 x 10^7 CFU group (**Figure 9A**). Compared to the PBS group, NcSAG1-specific IgG titers were significantly higher in Lm3Dx_SAG1 vaccinated animals of all dose groups from day 28 following primovaccination (**Figure 9A**). However, titers remained low compared to the positive control (2-15% of IgG titer in serum of Nc infected animals) and similar as the IFN-γ response, titers were variable between individuals.

Also in the pregnancy interference test (experiment 3), a mild increase of NcSAG1 IgG antibody titers was observed, but as opposed to experiment 1 only in animals following vaccination with 1 x 10^6 CFU/mouse (2.5% of IgG titer in serum of Nc infected animals, **Figure 9B**). The mean antibody titers that were determined in the 1 x 10^6 CFU groups in experiment 1 and 3 were similar (2.4 ± 3.4 and 2.7 ± 3.7 respectively) but differed in the 1 x10^7 CFU groups (14.7 ± 17.8 and 0.6 ± 2.6, respectively). Although the difference in antibody titers between offspring from

TABLE 2 | Data of the pregnancy outcome experiment (experiment 3). Mice received 3 doses of either 1 x 10^6 CFU Lm3Dx_SAG1, 1 x 10^7 CFU Lm3Dx_SAG1 or PBS.

Group	Pregnant mice	Fertility rate [%]	Litter size	Neonatal Mortality	Neonatal mortality rate [%]	Postnatal mortality	Postnatal mortality [%]	Postnatal survival [%]
10^6 CFU	4/6	66.7	28	2/28	7.1	0/26	0.0	100.0
10^7 CFU	3/6	50.0	21	3/21	14.3	0/18	0.0	100.0
PBS	3/6	50.0	21	1/21	4.8	0/20	0.0	100.0

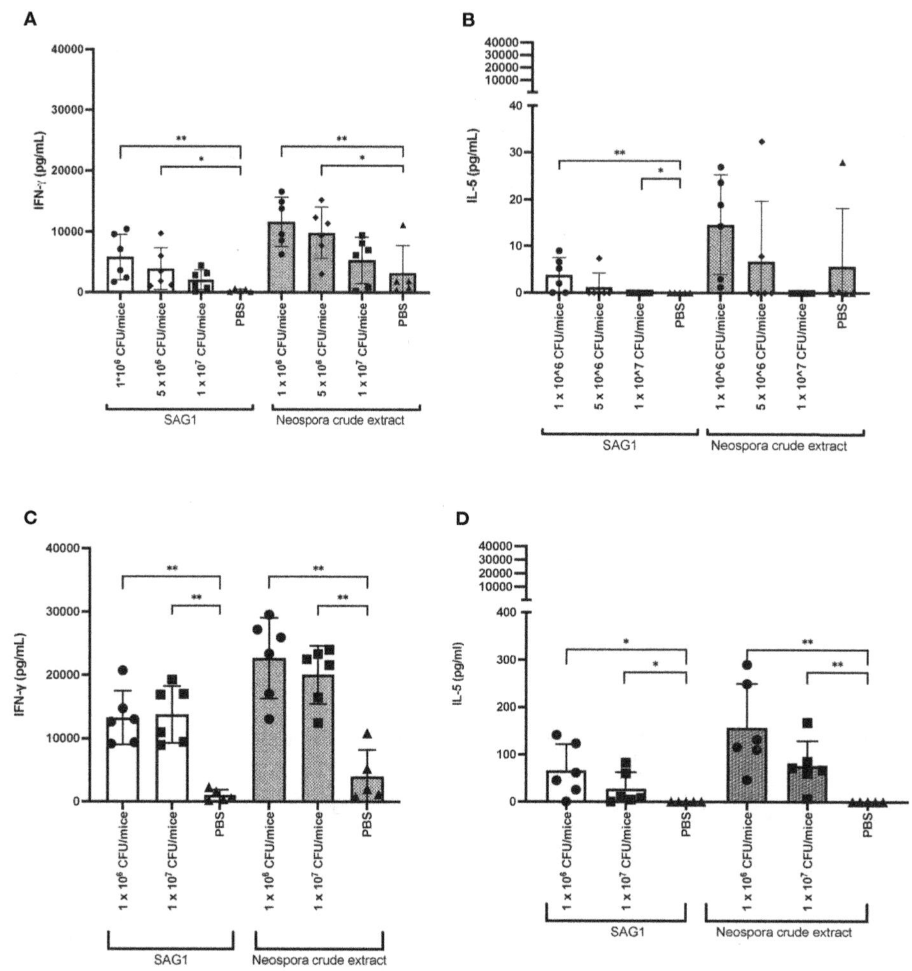

FIGURE 8 | IFN-γ and IL-5 response in Lm3Dx_SAG1-immunized mice. **(A)** IFN-γ and **(B)** IL-5 response of splenocytes isolated from spleens 14 days after the second boost of non-pregnant mice. Splenocytes were stimulated with recombinant NcSAG1 or Neospora caninum crude extract (grey bars). **(C)** IFN-γ and **(D)** IL-5 response upon stimulation in the pregnancy outcome model. In this experiment, splenocytes of mice were recovered 42 days after the second boost or sham (PBS) injection. Columns represent the median and whiskers the standard deviation. * indicate significant levels compared to the PBS group: *$P \leq 0.0332$, **$P \leq 0.0021$ (Mann Whitney-U test).

dams vaccinated with 1 x 10^6 CFU/mouse and from non-vaccinated dams was significant, the titers were very low compared to titers of Nc-infected animals (**Figure 9C**). In summary, the Nc specific IgG response was very low in all vaccinated animals.

DISCUSSION

Over the past 20 years, a growing body of evidence has shown that Lm modulates the immune response and is highly amenable to genetic manipulation, and thus constitutes a promising vaccine vector for prevention and therapy of cancer and infectious diseases (Flickinger et al., 2018). We demonstrate the safety of the highly attenuated Lm vaccine vector Lm3Dx_NcSAG1, which is devoid of any exogenous antibiotic resistance gene, in adult mice and provide first evidence of its immunogenicity.

Notwithstanding the claimed safety of previously developed Lm-based vaccine vectors with either single (Δ*actA*, Δ*prfA*) or double (Δ*actA*/Δ*inlB*) virulence gene deletions, several reports have indicated sporadic side effects post-vaccination, and isolated cases of vaccine-induced acute and delayed listeriosis have been described in humans and dogs (Maciag et al., 2009; Sacco et al., 2016; Denham et al., 2018; Fares et al., 2019). Indeed, even though *prfA* is the regulator of most of the virulence genes, *inlA* and *inlB* are also regulated by *sigB* (Kim et al., 2005), which may explain why the Δ*prfA knock-out* mutant used was not fully attenuated and may have been able to cause adverse effects upon infection. Therefore, we created an antibiotic-resistance-free triple deletion mutant devoid of *actA*, *inlA* and *inlB* to minimize the likelihood of systemic infection. Deletion of *actA* causes a 1000-fold LD_{50}

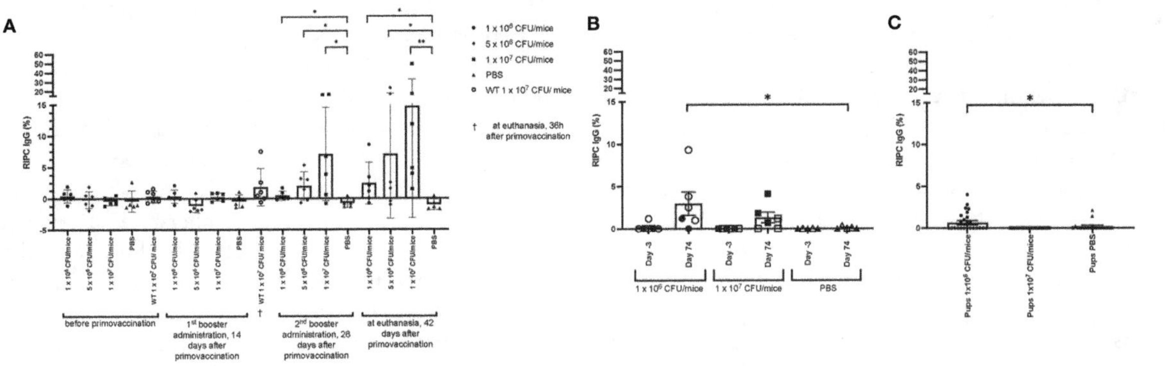

FIGURE 9 | Antibody titers in Lm3Dx_SAG1-immunized mice. **(A)** NcSAG1 IgG in Lm3Dx_SAG1-immunized non-pregnant mice (experiment 1; 1 x 10^6, 5 x 10^6 or 1 x 10^7 CFU/mice dose groups). Naïve mice (PBS) were included as negative control for each time point of measurement. **(B)** NcSAG1 IgG response in Lm3Dx_SAG1-immunized mice in the pregnancy outcome model (experiment 3; 1 x 10^6 and 1 x 10^7 CFU/mice dose groups, empty triangle, square or circle = non-pregnant mice, filled triangle, square or circle = pregnant mice). Naïve mice (PBS) were included as negative control for each time point of measurement. Sera were taken 3 days prior to primary vaccination (Day -3) and 42 days after the 2nd booster administration (74 days following primary vaccination, Day 74). **(C)** NcSAG1 IgG response in pups born from Lm3Dx_SAG1-immunized dams in the pregnancy outcome model (experiment 3; 1 x 10^6 and 1 x 10^7 CFU/mice dose groups). Sera were taken three weeks after birth during euthanasia and compared to sera from pups born from PBS vaccinated dams. Results are expressed as the mean of RIPC (relative index per cent) in relation to the positive control (serum of Nc infected mice), and error bars represent the standard error of the means (S.E.M) in each group. *P ≤ 0.0332, **P ≤ 0.0021 (Mann Whitney-U test).

increase of Lm *via* prevention of bacterial intercellular spread and, hence, systemic dissemination of infection, and additionally *via* promotion of autophagy (Flickinger et al., 2018; Radoshevich and Cossart, 2018; D'Orazio, 2019; Chávez Arroyo and Portnoy, 2020). Co-deletion of *actA* and *inlB* results in a safe vaccine vector by preventing hepatocyte infection and systemic spread while eliciting a potent immune reaction upon injection (Brockstedt et al., 2004; Flickinger et al., 2018). To further increase safety, we deleted two additional genes in Lm JF5203 generating the vector Lm3Dx: *inlA* to prevent infection of E-cadherin expressing tissues (Lecuit et al., 1997) and *fosX* to increase fosfomycin-sensitivity *in vitro* and *in vivo* (Scortti et al., 2018). *In vitro* fosfomycin resistance is an inherent feature of Lm and genetically encoded by *fosX* (Scortti et al., 2018). Therefore, *in vitro* sensitivity to fosfomycin can be used as a rapid phenotypical marker to discriminate the Lm3Dx vaccine vector lacking *fosX* from naturally occurring Lm. Moreover, *fosX* deletion further increases fosfomycin sensitivity of Lm *in vivo* (Scortti et al., 2018), and, therefore, fosfomycin becomes a potent alternative antibiotic to the commonly used ampicillin-gentamicin combination for elimination of potentially persisting bacteria after completion of the vaccination protocol and for therapy in case of post-vaccinal infection (Maciag et al., 2009; Basu et al., 2018; Safran et al., 2018).

Our *in vitro* results provided sufficient evidence of i) low risk of undesired systemic infection and persistence due to impaired epithelial cell infection and ii) sufficient APC targeting, to continue to test the vector safety *in vivo*. Additionally, we investigated the immune response against NcSAG1 in these experiments as a proof of concept by expressing the highly immunogenic *Neospora caninum* tachyzoite antigen in Lm3Dx. In contrast to most existing Lm vaccine platforms that rely on integration plasmids for antigen complementation (Lauer et al., 2002; Zebertavage et al., 2019), the gene coding for NcSAG1 was inserted by homologous recombination for two reasons. First, we wanted to avoid introduction of an exogenous antibiotic resistance gene. Although the use of integration plasmids allows rapid insertion of exogenous genes, the entire plasmid sequence containing antibiotic resistances genes allowing for selection is integrated into the vector genome at a predetermined site and retention in the bacterial genome requires propagation of the vaccine vector in selective media containing antibiotics or other selective components (Lauer et al., 2002). In contrast, when using suicidal homologous recombination plasmids, the antibiotic resistance gene is removed from the vaccine strain with the plasmid at the end of the cloning process. Furthermore, the use of a Lm vector lacking *fosX* such as Lm3Dx allows the complete abandonment of exogenous antibiotic resistance genes during cloning with recombination plasmids containing *fosX*. Secondly, we aimed to ensure insertion of the *sag1* gene into the *actA* locus, thus allowing for strong antigen expression *in vivo* to be regulated by the natural *actA* promotor, which is strongly activated by *prfA* during *in vivo* infection (Radoshevich and Cossart, 2018). Additionally, the gene integration is stable and does not require growth on selective media for maintenance. While others used homologous recombination plasmids for complementation (Frankel et al., 1995; Friedman et al., 2000), they did not insert the target antigen into the *actA* locus.

Throughout all *in vivo* studies employing the Lm3Dx_SAG1 vaccine, neither clinical signs nor adverse effects were observed, which was in contrast to WT injected mice. This is in accordance with the previously reported LD_{50} of 10^8 CFU in a $\Delta actA/\Delta inlB$ mutant (Brockstedt et al., 2004). Additionally, only few injected mice shed Lm3Dx_SAG1 in the feces, and only at a very low level. Furthermore, no lesions were detected in Lm target organs such as spleen or liver, and the local inflammation at the injection site in the thigh muscle resolved by itself within 6 weeks following the last injection as observed in histology and immunohistochemistry. Furthermore, transmission of Lm3Dx_SAG1 to sentinel mice was not observed. Altogether, these results suggest that Lm3Dx_SAG1 is not shed to a significant level into the environment *via* feces and does not persist in the immunocompetent host, which is of importance in the view of reported intravacuolar persistence and delayed infections following vaccination (Kortebi et al., 2017). Our observations including the extremely low shedding into the environment, absence of pregnancy interference, absence of clinical signs and target organ lesions as well as absence of persistent bacteria 42 days after the last boost indicates that the Lm3Dx vaccine vector exhibits a high safety level in adult non-lactating mice and, therefore, can be tested in other animal species including ruminants and dogs, susceptible hosts for *Neospora caninum*. It was surprising that Lm3Dx_SAG1 was excreted at considerable number into the milk when given to lactating mice. However, milk shedding was not associated with any clinical signs in neither dams nor pups, even though Lm3Dx_SAG1 was taken up by suckling pups with the milk. Crossing of the GIT barrier and colonization of internal organs was rarely observed in pups and only at very low levels. In line with these results, no histopathological lesions were observed in internal organs of pups. Sporadic crossing in some pups could be due to increased permeability of the GIT due to open tight-junctions at young age (Duffy, 2000; Nguyen et al., 2001; Gleeson et al., 2021). Alternatively, Lm3Dx_SAG1 might have reached internal organs *via* uptake into APCs and macrophages probing the GIT (Macpherson and Uhr, 2004). It was also surprising that while immunohistochemistry failed to detect Lm3Dx_SAG1 in the thigh muscle of non-lactating mice at 1.5d after vaccination, bacteria were still observed at day 4 in lactating mice, indicating impact of the physiological status on bacterial clearance. Milk contamination and prolonged persistence of bacteria in the muscle may be avoided by vaccinating lactating animals during the dry period or by implementing post-vaccination treatment with fosfomycin to ensure complete elimination of bacteria. However, our observations claim further investigations into mechanisms of milk excretion, impact of lactation on vector dynamics in the host and the safety of vector use during lactation before vaccination of lactating large animals is considered.

Lm infection triggers innate as well as adaptive immune responses (Wallecha et al., 2012; Flickinger et al., 2018; D'Orazio, 2019). Our preliminary data showing a strong IFN-γ production and low IgG responses point towards a Th1-biased immune response against NcSAG1. However, responses among individual mice of the same dose group varied, and not all mice developed immunity. External and internal factors such as those reported in humans (Zimmermann and Curtis, 2019) and mice (Franklin and Ericsson, 2017; Voelkl et al., 2020; Voelkl and Würbel, 2021; Zhang et al., 2021) (i.e. stress, microbiota diversity, variation in vaccination dose) may cause this variability and need to be further evaluated. Most studies showed Lm-induced immunity against foreign antigens including tumor associated antigens, HIV-1 gag, *Mycobacterium tuberculosis* and *Aeromonas hydrophila* (Friedman et al., 2000; Jia et al., 2017; Yin et al., 2017; Flickinger et al., 2018; Kim et al., 2019; Zeng et al., 2020), and they focused on the cellular immune response. One of the few studies that investigated both cellular and humoral immunity (Mahdy et al., 2019) observed rising antibody titers 14 days after the first vaccination with 1 x 10^6 bacteria. In contrast, even though relatively low in total numbers, we observed significantly increased antibody titers only after the third dose administration (6 weeks after the first vaccination) and with tenfold more bacteria. Differences in genetic content of the engineered vectors may account for these divergences and suggest the possibility to tailor immunogenicity of Lm vectors by removal of virulence genes. In addition, the intrinsic properties of the antigens under investigation can account for these differences. The aforementioned study used a Lm *ΔactA/ΔplcB* Lm strain, while Lm3Dx is deleted in *actA*, *inlA* and *inlB*. *PlcB* is involved in listerial vacuolar escape into the cytosol upon infection (Smith et al., 1995; Quereda et al., 2018). Removal of this gene potentially increases vacuolar retention and degradation of *Listeria*, hence stimulating the delivery of bacterial proteins to the class II MHC antigen presentation machinery and enforcing the humoral arm of the immune response (D'Orazio, 2019). Future investigations will evaluate the persistence of SAG1-specific antibodies and modulation of the humoral and cellular immune responses by vector dose and deletion of further virulence genes.

CONCLUSION

We here present an attenuated *Listeria* vaccine strain, Lm3Dx, which fulfills multiple safety requirements *in vitro* and *in vivo* in non-pregnant as well as pregnant BALB/c mice. However, its potential use in lactating animals needs to be further investigated. Lm3Dx is useful for stable expression of antigens of interest under the control of the *actA* promotor and is thus potentially applicable for the prevention and treatment of cancer as well as infectious diseases. Lm3Dx_SAG1 stimulates a Th1-biased immune response against NcSAG1, the major Nc tachyzoite surface protein, which is a promising neosporosis vaccine candidate. Considering the important protective role of Th1 immunity in the context of Nc infection, we suggest that Lm3Dx_SAG1 could be a potential live vaccine to be used for the prevention of neosporosis-induced fetal malformations and abortion. Thus, the safety and efficacy of the Lm3Dx_SAG1 vaccine will be further investigated in a pregnant neosporosis mouse model. In addition, since *N. caninum* is a member of the group of closely related apicomplexans including *T. gondii*, but also *Besnoitia besnoiti*, *Sarcocystis*, *Eimeria* and others, all of which impair human and/or animal health and which are bound to trigger similar immune responses (Innes and Vermeulen, 2006; Monney et al., 2011; Aguado-Martínez et al., 2017), our vaccine vector represents an interesting candidate for a wider range of applications.

AUTHOR CONTRIBUTIONS

WP, AO, and PP contributed to the conception of the study. WP, AO, DI, AH, PP, NT, SG-V, and FF contributed to the experimental design of the study. WP, DI, CM, NT, and AO performed the experiments. WP performed the statistical analysis. WP wrote the first draft of the manuscript. WP, DI, AH, and AO wrote sections of the manuscript. All authors contributed to the article and approved the submitted version.

ACKNOWLEDGMENTS

We would like to thank Prof. Joachim Frey for providing his expertise during the screening of alternative selection strategies for Listeria mutants. We would like to thank Prof. Gertraud Schüpbach for her support in the statistical evaluation of this paper. Also, we would like to thank all the members of the lab, and especially Marianne Wyss, for helping during specific steps of the Lm3Dx mutant cloning.

SUPPLEMENTARY MATERIAL

Supplementary File S1 | Plasmid map of pMAD_NactA100AA_SAG1. Image generated with Geneious (Geneious 8.1, Biomatters Inc.).

Supplementary File S2 | Names and origins of bacterial strains used in this study.

Supplementary File S3 | Names and origins of plasmids used in this study.

Supplementary File S4 | Sequences and names of primers used.

Supplementary File S5 | Number of generations during infection of MDCK and DH82 cells in the gentamicin protection assay.

Supplementary File S6 | Fosfomycin sensitivity of Lm3Dx. 10µL of WT (JF5203) or Lm3Dx were grown overnight at 37°C on a BHI-Agar plate supplemented with a fosfomycin E-Stripe. The WT strain is resistant to up to 1,024 µg/mL of fosfomycin (maximum concentration tested), while Lm3Dx is sensitive to fosfomycin from a concentration of 6 µg/mL as shown by the clear halo on the agar plate.

Supplementary File S7 | Immunofluorescence microscopy of MDCK cell infection with the parental WT, mutants and *Listeria (L.) innocua* over time. While the WT strain replicates efficiently in MDCK cells and clearly spreads between cells, the Δ*actA* mutant is able to invade cells, but clearly attenuated in intercellular spread. The Lm3Dx mutant and *L. innocua* are clearly attenuated in invasion efficiency with very low numbers of intracellular bacteria at 2h pi and in intracellular replication. Bacteria are labeled green, cellular and bacterial nuclei are stained with DAPI (Cyan) and cellular actin with phalloidin (red).

Supplementary File S8 | Immunofluorescence microscopy of DH82 cell infection with the parental WT, mutants and *Listeria (L.) innocua* over time. In DH82, the WT, Δ*actA* and Lm3Dx are readily phagocytosed by DH82 cells and increase in numbers until 6h. While the WT shows high numbers of bacteria until 24 h and appears to decrease at 48h, numbers in the Δ*actA* and Lm3Dx mutant appear to plateau or decrease earlier. In contrast, bacterial numbers of *L. innocua* remain very low over the entire experiment. Bacteria are labeled green, cellular and bacterial nuclei are stained with DAPI (Cyan) and cellular actin with phalloidin (red).

REFERENCES

1. Abdelhamed, H., Lawrence, M. L., and Karsi, A. (2015). A Novel Suicide Plasmid for Efficient Gene Mutation in Listeria Monocytogenes. *Plasmid* 81, 1–8. doi: 10.1016/j.plasmid.2015.05.003
2. Afghah, Z., Webb, B., Meng, X.-J., and Ramamoorthy, S. (2017). Ten Years of PCV2 Vaccines and Vaccination: Is Eradication a Possibility? *Vet. Microbiol.* 206, 21–28. doi: 10.1016/j.vetmic.2016.10.002
3. Aguado-Martınez, A., Basto, A. P., Leitão, A., and Hemphill, A. (2017). Neospora Caninum in Non-Pregnant and Pregnant Mouse Models: Cross-Talk Between Infection and Immunity. *Int. J. Parasitol* 47, 723–735. doi: 10.1016/j.ijpara.2017.09.001
4. Aguado-Martınez, A., Basto, A. P., Müller, J., Balmer, V., Manser, V., Leitão, A., et al. (2016a). N-Terminal Fusion of a Toll-Like Receptor 2-Ligand to a Neospora Caninum Chimeric Antigen Efficiently Modifies the Properties of the Specific Immune Response. *Parasitology* 143, 606–616. doi: 10.1017/S0031182016000056
5. Aguado-Martınez, A., Basto, A. P., Müller, J., Balmer, V., Manser, V., Leitão, A., et al. (2016b). N-Terminal Fusion of a Toll-Like Receptor 2-Ligand to a Neospora Caninum Chimeric Antigen Efficiently Modifies the Properties of the Specific Immune Response. *Parasitology* 143, 606–616. doi: 10.1017/ S0031182016000056
6. Aguado-Martın ez, A., Basto, A. P., Tanaka, S., Ryser, L. T., Nunes, T. P., Ortega-Mora, L. M., et al. (2019). Immunization With a Cocktail of Antigens Fused With OprI Reduces Neospora Caninum Vertical Transmission and Postnatal Mortality in Mice. *Vaccine* 37, 473–483. doi: 10.1016/j.vaccine.2018.11.060
7. Aguilar-Bultet, L., Nicholson, P., Rychener, L., Dreyer, M., Gözel, B., Origgi, F. C., et al. (2018). Genetic Separation of Listeria Monocytogenes Causing Central Nervous System Infections in Animals. *Front. Cell Infect. Microbiol.* 8:20. doi: 10.3389/fcimb.2018.00020
8. Anvari, D., Saberi, R., Sharif, M., Sarvi, S., Hosseini, S. A., Moosazadeh, M., et al. (2020). Seroprevalence of Neospora Caninum Infection in Dog Population Worldwide: A Systematic Review and Meta-Analysis. *Acta Parasitol.* 65, 273–290. doi: 10.2478/s11686-019-00163-4
9. Arnaud, M., Chastanet, A., and Debarbouille, M. (2004). New Vector for Efficient Allelic Replacement in Naturally Nontransformable, Low-GC-Content, Gram-Positive Bacteria. *Appl. Environ. Microbiol.* 70, 6887–6891. doi: 10.1128/ AEM.70.11.6887-6891.2004
10. Basu, P., Mehta, A., Jain, M., Gupta, S., Nagarkar, R. V., John, S., et al. (2018). A Randomized Phase 2 Study of ADXS11-001 Listeria Monocytogenes-Listeriolysin O Immunotherapy With or Without Cisplatin in Treatment of Advanced Cervical Cancer. *Int. J. Gynecol. Cancer* 28, 764–772. doi: 10.1097/ IGC.0000000000001235
11. Björkman, C., and Hemphill, A. (1998). Characterization of Neospora Caninum Iscom Antigens Using Monoclonal Antibodies. *Parasite Immunol.* 20, 73–80. doi: 10.1046/j.1365-3024.1998.00127.x
12. Brockstedt, D. G., Giedlin, M. A., Leong, M. L., Bahjat, K. S., Gao, Y., Luckett, W., et al. (2004). Listeria-Based Cancer Vaccines That Segregate Immunogenicity From Toxicity. *Proc. Natl. Acad. Sci.* 101, 13832–13837. doi: 10.1073/ pnas.0406035101
13. Chavez Arroyo, A., and Portnoy, D. A. (2020). Why is Listeria Monocytogenes Such a Potent Inducer of CD8+ T-Cells? *Cell. Microbiol.* 22, e13175. doi: 10.1111/cmi.13175
14. Cossart, P., and Lebreton, A. (2014). A Trip in the "New Microbiology" With the Bacterial Pathogen Listeria Monocytogenes. *FEBS Lett.* 588, 2437–2445. doi: 10.1016/j.febslet.2014.05.051

15. Davis-Wurzler, G. M. (2014). 2013 Update on Current Vaccination Strategies in Puppies and Kittens. The Veterinary Clinics of North America. *Small Anim. Pract.* 44, 235–263. doi: 10.1016/j.cvsm.2013.11.006
16. Debache, K., Guionaud, C., Alaeddine, F., Mevissen, M., and Hemphill, A. (2008). Vaccination of Mice With Recombinant NcROP2 Antigen Reduces Mortality and Cerebral Infection in Mice Infected With Neospora Caninum Tachyzoites. *Int. J. Parasitol* 38, 1455–1463. doi: 10.1016/j.ijpara.2008.04.001
17. Denham, J. D., Lee, D. H., Castro, M., Pandya, S., Aslam, S., Nanjappa, S., et al. (2018). Two Cases of Disseminated Infection Following Live Organism Anti- Cancer Vaccine Administration in Cancer Patients. *Int. J. Infect. Dis.* 72, 1–2. doi: 10.1016/j.ijid.2018.04.004
18. Di Pietrantonj, C., Rivetti, A., Marchione, P., Debalini, M. G., and Demicheli, V. (2020). Vaccines for Measles, Mumps, Rubella, and Varicella in Children. *Cochrane Database Systematic Rev.* 36, 381. doi: 10.1002/14651858. CD004407.pub4
19. D'Orazio, S. E. F. (2019). Innate and Adaptive Immune Responses During Listeria Monocytogenes Infection. *Microbiol. Spectr.* 7 (3), 1–40. doi: 10.1128/ microbiolspec.GPP3-0065-2019
20. Duffy, L. C. (2000). Interactions Mediating Bacterial Translocation in the Immature Intestine. *J. Nutr.* 130 (2), 432S–436S. doi: 10.1093/jn/130.2.432s
21. Fares, E., McCloskey, C. B., Gutierrez, A., Princiotta, M., Salinas, L. J., and Drevets, D. A. (2019). Vaccine Strain Listeria Monocytogenes Bacteremia Occurring 31 Months After Immunization. *Infection* 47, 489–492. doi: 10.1007/s15010-018-1249-7
22. Fischer, C. R., and Schnell, M. J. (2018). New Developments in Rabies Vaccination. *Rev. Sci. Tech.* 37, 657–672. doi: 10.20506/rst.37.2.2831
23. Flickinger, J. Jr., Rodeck, U., and Snook, A. (2018). Listeria Monocytogenes as a Vector for Cancer Immunotherapy: Current Understanding and Progress. *Vaccines (Basel)* 6, 48. doi: 10.3390/vaccines6030048
24. Frankel, F. R., Hegde, S., Lieberman, J., and Paterson, Y. (1995). Induction of Cell-Mediated Immune Responses to Human Immunodeficiency Virus Type 1 Gag Protein by Using Listeria Monocytogenes as a Live Vaccine Vector. *J. Immunol.* 155, 4775–4782.
25. Franklin, C. L., and Ericsson, A. C. (2017). Microbiota and Reproducibility of Rodent Models. *Lab. Anim.* 46, 114–122. doi: 10.1038/laban.1222
26. Friedman, R. S., Frankel, F. R., Xu, Z., and Lieberman, J. (2000). Induction of Human Immunodeficiency Virus (HIV)-Specific CD8 T-Cell Responses by Listeria Monocytogenes and a Hyperattenuated Listeria Strain Engineered to Express HIV Antigens. *J. Virol.* 74, 9987–9993. doi: 10.1128/jvi.74.21.9987- 9993.2000
27. Fukuhara, H., Ino, Y., and Todo, T. (2016). Oncolytic Virus Therapy: A New Era of Cancer Treatment at Dawn. *Cancer Sci.* 107, 1373–1379. doi: 10.1111/cas.13027 Gilbert, S. C. (2011). T-Cell-Inducing Vaccines - What's the Future. *Immunology* 135, 19–26. doi: 10.1111/j.1365-2567.2011.03517.x
28. Gleeson, J. P., Fein, K. C., Chaudhary, N., Doerfler, R., Newby, A. N., and Whitehead, K. A. (2021). The Enhanced Intestinal Permeability of Infant Mice Enables Oral Protein and Macromolecular Absorption Without Delivery Technology. *Int. J. Pharm.* 593, 120120. doi: 10.1016/j.ijpharm.2020.120120
29. Gray, J. I., Westerholf, L. M., and MacLeod, M. K. L. (2018). The Roles of Resident, Central and Effector Memory CD4 T-Cells in Protective Immunity Following Infection or Vaccination. *Immunology* 154, 574–581. doi: 10.1111/imm.12929
30. Griot, C., Moser, C., Cherpillod, P., Bruckner, L., Wittek, R., Zurbriggen, A., et al. (2004). Early DNA Vaccination of Puppies Against Canine Distemper in the Presence of Maternally Derived Immunity. *Vaccine* 22, 650–654. doi: 10.1016/ j.vaccine.2003.08.022
31. Hemphill, A., Aguado-Martinez, A., and Müller, J. (2016). Approaches for the Vaccination and Treatment of Neospora Caninum Infections in Mice and Ruminant Models. *Parasitology* 143, 245–259. doi: 10.1017/S0031182015001596
32. Hemphill, A., Felleisen, R., Connolly, B., Gottstein, B., Hentrich, B., and Müller, N. (1997). Characterization of a cDNA-Clone Encoding Nc-P43, a Major Neospora Caninum Tachyzoite Surface Protein. *Parasitology* 115, 581–590. doi: 10.1017/S0031182097001650
33. Hemphill, A., Von Laufen, N., and Naguleswaran, A. (2006). Cellular and Immunological Basis of the Host-Parasite Relationship During Infection With Neospora Caninum. *Parasitology* 133, 261–278. doi: 10.1017/S0031182006000485
34. Henao-Restrepo, A. M., Camacho, A., Longini, I. M., Watson, C. H., Edmunds, W. J., Egger, M., et al. (2017). Efficacy and Effectiveness of an rVSV-Vectored Vaccine in Preventing Ebola Virus Disease: Final Results From the Guinea Ring Vaccination, Open-Label, Cluster-Randomised Trial (Ebola Ç a Suffit!). *Lancet* 389, 505–518. doi: 10.1016/S0140-6736(16)32621-6
35. Henke, D., Rupp, S., Gaschen, V., Stoffel, M. H., Frey, J., Vandevelde, M., et al. (2015). Listeria Monocytogenes Spreads Within the Brain by Actin-Based Intra-Axonal Migration. *Infect. Immun.* 83, 2409–2419. doi: 10.1128/ IAI.00316-15
36. Ikonomidis, G., Paterson, Y., Kos, F. J., and Portnoy, D. A. (1994). Delivery of a Viral Antigen to the Class I Processing and Presentation Pathway by Listeria Monocytogenes. *J. Exp. Med.* 180, 2209–2218. doi: 10.1084/jem.180.6.2209
37. Innes, E. A., and Vermeulen, A. N. (2006). Vaccination as a Control Strategy Against the Coccidial Parasites Eimeria, Toxoplasma and Neospora. *Parasitology* 133, S145–S168. doi: 10.1017/S0031182006001855
38. Jameson, S. C., and Masopust, D. (2018). Understanding Subset Diversity in T Cell Memory. *Immunity* 48, 214–226. doi: 10.1016/j.immuni.2018.02.010
39. Jiang, Y., Jia, S., Zheng, D., Li, F., Wang, S., Wang, L., et al. (2019). Protective Immunity Against Canine Distemper Virus in Dogs Induced by Intranasal Immunization With a Recombinant Probiotic Expressing the Viral H Protein. *Vaccines (Basel)* 7, 213. doi: 10.3390/vaccines7040213
40. Jia, Y. Y., Tan, W. J., Duan, F. F., Pan, Z. M., Chen, X., Yin, Y. L., et al. (2017). A Genetically Modified Attenuated Listeria Vaccine Expressing HPV16 E7 Kill Tumor Cells in Direct and Antigen-Specific Manner. *Front. Cell Infect. Microbiol.* 7, 279. doi: 10.3389/fcimb.2017.00279
41. Johnson, P. V., Blair, B. M., Zeller, S., Kotton, C. N., and Hohmann, E. L. (2011). Attenuated Listeria Monocytogenes Vaccine Vectors Expressing Influenza A Nucleoprotein: Preclinical Evaluation and Oral Inoculation of Volunteers. *Microbiol. Immunol.* 55, 304–317. doi: 10.1111/j.1348-0421.2011.00322.x
42. Kim, V. M., Blair, A. B., Lauer, P., Foley, K., Che, X., Soares, K., et al. (2019). Anti- Pancreatic Tumor Efficacy of a Listeria-Based, Annexin A2-Targeting Immunotherapy in Combination With Anti-PD- 1 Antibodies. *J. ImmunoTher Cancer* 7, 132. doi: 10.1186/s40425-019-0601-5
43. Kim, H., Marquis, H., and Boor, K. J. (2005). SigmaB Contributes to Listeria Monocytogenes Invasion by Controlling Expression of inlA and Inlb. *Microbiol. (Reading Engl.)* 151, 3215–3222. doi: 10.1099/mic.0.28070-0
44. Kortebi, M., Milohanic, E., Mitchell, G., Pechoux, C., Prevost, M.-C., Cossart, P., et al. (2017). Listeria Monocytogenes Switches From Dissemination to Persistence by Adopting a Vacuolar Lifestyle in Epithelial Cells. *PLoS Pathog.* 13, e1006734. doi: 10.1371/journal.ppat.1006734
45. Lauer, P., Chow, M. Y. N., Loessner, M. J., Portnoy, D. A., and Calendar, R. (2002). Construction, Characterization, and Use of Two Listeria Monocytogenes Site- Specific Phage Integration Vectors. *J. Bacteriol* 184, 4177–4186. doi: 10.1128/ JB.184.15.4177-4186.2002
46. Lecuit, M., Ohayon, H., Braun, L., Mengaud, J., and Cossart, P. (1997). Internalin of Listeria Monocytogenes With an Intact Leucine-Rich Repeat Region Is Sufficient to Promote Internalization. *Infect. Immun.* 65, 5309–5319. doi: 10.1128/iai.65.12.5309-5319.1997
47. Leong, M. L., Hampl, J., Liu, W., Mathur, S., Bahjat, K. S., Luckett, W., et al. (2009). Impact of Preexisting Vector-Specific Immunity on Vaccine Potency: Characterization of Listeria Monocytogenes-Specific Humoral and Cellular Immunity in Humans and Modeling Studies Using Recombinant Vaccines in Mice. *Infect. Immun.* 77, 3958–3968. doi: 10.1128/IAI.01274-08

48. Liu, D. (2006). Listeria-Based Anti-Infective Vaccine Strategies. *Recent Pat. Antiinfect Drug Discov.* 1, 281–290. doi: 10.2174/157489106778777619
49. Liu, Y., Reichel, M. P., and Lo, W. C. (2020). Combined Control Evaluation for Neospora Caninum Infection in Dairy: Economic Point of View Coupled With Population Dynamics. *Veterinary Parasitol* 277, 108967. doi: 10.1016/j. vetpar. 2019.108967
50. Maciag, P. C., Radulovic, S., and Rothman, J. (2009). The First Clinical Use of a Live-Attenuated Listeria Monocytogenes Vaccine: A Phase I Safety Study of Lm-LLO-E7 in Patients With Advanced Carcinoma of the Cervix. *Vaccine* 27, 3975–3983. doi: 10.1016/j.vaccine.2009.04.041
51. Macpherson, A. J., and Uhr, T. (2004). Induction of Protective IgA by Intestinal Dendritic Cells Carrying Commensal Bacteria. *Science* 303, 1662–1665. doi: 10.1126/science.1091334
52. Mahdy, S. E., Liu, S., Su, L., Zhang, X., Chen, H., Pei, X., et al. (2019). Expression of the VP1 Protein of FMDV Integrated Chromosomally With Mutant Listeria Monocytogenes Strain Induced Both Humoral and Cellular Immune Responses. *Appl. Microbiol. Biotechnol.* 23, 77–11. doi: 10.1007/ s00253-018- 09605-x
53. Matle, I., Mbatha, K. R., and Madoroba, E. (2020). A Review of Listeria Monocytogenes From Meat and Meat Products: Epidemiology, Virulence Factors, Antimicrobial Resistance and Diagnosis. *Onderstepoort J. Veterinary Res.* 87, 29. doi: 10.4102/ojvr.v87i1.1869
54. McAllister, M. M., Dubey, J. P., Lindsay, D. S., Jolley, W. R., Wills, R. A., and McGuire, A. M. (1998). Rapid Communication: Dogs are Definitive Hosts of Neospora Caninum. *Int. J. Parasitol* 28, 1473–1479. doi: 10.1016/S0020-7519 (98)00138-6
55. Meyer, H., Ehmann, R., and Smith, G. L. (2020). Smallpox in the Post-Eradication Era. *Viruses 2014* 6, 2122–2137 12, 138. doi: 10.3390/v12020138
56. Monney, T., Debache, K., and Hemphill, A. (2011). Vaccines Against a Major Cause of Abortion in Cattle, Neospora Caninum Infection. *Anim. 2011* 1, 306– 325. doi: 10.3390/ani1030306. Pages 306-325 1.
57. Moreno, B., Collantes-Fernandez, E., Villa, A., Navarro, A., Regidor-Cerrillo, J., and Ortega-Mora, L. M. (2012). Occurrence of Neospora Caninum and Toxoplasma Gondii Infections in Ovine and Caprine Abortions. *Veterinary Parasitol* 187, 312–318. doi: 10.1016/j.vetpar.2011.12.034
58. Nguyen, D. A., Parlow, A. F., and Neville, M. C. (2001). Hormonal Regulation of Tight Junction Closure in the Mouse Mammary Epithelium During the Transition From Pregnancy to Lactation. *J. Endocrinol.* 170, 347–356. doi: 10.1677/joe.0.1700347
59. Nielsen, L., Jensen, T. H., Kristensen, B., Jensen, T. D., Karlskov-Mortensen, P., Lund, M., et al. (2012). DNA Vaccines Encoding Proteins From Wild-Type and Attenuated Canine Distemper Virus Protect Equally Well Against Wild-Type Virus Challenge. *Arch. Virol.* 157, 1887–1896. doi: 10.1007/ s00705-012-1375-y
60. Oevermann, A., Di Palma, S., Doherr, M. G., Abril, C., Zurbriggen, A., and Vandevelde, M. (2010). Neuropathogenesis of Naturally Occurring Encephalitis Caused by Listeria Monocytogenes in Ruminants. *Brain Pathol.* 20, 378–390. doi: 10.1111/j.1750-3639.2009.00292.x
61. Pamer, E. G. (2004). Immune Responses to Listeria Monocytogenes. *Nat. Rev. Immunol.* 4, 812–823. doi: 10.1038/nri1461
62. Peng, Y., Mentzer, A. J., Liu, G., Yao, X., Yin, Z., Dong, D., et al. (2020). Broad and Strong Memory $CD4^+$ and $CD8^+$ T Cells Induced by SARS-CoV-2 in UK Convalescent Individuals Following COVID-19. *Nat. Immunol.* 7, 1–10. doi: 10.1038/s41590-020-0782-6
63. Quereda, J. J., Andersson, C., Cossart, P., Johansson, J., and Pizarro-Cerdà, J. (2018). Role in Virulence of Phospholipases, Listeriolysin O and Listeriolysin S From Epidemic Listeria Monocytogenes Using the Chicken Embryo Infection Model. *Vet. Res.* 49, 1–9. doi: 10.1186/s13567-017-0496-4
64. Radoshevich, L., and Cossart, P. (2018). Listeria Monocytogenes: Towards a Complete Picture of its Physiology and Pathogenesis. *Nat. Rev. Microbiol.* 16, 32–46. doi: 10.1038/nrmicro.2017.126
65. Reichel, M. P., Alejandra Ayanegui-Alcerreca, M., Gondim, L. F. P., and Ellis, J. T. (2013). What is the Global Economic Impact of Neospora Caninum in Cattle – The Billion Dollar Question. *Int. J. Parasitol* 43, 133–142. doi: 10.1016/ j.ijpara.2012.10.022
66. Rupp, S., Aguilar-Bultet, L., Jagannathan, V., Guldimann, C., Drögemüller, C., Pfarrer, C., et al. (2015). A Naturally Occurring prfA Truncation in a Listeria Monocytogenes Field Strain Contributes to Reduced Replication and Cell-to- Cell Spread. *Vet. Microbiol.* 179, 91–101. doi: 10.1016/j.vetmic.2015.03.002
67. Sacco, J. J., Evans, M., Harrington, K. J., Man, S., Powell, N., Shaw, R. J., et al. (2016). Systemic Listeriosis Following Vaccination With the Attenuated Listeria Monocytogenes Therapeutic Vaccine, ADXS11-001. *Hum. Vaccin Immunother.* 12, 1085–1086. doi: 10.1080/21645515.2015.1121338
68. Safran, H., Leonard, K.-L., Perez, K., Vrees, M., Klipfel, A., Schechter, S., et al. (2018). Tolerability of ADXS11-001 Lm-LLO Listeria-Based Immunotherapy With Mitomycin, Fluorouracil, and Radiation for Anal Cancer. *Int. J. Radiat. Oncol. Biol. Phys.* 100, 1175–1178. doi: 10.1016/ j.ijrobp.2018.01.004
69. Schares, G., Peters, M., Wurm, R., Bärwald, A., and Conraths, F. J. (1998). The Efficiency of Vertical Transmission of Neospora Caninum in Dairy Cattle Analysed by Serological Techniques. *Veterinary Parasitol* 80, 87–98. doi: 10.1016/S0304-4017(98)00195-2
70. Schindelin, J., Arganda-Carreras, I., Frise, E., Kaynig, V., and Longair, M. (2012). Fiji: An Open-Source Platform for Biological-Image Analysis. *Nat Methods* 9, 676–682. Schlech, W. F. (2019). Epidemiology and Clinical Manifestations of Listeria Monocytogenes Infection. *Microbiol. Spectr.* 7 (3), 1–12. doi: 10.1128/microbiolspec.GPP3-0014-2018
71. Scortti, M., Han, L., Alvarez, S., Leclercq, A., Moura, A., Lecuit, M., et al. (2018). Epistatic Control of Intrinsic Resistance by Virulence Genes in Listeria. *PLoS Genet.* 14, e1007525. doi: 10.1371/journal.pgen.1007525
72. Scortti, M., Lacharme-Lora, L., Wagner, M., Chico-Calero, I., Losito, P., and Vazquez-Boland, J. A. (2006). Coexpression of Virulence and Fosfomycin Susceptibility in Listeria: Molecular Basis of an Antimicrobial *In Vitro-In Vivo* Paradox. *Nat. Med.* 5 (12), 515–517. doi: 10.1038/nm1396
73. Sewell, D. A., Pan, Z.-K., and Paterson, Y. (2008). Listeria-Based HPV-16 E7 Vaccines Limit Autochthonous Tumor Growth in a Transgenic Mouse Model for HPV-16 Transformed Tumors. *Vaccine* 26, 5315–5320. doi: 10.1016/ j.vaccine.2008.07.036
74. Sharma, O., Sultan, A. A., Ding, H., and Triggle, C. R. (2020). A Review of the Progress and Challenges of Developing a Vaccine for COVID-19. *Front. Immunol.* 11, 585354. doi: 10.3389/fimmu.2020.585354
75. Singh, R., and Wallecha, A. (2011). Cancer Immunotherapy Using Recombinant Listeria Monocytogenes: Transition From Bench to Clinic. *Hum. Vaccines* 7, 497–505. doi: 10.4161/hv.7.5.15132
76. Smith, G. A., Marquis, H., Jones, S., Johnston, N. C., Portnoy, D. A., and Goldfine, H. (1995). The Two Distinct Phospholipases C of Listeria Monocytogenes Have Overlapping Roles in Escape From a Vacuole and Cell-to-Cell Spread. *Infect. Immun.* 63, 4231–4237. doi: 10.1128/iai.63.11. 4231-4237.1995
77. Vetter, V., Denizer, G., Friedland, L. R., Krishnan, J., and Shapiro, M. (2018). Understanding Modern-Day Vaccines: What You Need to Know. *Ann. Med.* 50, 110–120. doi: 10.1080/07853890.2017.1407035
78. Voelkl, B., Altman, N. S., Forsman, A., Forstmeier, W., Gurevitch, J., Jaric, I., et al. (2020). Reproducibility of Animal Research in Light of Biological Variation. *Nat. Rev. Neurosci.* 21, 384–393. doi: 10.1038/s41583-020-0313-3
79. Voelkl, B., and Würbel, H. (2021). A Reaction Norm Perspective on Reproducibility. *Theor. Biosci.* 140, 169–176. doi: 10.1007/s12064-021-00340-y
80. Wallecha, A., Petit, R., French, C., and Rothman, J. (2012). Immune Response and Immunotherapy: Live Attenuated Listeria Monocytogenes (Lm)-LLO Immunotherapy for the Treatment of Prostate Cancer. *Curr. Cancer Ther. Rev.* 8, 254–263. doi: 10.2174/1573394711208040254
81. Wang, Z., Sun, H., and Yakisich, J. S. (2014). Overcoming the Blood-Brain Barrier for Chemotherapy: Limitations, Challenges and Rising Problems. *Anticancer Agents Med. Chem.* 14, 1085–1093. doi: 10.2174/18715206113139990029
82. Wendel Naumann, R., Leath, C. A. 3rd. (2020). Advances in Immunotherapy for Cervical Cancer. *Curr. Opin. Oncol.* 32 (5), 481–487. doi: 10.1097/ CCO.0000000000000663
83. Whitten, M. K. (1957). Effect of Exteroceptive Factors on the Oestrous Cycle of Mice. *Nature* 180, 1436–1436. doi: 10.1038/1801436a0
84. Wood, L. M., and Paterson, Y. (2014). Attenuated Listeria Monocytogenes: A Powerful and Versatile Vector for the Future of Tumor Immunotherapy. *Front. Cell Infect. Microbiol.* 4, 51. doi: 10.3389/fcimb.2014.00051
85. Yin, Y., Lian, K., Zhao, D., Tao, C., Chen, X., Tan, W., et al. (2017). A Promising Listeria-Vectored Vaccine Induces Th1-Type Immune Responses and Confers Protection Against Tuberculosis. *Front. Cell Infect. Microbiol.* 7, 407. doi: 10.3389/fcimb.2017.00407
86. Zebertavage, L., Bambina, S., Shugart, J., Alice, A., Zens, K. D., Lauer, P., et al. (2019). A Microbial-Based Cancer Vaccine for Induction of EGFRvIII-Specific $CD8^+$ T Cells and Anti-Tumor Immunity. *PLoS One* 14, e0209153. doi: 10.1371/journal.pone.0209153
87. Zeng, H., Xie, M., Ding, C., Ma, J., Xu, D., Wang, X., et al. (2020). Attenuated Listeria Monocytogenes as a Vaccine Vector for the Delivery of OMPW, the Outer Membrane Protein of Aeromonas Hydrophila. *Front. Microbiol.* 11, 70. doi: 10.3389/fmicb.2020.00070

88. Zhang, C., Franklin, C. L., and Ericsson, A. C. (2021). Consideration of Gut Microbiome in Murine Models of Diseases. *Microorganisms* 9, 1062. doi: 10.3390/microorganisms9051062

89. Zimmermann, P., and Curtis, N. (2019). Factors That Influence the Immune Response to Vaccination. *Clin. Microbiol. Rev.* 32 (2), e00084–18. doi: 10.1128/CMR.00084-18

10

Progress and Insights Toward an Effective Placental Malaria Vaccine

Benoît Gamain[1,2], Arnaud Chêne[1,2], Nicola K. Viebig[3], Nicaise Tuikue Ndam[4] and Morten A. Nielsen[5,6]*

[1] *Université de Paris, Inserm, Biologie Intégrée du Globule Rouge, Paris, France,* [2] *Institut National de la Transfusion Sanguine, Paris, France,* [3] *European Vaccine Initiative, UniversitätsKlinikum Heidelberg, Heidelberg, Germany,* [4] *Université de Paris, MERIT, IRD, Paris, France,* [5] *Centre for Medical Parasitology at Department of Immunology and Microbiology, Faculty of Health and Medical Sciences, University of Copenhagen, Copenhagen, Denmark,* [6] *Department of Infectious Diseases, Rigshospitalet, Copenhagen, Denmark*

Correspondence:
Benoît Gamain
benoit.gamain@inserm.fr

In areas where *Plasmodium falciparum* transmission is endemic, clinical immunity against malaria is progressively acquired during childhood and adults are usually protected against the severe clinical consequences of the disease. Nevertheless, pregnant women, notably during their first pregnancies, are susceptible to placental malaria and the associated serious clinical outcomes. Placental malaria is characterized by the massive accumulation of *P. falciparum* infected erythrocytes and monocytes in the placental intervillous spaces leading to maternal anaemia, hypertension, stillbirth and low birth weight due to premature delivery, and foetal growth retardation. Remarkably, the prevalence of placental malaria sharply decreases with successive pregnancies. This protection is associated with the development of antibodies directed towards the surface of *P. falciparum*-infected erythrocytes from placental origin. Placental sequestration is mediated by the interaction between VAR2CSA, a member of the *P. falciparum* erythrocyte membrane protein 1 family expressed on the infected erythrocytes surface, and the placental receptor chondroitin sulfate A. VAR2CSA stands today as the leading candidate for a placental malaria vaccine. We recently reported the safety and immunogenicity of two VAR2CSA-derived placental malaria vaccines (PRIMVAC and PAMVAC), spanning the chondroitin sulfate A-binding region of VAR2CSA, in both malaria-naïve and *P. falciparum*-exposed non-pregnant women in two distinct Phase I clinical trials (ClinicalTrials.gov, NCT02658253 and NCT02647489). This review discusses recent advances in placental malaria vaccine development, with a focus on the recent clinical data, and discusses the next clinical steps to undertake in order to better comprehend vaccine-induced immunity and accelerate vaccine development.

Keywords: *Plasmodium falciparum*, placental malaria, VAR2CSA, PfEMP1, vaccine, pregnancy

INTRODUCTION

In 2019, approximately 11 million pregnant women were exposed to the risk of *P. falciparum* infection (1). Malaria contracted during pregnancy can lead to significant clinical complications for the mother, including anaemia (2, 3) and hypertension (4, 5), but also for the child. Indeed, malaria in pregnancy may account for over 200,000 stillbirths each year (6) and for the delivery of over 800,000 low birth weight babies (1). This clinical picture varies depending on the parity status and intensity of *P. falciparum* transmission in a given geographical area (7). Primigravid women are highly susceptible to develop severe clinical outcomes following *P. falciparum* infection. However, in high endemicity area, the incidence of illness sharply drops after successive pregnancies (7), demonstrating that protective immunity can be naturally acquired. These observations raised the hope of developing a vaccine that could protect pregnant women against the serious clinical manifestations of malaria in pregnancy.

P. falciparum infection in pregnancy can cause substantial morphological and immunological changes in the placenta, where a massive accumulation of infected erythrocytes (IEs) takes place (8–10), reshaping the cytokine profile of the local environment (11–13) and altering the maternofoetal exchanges (14). IEs from placental origin present a unique adhesive phenotype and do not bind to the host receptors (CD36, CD31, EPCR) commonly used by the parasite to cytoadhere to the microvasculature lining (15–17). Instead, placental IEs interact with a low-sulphated sugar only present at the surface of syncytiotrophoblasts, the chondroitin sulphate A (CSA) (18–21). This low-sulphated placental CSA is structurally distinct from CSA present in other organs or secreted into the extracellular matrix and body fluids (21). A single member of the *P. falciparum* Erythrocyte Membrane Protein 1 (PfEMP1) family, named VAR2CSA, has been identified as the main parasite-derived ligand mediating the interaction of IEs with placental CSA (22–27). Numerous studies have correlated the presence of antibodies reacting to VAR2CSA with protection against placental malaria (PM) (28–30). In a recent systematic review and meta-analysis, Cutts et al. showed that VAR2CSA derived antigens were positively associated with the presence of placental infections. However, they could not identify evidence that antibody response towards a specific VAR2CSA antigen is associated with protection from PM (31). The capacity of anti-VAR2CSA antibodies to block the adhesion of IEs to CSA is thought to play a major role in protection (32) but accumulating evidence suggests that other antibody-dependent effector mechanisms, such as opsonic phagocytosis (33–35), could also actively participate in parasite clearance.

Current malaria control strategies during pregnancy mainly consist in the use of long-lasting insecticidal bed nets and the administration of intermittent preventive treatments based on sulphadoxine-pyrimethamine (IPT-SP) as well as iron and folic acid supplementation [reviewed in (36, 37)]. Even if effective in reducing the malaria burden in pregnant women living in endemic areas (1), the global implementation of such approaches is threatened by the emergence of widespread resistance of both anopheles mosquitoes to insecticides (38) and of parasites to anti-malarial drugs (39). Furthermore, since IPT-SP is only initiated at the first antenatal care visit, usually in the second trimester, and that increasing evidence suggests that *P. falciparum* infection is particularly frequent and detrimental in the first trimester of pregnancy (40–43), complementary intervention regimens such as vaccines would therefore be extremely valuable. In the current global malaria vaccine landscape, predominated by anti-infection/transmission approaches, VAR2CSA-based PM vaccines stand as the main anti-disease strategy to reduce placental malaria morbidity and mortality.

IDENTIFYING THE BEST VAR2CSA-DERIVED VACCINE CANDIDATE

Prevention of placental infection in first pregnancies is not bestowed by the naturally acquired immune responses from previous *P. falciparum* infections, i.e., prior to pregnancy. Nevertheless, natural and protective immunity develops after one or two pregnancies (7, 44, 45). Vaccine candidates aiming to protect against PM should mimic, at least in part, the naturally acquired antibody response associated with protection (32). Ideally, the vaccine-induced immune responses should be boosted and even substantiated by natural infections.

Following the identification of VAR2CSA and the determination of its role in PM pathogenesis and immunity, researchers have been trying to identify the best VAR2CSA-derived antigen to include in a PM vaccine (27). Indeed, VAR2CSA is a complex cysteine-rich 350 kDa protein composed of an N-terminal segment (NTS) followed by six Duffy-binding like (DBL) domains interspaced by four inter-domains (ID) with less defined structures, a transmembrane region and a cytoplasmic ATS region (**Figure 1**). This complexity, associated to the difficulty in expressing sufficient material of the full-length VAR2CSA extracellular region to proceed to clinical trial, have spurred researchers to characterize and identify a subunit VAR2CSA vaccine. All *P. falciparum* genomes carry one or several *var2csa* genes (46, 47). *Var2csa* has also been identified in the genomes of *P. reichenowi*, which infects the chimpanzee, indicating that the CSA-binding phenotype has an ancient origin and that protein functionality might exert some degree of constraint on sequence variation (48). Among the various VAR2CSA variants, most of the functional studies have been performed on VAR2CSA derived from 3D7 and FCR3 laboratory strains. The secondary structure of the DBL fold is conserved, and variable regions are scattered in the primary sequence as mosaic blocks, which are generally the prime target of anti-VAR2CSA antibodies (49–51). The assumption that a structurally constrained adhesion-mediating region within VAR2CSA could be more conserved than others, led early research to focus on the determination of the single DBL domain(s) involved in CSA-binding (25, 51–57). The finding that single DBL domains, which appeared not to bind CSA, could induce inhibitory antibodies was a primary indication that the tertiary structure of the protein was not like DBL-pearls on a string (58, 59). When full-length recombinant VAR2CSA proteins became available, low-resolution structures obtained by small-angle X-ray scattering (SAXS) and CSA-binding kinetics of the full-length

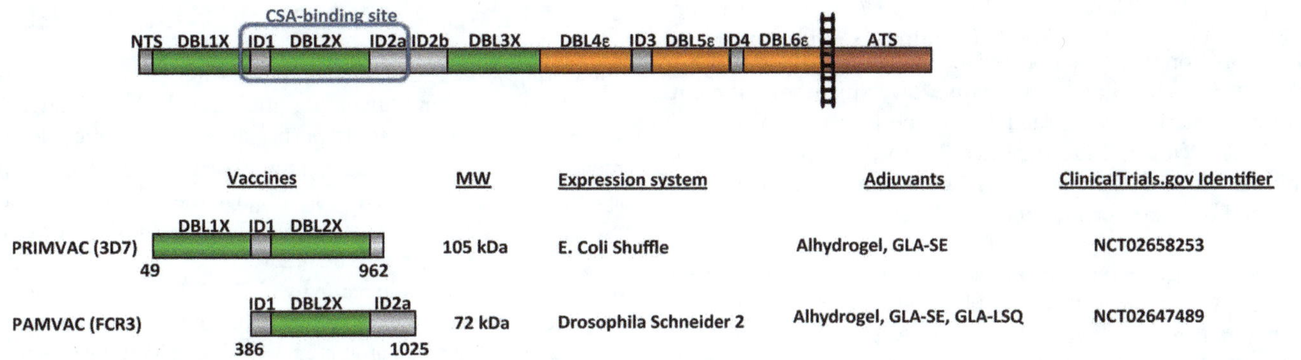

FIGURE 1 | Schematic representation of VAR2CSA and vaccines tested in clinical trials. VAR2CSA is a 350-kDa transmembrane protein composed of an N-terminal segment (NTS) followed by six Duffy-binding like (DBL) domains interspaced by 4 inter-domains (ID), a transmembrane region and a cytoplasmic Acidic C terminus sequence (ATS). PRIMVAC and PAMVAC schematic representation with sequences boundaries, predicted molecular weight, expression systems, and adjuvants used for the Phase I clinical trials. ClinicalTrials identifier for both Phase I are indicated.

recombinant proteins indicated that VAR2CSA harboured a globular conformation rather than a linear-shaped structure (60, 61). The determination of the CSA-binding kinetics of the full-length recombinant VAR2CSA also revealed that the full-length protein was able to interact with CSA with high specificity and high affinity, yielding nano-molar affinity constants. This was markedly different to those obtained for single-domain constructs in the micromolar range (60, 61). Using SAXS and single particle reconstruction from negative stained electron micrographs, a recent study confirmed the globular conformation of VAR2CSA and suggested a model for CSA-binding (62). Dissection of the CSA-binding affinities of recombinant truncations of full-length VAR2CSA, as opposed to single DBL domains, identified the N-terminal part of VAR2CSA as the CSA-binding region (63–65). While for the 3D7 variant, a more specific binding to CSA was observed using the DBL1x-DBL3x multidomain protein (64), the DBL1x and DBL3x domains did not appear as essential for high affinity CSA binding for the FCR3 variant (65). The binding affinity of FCR3 DBL2x including small N and C terminal flanking ID1 and ID2 inter-domains was similar to the autologous full-length VAR2CSA. Thus, the minimal binding region of FCR3-VAR2CSA was designated as ID1-DBL2x-ID2a (65).

Although the identification of the high affinity CSA-binding site has orientated researchers to target this region to induce inhibitory antibodies, many studies have looked at the quality of the immune response generated by the different single DBL domains and multiple domains, including the full-length extracellular region of VAR2CSA. Indeed, due to the globular fold of the full-length molecule it appears possible that antibodies directed towards residues not directly involved in CSA-binding could i) be cross-reactive against different variants and/or ii) affect the molecular interaction of VAR2CSA with CSA by steric hindrance.

Interestingly, the generation of single domain nanobodies following immunization of camelids with the full-length VAR2CSA recombinant protein revealed a preferential targeting of the DBL1x domain and, to a lower extent, of DBL4ϵ, DBL5ϵ, and DBL6ϵ (66) suggesting the existence of immunodominant epitopes outside the CSA-binding region of the protein. This assumption is also strengthened by another study showing that monoclonal antibodies generated from naturally infected women are predominantly directed against DBL3x and DBL5x (67). Remarkably, none of these nanobodies and monoclonal antibodies presented CSA-binding inhibitory capability, which indicates that a single molecule targeting an epitope outside the binding region is unlikely to inhibit the adhesion of IEs to CSA.

Several small animal immunization studies, many of which have been carried out in collaboration between different laboratories, have established that the generation of antibodies targeting epitopes shared between different parasite lines could be achieved using various VAR2CSA domains (68–75). Although antibodies raised against the full-length VAR2CSA may not be cross-inhibitory (76), several studies performed in rodents have shown that shorter constructs including the N-terminal region of VAR2CSA are able to induce cross-inhibitory antibodies preventing IEs from binding to CSA (77–81).

Taken together, these data have evolved the rationale for developing a vaccine against PM based on the CSA binding N-terminal region, in the hope that it will prime the immune response towards semi-conserved antigenic determinants and then mimic the antibody repertoire acquired through natural exposure in first pregnancy (32).

PRIMVAC AND PAMVAC PHASE I CLINICAL TRIALS

VAR2CSA-based vaccines spanning the CSA-binding region (PRIMVAC and PAMVAC), designed to generate antibodies capable of inhibiting IEs adhesion to placental cells, have recently been assessed in two separate phase I clinical trials (ClinicalTrials.gov identifiers NCT02658253 and NCT02647489, respectively) (**Figure 1**). Together they represent an attractive intervention strategy to protect primigravid women from the serious clinical outcomes of PM. PAMVAC expressed in a Drosophila Schneider 2-derived cell line spans the interdomain region 1 through Duffy binding-like domain 2 to inter-domains 2 (ID1-DBL2x-ID2a) of the FCR3 variant of VAR2CSA (82), while PRIMVAC expressed in *E. coli* SHuffle® is based on the DBL1x-2x multidomain of VAR2CSA from the *P. falciparum* 3D7 strain (**Figure 1**) (79, 80 83). In order to allow comparative assessment of different placental malaria vaccine candidates, especially PRIMVAC and PAMVAC, two workshops hosted by the European Vaccine Initiative allowed the harmonization of clinical development plans and of assays for immunological assessment (84).

Based on these recommendations, both clinical trials were designed as randomized, double-blind, placebo-controlled, dose escalation trials and were meant to evaluate the safety and immunogenicity of three intramuscular vaccinations with progressively higher doses. PRIMVAC was adjuvanted with Alhydrogel or glucopyranosyl lipid A adjuvant in stable emulsion (GLA-SE) whereas PAMVAC was adjuvanted with Alhydrogel or GLA-SE or injected as a liposomal formulation in combination with QS21 (GLA-LSQ) (**Figure 1**). Volunteers were recruited into sequential cohorts receiving 20 μg, 50 μg, or 100 μg of vaccines at day 0, 28, and 56. PAMVAC volunteers were observed for 6 months following last immunization, while PRIMVAC volunteers were followed for one year after the last vaccination. While the safety and immunogenicity of PRIMVAC has been recently published in both malaria naïve (French volunteers) and *P. falciparum*-exposed non-pregnant women (Burkinabe women) (83), only the clinical evaluation of PAMVAC in malaria naïve volunteers (German volunteers) has been so far reported (82). All PAMVAC and PRIMVAC formulations were safe and well tolerated and none of the vaccines induced serious adverse events (82, 83).

PAMVAC and PRIMVAC were immunogenic in all participants and antibody levels were usually higher for both vaccines when adjuvanted with GLA-SE as compared to Alhydrogel and GLA-LSQ, at all dosages. In the case of PRIMVAC, all the volunteers seroconverted after two vaccine doses and a high proportion of them were still seroconverted one year after the third vaccination, which is indicative of a long-lasting immunity. Interestingly, IgG subclass analysis revealed that the induced antibodies were mostly IgG1 and IgG3 for PRIMVAC vaccinated volunteers. Therefore, the PRIMVAC-induced antibody response seems to mimic the naturally acquired immune response observed in multigravid women (85, 86).

Both vaccines generated antibodies reacting with the homologous VAR2CSA expressing parasites (NF54 for PRIMVAC and FCR3 for PAMVAC), however limited cross-reactivity was observed against heterologous VAR2CSA variants either recombinantly expressed (PAMVAC trial) or expressed on the surface of FCR3-CSA and 7G8-CSA IEs (PRIMVAC trial). The highest cross-reactivity was observed in sera collected from women that received the 100 μ PRIMVAC dose. Both vaccines induced functionally active antibodies inhibiting the interaction of their corresponding homologous VAR2CSA expressing IEs to CSA but low or no CSA-binding inhibition was observed for IEs expressing heterologous VAR2CSA variants (82, 83).

DISCREPANCIES BETWEEN PRECLINICAL AND CLINICAL STUDIES

Interestingly, the PAMVAC and PRIMVAC vaccines were able to induce antibodies in humans at significantly high titers after three doses received by the study participants. These antibodies were mainly vaccine-specific and mainly possessed functional activity against the homologous strains. Although these antibodies made it possible to describe a cross-reactivity with the constructs originating from other parasite variants, in particular those induced by vaccines adjuvanted with GLA-SE (82, 83), the lower cross-reactivity and the lack of cross-inhibition contrasts with the data generated in small animal models that guided the selection of these vaccine candidates (63, 77, 79, 80).

The observation that the responses in humans appear less cross-reactive than in rodents clearly raises the question of the transferability of the data generated in small animal models to humans. One confounding effect could be that the rodents received a higher dose per bodyweight than humans, so that the induced antibody titers are overall lower in humans compared to small animal models. A lower antibody titer would then possess less cross-reactive antibodies and then explain the lowest observed cross-reactivity. It is also possible that there is species-specific selection for cross-reactive epitopes in rodents versus humans. This would be a major obstacle in the placental malaria vaccine development process where the lack of an appropriate animal model remains. An animal model that would be as close as possible to humans, like non-human primates could be an asset in the preclinical validation phases. Efforts to develop such a model in the Aotus monkey is currently underway and could offer an interesting track in this perspective.

Interestingly, it was noted that some nulligravid women participating in the study in Burkina Faso to receive the PRIMVAC vaccine, possessed VAR2CSA antibodies before the administration of the vaccine doses (83). While these observations corroborate those of a few studies which have shown the presence of antibodies reacting with certain VAR2CSA antigens in some non-pregnant or male subjects living in endemic regions (87–89), their potential interference or benefit with vaccination deserves to be considered.

CURRENT VACCINE DEVELOPMENT GAPS AND POTENTIAL FUTURE DEVELOPMENTS

The preclinical and phase I clinical trial results for PAMVAC and PRIMVAC are highly encouraging and confirm the feasibility of developing a PM vaccine through further clinical testing. However, prior to embarking on costly, large-scale phase II clinical trials, it is essential to further evaluate the longevity of the immune response in vaccinated women and meanwhile assess its development upon natural infections. Novel strategies to enhance the immunogenicity of the PM vaccine candidates and to maximize the antibody cross-reactivity against different VAR2CSA variants could also be envisaged.

Longevity

Longevity of the vaccine-induced immune response is an essential element in placental malaria vaccine development, since nulligravid women will be vaccinated many months or years prior to their first pregnancy. In 2012, Fowkes et al. suggested that half-lives of antibody responses in pregnant women induced by natural *P. falciparum* infection were in general relatively short for merozoite antigens (0.8–7.6 years) (90). However, half-lives of antibodies to VAR2CSA were significantly longer (36–157 years), suggesting that antibodies acquired in one pregnancy may be maintained to protect subsequent pregnancies (90). This raises hope for PM vaccine development, a hope that is further bolstered by the results obtained in the pre-clinical and clinical PM vaccination studies. The PM vaccine candidates, especially PRIMVAC, produced a long-lasting immune response in PRIMVAC vaccinated women who developed an immune response that lasted for more than a year (83). To further characterize the longevity of the PRIMVAC-induced immune response in women in malaria-endemic areas and to define vaccination age and frequency of booster vaccinations, follow-up of the vaccinated women for several years will be crucial. Additionally, the capacity of the vaccine candidates to boost and broaden a naturally acquired immune response would provide valuable insight.

Immunogenicity

Recombinant soluble proteins are often thought to induce an immune response of insufficient strength and breadth to confer full protection. Therefore, alternative approaches for the presentation of the VAR2CSA antigens are considered. The most advanced approach is using a capsid-like particle (CLP) that has been added as a backbone to the PM antigen, thereby possibly inducing a stronger immune response than a vaccine based on soluble recombinant protein and thus potentially improving immunogenicity, cross-reactivity and longevity of the induced immune response (91, 92).

Cross-Reactivity

Each vaccine candidate, PAMVAC and PRIMVAC, consists of a single recombinant protein. However, VAR2CSA is a diverse antigen and in Benin alone, 57 haplotypes of the vaccine target were identified which phylogenetically cluster into five clades (93). The PM vaccine candidates PRIMVAC and PAMVAC are from two distinct clades; 3D7 (clade 1) and FCR3 (clade 2) respectively. Interestingly, the authors found an association between the 3D7-like clade and low birthweight (93). Because of the extensive VAR2CSA polymorphism, the development of a PM vaccine is challenging. While the correct part of VAR2CSA to target appears established, it may be needed to generate second-generation vaccines, which expands the possibility of immunizing against several variants to improve cross-reactivity.

Different approaches may be evaluated: 1) prime - boost vaccination using VAR2CSA variants from different clades, 2) combination vaccination approaches either using, e.g., soluble recombinant proteins or multi-VAR2CSA-CLPs, 3) chimeric VAR2CSA variants, either based on the PAMVAC or PRIMVAC protein boundaries or rational structure-based designs. Finally, the recently hyped mRNA vaccine technology deployed against Covid-19 may be a way to incorporate several variants due to the ease and low cost of manufacture (94).

CONCLUSION

Over the past years, a promising portfolio of PM vaccine candidates was developed and two VAR2CSA-derived vaccines were brought to clinical evaluation, confirming the feasibility of developing a PM vaccine. However, to evaluate and compare the results of the various PM vaccine approaches, the harmonization of clinical trial procedures and the standardization of immunoassays that was initiated before the start of the phase I clinical trials (84) has to be further strengthened. Stringent go/no-go criteria will be required to decide to enter in the next development stages based on production feasibility, safety, and induction of cross-reactive and functional immune responses. A major obstacle to transitioning a PM vaccine from preclinic to clinic is the lack of a suitable animal model (95). Evaluation of PM vaccine efficacy is particularly complex. Indeed, the lack of surrogates to predict PM vaccine-induced protection limits the potential of early clinical trials to provide indications on vaccine efficacy. The amplitude of the antibody response resulting from vaccination appears today as an indicator of putative efficacy, although the threshold levels of antibodies required for protection are undetermined. The lowest cross-reactivity observed during the clinical trials in comparison to the preclinical evaluation could be the consequence of a lower amplitude of the immune response upon antigen exposure in humans compared to rodents. Since sterile immunity is not required for a PM vaccine, the hope is that the vaccine-induced response will be boosted and even broadened by natural infection. Alternate schedules of immunization, antigen dosage, and combinations with other VAR2CSA-based vaccines are under development and will be assessed in future studies for their capacities to broaden the cross-reactivity of the induced immunity against heterologous VAR2CSA variants and then fully protect women from the negative outcomes of PM.

AUTHOR CONTRIBUTIONS

BG, AC, NV, NTN, and MN wrote the manuscript. All authors contributed to the article and approved the submitted version.

REFERENCES

1. World Health Organization, Geneva. *World Malaria Report 2019.* (2019) (World malaria report 2019 (who.int)).
2. Verhoeff FH, Brabin BJ, Chimsuku L, Kazembe P, Broadhead RL. An analysis of the determinants of anaemia in pregnant women in rural Malawi–a basis for action. *Ann Trop Med Parasitol* (1999) 93(2):119–33. doi: 10.1080/00034989958609
3. Shulman CE, Graham WJ, Jilo H, Lowe BS, New L, Obiero J, et al. Malaria is an important cause of anaemia in primigravidae: evidence from a district hospital in coastal Kenya. *Trans R Soc Trop Med Hyg* (1996) 90(5):535–9. doi: 10.1016/s0035-9203(96)90312-0

4. Ndao CT, Dumont A, Fievet N, Doucoure S, Gaye A, Lehesran JY. Placental malarial infection as a risk factor for hypertensive disorders during pregnancy in Africa: a case-control study in an urban area of Senegal, West Africa. *Am J Epidemiol* (2009) 170(7):847–53. doi: 10.1093/aje/kwp207
5. Muehlenbachs A, Mutabingwa TK, Edmonds S, Fried M, Duffy PE. Hypertension and maternal-fetal conflict during placental malaria. *PLoS Med* (2006) 3(11):e446. doi: 10.1371/journal.pmed.0030446
6. Moore KA, Simpson JA, Scoullar MJL, McGready R, Fowkes FJI. Quantification of the association between malaria in pregnancy and stillbirth: a systematic review and meta-analysis. *Lancet Glob Health* (2017) 5(11):e1101–e12. doi: 10.1016/S2214-109X(17)30340-6
7. Desai M, ter Kuile FO, Nosten F, McGready R, Asamoa K, Brabin B, et al. Epidemiology and burden of malaria in pregnancy. *Lancet Infect Dis* (2007) 7 (2):93–104. doi: 10.1016/S1473-3099(07)70021-X
8. Galbraith RM, Fox H, Hsi B, Galbraith GM, Bray RS, Faulk WP. The human materno-foetal relationship in malaria. II. Histological, ultrastructural and immunopathological studies of the placenta. *Trans R Soc Trop Med Hyg* (1980) 74(1):61–72. doi: 10.1016/0035-9203(80)90012-7
9. Walter PR, Garin Y, Blot P. Placental pathologic changes in malaria. A histologic and ultrastructural study. *Am J Pathol* (1982) 109(3):330–42.
10. Ismail MR, Ordi J, Menendez C, Ventura PJ, Aponte JJ, Kahigwa E, et al. Placental pathology in malaria: a histological, immunohistochemical, and quantitative study. *Hum Pathol* (2000) 31(1):85–93. doi: 10.1016/s0046-8177 (00)80203-8
11. Fried M, Muga RO, Misore AO, Duffy PE. Malaria elicits type 1 cytokines in the human placenta: IFN-gamma and TNF-alpha associated with pregnancy outcomes. *J Immunol* (1998) 160(5):2523–30.
12. Moormann AM, Sullivan AD, Rochford RA, Chensue SW, Bock PJ, Nyirenda T, et al. Malaria and pregnancy: placental cytokine expression and its relationship to intrauterine growth retardation. *J Infect Dis* (1999) 180(6):1987–93. doi: 10.1086/315135
13. Fievet N, Moussa M, Tami G, Maubert B, Cot M, Deloron P, et al. Plasmodium falciparum induces a Th1/Th2 disequilibrium, favoring the Th1-type pathway, in the human placenta. *J Infect Dis* (2001) 183 (10):1530–4. doi: 10.1086/320201
14. Umbers AJ, Boeuf P, Clapham C, Stanisic DI, Baiwog F, Mueller I, et al. Placental malaria-associated inflammation disturbs the insulin-like growth factor axis of fetal growth regulation. *J Infect Dis* (2011) 203(4):561–9. doi: 10.1093/infdis/jiq080
15. Smith JD, Chitnis CE, Craig AG, Roberts DJ, Hudson-Taylor DE, Peterson DS, et al. Switches in expression of Plasmodium falciparum var genes correlate with changes in antigenic and cytoadherent phenotypes of infected erythrocytes. *Cell* (1995) 82(1):101–10. doi: 10.1016/0092-8674(95)90056-x
16. Baruch DI, Pasloske BL, Singh HB, Bi X, Ma XC, Feldman M, et al. Cloning the P. falciparum gene encoding PfEMP1, a malarial variant antigen and adherence receptor on the surface of parasitized human erythrocytes. *Cell* (1995) 82(1):77–87. doi: 10.1016/0092-8674(95)90054-3
17. Turner L, Lavstsen T, Berger SS, Wang CW, Petersen JE, Avril M, et al. Severe malaria is associated with parasite binding to endothelial protein C receptor. *Nature* (2013) 498(7455):502–5. doi: 10.1038/nature12216
18. Fried M, Duffy PE. Adherence of Plasmodium falciparum to chondroitin sulfate A in the human placenta. *Science* (1996) 272(5267):1502–4. doi: 10.1126/science.272.5267.1502
19. Gysin J, Pouvelle B, Fievet N, Scherf A, Lepolard C. Ex vivo desequestration of Plasmodium falciparum-infected erythrocytes from human placenta by chondroitin sulfate A. *Infect Immun* (1999) 67(12):6596–602.
20. Maubert B, Guilbert LJ, Deloron P. Cytoadherence of Plasmodium falciparum to intercellular adhesion molecule 1 and chondroitin-4-sulfate expressed by the syncytiotrophoblast in the human placenta. *Infect Immun* (1997) 65 (4):1251–7. doi: 10.1128/IAI.65.4.1251-1257.1997
21. Achur RN, Valiyaveettil M, Alkhalil A, Ockenhouse CF, Gowda DC. Characterization of proteoglycans of human placenta and identification of unique chondroitin sulfate proteoglycans of the intervillous spaces that mediate the adherence of Plasmodium falciparum-infected erythrocytes to the placenta. *J Biol Chem* (2000) 275(51):40344–56. doi: 10.1074/jbc.M006398200
22. Viebig NK, Gamain B, Scheidig C, Lepolard C, Przyborski J, Lanzer M, et al. A single member of the Plasmodium falciparum var multigene family determines cytoadhesion to the placental receptor chondroitin sulphate A. *EMBO Rep* (2005) 6(8):775–81. doi: 10.1038/sj.embor.7400466
23. Elliott SR, Duffy MF, Byrne TJ, Beeson JG, Mann EJ, Wilson DW, et al. Cross-reactive surface epitopes on chondroitin sulfate A-adherent Plasmodium falciparum-infected erythrocytes are associated with transcription of var2csa. *Infect Immun* (2005) 73(5):2848–56. doi: 10.1128/IAI.73.5.2848-2856.2005
24. Duffy MF, Byrne TJ, Elliott SR, Wilson DW, Rogerson SJ, Beeson JG, et al. Broad analysis reveals a consistent pattern of var gene transcription in Plasmodium falciparum repeatedly selected for a defined adhesion phenotype. *Mol Microbiol* (2005) 56(3):774–88. doi: 10.1111/j.1365-2958.2005.04577.x
25. Gamain B, Trimnell AR, Scheidig C, Scherf A, Miller LH, Smith JD. Identification of multiple chondroitin sulfate A (CSA)-binding domains in the var2CSA gene transcribed in CSA-binding parasites. *J Infect Dis* (2005) 191(6):1010–3. doi: 10.1086/428137
26. Salanti A, Dahlback M, Turner L, Nielsen MA, Barfod L, Magistrado P, et al. Evidence for the involvement of VAR2CSA in pregnancy-associated malaria. *J Exp Med* (2004) 200(9):1197–203. doi: 10.1084/jem.20041579
27. Salanti A, Staalsoe T, Lavstsen T, Jensen AT, Sowa MP, Arnot DE, et al. Selective upregulation of a single distinctly structured var gene in chondroitin sulphate A-adhering Plasmodium falciparum involved in pregnancy-associated malaria. *Mol Microbiol* (2003) 49(1):179–91. doi: 10.1046/j.1365-2958.2003.03570.x
28. Babakhanyan A, Leke RG, Salanti A, Bobbili N, Gwanmesia P, Leke RJ, et al. The antibody response of pregnant Cameroonian women to VAR2CSA ID1-ID2a, a small recombinant protein containing the CSA-binding site. *PLoS One* (2014) 9(2):e88173. doi: 10.1371/journal.pone.0088173
29. Dechavanne S, Srivastava A, Gangnard S, Nunes-Silva S, Dechavanne C, Fievet N, et al. Parity-dependent recognition of DBL1X-3X suggests an important role of the VAR2CSA high-affinity CSA-binding region in the development of the humoral response against placental malaria. *Infect Immun* (2015) 83(6):2466–74. doi: 10.1128/IAI.03116-14
30. Tutterrow YL, Salanti A, Avril M, Smith JD, Pagano IS, Ako S, et al. High avidity antibodies to full-length VAR2CSA correlate with absence of placental malaria. *PLoS One* (2012) 7(6):e40049. doi: 10.1371/journal.pone.0040049
31. Cutts JC, Agius PA, Zaw L, Powell R, Moore K, Draper B, et al. Pregnancy-specific malarial immunity and risk of malaria in pregnancy and adverse birth outcomes: a systematic review. *BMC Med* (2020) 18(1):14. doi: 10.1186/s12916-019-1467-6
32. Fried M, Nosten F, Brockman A, Brabin BJ, Duffy PE. Maternal antibodies block malaria. *Nature* (1998) 395(6705):851–2. doi: 10.1038/27570
33. Keen J, Serghides L, Ayi K, Patel SN, Ayisi J, van Eijk A, et al. HIV impairs opsonic phagocytic clearance of pregnancy-associated malaria parasites. *PLoS Med* (2007) 4(5):e181. doi: 10.1371/journal.pmed.0040181
34. Ataide R, Mwapasa V, Molyneux ME, Meshnick SR, Rogerson SJ. Antibodies that induce phagocytosis of malaria infected erythrocytes: effect of HIV infection and correlation with clinical outcomes. *PLoS One* (2011) 6(7): e22491. doi: 10.1371/journal.pone.0022491
35. Jaworowski A, Fernandes LA, Yosaatmadja F, Feng G, Mwapasa V, Molyneux ME, et al. Relationship between human immunodeficiency virus type 1 coinfection, anemia, and levels and function of antibodies to variant surface antigens in pregnancy-associated malaria. *Clin Vaccine Immunol* (2009) 16 (3):312–9. doi: 10.1128/CVI.00356-08
36. Saito M, Briand V, Min AM, McGready R. Deleterious effects of malaria in pregnancy on the developing fetus: a review on prevention and treatment with antimalarial drugs. *Lancet Child Adolesc Health* (2020) 4(10):761–74. doi: 10.1016/S2352-4642(20)30099-7
37. Desai M, Hill J, Fernandes S, Walker P, Pell C, Gutman J, et al. Prevention of malaria in pregnancy. *Lancet Infect Dis* (2018) 18(4):e119–e32. doi: 10.1016/S1473-3099(18)30064-1
38. World Health Organization, Geneva. *Global report on insecticide resistance in malaria vectors: 2010–2016.* (2018).
39. van Eijk AM, Larsen DA, Kayentao K, Koshy G, Slaughter DEC, Roper C, et al. Effect of Plasmodium falciparum sulfadoxine-pyrimethamine resistance on the effectiveness of intermittent preventive therapy for malaria in pregnancy in Africa: a systematic review and meta-analysis. *Lancet Infect Dis* (2019) 19 (5):546–56. doi: 10.1016/S1473-3099(18)30732-1

40. Accrombessi M, Fievet N, Yovo E, Cottrell G, Agbota G, Massougbodji A, et al. Prevalence and Associated Risk Factors of Malaria in the First Trimester of Pregnancy: A Preconceptional Cohort Study in Benin. *J Infect Dis* (2018) 217(8):1309–17. doi: 10.1093/infdis/jiy009
41. Accrombessi M, Yovo E, Fievet N, Cottrell G, Agbota G, Gartner A, et al. Effects of Malaria in the First Trimester of Pregnancy on Poor Maternal and Birth Outcomes in Benin. *Clin Infect Dis* (2019) 69(8):1385–93. doi: 10.1093/cid/ciy1073
42. Hounkonnou CPA, Briand V, Fievet N, Accrombessi M, Yovo E, Mama A, et al. Dynamics of Submicroscopic Plasmodium falciparum Infections Throughout Pregnancy: A Preconception Cohort Study in Benin. *Clin Infect Dis* (2020) 71(1):166–74. doi: 10.1093/cid/ciz748
43. Jafari-Guemouri S, Courtois L, Mama A, Rouas B, Neto Braga G, Accrombessi M, et al. Genotyping Study in Benin Comparing the Carriage of Plasmodium falciparum Infections Before Pregnancy and in Early Pregnancy: Story of a Persistent Infection. *Clin Infect Dis* (2020). doi: 10.1093/cid/ciaa841
44. Fried M, Duffy PE. Maternal malaria and parasite adhesion. *J Mol Med (Berl)* (1998) 76(3-4):162–71. doi: 10.1007/s001090050205
45. Walker PG, ter Kuile FO, Garske T, Menendez C, Ghani AC. Estimated risk of placental infection and low birthweight attributable to Plasmodium falciparum malaria in Africa in 2010: a modelling study. *Lancet Glob Health* (2014) 2(8):e460–7. doi: 10.1016/S2214-109X(14)70256-6
46. Tuikue Ndam NG, Salanti A, Bertin G, Dahlback M, Fievet N, Turner L, et al. High level of var2csa transcription by Plasmodium falciparum isolated from the placenta. *J Infect Dis* (2005) 192(2):331–5. doi: 10.1086/430933
47. Sander AF, Salanti A, Lavstsen T, Nielsen MA, Theander TG, Leke RG, et al. Positive selection of Plasmodium falciparum parasites with multiple var2csa-type PfEMP1 genes during the course of infection in pregnant women. *J Infect Dis* (2011) 203(11):1679–85. doi: 10.1093/infdis/jir168
48. Gangnard S, Chene A, Dechavanne S, Srivastava A, Avril M, Smith JD, et al. VAR2CSA binding phenotype has ancient origin and arose before Plasmodium falciparum crossed to humans: implications in placental malaria vaccine design. *Sci Rep* (2019) 9(1):16978. doi: 10.1038/s41598-019-53334-8
49. Gangnard S, Lewit-Bentley A, Dechavanne S, Srivastava A, Amirat F, Bentley GA, et al. Structure of the DBL3X-DBL4epsilon region of the VAR2CSA placental malaria vaccine candidate: insight into DBL domain interactions. *Sci Rep* (2015) 5:14868. doi: 10.1038/srep14868
50. Khunrae P, Philip JM, Bull DR, Higgins MK. Structural comparison of two CSPG-binding DBL domains from the VAR2CSA protein important in malaria during pregnancy. *J Mol Biol* (2009) 393(1):202–13. doi: 10.1016/j.jmb.2009.08.027
51. Dahlback M, Rask TS, Andersen PH, Nielsen MA, Ndam NT, Resende M, et al. Epitope mapping and topographic analysis of VAR2CSA DBL3X involved in P. falciparum placental sequestration. *PLoS Pathog* (2006) 2(11): e124. doi: 10.1371/journal.ppat.0020124
52. Avril M, Gamain B, Lepolard C, Viaud N, Scherf A, Gysin J. Characterization of anti-var2CSA-PfEMP1 cytoadhesion inhibitory mouse monoclonal antibodies. *Microbes Infect* (2006) 8(14-15):2863–71. doi: 10.1016/j.micinf.2006.09.005
53. Bir N, Yazdani SS, Avril M, Layez C, Gysin J, Chitnis CE. Immunogenicity of Duffy binding-like domains that bind chondroitin sulfate A and protection against pregnancy-associated malaria. *Infect Immun* (2006) 74(10):5955–63. doi: 10.1128/IAI.00481-06
54. Higgins MK. The structure of a chondroitin sulfate-binding domain important in placental malaria. *J Biol Chem* (2008) 283(32):21842–6. doi: 10.1074/jbc.C800086200
55. Resende M, Ditlev SB, Nielsen MA, Bodevin S, Bruun S, Pinto VV, et al. Chondroitin sulphate A (CSA)-binding of single recombinant Duffy-binding-like domains is not restricted to Plasmodium falciparum Erythrocyte Membrane Protein 1 expressed by CSA-binding parasites. *Int J Parasitol* (2009) 39(11):1195–204. doi: 10.1016/j.ijpara.2009.02.022
56. Singh K, Gittis AG, Nguyen P, Gowda DC, Miller LH, Garboczi DN. Structure of the DBL3x domain of pregnancy-associated malaria protein VAR2CSA complexed with chondroitin sulfate A. *Nat Struct Mol Biol* (2008) 15(9):932–8. doi: 10.1038/nsmb.1479
57. Singh K, Gitti RK, Diouf A, Zhou H, Gowda DC, Miura K, et al. Subdomain 3 of Plasmodium falciparum VAR2CSA DBL3x is identified as a minimal chondroitin sulfate A-binding region. *J Biol Chem* (2010) 285(32):24855–62. doi: 10.1074/jbc.M110.118612
58. Salanti A, Resende M, Ditlev SB, Pinto VV, Dahlback M, Andersen G, et al. Several domains from VAR2CSA can induce Plasmodium falciparum adhesion-blocking antibodies. *Malar J* (2010) 9:11. doi: 10.1186/1475-2875-9-11
59. Pinto VV, Ditlev SB, Jensen KE, Resende M, Dahlback M, Andersen G, et al. Differential induction of functional IgG using the Plasmodium falciparum placental malaria vaccine candidate VAR2CSA. *PLoS One* (2011) 6(3):e17942. doi: 10.1371/journal.pone.0017942
60. Khunrae P, Dahlback M, Nielsen MA, Andersen G, Ditlev SB, Resende M, et al. Full-length recombinant Plasmodium falciparum VAR2CSA binds specifically to CSPG and induces potent parasite adhesion-blocking antibodies. *J Mol Biol* (2010) 397(3):826–34. doi: 10.1016/j.jmb.2010.01.040
61. Srivastava A, Gangnard S, Round A, Dechavanne S, Juillerat A, Raynal B, et al. Full-length extracellular region of the var2CSA variant of PfEMP1 is required for specific, high-affinity binding to CSA. *Proc Natl Acad Sci U S A* (2010) 107 (11):4884–9. doi: 10.1073/pnas.1000951107
62. Bewley MC, Gautam L, Jagadeeshaprasad MG, Gowda DC, Flanagan JM. Molecular architecture and domain arrangement of the placental malaria protein VAR2CSA suggests a model for carbohydrate binding. *J Biol Chem* (2020) 295(52):18589–603. doi: 10.1074/jbc.RA120.014676
63. Dahlback M, Jorgensen LM, Nielsen MA, Clausen TM, Ditlev SB, Resende M, et al. The chondroitin sulfate A-binding site of the VAR2CSA protein involves multiple N-terminal domains. *J Biol Chem* (2011) 286(18):15908–17. doi: 10.1074/jbc.M110.191510
64. Srivastava A, Gangnard S, Dechavanne S, Amirat F, Lewit Bentley A, Bentley GA, et al. Var2CSA minimal CSA binding region is located within the N-terminal region. *PLoS One* (2011) 6(5):e20270. doi: 10.1371/journal.pone.0020270
65. Clausen TM, Christoffersen S, Dahlback M, Langkilde AE, Jensen KE, Resende M, et al. Structural and functional insight into how the Plasmodium falciparum VAR2CSA protein mediates binding to chondroitin sulfate A in placental malaria. *J Biol Chem* (2012) 287(28):23332–45. doi: 10.1074/jbc.M112.348839
66. Nunes-Silva S, Gangnard S, Vidal M, Vuchelen A, Dechavanne S, Chan S, et al. Llama immunization with full-length VAR2CSA generates cross-reactive and inhibitory single-domain antibodies against the DBL1X domain. *Sci Rep* (2014) 4:7373. doi: 10.1038/srep07373
67. Barfod L, Bernasconi NL, Dahlback M, Jarrossay D, Andersen PH, Salanti A, et al. Human pregnancy-associated malaria-specific B cells target polymorphic, conformational epitopes in VAR2CSA. *Mol Microbiol* (2007) 63(2):335–47. doi: 10.1111/j.1365-2958.2006.05503.x
68. Avril M, Kulasekara BR, Gose SO, Rowe C, Dahlback M, Duffy PE, et al. Evidence for globally shared, cross-reacting polymorphic epitopes in the pregnancy-associated malaria vaccine candidate VAR2CSA. *Infect Immun* (2008) 76(4):1791–800. doi: 10.1128/IAI.01470-07
69. Barfod L, Dobrilovic T, Magistrado P, Khunrae P, Viwami F, Bruun J, et al. Chondroitin sulfate A-adhering Plasmodium falciparum-infected erythrocytes express functionally important antibody epitopes shared by multiple variants. *J Immunol* (2010) 185(12):7553–61. doi: 10.4049/jimmunol.1002390
70. Doritchamou JY, Herrera R, Aebig JA, Morrison R, Nguyen V, Reiter K, et al. VAR2CSA Domain-Specific Analysis of Naturally Acquired Functional Antibodies to Plasmodium falciparum Placental Malaria. *J Infect Dis* (2016) 214(4):577–86. doi: 10.1093/infdis/jiw197
71. Fried M, Avril M, Chaturvedi R, Fernandez P, Lograsso J, Narum D, et al. Multilaboratory approach to preclinical evaluation of vaccine immunogens for placental malaria. *Infect Immun* (2013) 81(2):487–95. doi: 10.1128/IAI.01106-12
72. Magistrado PA, Minja D, Doritchamou J, Ndam NT, John D, Schmiegelow C, et al. High efficacy of anti DBL4varepsilon-VAR2CSA antibodies in inhibition of CSA-binding Plasmodium falciparum-infected erythrocytes from pregnant women. *Vaccine* (2011) 29(3):437–43. doi: 10.1016/j.vaccine.2010.10.080
73. Nielsen MA, Pinto VV, Resende M, Dahlback M, Ditlev SB, Theander TG, et al. Induction of adhesion-inhibitory antibodies against placental Plasmodium falciparum parasites by using single domains of VAR2CSA. *Infect Immun* (2009) 77(6):2482–7. doi: 10.1128/IAI.00159-09
74. Nielsen MA, Resende M, de Jongh WA, Ditlev SB, Mordmuller B, Houard S, et al. The Influence of Sub-Unit Composition and Expression System on the Functional Antibody Response in the Development of a VAR2CSA Based

Plasmodium falciparum Placental Malaria Vaccine. *PLoS One* (2015) 10(9): e0135406. doi: 10.1371/journal.pone.0135406
75. Obiakor H, Avril M, Macdonald NJ, Srinivasan P, Reiter K, Anderson C, et al. Identification of VAR2CSA domain-specific inhibitory antibodies of the Plasmodium falciparum erythrocyte membrane protein 1 using a novel flow cytometry assay. *Clin Vaccine Immunol* (2013) 20(3):433–42. doi: 10.1128/CVI.00638-12
76. Avril M, Hathaway MJ, Srivastava A, Dechavanne S, Hommel M, Beeson JG, et al. Antibodies to a full-length VAR2CSA immunogen are broadly strain-transcendent but do not cross-inhibit different placental-type parasite isolates. *PLoS One* (2011) 6(2):e16622. doi: 10.1371/journal.pone.0016622
77. Bigey P, Gnidehou S, Doritchamou J, Quiviger M, Viwami F, Couturier A, et al. The NTS-DBL2X region of VAR2CSA induces cross-reactive antibodies that inhibit adhesion of several Plasmodium falciparum isolates to chondroitin sulfate A. *J Infect Dis* (2011) 204(7):1125–33. doi: 10.1093/infdis/jir499
78. Bordbar B, Tuikue-Ndam N, Bigey P, Doritchamou J, Scherman D, Deloron P. Identification of Id1-DBL2X of VAR2CSA as a key domain inducing highly inhibitory and cross-reactive antibodies. *Vaccine* (2012) 30(7):1343–8. doi: 10.1016/j.vaccine.2011.12.065
79. Chene A, Gangnard S, Dechavanne C, Dechavanne S, Srivastava A, Tetard M, et al. Down-selection of the VAR2CSA DBL1-2 expressed in E. coli as a lead antigen for placental malaria vaccine development. *NPJ Vaccines* (2018) 3:28. doi: 10.1038/s41541-018-0064-6
80. Chene A, Gangnard S, Guadall A, Ginisty H, Leroy O, Havelange N, et al. Preclinical immunogenicity and safety of the cGMP-grade placental malaria vaccine PRIMVAC. *EBioMedicine* (2019) 42:145–56. doi: 10.1016/j.ebiom.2019.03.010
81. Doritchamou J, Bigey P, Nielsen MA, Gnidehou S, Ezinmegnon S, Burgain A, et al. Differential adhesion-inhibitory patterns of antibodies raised against two major variants of the NTS-DBL2X region of VAR2CSA. *Vaccine* (2013) 31 (41):4516–22. doi: 10.1016/j.vaccine.2013.07.072
82. Mordmuller B, Sulyok M, Egger-Adam D, Resende M, de Jongh WA, Jensen MH, et al. First-in-human, Randomized, Double-blind Clinical Trial of Differentially Adjuvanted PAMVAC, A Vaccine Candidate to Prevent Pregnancy-associated Malaria. *Clin Infect Dis* (2019) 69(9):1509–16. doi: 10.1093/cid/ciy1140
83. Sirima SB, Richert L, Chene A, Konate AT, Campion C, Dechavanne S, et al. PRIMVAC vaccine adjuvanted with Alhydrogel or GLA-SE to prevent placental malaria: a first-in-human, randomised, double-blind, placebo-controlled study. *Lancet Infect Dis* (2020) 20(5):585–97. doi: 10.1016/S1473-3099(19)30739-X
84. Chene A, Houard S, Nielsen MA, Hundt S, D'Alessio F, Sirima SB, et al. Clinical development of placental malaria vaccines and immunoassays harmonization: a workshop report. *Malar J* (2016) 15:476. doi: 10.1186/s12936-016-1527-8
85. Elliott SR, Brennan AK, Beeson JG, Tadesse E, Molyneux ME, Brown GV, et al. Placental malaria induces variant-specific antibodies of the cytophilic subtypes immunoglobulin G1 (IgG1) and IgG3 that correlate with adhesion inhibitory activity. *Infect Immun* (2005) 73(9):5903–7. doi: 10.1128/IAI.73.9.5903-5907.2005
86. Megnekou R, Staalsoe T, Taylor DW, Leke R, Hviid L. Effects of pregnancy and intensity of Plasmodium falciparum transmission on immunoglobulin G subclass responses to variant surface antigens. *Infect Immun* (2005) 73 (7):4112–8. doi: 10.1128/IAI.73.7.4112-4118.2005
87. Beeson JG, Ndungu F, Persson KE, Chesson JM, Kelly GL, Uyoga S, et al. Antibodies among men and children to placental-binding Plasmodium falciparum-infected erythrocytes that express var2csa. *Am J Trop Med Hyg* (2007) 77(1):22–8.
88. Fodjo BA, Atemnkeng N, Esemu L, Yuosembom EK, Quakyi IA, Tchinda VH, et al. Antibody responses to the full-length VAR2CSA and its DBL domains in Cameroonian children and teenagers. *Malar J* (2016) 15(1):532. doi: 10.1186/s12936-016-1585-y
89. Gnidehou S, Doritchamou J, Arango EM, Cabrera A, Arroyo MI, Kain KC, et al. Functional antibodies against VAR2CSA in nonpregnant populations from colombia exposed to Plasmodium falciparum and Plasmodium vivax. *Infect Immun* (2014) 82(6):2565–73. doi: 10.1128/IAI.01594-14
90. Fowkes FJ, McGready R, Cross NJ, Hommel M, Simpson JA, Elliott SR, et al. New insights into acquisition, boosting, and longevity of immunity to malaria in pregnant women. *J Infect Dis* (2012) 206(10):1612–21. doi: 10.1093/infdis/jis566
91. Thrane S, Janitzek CM, Matondo S, Resende M, Gustavsson T, de Jongh WA, et al. Bacterial superglue enables easy development of efficient virus-like particle based vaccines. *J Nanobiotechnology* (2016) 14:30. doi: 10.1186/s12951-016-0181-1
92. Janitzek CM, Peabody J, Thrane S, P HRC, T GT, Salanti A, et al. A proof-of-concept study for the design of a VLP-based combinatorial HPV and placental malaria vaccine. *Sci Rep* (2019) 9(1):5260. doi: 10.1038/s41598-019-41522-5
93. Patel JC, Hathaway NJ, Parobek CM, Thwai KL, Madanitsa M, Khairallah C, et al. Increased risk of low birth weight in women with placental malaria associated with P. falciparum VAR2CSA clade. *Sci Rep* (2017) 7(1):7768. doi: 10.1038/s41598-017-04737-y
94. Rele S. COVID-19 vaccine development during pandemic: gap analysis, opportunities, and impact on future emerging infectious disease development strategies. *Hum Vaccin Immunother* (2020), 1–6. doi: 10.1080/21645515.2020.1822136
95. Doritchamou J, Teo A, Fried M, Duffy PE. Malaria in pregnancy: the relevance of animal models for vaccine development. *Lab Anim (NY)* (2017) 46 (10):388–98. doi: 10.1038/laban.1349

11

VAR2CSA-Mediated Host Defense Evasion of *Plasmodium falciparum* Infected Erythrocytes in Placental Malaria

Alice Tomlinson[1,2,3]*, Jean-Philippe Semblat*[1,2,3]*, Benoît Gamain*[1,2,3] *and Arnaud Chêne*[1,2,3*]

[1] *Université de Paris, Biologie Intégrée du Globule Rouge, UMR_S1134, BIGR, INSERM, Paris, France,* [2] *Institut National de la Transfusion Sanguine, Paris, France,* [3] *Laboratory of Excellence GR-Ex, Paris, France*

***Correspondence:**
Arnaud Chêne
arnaud.chene@inserm.fr

Over 30 million women living in *P. falciparum* endemic areas are at risk of developing malaria during pregnancy every year. Placental malaria is characterized by massive accumulation of infected erythrocytes in the intervillous space of the placenta, accompanied by infiltration of immune cells, particularly monocytes. The consequent local inflammation and the obstruction of the maternofetal exchanges can lead to severe clinical outcomes for both mother and child. Even if protection against the disease can gradually be acquired following successive pregnancies, the malaria parasite has developed a large panel of evasion mechanisms to escape from host defense mechanisms and manipulate the immune system to its advantage. Infected erythrocytes isolated from placentas of women suffering from placental malaria present a unique phenotype and express the pregnancy-specific variant VAR2CSA of the *Plasmodium falciparum* Erythrocyte Membrane Protein (PfEMP1) family at their surface. The polymorphic VAR2CSA protein is able to mediate the interaction of infected erythrocytes with a variety of host cells including placental syncytiotrophoblasts and leukocytes but also with components of the immune system such as non-specific IgM. This review summarizes the described VAR2CSA-mediated host defense evasion mechanisms employed by the parasite during placental malaria to ensure its survival and persistence.

Keywords: *Plasmodium falciparum*, placental malaria, VAR2CSA, PfEMP1, immune evasion, immuno-modulation, VAR2CSA polymorphism

INTRODUCTION

Nearly half the world's population, implicating 90 countries, lives in areas at risk of malaria transmission. In 2019, an estimated 11 million pregnant women were infected by *Plasmodium* in sub-Saharan Africa, where *P. falciparum* is the most prevalent parasite species, accounting for 99.7% of estimated malaria cases (1). *P. falciparum* infection contracted during pregnancy can lead to placental malaria (PM), a condition that could cause very serious clinical outcomes for both mother and child, including maternal anemia (2, 3), hypertension (4, 5), stillbirth (6, 7) as well as low birth-weight infants, which affected over 800,000 children in 2019 (1).

PM may result in significant morphological and immunological changes in the placenta. Focal syncytial necrosis, loss of syncytial microvilli, and proliferation of cytotrophoblastic cells are frequently observed as well as thickening of trophoblastic basement membranes together with the apparition of syncytial knots (8–10). Acute infection is also characterized by the substantial presence of infected erythrocytes (IEs) in the intervillous spaces of the placenta (**Figure 1A**).

Several transcriptomic and proteomic studies revealed that parasitized red blood cells isolated from *P. falciparum*-infected pregnant women display specific signatures, over-expressing a variety of different genes (11–13) and proteins (14–16) as compared to non-pregnancy-specific parasites. They also present a unique adhesive phenotype, interacting with chondroitin sulfate A (CSA), a low-sulfated glycosaminoglycan (GAG), which is the major host receptor involved in the adhesion of IEs to syncytiotrophoblastic cells (17–21) (**Figure 1B**). Chondroitin sulfate-proteoglycans (CSPGs) are present in the intervillous space of the placenta during the entire second and third trimesters and possibly during the latter part of the first trimester (22).

To date, the pregnancy-specific variant of the *Plasmodium falciparum* erythrocyte membrane protein 1 family (PfEMP1) VAR2CSA has been identified as the sole parasite-derived protein interacting with placental CSA (23–28).

This review focuses on the roles played by VAR2CSA in PM pathogenesis and introduces the latest information on its involvement in host defense evasion mechanisms ranging from cytoadhesion in the placenta, modulation of the placental microenvironment to escape of pregnancy-specific IEs from recognition by protective antibodies.

VAR2CSA STRUCTURE AND CHONDROITIN SULFATE A (CSA)-BINDING

VAR2CSA is a large protein of 350 kDa, with an extracellular region of approximately 300 kDa, displayed at the surface of IEs on membrane protrusions called knobs (29). PfEMP1 clustering

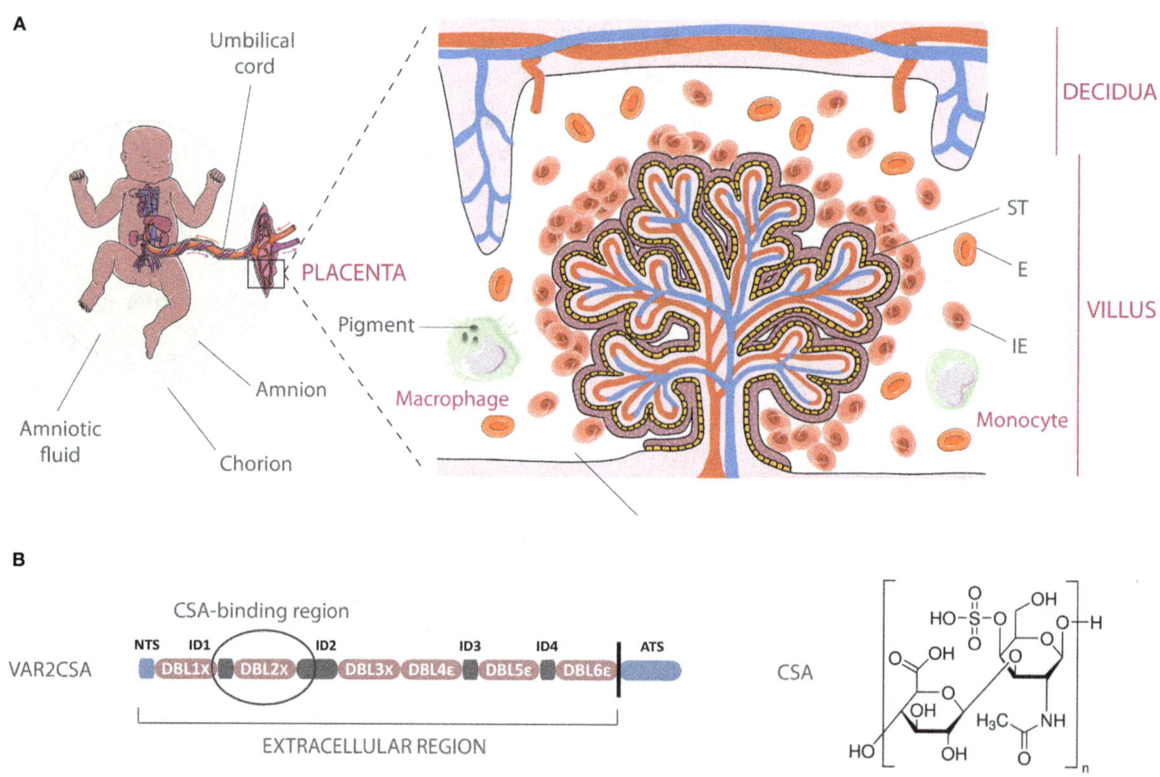

FIGURE 1 | Infected erythrocyte sequestration within the intervillous space of the placenta. **(A)** Schematic representation of infected erythrocytes (IE) adhering to the syncytiotrophoblastic lining of the fetal villus, with increased presence of macrophages and monocytes in the maternal blood. Parasite pigments (hemozoin) remain visible in macrophages following IEs phagocytosis. The natural transfer of gases and nutrients between maternal blood in the intervillous space and fetal blood circulating in the villi is impaired by IEs sequestration. E, Erythrocyte; ST, syncytiotrophoblast. **(B)** Architecture of the VAR2CSA protein and chemical structure of chondroitin-4-sulfate A. The circled region within VAR2CSA (ID1-ID2a) represents the CSA-binding region. The art pieces used in this figure were modified from Servier Medical Art by Servier, licensed under a Creative Commons Attribution 3.0 Unported License (https://smart.servier.com/).

on knob structures is thought to maximize cytoadhesion under flow conditions but also to act as an immune evasion mechanism, impairing antibody accessibility to key residues involved in CSA-binding (30, 31). Quantitative studies report an estimate of 3 to 80 VAR2CSA molecules per knob (32, 33). Knob density at the IEs surface has been shown to be linked to the PfEMP1 variant expressed by the parasite (34) and IEs stained by the monoclonal antibody PAM1.4 revealed that erythrocytes infected by the FCR3 parasite strains displayed more VAR2CSA clusters at the cell surface than erythrocytes infected by NF54 (35). Even if further studies are needed to precisely determine how these differences in PfEMP1 presentation impact antibody recognition, these observations highlight that *P. falciparum* is capable of complex variations at both intra- and inter-strain levels.

The cysteine-rich extracellular region of VAR2CSA has a complex architecture and is composed of six Duffy-Binding Like domains (DBLs), which are interspaced by four inter-domain regions (IDs) (**Figure 1B**). High-resolution structures have been obtained for the individual domains DBL3x, DBL6ϵ (36–40) as well as for the multidomain DBL3x-DBL4ϵ (41), providing a first step towards the definition of inter-domain interfaces and of the overall structure of the extracellular part of VAR2CSA. Low-resolution structures of the full-length extracellular part of VAR2CSA, obtained by small-angle X-ray scattering or single particle electron microscopy, reveal a compact organization of the protein maintained by specific inter-domain interactions (42–44). Nevertheless, the relative locations of the DBL domains within the overall structure of VAR2CSA significantly differ from one study to another (43, 44). In the recent work from Bewley et al., the VAR2CSA ectodomain low resolution structure appears as a duck-like shape with a packing of three tandem domains (DBL1x/DBL2x, DBL3x/DBL4ϵ, and DBL5ϵ/DBL6ϵ), which would form two pores, each theoretically susceptible to accommodate a 10-12-mer CSA molecule (44). This model suggests that the higher-order structural organization of VAR2CSA is most likely allowing the formation of one, or maybe two, CSA-binding site(s), which comprise(s) several domains. The current definition of the boundaries of the core binding region, established using truncated fragments of recombinant VAR2CSA, localizes the high affinity CSA-binding site within the N-terminal part of the protein (45) between the ID1-ID2a section (46) even-though the accessory implication of other domains such as DBL4ϵ cannot be excluded (44). Additional VAR2CSA structural data at high resolution, ideally in complex with CSA, is still required to determine the precise determinants of CSA-binding, which might also include post-translational modifications (47).

VAR2CSA-MEDIATED INFECTED ERYTHROCYTES CYTOADHESION IN THE PLACENTA AND EVASION FROM SPLENIC FILTRATION

As parasites develop from ring stage to schizont stage within erythrocytes, the biomechanical properties of the host cells are subjected to considerable modifications, leading to decreased cellular deformability and loss of membrane elasticity [Reviewed in (48)]. Cytoadhesion of mature pregnancy-specific IEs to syncytiotrophoblasts leads to their sequestration in the intervillous spaces of the placenta. By sequestering in the placenta, biomechanically altered IEs avoid splenic retention at the level of the reticular mesh of the red pulp or during the challenging passage through the inter-endothelial slits of the organ (49–52). *P. falciparum* has therefore developed an efficient host defense evasion mechanism, which relies on a tight interaction between IEs and the syncytiotrophoblastic lining delimiting the intervillous spaces of the maternal portion of the placenta. As CSPGs are also present within the micro-vascular system, notably in the lungs and brain (53), the reason for exclusive placental sequestration of VAR2CSA-expressing IEs remains unclear. A body of work elucidated some comprehensive elements by demonstrating that the interaction of VAR2CSA with CSA is highly correlated with the degree of C-4 sulfation and the length of the CS chain (54–56), which may vary in different tissues. CSA density and wall shear stress also appear as two components influencing the IEs binding to CSA (57). CSA density on syncytiotrophoblasts and forces acting upon placental tissues could thus determine the selective cytoadhesion of IEs in the organ. If placental sequestration of IEs represents an effective immune evasion mechanism employed by *P. falciparum* to avoid its clearance by the spleen, this is not without harmful consequences for the women and the fetus. Sequestration is thought to be one of the prime mediators of biological alterations leading to placental insufficiency and subsequently to fetal growth restriction and poor birth outcomes [Reviewed in (58, 59)].

VAR2CSA-MEDIATED MODULATION OF THE PLACENTAL MICROENVIRONMENT

The placenta is a tightly controlled pro-inflammatory and anti-inflammatory environment, depending upon the stage of gestation. In healthy pregnancies, a pro-inflammatory milieu is required for fetal implantation, notably by promoting trophoblast invasion. A shift toward a type 2 cytokine/chemokine milieu gradually occurs during gestation favoring pregnancy maintenance and rapid fetal growth and development [reviewed in (60)]. *P. falciparum* infection during pregnancy can affect the placental environment, notably promoting inflammatory responses (61–65), some of which are associated with fetal growth retardation, low birth-weight babies, and in more extreme cases, poor pregnancy outcomes, such as preterm delivery and pregnancy loss (66–71). *P. falciparum* is thus able to upset the fine equilibrium between pro-inflammatory and anti-inflammatory responses, deregulating the immune system, with detrimental consequences for the human host.

Syncytiotrophoblast Activation

The syncytiotrophoblasts covering the placental villi are terminally differentiated cells, which result from the syncytialization of underlying villous cytotrophoblasts. They exhibit high metabolic activity and are involved in many physiological processes such as the active transport of molecules, the diffusion of gases, and the synthesis and secretion of large amounts of hormones, including steroids [Reviewed in (72)]. Experiments performed using primary placental cells, as well as the widely used choriocarcinoma cell line BeWo, revealed that VAR2CSA-dependent binding of IEs to syncytiotrophoblasts induces a broad range of cellular responses, notably activating MAPK pathways (73, 74). Activation of syncytiotrophoblasts leads to the secretion of pro-inflammatory cytokines/chemokines such as macrophage inflammatory protein (MIP), the neutrophil chemotactic factor interleukin (IL) 8 and IL-6 (74, 75), but also to the production of soluble ICAM-1 (75), which may act as a protection mechanism to regulate the inflammatory response (76). The interaction of syncytiotrophoblasts with VAR2CSA-expressing IEs might therefore participate in the immunological shaping of the local environment, establishing a complex network of factors which could promote the migration of immune cells to the intervillous space (74), as well as the *in situ* modulation of their activity.

Macrophage and Monocyte Immunomodulation

Sections taken from healthy placenta at different time-points throughout normal pregnancy showed that nearly half of the decidual cells are of bone marrow origin, comprising 18–20% macrophages (77, 78). Polarization of decidual macrophages varies with gestational age, shifting from an M1 polarization during fetal implantation, towards a mixed M1/M2 profile which remains until mid-pregnancy (79). After the placental development is completed, decidual macrophages are predominantly of the M2 phenotype, contributing to a tolerant immune environment and to fetal immunoprotection (80, 81).

PM is characterized by a significant increase in the number of monocytes and macrophages in the intervillous space (8–10, 82, 83), which is notably associated with elevated expression of the β chemokines IL-8 and MIP-1 (84). *In vitro* co-incubation experiments, performed in absence of human plasma/serum, i.e. in absence of opsonic antibodies, showed that VAR2CSA-expressing IEs are able to modulate specific transcription factor activation in RAW-macrophages, as compared to erythrocytes infected with genetically modified parasites presenting a deficiency in the export of PfEMP1 at the cell surface (PfEMP1-null) (85). The decreased activation of NF-κB-, CREB-, and GAS/ISRE-binding factors is accompanied by reduced production of TNF and IL-10. Similar experiments using human primary monocytes also revealed that VAR2CSA-expressing IEs are able to alter the production profiles of other cytokines/chemokines, limiting the release of IL-1β, IL-6, IL-10, MCP-1, MIP-1α, and MIP-1β, as compared to cells infected withfimmu.2020.624126 PfEMP1-null parasites (85). Although the precise nature of the monocyte receptor(s) involved still remains to be elucidated, these observations highlight how *P. falciparum* could exploit the host cellular pathways to modulate the immune response.

Interestingly, a study performed in an area of low prevalence of malaria, revealed gravidity-dependent differences in the capacity of peripheral blood mononuclear cells (PBMCs) to produce cytokines and chemokines in response to pregnancy-specific IEs (86). Despite no differences in opsonic antibody levels, cellular immune responses differed between women in their second to fourth pregnancy (G2-4) and grand multigravida (G5-G7). Indeed, more IL-10, IL-1β, IL-6, tumor necrosis factor (TNF) but less CXCL-8, CCL-8, IFNγ, and CXCL-10 were detected in G2-4 compared to G5-7, highlighting the modulation of immune cell function occurring during PM (86).

VAR2CSA BINDING TO NON-SPECIFIC IGM AND DIVERSION OF THE IMMUNE RESPONSE

PM induces VAR2CSA-specific immunoglobulin Gs (IgGs) belonging to the IgG1 subclass, and to a lower extent the IgG3 subclass (87, 88), both highly potent at interacting with Fcγ receptors present at the surface of phagocytic cells. Concordantly, women living in areas where malaria is endemic naturally acquire specific antibodies that promote the phagocytosis of VAR2CSA-expressing IEs (89–91), thus participating in parasite clearance. Binding of non-specific IgM on the surface of IEs was first demonstrated on rosetting parasites (92–94) and subsequently on VAR2CSA-expressing red blood cells (95). Following these observations, the function of IgM binding to VAR2CSA has been uncertain for several years. In 2011, a study performed by Barfod et al. showed that non-specific IgM binding participates in the masking of protective epitopes on VAR2CSA, leading to IE evasion of macrophage-mediated opsonic phagocytosis (96). The same study revealed that non-specific IgM binding to VAR2CSA-expressing IEs did not interfere with their capacity to adhere to CSA and did not increase their susceptibility to undergo complement-mediated lysis (96). The extensive analysis of non-specific IgM binding to large panels of PfEMP1 members demonstrated that IgM binding is a common functional phenotype found in multiple PfEMP1 variants across various parasite strains, thus providing a better understanding of the underlying molecular mechanisms (97–99). Although the CSA-binding site of VAR2CSA resides within the N-terminal region of the protein (100, 101), the IgM interacting residues appear to be mainly located within the C-terminal section, at the level of the DBL5ε or DBL6ε domains in VAR2CSA variants carried by the 3D7 and FCR3/IT parasite strains, respectively (102, 103) as well as in DBLε and DBLζ domains near the C-terminus of other PfEMP1 variants (98, 99, 104, 105).

The PfEMP1 binding sites on IgM have been located within the μ region of the fragment crystallizable (Fcμ) of polymeric immunoglobulins (97), and more precisely in the Cμ4 domain for the DBL4β domain of PfEMP1-VAR1 of the TM284 strain (106). These observations, together with the additional definition of the architecture of the IgM/PfEMP1 complex (107), provide critical molecular elements which could explain how PfEMP1s interfere with the binding of the complement component C1q to the adjacent Cμ3 domain, thus inhibiting complement-mediated lysis. Furthermore, these findings demonstrate how IgMs participate in PfEMP1 clustering on the cell surface, strengthening the interactions with host receptors (107–109). PfEMP1 binding to IgM has also been proposed as a non-exclusive molecular mechanism involved in the triggering of polyclonal B cell activation, a hall mark of malaria (110, 111). This activation would lead to hyper-gamma-immunoglobulinemia and the subsequent diversion of the specific humoral immune response towards antigens relevant for protection.

VAR2CSA POLYMORPHISM

All the *P. falciparum* genomes sequenced to date reveal the presence of one or more *var2csa* gene copies (112–114). VAR2CSA is a highly polymorphic multidomain protein, usually consisting of six DBL domains; the first three DBL domains belong to the DBLx subtype and the three others to the DBLϵ subtype. The protein also contains a $CIDR_{PAM}$ domain (also referred to as ID2) between the DBL2x and DBL3x domains. A recent study has identified atypical extended or truncated VAR2CSA structures (115). Extended structures include one or two additional DBLε domains downstream of the conventional DBL1x-6ε domain structure (115). Within the conventional six DBL domain structure, DBL4ε is the most conserved DBL domain while DBL6ε is the most polymorphic DBL domain (112). *Var2csa* is present in all genomes of known *Laverania* sub-genus members (116). One of the closest *P. falciparum* relatives, the chimpanzee parasite *Plasmodium reichenowi*, possesses a *var2csa*-like gene which is annotated as a pseudogene and encodes a functional truncated protein (NTS-DBL1x-ID1-DBL2x-truncated ID2) (117).

Global sequence diversity and analysis of *var2csa* have been reported in different studies (118–121) and more recently for 1,249 sequences spanning 7 Kb of *var2csa* (NTS-DBL5ε) from various strains and field isolates (122). Although it was previously shown that the DBL6ε domain is the most polymorphic domain (112), this latest study, which does not include DBL6ε, demonstrates that the nucleotide diversity is higher towards the N-terminus of the protein and that the

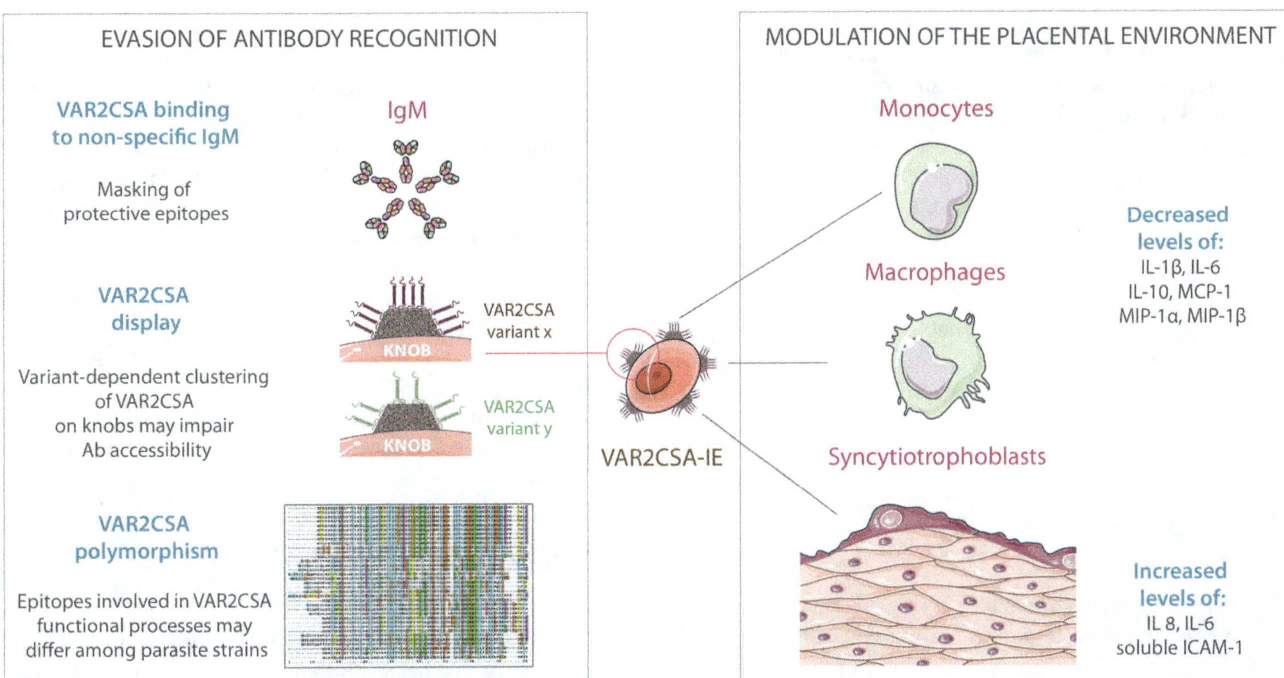

FIGURE 2 | Evasion of antibody recognition and modulation of the placental environment by VAR2CSA-expressing infected erythrocytes. IgM binding to VAR2CSA could mask protein epitopes recognized by anti-VAR2CSA IgGs and consequently alter opsonic phagocytosis of IEs. PfEMP1 clustering on knob structures may act as an immune evasion mechanism, impairing antibody accessibility to key residues involved in CSA-binding. Due to extensive polymorphism, epitopes involved in each VAR2CSA functional process may differ among parasite strains. Furthermore, multiplicity of *var2csa* genes within the parasite genome may also confer a greater capacity for antigenic variation and evasion of variant-specific immune responses. The presence of VAR2CSA on the IEs surface could lead to decreased production of IL-1β, IL-6, IL-10, MCP-1, MIP-1α, and MIP-1β by monocytes and macrophages. VAR2CSA-dependent binding of IEs to syncytiotrophoblasts is able to activate MAPK pathways and lead to increased secretion of IL-8, IL-6, and soluble ICAM-1. The art pieces used in this figure were modified from Servier Medical Art by Servier, licensed under a Creative Commons Attribution 3.0 Unported License (https://smart.servier.com/). The illustration of the protein sequence alignment is licensed under a Creative Commons Attribution, CC BY-SA 3.0 (https://creativecommons.org/licenses/by-sa/3.0/).

diversity is generally higher in African parasite populations than in South East Asian populations. While the DBL2x domain has the lowest nucleotide diversity (122), it possesses the highest density of insertions and deletions, with sequence length across samples ranging from 430 to 550 amino acids (122). In a population structure analysis performed on *var2csa* sequences from Benin and Malawi, five different clades of ID1-DBL2x (encoding for the CSA-binding region) were identified and the authors found an association between the 3D7-like clade and low birth-weight (120). Only four clades were identified, including a 3D7-like clade (clade 1) and an FCR3-like clade (clade 2) (120). Indeed, two of the previously identified clades could not be separated using this much larger dataset. Clades 1, 2, and 4 were present across all the *P. falciparum* malaria endemic areas and clade 1, which is associated with low birth-weight, is highly represented in the West African populations (41.7%), followed by East Africa (27.5%), South East Asia (23.5%), and South America (21.1%). However, clade 3 is exclusively found in African parasite populations but appears to represent less than 1% of the *var2csa* sequences.

A recent study, which used plasma obtained from Tanzanian and Malian women at the time of delivery, simultaneously examined the capability of antibodies to recognize native VAR2CSA expressed by either NF54 or FCR3, to inhibit the binding of IEs to CSA and to promote phagocytosis by THP1 cells. Plasma from Malian women reacted more strongly with VAR2CSA-expressing erythrocytes infected by the FCR3 parasite strain whereas Tanzanian plasma preferentially reacted with erythrocytes infected by NF54 (35). Analysis of antibody functionality showed that the balance between binding inhibition capability and opsonizing activity could be biased depending on the expressed VAR2CSA variant and on the geographical location (35), suggesting that epitopes involved in each functional process may differ among parasite strains and that parasite transmission in a given place could therefore shape antibody profiles. In addition, the multiplicity of *var2csa* genes within the parasite genome may also confer a greater capacity for antigenic variation and evasion of variant-specific immune responses (114).

CONCLUDING REMARKS

P. falciparum infection contracted during pregnancy elicits a broad range of immune responses, combining components of both the innate and the adaptive immunity, orchestrated by a complex network of pro- and anti-inflammatory cytokines (**Figure 2**). *P. falciparum* has developed the ability to manipulate the immune system to its advantage to ensure its survival and persistence within the human host.

Although the parasite is able to escape host defense processes and manipulate the induced immune response using a variety of mechanisms described herein, women living in malaria endemic areas can gradually acquire protective clinical immunity against PM, depending on the intensity of parasite transmission (123). In moderate malaria transmission. PM adverse clinical outcomes can be seen in women of all parity status (124), whereas protection appears to develop in a more marked parity-dependent manner in high transmission settings (125). Importantly, PM protection has been linked to the presence of antibodies targeting PM-specific variant surface antigens (126) and more specifically VAR2CSA (127–129). These observations led to the belief that a VAR2CSA-based vaccine against PM could potentially be achieved. However, the high degree of sequence diversity within VAR2CSA represents a major hurdle for vaccine design.

Following extensive preclinical evaluation, two recombinant vaccine candidates PRIMVAC and PAMVAC, comprising the CSA-binding region of VAR2CSA from the 3D7 (clade 1) and FCR3 (clade 2) strains respectively, have been assessed in Phase I clinical trials in Europe and Africa (ClinicalTrials.gov identifiers NCT02658253 and NCT02647489, respectively) (130–134). The identification of immunological correlates of protection against PM being complex, there is to date no clear surrogate allowing an easy evaluation of the protective effects of vaccines in early clinical trials (135). Exploratory analyses performed for the PRIMVAC and PAMVAC trials nevertheless revealed that vaccine-induced antibodies had a limited capability to cross-react with VAR2CSA originating from heterologous parasite strains (133, 134), highlighting the difficulty to compose with the high degree of polymorphisms of the protein when designing vaccines. Alternative vaccine approaches, using VAR2CSA in combination with other *P. falciparum* antigens, such as the circumsporozoite protein (CSP) (136), or virus-like particles (VLPs) to display VAR2CSA-derived antigens are also currently under investigation (137–139).

Improving our understanding on how *P. falciparum* escapes host defenses, modulates the immune system and on how natural immunity develops during PM despite VAR2CSA polymorphisms is therefore crucial to design efficient and effective immuno-therapeutic approaches but also to appropriately evaluate them.

AUTHOR CONTRIBUTIONS

AT, J-PS, BG, and AC wrote the manuscript. All authors contributed to the article and approved the submitted version.

ACKNOWLEDGMENTS

We would like to thank Auria Godard for creating the illustration of the placental villus presented in **Figure 1A**. We also thank the peer-reviewers for critical review of the former version of the manuscript.

REFERENCES

1. World Health Organization. *World Malaria Report 2019*. Geneva: World Health Organization (2019) Licence: CC BY-NC-SA 3.0 IGO.
2. Verhoeff FH, Brabin BJ, Chimsuku L, Kazembe P, Broadhead RL. An analysis of the determinants of anaemia in pregnant women in rural Malawi–a basis for action. *Ann Trop Med Parasitol* (1999) 93:119–33. doi: 10.1080/00034989958609
3. Shulman CE, Graham WJ, Jilo H, Lowe BS, New L, Obiero J, et al. Malaria is an important cause of anaemia in primigravidae: evidence from a district hospital in coastal Kenya. *Trans R Soc Trop Med Hyg* (1996) 90:535–9. doi: 10.1016/s0035-9203(96)90312-0
4. Ndao CT, Dumont A, Fievet N, Doucoure S, Gaye A, Lehesran JY. Placental malarial infection as a risk factor for hypertensive disorders during pregnancy in Africa: a case-control study in an urban area of Senegal, West Africa. *Am J Epidemiol* (2009) 170:847–53. doi: 10.1093/aje/kwp207
5. Muehlenbachs A, Mutabingwa TK, Edmonds S, Fried M, Duffy PE. Hypertension and maternal-fetal conflict during placental malaria. *PLoS Med* (2006) 3:e446. doi: 10.1371/journal.pmed.0030446
6. Akuze J, Blencowe H, Waiswa P, Baschieri A, Gordeev VS, Kwesiga D, et al. Randomised comparison of two household survey modules for measuring stillbirths and neonatal deaths in five countries: the Every Newborn-INDEPTH study. *Lancet Glob Health* (2020) 8:e555–66. doi: 10.1016/S2214-109X(20)30044-9
7. Moore KA, Simpson JA, Scoullar MJL, McGready R, Fowkes FJI. Quantification of the association between malaria in pregnancy and stillbirth: a systematic review and meta-analysis. *Lancet Glob Health* (2017) 5:e1101–12. doi: 10.1016/S2214-109X(17)30340-6
8. Galbraith RM, Fox H, Hsi B, Galbraith GM, Bray RS, Faulk WP. The human materno-foetal relationship in malaria. II. Histological, ultrastructural and immunopathological studies of the placenta. *Trans R Soc Trop Med Hyg* (1980) 74:61–72. doi: 10.1016/0035-9203(80)90012-7
9. Walter PR, Garin Y, Blot P. Placental pathologic changes in malaria. A histologic and ultrastructural study. *Am J Pathol* (1982) 109:330–42.
10. Ismail MR, Ordi J, Menendez C, Ventura PJ, Aponte JJ, Kahigwa E, et al. Placental pathology in malaria: a histological, immunohistochemical, and quantitative study. *Hum Pathol* (2000) 31:85–93. doi: 10.1016/s0046-8177(00)80203-8
11. Tuikue Ndam N, Bischoff E, Proux C, Lavstsen T, Salanti A, Guitard J, et al. Plasmodium falciparum transcriptome analysis reveals pregnancy malaria associated gene expression. *PLoS One* (2008) 3:e1855. doi: 10.1371/journal.pone.0001855
12. Francis SE, Malkov VA, Oleinikov AV, Rossnagle E, Wendler JP, Mutabingwa TK, et al. Six genes are preferentially transcribed by the circulating and sequestered forms of Plasmodium falciparum parasites that infect pregnant women. *Infect Immun* (2007) 75:4838–50. doi: 10.1128/IAI.00635-07
13. Tuikue Ndam NG, Salanti A, Bertin G, Dahlbäck M, Fievet N, Turner L, et al. High level of var2csa transcription by Plasmodium falciparum isolated from the placenta. *J Infect Dis* (2005) 192:331–5. doi: 10.1086/430933
14. Kamaliddin C, Salnot V, Leduc M, Ezinmegnon S, Broussard C, Fievet N, et al. PFI1785w: A highly conserved protein associated with pregnancy associated malaria. *PLoS One* (2017) 12:e0187817. doi: 10.1371/journal.pone.0187817
15. Bertin GI, Sabbagh A, Guillonneau F, Jafari-Guemouri S, Ezinmegnon S, Federici C, et al. Differential protein expression profiles between Plasmodium falciparum parasites isolated from subjects presenting with pregnancy-associated malaria and uncomplicated malaria in Benin. *J Infect Dis* (2013) 208:1987–97. doi: 10.1093/infdis/jit377
16. Fried M, Hixson KK, Anderson L, Ogata Y, Mutabingwa TK, Duffy PE. The distinct proteome of placental malaria parasites. *Mol Biochem Parasitol* (2007) 155:57–65. doi: 10.1016/j.molbiopara.2007.05.010
17. Fried M, Duffy PE. Adherence of Plasmodium falciparum to Chondroitin Sulfate A in the Human Placenta. *Science* (1996) 272:1502–4. doi: 10.1126/science.272.5267.1502
18. Achur RN, Valiyaveettil M, Alkhalil A, Ockenhouse CF, Gowda DC. Characterization of proteoglycans of human placenta and identification of unique chondroitin sulfate proteoglycans of the intervillous spaces that mediate the adherence of Plasmodium falciparum-infected erythrocytes to the placenta. *J Biol Chem* (2000) 275:40344–56. doi: 10.1074/jbc.M006398200
19. Gysin J, Pouvelle B, Fievet N, Scherf A, Lépolard C. Ex vivo desequestration of Plasmodium falciparum-infected erythrocytes from human placenta by chondroitin sulfate A. *Infect Immun* (1999) 67:6596–602. doi: 10.1128/IAI.67.12.6596-6602
20. Maubert B, Guilbert LJ, Deloron P. Cytoadherence of Plasmodium falciparum to intercellular adhesion molecule 1 and chondroitin-4-sulfate expressed by the syncytiotrophoblast in the human placenta. *Infect Immun* (1997) 65:1251–7. doi: 10.1128/IAI.65.4.1251-1257.1997
21. Maubert B, Fievet N, Tami G, Boudin C, Deloron P. Cytoadherence of Plasmodium falciparum-infected erythrocytes in the human placenta. *Parasite Immunol* (2000) 22:191–9. doi: 10.1046/j.1365-3024.2000.00292.x
22. Agbor-Enoh ST, Achur RN, Valiyaveettil M, Leke R, Taylor DW, Gowda DC. Chondroitin Sulfate Proteoglycan Expression and Binding of Plasmodium falciparum-Infected Erythrocytes in the Human Placenta during Pregnancy. *IAI* (2003) 71:2455–61. doi: 10.1128/IAI.71.5.2455-2461.2003
23. Viebig NK, Gamain B, Scheidig C, Lépolard C, Przyborski J, Lanzer M, et al. A single member of the Plasmodium falciparum var multigene family determines cytoadhesion to the placental receptor chondroitin sulphate A. *EMBO Rep* (2005) 6:775–81. doi: 10.1038/sj.embor.7400466
24. Duffy MF, Byrne TJ, Elliott SR, Wilson DW, Rogerson SJ, Beeson JG, et al. Broad analysis reveals a consistent pattern of var gene transcription in Plasmodium falciparum repeatedly selected for a defined adhesion phenotype. *Mol Microbiol* (2005) 56:774–88. doi: 10.1111/j.1365-2958.2005.04577.x
25. Elliott SR, Duffy MF, Byrne TJ, Beeson JG, Mann EJ, Wilson DW, et al. Cross-reactive surface epitopes on chondroitin sulfate A-adherent Plasmodium falciparum-infected erythrocytes are associated with transcription of var2csa. *Infect Immun* (2005) 73:2848–56. doi: 10.1128/IAI.73.5.2848-2856.2005
26. Gamain B, Trimnell AR, Scheidig C, Scherf A, Miller LH, Smith JD. Identification of multiple chondroitin sulfate A (CSA)-binding domains in the var2CSA gene transcribed in CSA-binding parasites. *J Infect Dis* (2005) 191:1010–3. doi: 10.1086/428137
27. Salanti A, Dahlbäck M, Turner L, Nielsen MA, Barfod L, Magistrado P, et al. Evidence for the involvement of VAR2CSA in pregnancy-associated malaria. *J Exp Med* (2004) 200:1197–203. doi: 10.1084/jem.20041579
28. Salanti A, Staalsoe T, Lavstsen T, Jensen ATR, Sowa MPK, Arnot DE, et al. Selective upregulation of a single distinctly structured var gene in chondroitin sulphate A-adhering Plasmodium falciparum involved in pregnancy-associated malaria. *Mol Microbiol* (2003) 49:179–91. doi: 10.1046/j.1365-2958.2003.03570.x
29. Gruenberg J, Allred DR, Sherman IW. Scanning electron microscope-analysis of the protrusions (knobs) present on the surface of Plasmodium falciparum-infected erythrocytes. *J Cell Biol* (1983) 97:795–802. doi: 10.1083/jcb.97.3.795
30. Crabb BS, Cooke BM, Reeder JC, Waller RF, Caruana SR, Davern KM, et al. Targeted gene disruption shows that knobs enable malaria-infected red cells to cytoadhere under physiological shear stress. *Cell* (1997) 89:287–96. doi: 10.1016/s0092-8674(00)80207-x
31. Raventos-Suarez C, Kaul DK, Macaluso F, Nagel RL. Membrane knobs are required for the microcirculatory obstruction induced by Plasmodium falciparum-infected erythrocytes. *Proc Natl Acad Sci U S A* (1985) 82:3829–33. doi: 10.1073/pnas.82.11.3829
32. Joergensen LM, Salanti A, Dobrilovic T, Barfod L, Hassenkam T, Theander TG, et al. The kinetics of antibody binding to Plasmodium falciparum VAR2CSA PfEMP1 antigen and modelling of PfEMP1 antigen packing on the membrane knobs. *Malar J* (2010) 9:100. doi: 10.1186/1475-2875-9-100
33. Sanchez CP, Karathanasis C, Sanchez R, Cyrklaff M, Jäger J, Buchholz B, et al. Single-molecule imaging and quantification of the immune-variant adhesin VAR2CSA on knobs of Plasmodium falciparum-infected erythrocytes. *Commun Biol* (2019) 2:172. doi: 10.1038/s42003-019-0429-z
34. Subramani R, Quadt K, Jeppesen AE, Hempel C, Petersen JEV, Hassenkam T, et al. Plasmodium falciparum-infected erythrocyte knob density is linked to the PfEMP1 variant expressed. *mBio* (2015) 6:e01456–01415. doi: 10.1128/mBio.01456-15
35. Doritchamou J, Teo A, Morrison R, Arora G, Kwan J, Manzella-Lapeira J, et al. Functional Antibodies against Placental Malaria Parasites Are Variant

Dependent and Differ by Geographic Region. *Infect Immun* (2019) 87(7): e00865-18. doi: 10.1128/IAI.00865-18
36. Singh K, Gitti RK, Diouf A, Zhou H, Gowda DC, Miura K, et al. Subdomain 3 of Plasmodium falciparum VAR2CSA DBL3x is identified as a minimal chondroitin sulfate A-binding region. *J Biol Chem* (2010) 285:24855–62. doi: 10.1074/jbc.M110.118612
37. Vuchelen A, Pardon E, Steyaert J, Gamain B, Loris R, van Nuland NAJ, et al. Production, crystallization and X-ray diffraction analysis of two nanobodies against the Duffy binding-like (DBL) domain DBL6ϵ-FCR3 of the Plasmodium falciparum VAR2CSA protein. *Acta Crystallogr Sect F Struct Biol Cryst Commun* (2013) 69:270–4. doi: 10.1107/S1744309113001917
38. Gangnard S, Badaut C, Ramboarina S, Baron B, Ramdani T, Gamain B, et al. Structural and immunological correlations between the variable blocks of the VAR2CSA domain DBL6ϵ from two Plasmodium falciparum parasite lines. *J Mol Biol* (2013) 425:1697–711. doi: 10.1016/j.jmb.2013.02.014
39. Singh K, Gittis AG, Nguyen P, Gowda DC, Miller LH, Garboczi DN. Structure of the DBL3x domain of pregnancy-associated malaria protein VAR2CSA complexed with chondroitin sulfate A. *Nat Struct Mol Biol* (2008) 15:932–8. doi: 10.1038/nsmb.1479
40. Khunrae P, Philip JMD, Bull DR, Higgins MK. Structural comparison of two CSPG-binding DBL domains from the VAR2CSA protein important in malaria during pregnancy. *J Mol Biol* (2009) 393:202–13. doi: 10.1016/j.jmb.2009.08.027
41. Gangnard S, Lewit-Bentley A, Dechavanne S, Srivastava A, Amirat F, Bentley GA, et al. Structure of the DBL3X-DBL4ϵ region of the VAR2CSA placental malaria vaccine candidate: insight into DBL domain interactions. *Sci Rep* (2015) 5:14868. doi: 10.1038/srep14868
42. Srivastava A, Gangnard S, Round A, Dechavanne S, Juillerat A, Raynal B, et al. Full-length extracellular region of the var2CSA variant of PfEMP1 is required for specific, high-affinity binding to CSA. *Proc Natl Acad Sci U S A* (2010) 107:4884–9. doi: 10.1073/pnas.1000951107
43. Clausen TM, Christoffersen S, Dahlbäck M, Langkilde AE, Jensen KE, Resende M, et al. Structural and functional insight into how the Plasmodium falciparum VAR2CSA protein mediates binding to chondroitin sulfate A in placental malaria. *J Biol Chem* (2012) 287:23332–45. doi: 10.1074/jbc.M112.348839
44. Bewley MC, Gautam L, Jagadeeshaprasad MG, Gowda DC, Flanagan JM. Molecular architecture and domain arrangement of the placental malaria protein VAR2CSA suggests a model for carbohydrate binding. *J Biol Chem* (2020) 295(52):18589–603. doi: 10.1074/jbc.RA120.014676
45. Srivastava A, Gangnard S, Dechavanne S, Amirat F, Lewit Bentley A, Bentley GA, et al. Var2CSA minimal CSA binding region is located within the N-terminal region. *PLoS One* (2011) 6:e20270. doi: 10.1371/journal.pone.0020270
46. Dahlbäck M, Jørgensen LM, Nielsen MA, Clausen TM, Ditlev SB, Resende M, et al. The chondroitin sulfate A-binding site of the VAR2CSA protein involves multiple N-terminal domains. *J Biol Chem* (2011) 286:15908–17. doi: 10.1074/jbc.M110.191510
47. Dorin-Semblat D, Tétard M, Claës A, Semblat J-P, Dechavanne S, Fourati Z, et al. Phosphorylation of the VAR2CSA extracellular region is associated with enhanced adhesive properties to the placental receptor CSA. *PLoS Biol* (2019) 17:e3000308. doi: 10.1371/journal.pbio.3000308
48. Lavazec C. Molecular mechanisms of deformability of Plasmodium-infected erythrocytes. *Curr Opin Microbiol* (2017) 40:138–44. doi: 10.1016/j.mib.2017.11.011
49. Nash GB, O'Brien E, Gordon-Smith EC, Dormandy JA. Abnormalities in the mechanical properties of red blood cells caused by Plasmodium falciparum. *Blood* (1989) 74:855–61. doi: 10.1182/blood.V74.2.855.855
50. Herricks T, Antia M, Rathod PK. Deformability limits of Plasmodium falciparum-infected red blood cells. *Cell Microbiol* (2009) 11:1340–53. doi: 10.1111/j.1462-5822.2009.01334.x
51. Herricks T, Seydel KB, Molyneux M, Taylor T, Rathod PK. Estimating physical splenic filtration of Plasmodium falciparum-infected red blood cells in malaria patients. *Cell Microbiol* (2012) 14:1880–91. doi: 10.1111/cmi.12007
52. Lavazec C, Deplaine G, Safeukui I, Perrot S, Milon G, Mercereau-Puijalon O, et al. Microsphiltration: a microsphere matrix to explore erythrocyte deformability. *Methods Mol Biol* (2013) 923:291–7. doi: 10.1007/978-1-62703-026-7_20
53. Robert C, Pouvelle B, Meyer P, Muanza K, Fujioka H, Aikawa M, et al. Chondroitin-4-sulphate (proteoglycan), a receptor for Plasmodium falciparum-infected erythrocyte adherence on brain microvascular endothelial cells. *Res Immunol* (1995) 146:383–93. doi: 10.1016/0923-2494(96)81042-x
54. Alkhalil A, Achur RN, Valiyaveettil M, Ockenhouse CF, Gowda DC. Structural requirements for the adherence of Plasmodium falciparum-infected erythrocytes to chondroitin sulfate proteoglycans of human placenta. *J Biol Chem* (2000) 275:40357–64. doi: 10.1074/jbc.M006399200
55. Chai W, Beeson JG, Lawson AM. The structural motif in chondroitin sulfate for adhesion of Plasmodium falciparum-infected erythrocytes comprises disaccharide units of 4-O-sulfated and non-sulfated N-acetylgalactosamine linked to glucuronic acid. *J Biol Chem* (2002) 277:22438–46. doi: 10.1074/jbc.M111401200
56. Sugiura N, Clausen TM, Shioiri T, Gustavsson T, Watanabe H, Salanti A. Molecular dissection of placental malaria protein VAR2CSA interaction with a chemo-enzymatically synthesized chondroitin sulfate library. *Glycoconj J* (2016) 33:985–94. doi: 10.1007/s10719-016-9685-z
57. Rieger H, Yoshikawa HY, Quadt K, Nielsen MA, Sanchez CP, Salanti A, et al. Cytoadhesion of Plasmodium falciparum-infected erythrocytes to chondroitin-4-sulfate is cooperative and shear enhanced. *Blood* (2015) 125:383–91. doi: 10.1182/blood-2014-03-561019
58. Ngai M, Weckman AM, Erice C, McDonald CR, Cahill LS, Sled JG, et al. Malaria in Pregnancy and Adverse Birth Outcomes: New Mechanisms and Therapeutic Opportunities. *Trends Parasitol* (2020) 36:127–37. doi: 10.1016/j.pt.2019.12.005
59. Umbers AJ, Aitken EH, Rogerson SJ. Malaria in pregnancy: small babies, big problem. *Trends Parasitol* (2011) 27:168–75. doi: 10.1016/j.pt.2011.01.007
60. Yockey LJ, Iwasaki A. Interferons and Proinflammatory Cytokines in Pregnancy and Fetal Development. *Immunity* (2018) 49:397–412. doi: 10.1016/j.immuni.2018.07.017
61. Fievet N, Moussa M, Tami G, Maubert B, Cot M, Deloron P, et al. Plasmodium falciparum induces a Thl/Th2 disequilibrium, favoring the Thl-type pathway, in the human placenta. *J Infect Dis* (2001) 183:1530–4. doi: 10.1086/320201
62. Suguitan AL, Leke RGF, Fouda G, Zhou A, Thuita L, Metenou S, et al. Changes in the levels of chemokines and cytokines in the placentas of women with Plasmodium falciparum malaria. *J Infect Dis* (2003) 188:1074–82. doi: 10.1086/378500
63. Diouf I, Fievet N, Doucouré S, Ngom M, Andrieu M, Mathieu J-F, et al. IL-12 producing monocytes and IFN-gamma and TNF-alpha producing T-lymphocytes are increased in placentas infected by Plasmodium falciparum. *J Reprod Immunol* (2007) 74:152–62. doi: 10.1016/j.jri.2006.10.001
64. Kabyemela ER, Muehlenbachs A, Fried M, Kurtis JD, Mutabingwa TK, Duffy PE. Maternal peripheral blood level of IL-10 as a marker for inflammatory placental malaria. *Malar J* (2008) 7:26. doi: 10.1186/1475-2875-7-26
65. Boström S, Ibitokou S, Oesterholt M, Schmiegelow C, Persson J-O, Minja D, et al. Biomarkers of Plasmodium falciparum infection during pregnancy in women living in northeastern Tanzania. *PLoS One* (2012) 7:e48763. doi: 10.1371/journal.pone.0048763
66. Chêne A, Briand V, Ibitokou S, Dechavanne S, Massougbodji A, Deloron P, et al. Placental cytokine and chemokine profiles reflect pregnancy outcomes in women exposed to Plasmodium falciparum infection. *Infect Immun* (2014) 82:3783–9. doi: 10.1128/IAI.01922-14
67. Umbers AJ, Boeuf P, Clapham C, Stanisic DI, Baiwog F, Mueller I, et al. Placental malaria-associated inflammation disturbs the insulin-like growth factor axis of fetal growth regulation. *J Infect Dis* (2011) 203:561–9. doi: 10.1093/infdis/jiq080
68. Silver KL, Conroy AL, Leke RGF, Leke RJI, Gwanmesia P, Molyneux ME, et al. Circulating soluble endoglin levels in pregnant women in Cameroon and Malawi–associations with placental malaria and fetal growth restriction. *PLoS One* (2011) 6:e24985. doi: 10.1371/journal.pone.0024985
69. Dong S, Kurtis JD, Pond-Tor S, Kabyemela E, Duffy PE, Fried M. CXC ligand 9 response to malaria during pregnancy is associated with low-birth-weight deliveries. *Infect Immun* (2012) 80:3034–8. doi: 10.1128/IAI.00220-12
70. Fried M, Muga RO, Misore AO, Duffy PE. Malaria elicits type 1 cytokines in the human placenta: IFN-gamma and TNF-alpha associated with pregnancy outcomes. *J Immunol* (1998) 160:2523–30.
71. Moormann AM, Sullivan AD, Rochford RA, Chensue SW, Bock PJ, Nyirenda T, et al. Malaria and pregnancy: placental cytokine expression

and its relationship to intrauterine growth retardation. *J Infect Dis* (1999) 180:1987–93. doi: 10.1086/315135

72. Burton GJ, Fowden AL. The placenta: a multifaceted, transient organ. *Philos Trans R Soc Lond B Biol Sci* (2015) 370:20140066. doi: 10.1098/rstb.2014.0066
73. Lucchi NW, Koopman R, Peterson DS, Moore JM. Plasmodium falciparum-infected red blood cells selected for binding to cultured syncytiotrophoblast bind to chondroitin sulfate A and induce tyrosine phosphorylation in the syncytiotrophoblast. *Placenta* (2006) 27:384–94. doi: 10.1016/j.placenta.2005.04.009
74. Lucchi NW, Peterson DS, Moore JM. Immunologic activation of human syncytiotrophoblast by Plasmodium falciparum. *Malar J* (2008) 7:42. doi: 10.1186/1475-2875-7-42
75. Vásquez AM, Segura C, Blair S. Induction of pro-inflammatory response of the placental trophoblast by Plasmodium falciparum infected erythrocytes and TNF. *Malar J* (2013) 12:421. doi: 10.1186/1475-2875-12-421
76. Witkowska AM, Borawska MH. Soluble intercellular adhesion molecule-1 (sICAM-1): an overview. *Eur Cytokine Netw* (2004) 15:91–8.
77. Mues B, Langer D, Zwadlo G, Sorg C. Phenotypic characterization of macrophages in human term placenta. *Immunology* (1989) 67:303–7.
78. Vince GS, Starkey PM, Jackson MC, Sargent IL, Redman CW. Flow cytometric characterisation of cell populations in human pregnancy decidua and isolation of decidual macrophages. *J Immunol Methods* (1990) 132:181–9. doi: 10.1016/0022-1759(90)90028-t
79. Jaiswal MK, Mallers TM, Larsen B, Kwak-Kim J, Chaouat G, Gilman-Sachs A, et al. V-ATPase upregulation during early pregnancy: a possible link to establishment of an inflammatory response during preimplantation period of pregnancy. *Reproduction* (2012) 143:713–25. doi: 10.1530/REP-12-0036
80. Svensson J, Jenmalm MC, Matussek A, Geffers R, Berg G, Ernerudh J. Macrophages at the fetal-maternal interface express markers of alternative activation and are induced by M-CSF and IL-10. *J Immunol* (2011) 187:3671–82. doi: 10.4049/jimmunol.1100130
81. Gustafsson C, Mjösberg J, Matussek A, Geffers R, Matthiesen L, Berg G, et al. Gene expression profiling of human decidual macrophages: evidence for immunosuppressive phenotype. *PLoS One* (2008) 3:e2078. doi: 10.1371/journal.pone.0002078
82. Ordi J, Ismail MR, Ventura PJ, Kahigwa E, Hirt R, Cardesa A, et al. Massive chronic intervillositis of the placenta associated with malaria infection. *Am J Surg Pathol* (1998) 22:1006–11. doi: 10.1097/00000478-199808000-00011
83. Ordi J, Menendez C, Ismail MR, Ventura PJ, Palacín A, Kahigwa E, et al. Placental malaria is associated with cell-mediated inflammatory responses with selective absence of natural killer cells. *J Infect Dis* (2001) 183:1100–7. doi: 10.1086/319295
84. Abrams ET, Brown H, Chensue SW, Turner GDH, Tadesse E, Lema VM, et al. Host response to malaria during pregnancy: placental monocyte recruitment is associated with elevated beta chemokine expression. *J Immunol* (2003) 170:2759–64. doi: 10.4049/jimmunol.170.5.2759
85. Sampaio NG, Eriksson EM, Schofield L. Plasmodium falciparum PfEMP1 Modulates Monocyte/Macrophage Transcription Factor Activation and Cytokine and Chemokine Responses. *Infect Immun* (2018) 86(1):e00447-17. doi: 10.1128/IAI.00447-17
86. Ludlow LE, Hasang W, Umbers AJ, Forbes EK, Ome M, Unger HW, et al. Peripheral blood mononuclear cells derived from grand multigravidae display a distinct cytokine profile in response to P. falciparum infected erythrocytes. *PLoS One* (2014) 9:e86160. doi: 10.1371/journal.pone.0086160
87. Elliott SR, Brennan AK, Beeson JG, Tadesse E, Molyneux ME, Brown GV, et al. Placental malaria induces variant-specific antibodies of the cytophilic subtypes immunoglobulin G1 (IgG1) and IgG3 that correlate with adhesion inhibitory activity. *Infect Immun* (2005) 73:5903–7. doi: 10.1128/IAI.73.9.5903-5907.2005
88. Megnekou R, Staalsoe T, Taylor DW, Leke R, Hviid L. Effects of pregnancy and intensity of Plasmodium falciparum transmission on immunoglobulin G subclass responses to variant surface antigens. *Infect Immun* (2005) 73:4112–8. doi: 10.1128/IAI.73.7.4112-4118.2005
89. Keen J, Serghides L, Ayi K, Patel SN, Ayisi J, van Eijk A, et al. HIV impairs opsonic phagocytic clearance of pregnancy-associated malaria parasites. *PLoS Med* (2007) 4:e181. doi: 10.1371/journal.pmed.0040181
90. Ataíde R, Mwapasa V, Molyneux ME, Meshnick SR, Rogerson SJ. Antibodies that induce phagocytosis of malaria infected erythrocytes: effect of HIV infection and correlation with clinical outcomes. *PLoS One* (2011) 6:e22491. doi: 10.1371/journal.pone.0022491
91. Jaworowski A, Fernandes LA, Yosaatmadja F, Feng G, Mwapasa V, Molyneux ME, et al. Relationship between human immunodeficiency virus type 1 coinfection, anemia, and levels and function of antibodies to variant surface antigens in pregnancy-associated malaria. *Clin Vaccine Immunol* (2009) 16:312–9. doi: 10.1128/CVI.00356-08
92. Clough B, Atilola FA, Black J, Pasvol G. Plasmodium falciparum: the importance of IgM in the rosetting of parasite-infected erythrocytes. *Exp Parasitol* (1998) 89:129–32. doi: 10.1006/expr.1998.4275
93. Scholander C, Treutiger CJ, Hultenby K, Wahlgren M. Novel fibrillar structure confers adhesive property to malaria-infected erythrocytes. *Nat Med* (1996) 2:204–8. doi: 10.1038/nm0296-204
94. Rowe JA, Shafi J, Kai OK, Marsh K, Raza A. Nonimmune IgM, but not IgG binds to the surface of Plasmodium falciparum-infected erythrocytes and correlates with rosetting and severe malaria. *Am J Trop Med Hyg* (2002) 66:692–9. doi: 10.4269/ajtmh.2002.66.692
95. Creasey AM, Staalsoe T, Raza A, Arnot DE, Rowe JA. Nonspecific immunoglobulin M binding and chondroitin sulfate A binding are linked phenotypes of Plasmodium falciparum isolates implicated in malaria during pregnancy. *Infect Immun* (2003) 71:4767–71. doi: 10.1128/iai.71.8.4767-4771.2003
96. Barfod L, Dalgaard MB, Pleman ST, Ofori MF, Pleass RJ, Hviid L. Evasion of immunity to Plasmodium falciparum malaria by IgM masking of protective IgG epitopes in infected erythrocyte surface-exposed PfEMP1. *Proc Natl Acad Sci U S A* (2011) 108:12485–90. doi: 10.1073/pnas.1103708108
97. Jeppesen A, Ditlev SB, Soroka V, Stevenson L, Turner L, Dzikowski R, et al. Multiple Plasmodium falciparum Erythrocyte Membrane Protein 1 Variants per Genome Can Bind IgM via Its Fc Fragment Fcμ. *Infect Immun* (2015) 83:3972–81. doi: 10.1128/IAI.00337-15
98. Stevenson L, Huda P, Jeppesen A, Laursen E, Rowe JA, Craig A, et al. Investigating the function of Fc-specific binding of IgM to Plasmodium falciparum erythrocyte membrane protein 1 mediating erythrocyte rosetting. *Cell Microbiol* (2015) 17:819–31. doi: 10.1111/cmi.12403
99. Quintana MDP, Ecklu-Mensah G, Tcherniuk SO, Ditlev SB, Oleinikov AV, Hviid L, et al. Comprehensive analysis of Fc-mediated IgM binding to the Plasmodium falciparum erythrocyte membrane protein 1 family in three parasite clones. *Sci Rep* (2019) 9:6050. doi: 10.1038/s41598-019-42585-0
100. Srivastava A, Gangnard S, Dechavanne S, Amirat F, Lewit Bentley A, Bentley GA, et al. Var2CSA minimal CSA binding region is located within the N-terminal region. *PLoS One* (2011) 6:e20270. doi: 10.1371/journal.pone.0020270
101. Dahlbäck M, Jørgensen LM, Nielsen MA, Clausen TM, Ditlev SB, Resende M, et al. The chondroitin sulfate A-binding site of the VAR2CSA protein involves multiple N-terminal domains. *J Biol Chem* (2011) 286:15908–17. doi: 10.1074/jbc.M110.191510
102. Rasti N, Namusoke F, Chêne A, Chen Q, Staalsoe T, Klinkert M-Q, et al. Nonimmune immunoglobulin binding and multiple adhesion characterize Plasmodium falciparum-infected erythrocytes of placental origin. *Proc Natl Acad Sci U S A* (2006) 103:13795–800. doi: 10.1073/pnas.0601519103
103. Semblat J-P, Raza A, Kyes SA, Rowe JA. Identification of Plasmodium falciparum var1CSA and var2CSA domains that bind IgM natural antibodies. *Mol Biochem Parasitol* (2006) 146:192–7. doi: 10.1016/j.molbiopara.2005.12.007
104. Jeppesen A, Ditlev SB, Soroka V, Stevenson L, Turner L, Dzikowski R, et al. Multiple Plasmodium falciparum Erythrocyte Membrane Protein 1 Variants per Genome Can Bind IgM via Its Fc Fragment Fcμ. *Infect Immun* (2015) 83:3972–81. doi: 10.1128/IAI.00337-15
105. Akhouri RR, Goel S, Furusho H, Skoglund U, Wahlgren M. Architecture of Human IgM in Complex with P. falciparum Erythrocyte Membrane Protein 1. *Cell Rep* (2016) 14:723–36. doi: 10.1016/j.celrep.2015.12.067
106. Ghumra A, Semblat J-P, McIntosh RS, Raza A, Rasmussen IB, Braathen R, et al. Identification of residues in the Cmu4 domain of polymeric IgM essential for interaction with Plasmodium falciparum erythrocyte membrane protein 1 (PfEMP1). *J Immunol* (2008) 181:1988–2000. doi: 10.4049/jimmunol.181.3.1988
107. Akhouri RR, Goel S, Furusho H, Skoglund U, Wahlgren M. Architecture of Human IgM in Complex with P. falciparum Erythrocyte Membrane Protein 1. *Cell Rep* (2016) 14:723–36. doi: 10.1016/j.celrep.2015.12.067

108. Stevenson L, Huda P, Jeppesen A, Laursen E, Rowe JA, Craig A, et al. Investigating the function of Fc-specific binding of IgM to Plasmodium falciparum erythrocyte membrane protein 1 mediating erythrocyte rosetting. *Cell Microbiol* (2015) 17:819–31. doi: 10.1111/cmi.12403
109. Stevenson L, Laursen E, Cowan GJ, Bandoh B, Barfod L, Cavanagh DR, et al. α2-Macroglobulin Can Crosslink Multiple Plasmodium falciparum Erythrocyte Membrane Protein 1 (PfEMP1) Molecules and May Facilitate Adhesion of Parasitized Erythrocytes. *PLoS Pathog* (2015) 11:e1005022. doi: 10.1371/journal.ppat.1005022
110. Donati D, Zhang LP, Chêne A, Chen Q, Flick K, Nyström M, et al. Identification of a polyclonal B-cell activator in Plasmodium falciparum. *Infect Immun* (2004) 72:5412–8. doi: 10.1128/IAI.72.9.5412-5418.2004
111. Donati D, Mok B, Chêne A, Xu H, Thangarajh M, Glas R, et al. Increased B cell survival and preferential activation of the memory compartment by a malaria polyclonal B cell activator. *J Immunol* (2006) 177:3035–44. doi: 10.4049/jimmunol.177.5.3035
112. Bockhorst J, Lu F, Janes JH, Keebler J, Gamain B, Awadalla P, et al. Structural polymorphism and diversifying selection on the pregnancy malaria vaccine candidate VAR2CSA. *Mol Biochem Parasitol* (2007) 155:103–12. doi: 10.1016/j.molbiopara.2007.06.007
113. Sander AF, Salanti A, Lavstsen T, Nielsen MA, Magistrado P, Lusingu J, et al. Multiple var2csa-type PfEMP1 genes located at different chromosomal loci occur in many Plasmodium falciparum isolates. *PLoS One* (2009) 4:e6667. doi: 10.1371/journal.pone.0006667
114. Sander AF, Salanti A, Lavstsen T, Nielsen MA, Theander TG, Leke RGF, et al. Positive selection of Plasmodium falciparum parasites with multiple var2csa-type PfEMP1 genes during the course of infection in pregnant women. *J Infect Dis* (2011) 203:1679–85. doi: 10.1093/infdis/jir168
115. Doritchamou JYA, Morrison R, Renn JP, Ribeiro J, Duan J, Fried M, et al. Placental malaria vaccine candidate antigen VAR2CSA displays atypical domain architecture in some Plasmodium falciparum strains. *Commun Biol* (2019) 2:457. doi: 10.1038/s42003-019-0704-z
116. Otto TD, Gilabert A, Crellen T, Böhme U, Arnathau C, Sanders M, et al. Genomes of all known members of a Plasmodium subgenus reveal paths to virulent human malaria. *Nat Microbiol* (2018) 3:687–97. doi: 10.1038/s41564-018-0162-2
117. Larremore DB, Sundararaman SA, Liu W, Proto WR, Clauset A, Loy DE, et al. Ape parasite origins of human malaria virulence genes. *Nat Commun* (2015) 6:8368. doi: 10.1038/ncomms9368
118. Bordbar B, Tuikue Ndam N, Renard E, Jafari-Guemouri S, Tavul L, Jennison C, et al. Genetic diversity of VAR2CSA ID1-DBL2Xb in worldwide Plasmodium falciparum populations: impact on vaccine design for placental malaria. *Infect Genet Evol* (2014) 25:81–92. doi: 10.1016/j.meegid.2014.04.010
119. Doritchamou J, Sabbagh A, Jespersen JS, Renard E, Salanti A, Nielsen MA, et al. Identification of a Major Dimorphic Region in the Functionally Critical N-Terminal ID1 Domain of VAR2CSA. *PLoS One* (2015) 10:e0137695. doi: 10.1371/journal.pone.0137695
120. Patel JC, Hathaway NJ, Parobek CM, Thwai KL, Madanitsa M, Khairallah C, et al. Increased risk of low birth weight in women with placental malaria associated with P. falciparum VAR2CSA clade. *Sci Rep* (2017) 7:7768. doi: 10.1038/s41598-017-04737-y
121. Verity R, Hathaway NJ, Waltmann A, Doctor SM, Watson OJ, Patel JC, et al. Plasmodium falciparum genetic variation of var2csa in the Democratic Republic of the Congo. *Malar J* (2018) 17:46. doi: 10.1186/s12936-018-2193-9
122. Benavente ED, Oresegun DR, de Sessions PF, Walker EM, Roper C, Dombrowski JG, et al. Global genetic diversity of var2csa in Plasmodium falciparum with implications for malaria in pregnancy and vaccine development. *Sci Rep* (2018) 8:15429. doi: 10.1038/s41598-018-33767-3
123. Mayor A, Bardají A, Macete E, Nhampossa T, Fonseca AM, González R, et al. Changing Trends in P. falciparum Burden, Immunity, and Disease in Pregnancy. *N Engl J Med* (2015) 373:1607–17. doi: 10.1056/NEJMoa1406459
124. Shulman CE, Marshall T, Dorman EK, Bulmer JN, Cutts F, Peshu N, et al. Malaria in pregnancy: adverse effects on haemoglobin levels and birthweight in primigravidae and multigravidae. *Trop Med Int Health* (2001) 6:770–8. doi: 10.1046/j.1365-3156.2001.00786.x
125. Walker PGT, ter Kuile FO, Garske T, Menendez C, Ghani AC. Estimated risk of placental infection and low birthweight attributable to Plasmodium falciparum malaria in Africa in 2010: a modelling study. *Lancet Glob Health* (2014) 2:e460–467. doi: 10.1016/S2214-109X(14)70256-6
126. Staalsoe T, Shulman CE, Bulmer JN, Kawuondo K, Marsh K, Hviid L. Variant surface antigen-specific IgG and protection against clinical consequences of pregnancy-associated Plasmodium falciparum malaria. *Lancet* (2004) 363:283–9. doi: 10.1016/S0140-6736(03)15386-X
127. Gavina K, Gnidehou S, Arango E, Hamel-Martineau C, Mitran C, Agudelo O, et al. Clinical Outcomes of Submicroscopic Infections and Correlates of Protection of VAR2CSA Antibodies in a Longitudinal Study of Pregnant Women in Colombia. *Infect Immun* (2018) 86(4):e00797-17. doi: 10.1128/IAI.00797-17
128. Ndam NT, Denoeud-Ndam L, Doritchamou J, Viwami F, Salanti A, Nielsen MA, et al. Protective Antibodies against Placental Malaria and Poor Outcomes during Pregnancy, Benin. *Emerg Infect Dis* (2015) 21:813–23. doi: 10.3201/eid2105.141626
129. Tutterrow YL, Salanti A, Avril M, Smith JD, Pagano IS, Ako S, et al. High avidity antibodies to full-length VAR2CSA correlate with absence of placental malaria. *PLoS One* (2012) 7:e40049. doi: 10.1371/journal.pone.0040049
130. Chêne A, Gangnard S, Dechavanne C, Dechavanne S, Srivastava A, Tétard M, et al. Down-selection of the VAR2CSA DBL1-2 expressed in E. coli as a lead antigen for placental malaria vaccine development. *NPJ Vaccines* (2018) 3:28. doi: 10.1038/s41541-018-0064-6
131. Chêne A, Gangnard S, Guadall A, Ginisty H, Leroy O, Havelange N, et al. Preclinical immunogenicity and safety of the cGMP-grade placental malaria vaccine PRIMVAC. *EBioMedicine* (2019) 42:145–56. doi: 10.1016/j.ebiom.2019.03.010
132. Nielsen MA, Resende M, de Jongh WA, Ditlev SB, Mordmüller B, Houard S, et al. The Influence of Sub-Unit Composition and Expression System on the Functional Antibody Response in the Development of a VAR2CSA Based Plasmodium falciparum Placental Malaria Vaccine. *PLoS One* (2015) 10: e0135406. doi: 10.1371/journal.pone.0135406
133. Sirima SB, Richert L, Chêne A, Konate AT, Campion C, Dechavanne S, et al. PRIMVAC vaccine adjuvanted with Alhydrogel or GLA-SE to prevent placental malaria: a first-in-human, randomised, double-blind, placebo-controlled study. *Lancet Infect Dis* (2020) 20:585–97. doi: 10.1016/S1473-3099(19)30739-X
134. Mordmüller B, Sulyok M, Egger-Adam D, Resende M, de Jongh WA, Jensen MH, et al. First-in-human, Randomized, Double-blind Clinical Trial of Differentially Adjuvanted PAMVAC, A Vaccine Candidate to Prevent Pregnancy-associated Malaria. *Clin Infect Dis* (2019) 69:1509–16. doi: 10.1093/cid/ciy1140
135. McCall MBB, Kremsner PG, Mordmüller B. Correlating efficacy and immunogenicity in malaria vaccine trials. *Semin Immunol* (2018) 39:52–64. doi: 10.1016/j.smim.2018.08.002
136. Sungwa M, Susan T, Mikkel JC, Adolph KR, Boniface MS, Grundtvig TT, et al. A VAR2CSA:CSP conjugate capable of inducing dual specificity antibody responses. *Afr Health Sci* (2017) 17:373–81. doi: 10.4314/ahs.v17i2.11
137. Janitzek CM, Peabody J, Thrane S, Carlsen P HR, Theander T G, Salanti A, et al. A proof-of-concept study for the design of a VLP-based combinatorial HPV and placental malaria vaccine. *Sci Rep* (2019) 9:5260. doi: 10.1038/s41598-019-41522-5
138. Andersson A-MC, Resende M, Salanti A, Nielsen MA, Holst PJ. Novel adenovirus encoded virus-like particles displaying the placental malaria associated VAR2CSA antigen. *Vaccine* (2017) 35:1140–7. doi: 10.1016/j.vaccine.2017.01.016
139. Thrane S, Janitzek CM, Agerbæk MØ, Ditlev SB, Resende M, Nielsen MA, et al. A Novel Virus-Like Particle Based Vaccine Platform Displaying the Placental Malaria Antigen VAR2CSA. *PLoS One* (2015) 10:e0143071. doi: 10.1371/journal.pone.0143071

12

Maternal and Foetal Cellular Immune Responses in Dams Infected with High- and Low-Virulence Isolates of *Neospora caninum* at Mid-Gestation

Marta García-Sánchez[1†], Laura Jiménez-Pelayo[1†], Patricia Vázquez[1], Pilar Horcajo[1], Javier Regidor-Cerrillo[1], Alejandro Jiménez-Meléndez[1], Koldo Osoro[2], Luis Miguel Ortega-Mora[1*] and Esther Collantes-Fernández[1*]

[1] Saluvet, Animal Health Department, Complutense University of Madrid, Madrid, Spain, [2] Regional Service for Research and Agri-Food Development (SERIDA), Villaviciosa, Spain

***Correspondence:**
Luis Miguel Ortega-Mora
luis.ortega@ucm.es
Esther Collantes-Fernández
esthercf@ucm.es

[†]These authors have contributed equally to this work and share first authorship

Bovine neosporosis is currently considered one of the main causes of abortion in cattle worldwide and the outcome of the infection is, in part, determined by *Neospora caninum* isolate virulence. However, the dam and foetal immune responses associated with this factor are largely unknown. We used a model of bovine infection at day 110 of gestation to study the early infection dynamics (10- and 20-days post-infection, dpi) after experimental challenge with high- and low-virulence isolates of *N. caninum* (Nc-Spain7 and Nc-Spain1H, respectively). In the present work, dam peripheral cellular immune responses were monitored twice a week from -1 to 20 dpi. At different time points, IFN-γ and IL-4 production was investigated in stimulated dam blood and the percentage of monocytes, NK cells, B cells and T cells (CD4+, CD8+ and $\gamma\delta$) in peripheral blood mononuclear cells (PBMC) were determined by flow cytometry. In addition, maternal iliofemoral lymph nodes and foetal spleen and thymus were collected at 10 and 20 dpi for the study of the same cell subpopulations. Peripheral immune response dynamics were similar after the infection with both isolates, with a significant increase in the percentage of CD4+ T cells at 6 and 9 dpi in PBMC, coincident with the higher levels of IFN-γ and IL-4 release. However, the levels of IFN-γ were significantly higher and an increase in CD8+ T cells at 9, 13 and 20 dpi was observed in the dams infected with Nc-Spain7. Nc-Spain1H infection induced higher IL4 levels in stimulated blood and a higher CD4+/CD8+ ratio in PBMC. The analysis of the maternal iliofemoral lymph node showed a significant enhancement in the percentage of NK, CD4+ and CD8+ T cells for the animals infected with the highly virulent isolate and euthanized at 20 dpi. Regarding the foetal responses, the most remarkable result was an increase in the percentage of monocytes at 20 dpi in the spleen of foetuses from both infected groups, which suggests that foetuses were able to respond to *N. caninum* infection at mid gestation. This work provides insights into how isolate virulence affects the maternal and foetal immune responses generated against *N. caninum*, which may influence the course of infection.

Keywords: *Neospora caninum*, virulence, pregnant cattle, cellular immune responses, pathogenesis

INTRODUCTION

Neospora caninum infection is a major cause of bovine abortion worldwide. Over the last few years, bovine neosporosis has been studied intensively, but the pathogenesis is complex and poorly understood. Previous studies have demonstrated the influence of timing of the infection during pregnancy (Benavides et al., 2014; Almería et al., 2017) and the *N. caninum* isolate (Rojo-Montejo et al., 2009; Goodswen et al., 2013; Regidor-Cerrillo et al., 2014; Jiménez-Pelayo et al., 2019) on the outcome of infection in cattle. Specifically, *in vivo* studies in pregnant cattle carried out by our group have shown a high percentage of abortion upon Nc-Spain7 infection with foetal death estimated to occur between 24 and 49 dpi (Caspe et al., 2012; Regidor-Cerrillo et al., 2014; Vázquez et al., 2019). In contrast no foetal death occurs in pregnant cattle experimentally infected with the Nc-Spain1H isolate (Rojo-Montejo et al., 2009). Recently, with the aim of exploring in more depth the mechanisms involved in the pathogenesis of abortion or vertical transmission, we used a pregnant bovine model of infection at mid-gestation, in which early infection dynamics (10- and 20-days post-infection, dpi) were compared after inoculation with the high-virulence Nc-Spain7 and the low-virulence Nc-Spain1H isolates. The results showed parasite presence and severe necrosis in placental tissues, as well as foetal mortality in Nc-Spain7-infected heifers. In contrast, Nc-Spain1H infection did not result in lesion development or foetal death (Jiménez-Pelayo et al., 2019). These results were associated with a differential pattern in the local immune response at the placental level, particularly in the early stages of infection. The low-virulence isolate Nc-Spain1H elicited an early and robust immune response characterized by a mixed Th1/Th2 profile, whereas a more predominantly pro-inflammatory Th1-based response was induced in Nc-Spain7-infected placentomes (Jiménez-Pelayo et al., 2020).

Cell-mediated immune (CMI) responses involving innate immune cells such as monocytes, natural killer cells, and adaptive immune cells including T and B lymphocyte subsets, as well as the production of cytokines such as IFN-γ and IL-4 are thought to be determinant factors for bovine neosporosis pathogenesis (Innes et al., 2002; Almeria et al., 2003; Rosbottom et al., 2007; Bartley et al., 2012; Bartley et al., 2013; Almería et al., 2017). The aim of this study was to determine how *N. caninum* isolate virulence may influence peripheral maternal and foetal cellular immune responses during the initial events of infection (10 and 20 dpi) at mid-gestation. This research may help to identify key immune components that could influence the outcome of infection.

MATERIALS AND METHODS

Ethics Statement

All protocols involving animals were approved by the Animal Research Ethics (reference number PROAE 25/2016), following the proceedings described in Spanish and EU legislations (Law 32/2007, R.D. 53/2013, and Council Directive 2010/63/EU). All animals were handled in strict accordance with good clinical practices and all efforts were made to minimize suffering.

Experimental Design and Sampling

The experimental design has been described in detail in a previous publication (Jiménez-Pelayo et al., 2019). Briefly, pregnant Asturian heifers (n=24) were randomly distributed into three experimental groups. At 110 days of gestation, animals were inoculated intravenously (IV) with phosphate buffered saline (PBS; G-Control, n=6) or 10^7 tachyzoites of *N. caninum* Nc-Spain7 isolate (G-NcSpain7, n=9) or Nc-Spain1H isolate (G-NcSpain1H, n=9). Three animals from G-Control and four animals from G-NcSpain7 and G-NcSpain1H were culled at 10 days dpi. The remaining heifers from each group were culled at 20 dpi.

Blood samples were collected by coccygeal venipuncture into EDTA- and lithium heparin-coated tubes (Becton–Dickinson and Company, UK) for the flow cytometry and lymphoproliferation assays, described in sections 2.4 and 2.5 respectively. The time schedule for the samplings was as follows: -1, 2, 6 and 9 dpi for all heifers used in the experiment and culled at 10 or 20 dpi (n=24), and 13, 16 and 20 dpi only for those heifers culled at 20 dpi (n=13). Animals were euthanized by an IV overdose of embutramide and mebezodium iodide (T61; Intervet, Spain) after sedation by the intramuscular injection of xylazine (Rompun; Bayer, Germany). At necropsy, maternal iliofemoral lymph nodes, and foetal thymus and spleen were collected and maintained fresh in RPMI 1640 medium (Gibco, UK) until further assay. Two heifers (3581 and 7934) from G-NcSpain7 that were culled at 20 dpi presented foetal mortality (Jiménez-Pelayo et al., 2019).

Parasite Inocula

Neospora caninum tachyzoites of Nc-Spain7 and Nc-Spain1H isolates were routinely maintained in a MARC-145 cell line culture as previously described (Regidor-Cerrillo et al., 2008). Tachyzoites were collected by cell scraping from three-day growth cultures, and at least 80% of the parasitophorous vacuoles were undisrupted. Parasites were counted in a Neubauer chamber by Trypan blue exclusion and resuspended in PBS, preparing the inocula at the required dose of 10^7 tachyzoites in a final volume of 2 mL. Animals were infected before one hour of parasite harvest to minimize loss of viability.

Peripheral Blood Stimulation Assay and Quantification of IFN-γ and IL-4 Release

A total of 500 mL of heparinized blood samples was cultured in triplicate within two hours of collection in 24-well plates (Thermo Fisher Scientific, USA) with 500 mL RPMI supplemented with 10% foetal bovine serum (Thermo Fisher Scientific, Waltham, USA) and 1% penicillin-streptomycin-amphotericin B mixture (Lonza, Belgium) referred to as complete medium (CM), as described previously (Vázquez et al., 2019). Each blood replicate was also supplemented with *N. caninum* soluble extract antigen obtained from Nc-Spain7 tachyzoites (Alvarez-García et al., 2003) at 5 μg/mL, concanavalin (ConA) (Sigma-Aldrich, Spain) at 5 μg/mL as a positive control, and PBS as negative control. After 24 h of incubation (37°C, 5% CO_2), culture supernatants were collected by centrifugation of plates at 1000 × g for 10 min at 4°C and stored at −80 °C until laboratory analysis for the evaluation of IFN-γ and IL-4 release.

Cytokine release was measured with commercial bovine IFN-γ and bovine IL-4 ELISA kits (Mabtech AB, Nacka Strand, Sweden) following the manufacturer's guidelines. The cytokine concentrations were calculated by interpolation from a standard curve produced with recombinant cytokines provided with the kits. The colour reaction was developed by the addition of 3,3',5,5'-tetramethylbenzidine substrate (TMB, Sigma-Aldrich, Spain). Plates were read at 450 nm.

Phenotypic Analysis of Immune Cells by Flow Cytometry

For the analysis of immune cell subpopulations from peripheral blood mononuclear cells (PBMC), a total of 20 mL of bovine peripheral blood collected in EDTA-coated tubes was mixed with 20 mL of PBS and centrifuged at 650 g for 30 min at room temperature (RT). PBMC were separated by gradient density centrifugation (800 g for 30 min at RT) on Histopaque 1077 (Sigma-Aldrich, USA).

For the analysis of immune cell subpopulations from the maternal iliofemoral lymph node and foetal thymus and spleen, the organs were mechanically disaggregated with Polytron® PT 1600E (Kinematica AG, Lucerne, USA) in 20 mL of CM. The mixture was filtered through 100 μm nylon cell strainers followed by 40 μm nylon cell strainers (VWR, Radnor, PA, USA) and centrifuged at 350 g for 10 min at 4°C. The obtained pellet was resuspended in 5 mL PBS and mononuclear cells were separated by gradient density centrifugation on Histopaque 1077 as described above.

Mononuclear cells obtained from peripheral blood or organs were incubated with a sodium bicarbonate solution (0.01 M) for 5 min to lyse the erythrocytes followed by washing with cold PBS. Then, the cells were pelleted in a V-bottom 96-well plate at a density of 2×10^5 cells/well and incubated with 50 μL of diluted antibody (1:100) or PBS for 30 min on ice and protected from light. After incubation, the samples were washed with PBS and fixed with BD Cellfix (BD Bioscience, USA).

The percentages of helper (CD4+), cytotoxic (CD8+) and γδ (WC1+) T cells, B lymphocytes (CD21+), NK cells (CD335+) and monocytes (CD14+) were analysed using flow cytometry after staining with antibodies specific for bovine leucocyte subpopulations (**Table 1**). The percentage of positive cells for each marker was determined using a Becton Dickinson FACSCalibur cytometer (BD Bioscience, USA), by calculating the proportion of the subpopulation reactive with each specific antibody in relation to the total mononuclear cell number.

Statistical Analysis

A repeated measures ANOVA test, followed by Tukey´s multiple comparisons test, was performed to compare cytokine levels in culture supernatants and the percentage of immune cell subsets in PBMC. Due to the differences in the number of animals before and after sacrifice at 10 dpi, days -1 to 9 dpi and 13 to 20 dpi were analysed separately. Dunnett´s multiple comparisons post-test was used to compare cell subsets in PBMC at each time point *versus* -1 dpi (preinfection day) for each group. A difference in the percentage of cell subsets in PBMC between infected and pre-infection values was considered valid only if no similar changes were seen in control animals. Differences in immune cell subsets in the thymus, spleen and maternal iliofemoral lymph nodes at 10 and 20 dpi were evaluated using the non-parametric Kruskal-Wallis followed by Dunn's multiple range test to compare groups. Statistical significance for all analyses was established with $P < 0.05$. All statistical analyses were carried out using GraphPad Prism 7 v.7.03 (San Diego, CA, USA) software.

RESULTS

Nc-Spain7 Induced Higher and Earlier IFN-γ Production, but Nc-Spain1H Infection Led to Higher IL-4 Levels in Stimulated Blood

The levels of IFN-γ and IL-4 were measured in stimulated blood by ELISA, and there was no antigen-specific IFN-γ or IL-4 secretion in the PBMC of the control animals (**Figure 1**). IFN-γ production increased faster and more markedly in G-NcSpain7, reaching the peak of production at 6 dpi (P<0.0001 *versus* G-Control), with differences observed at this time-point in relation to G-NcSpain1H (P < 0.05). For G-Nc-Spain1H the highest levels were observed at 9 dpi (P<0.01 *versus* G-Control), and the production was maintained over time (6-13 dpi) (**Figure 1A**). Then, IFN-γ decreased in both

TABLE 1 | List of antibodies used for analysis of cell subsets in PBMC, ileofemoral lymph node, fetal thymus and spleen.

Antibody	Conjugate	Supplier	Species	Type	Clone	Reference
CD14	FITC	Bio-Rad Laboratories (Pleasanton, CA, USA)	Mouse anti-bovine	Monoclonal	CC-G33	MCA2678F
CD4	Alexa Fluor 647				CC8	MCA1653A647
CD8	RPE				CC63	MCA837PE
CD335	Alexa Fluor 488				AKS1	MCA2365A488
WC1	FITC				CC15	MCA838F
CD21	FITC		Mouse anti-human		LB21	MCA1195F

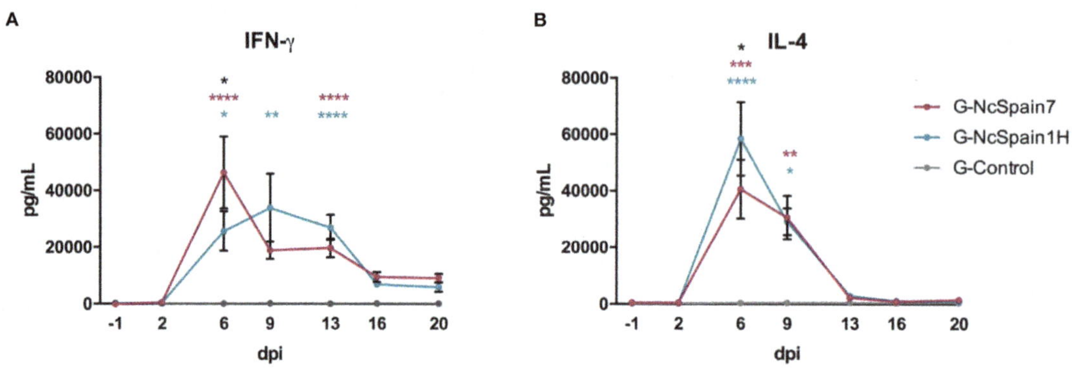

FIGURE 1 | IFN-γ and IL-4 production after Nc-Spain7 and Nc-Spain1H infection. Concentrations of **(A)** IFN-γ and **(B)** IL-4 in response to *N. caninum* soluble extract antigen, in peripheral blood culture supernatants of heifers challenged with Nc-Spain7 (G-NcSpain7) and Nc-Spain1H (G-NcSpain1H) tachyzoites and the uninfected control group (G-Control). Each point represents the mean + SD at different sampling times. Asterisks indicate significant differences in G-NcSpain1H *versus* G-Control comparison (blue), G-NcSpain7 versus G-Control (red) and G-NcSpain1H *versus* G-NcSpain7 (black). ****$P < 0.0001$, ***$P < 0.001$, **$P < 0.01$, *$P < 0.05$.

infected groups and significant differences were not found. Regarding IL-4, significantly higher levels were observed in the infected groups than in G-control at 6 and 9 dpi (P < 0.05-0.0001), but afterwards, the IL-4 levels returned to basal levels. The peak of production was observed at 6 dpi for both infected groups, being higher in the G-NcSpain1H (P < 0.05) (**Figure 1B**).

Nc-Spain7 Triggered a Higher CD8+ Cells Percentage Whereas a Higher CD4+/CD8+ Ratio Was Induced by Nc-Spain1H Infection in PBMC

The percentages of CD21+ (B cells), WC1+ (γδ-T cells), CD4+ (helper T cells), CD8+ (cytotoxic T cells), CD14+ (monocytes/macrophages) and CD335+ (NK) cells were studied in the population of PBMC from G-NcSpain7, G-NcSpain1H and G-Control by flow cytometry at different times post-infection (**Figure 2** and **Supplementary S1**). All values were within reference ranges, and there were no consistent changes over time in control animals (**Supplementary S1**). Significant differences with respect to the control group were observed in infected animals, mainly at 6 and 9 dpi. One of the most notable changes in PBMC subpopulations following *N. caninum* infection was an abrupt decrease in the relative percentage of the B lymphocyte subset (CD21+ cells) from 6 to 9 dpi *versus* uninfected animals (P < 0.05) and preinfection values (P < 0.001-0.0001). Then, relative percentages remained close to uninfected levels towards the end of the study. Similarly, in the infected groups, the relative percentages of γδ-T cells (WC1+) decreased gradually from 2 dpi, being significantly lower than those of non-infected animals at 6 dpi for G-NcSpain1H and 9 dpi for G-NcSpain7 (P < 0.05). In contrast, *N. caninum* infection induced a significant increase in the proportion of circulating CD4+, and CD8+ cells. In addition, the percentage of CD14+ cells was higher at 2 dpi in G-NcSpain1H (P < 0.05) and in both infected groups at 6 dpi (P < 0.01-0.001) *versus* G-control. However, CD14+ cell percentages were variable during the study period in both the control and infected animals, and we did not observe significant differences on day -1 *versus* 2 and 6 dpi in infected groups (**Supplementary S1**). The percentage of CD4+ cells also suffered an increase at 6 and 9 dpi for G-NcSpain1H (P < 0.01) and only at 9 dpi for G-NcSpain7 (P < 0.01) *versus* uninfected animals. When comparing with pre-infection values, the increase was statistically significant at 6 and 9 dpi for G-NcSpain7 (P < 0.001-0.0001) and at 6, 9 and 13 dpi for G-NcSpain1H (P < 0.05-0.0001). In general, the kinetics of immune cell subsets were essentially the same between G-NcSpain7 and G-NcSpain1H after inoculation. However, in G-NcSpain7, the CD8+ values increased at 9 dpi with respect to G-control (P < 0.05-0.01) and its own values before infection (P < 0.05-0.0001) remaining high until the end of the experiment, and the percentages were also higher *versus* G-NcSpain1H at 9 (P < 0.0001) and 13 dpi (P < 0.01). Nc-Spain1H induced only a modest CD8+ increase at 16 dpi (P < 0.05), which was only significant compared to the control group. Unlike the other cell subpopulations studied, there were no obvious changes in the relative percentage of the CD335+ (NK) subpopulation.

The ratio between helper (CD4+) and cytotoxic (CD8+) T cells was calculated to assess the immunoregulatory balance of T cells. In G-Control, the CD4+/CD8+ ratio was ~2.5 during the experimental period. For G-NcSpain1H, the ratio significantly increased from 6 dpi (~4.7) to 9 dpi (~4.9) due to the increase in CD4+ T cells in circulating blood (G-NcSpain1H versus G-Control: P < 0.001-0.0001; G-NcSpain1H *versus* G-NcSpain7: P < 0.05-0.0001). From 13 dpi onwards, the CD4+/CD8+ ratio decreased following a similar profile to that observed for G-NcSpain7, which was lower than the value observed in the uninfected animals. The ratio was significantly lower for G-NcSpain7 from 13 to 20 dpi (P < 0.05-0.001) and for G-NcSpain1H only at 16 dpi (P < 0.001) due to the increase in CD8+ percentages in relation to G-Control.

Nc-Spain7 Infection Induced Changes in Immune Cell Percentages From Maternal Iliofemoral Lymph Nodes at 20 dpi

The same immune cell populations studied in PBMC were analysed in the iliofemoral lymph nodes of heifers infected

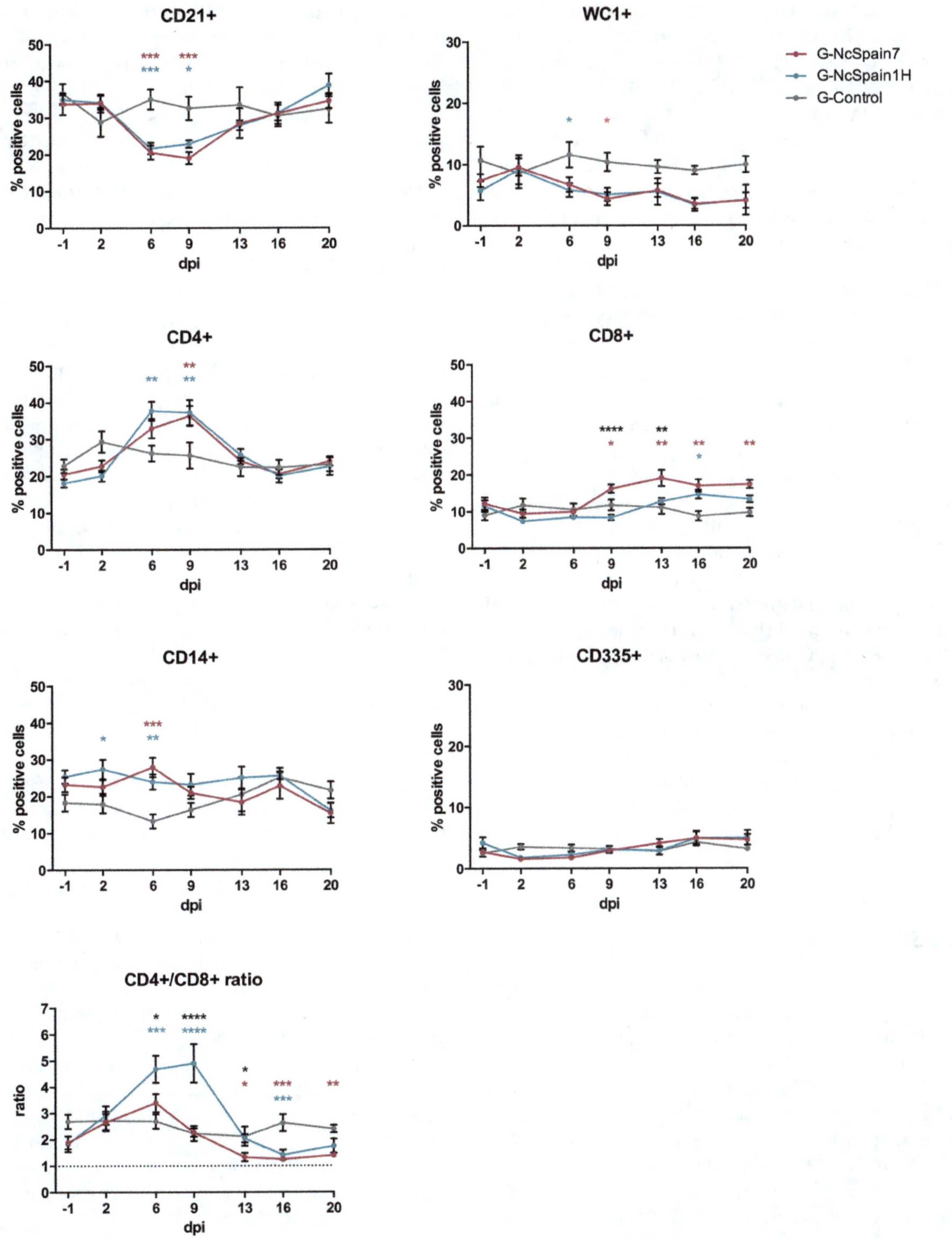

FIGURE 2 | Relative percentage of immune cells in a PBMC population from Nc-Spain7- and Nc-Spain1H-infected heifers. Graphs indicate the relative percentage of cells positive for CD21, WC1, CD4, CD8, CD14 and CD335 surface markers, and CD4+/CD8+ ratio in PBMC obtained from uninfected heifers (G-Control) and heifers challenged with Nc-Spain7 (G-NcSpain7) and Nc-Spain1H (G-NcSpain1H) tachyzoites. The results are represented as the mean + SD. Asterisks indicate significant differences in G-NcSpain1H *versus* G-Control comparison (blue), G-NcSpain7 *versus* G-Control (red) and G-NcSpain1H *versus* G-NcSpain7 (black). ****$P < 0.0001$, ***$P < 0.001$, **$P < 0.01$, *$P < 0.05$.

with Nc-Spain7 and Nc-Spain1H and culled at 10 dpi or 20 dpi (**Figure 3**). Nc-Spain7-infected dams showed significantly lower percentages of CD21+ populations at 20 dpi (P<0.01), than uninfected dams. In addition, an increase in the CD4+ (P<0.05), CD8+ (P<0.05) and CD335+ (P<0.01) percentages in G-NcSpain7 *versus* G-control was found at 20 dpi. A higher CD4+ cell percentage was detected in G-NcSpain1H at 10 dpi, but the differences were not statistically significant due to a high variability observed between animals of this infection group. *Neospora caninum* infection had no impact on the percentage of CD14+, WC1+ cells or CD4+/CD8+ ratio for either of the isolates or time points assayed.

Foetal Immune System Responded to Infection by *N. caninum* Isolates of High and Low Virulence

Foetal immune responses to *N. caninum* infection were studied by the analysis of immune cells in the spleen (**Figure 4**) and thymus (**Figure 5**). In both organs, we found cells double positive for CD4 and CD8 (up to 12% in the spleen and 70% in the thymus) in foetuses from infected and non-infected animals. In the foetal spleen, an increase in CD14+ cells in G-NcSpain7 (P < 0.01) and G-NcSpain1H (P < 0.05) was found at 20 dpi. In contrast, G-NcSpain7 induced a reduction in the percentage of CD21+ cells at 10 (P < 0.05) and 20 dpi (P < 0.01). In addition, the WC1+ cell percentage decreased at 10 dpi for G-NcSpain1H and at 20 dpi for G-NcSpain7 (P < 0.05). There were no changes in the CD4+, CD8+ and CD335+ subpopulation percentages or CD4+/CD8+ ratios.

In the thymus, an increase in the percentage of double CD4+CD8+ cells was observed for both isolates at 20 dpi, although this increase was only statistically significant for G-NcSpain7 (P < 0.05). In contrast, a reduction in the percentage of CD335+ cells in G-NcSpain1H foetuses at 10 and 20 dpi (P < 0.05) was observed.

DISCUSSION

In the present study, cellular immune response to *N. caninum* infection at mid gestation was studied with the aim of unravelling the immunological regulation that takes place at the initial events of infection (10 and 20 dpi) in pregnant cattle and their foetuses. We observed that independent of the isolate, dams mounted an early specific CMI response characterized mainly by an increase in the proportion of helper (CD4+) T cells at early infection (6 to 9 dpi) and cytotoxic (CD8+) T cells at late infection (9 to 20 dpi for Nc-Spain7 and 16 dpi for Nc-Spain1H). Previous studies also reported an increase in the percentages of CD4+ and CD8+ T cells in blood (Rosbottom et al., 2007) and lymph nodes (Almeria et al., 2003) after *Neospora* experimental infection in cattle. In addition it was demonstrated that T lymphocytes were able to recognize and respond to parasite-infected cells by producing IFN-γ, which is crucial for host defence against *N. caninum* (Innes et al., 2002; Innes et al., 2005; Williams et al., 2007). In the present study, following stimulation with *N. caninum* antigen, peripheral blood cells obtained from the infected cows were able to produce both IFN-γ and IL-4 from the end of the first week post-infection. In the same groups of animals as described here, we also reported a peak in IFN-γ levels in sera as early as 2 dpi in infected animals (Jiménez-Pelayo et al., 2019). According to our results, a very similar time course of cytokine production was observed previously (Rosbottom et al., 2007; Regidor-Cerrillo et al., 2014; Vázquez et al., 2019). In contrast, a decrease in the relative percentage of the B lymphocyte subset (CD21+) was observed in both infected groups. Previously, a decline in lymphocyte subpopulations after experimental *Neospora* infection in heifers at day 110 of gestation was also described (Almeria et al., 2003). Our finding may be a consequence of the increase in T cell populations, as an almost identical but inversely proportional profile was observed for CD21+ cells in relation to CD4+ T cells. Regarding γδ-T cells, previous *in vitro* studies have suggested that these cells may act as a short-term or innate response to *N. caninum* infection based on the capability of these cells to kill infected target cells upon cytokine stimulation (Peckham et al., 2014). Although *in vivo* studies have also demonstrated infiltration of γδ-T cells in placental tissues (Cantón et al., 2014; Hecker et al., 2015), our results suggest that γδ-T cells are not a main immune cell implicated in bovine peripheral immune responses against this parasite. In addition, NK cells did not experience any important changes after infection in our study. NK cells are important in innate defence against intracellular pathogens and act as early responders in *N. caninum* infections in bovine models (Klevar et al., 2007). Further investigations are necessary to investigate the potential role of γδ-T cells and NK cells in bovine neosporosis.

The ability of the foetal immune system to respond effectively to the parasite could be also of critical importance in determining the outcome of infection. However, the results from our study did not allow us to draw relevant conclusions, probably due to immaturity of the developing foetus at mid-gestation and the high variability between animals. Notably, a higher percentage of CD4+CD8+ double-positive cells was found in the thymus of *N. caninum*-infected fetuses at 10 dpi, indicating an active response against an ongoing infection. At 20 dpi, there was a reduction in the percentage of CD4+CD8+ double-positive cells in all the groups, possibly due to a higher level of maturation of the thymus at 130 days of gestation. In the spleen, the most remarkable result was an increase in the percentage of CD14+ cells at 20 dpi in fetuses from both infected groups. These findings again suggest that fetuses were able to respond to *N. caninum* infection at mid-gestation and that the spleen may have a greater responsiveness at this stage of pregnancy as has been previously suggested (Almeria et al., 2016).

When we compared the differential induction of maternal CMI response by infection with two *N. caninum* isolates showing marked differences in virulence traits (Jiménez-Pelayo et al., 2019; Jiménez-Pelayo et al., 2020), the results were rather similar but some differences were found. First, infection with the low-virulence Nc-Spain1H isolate induced an

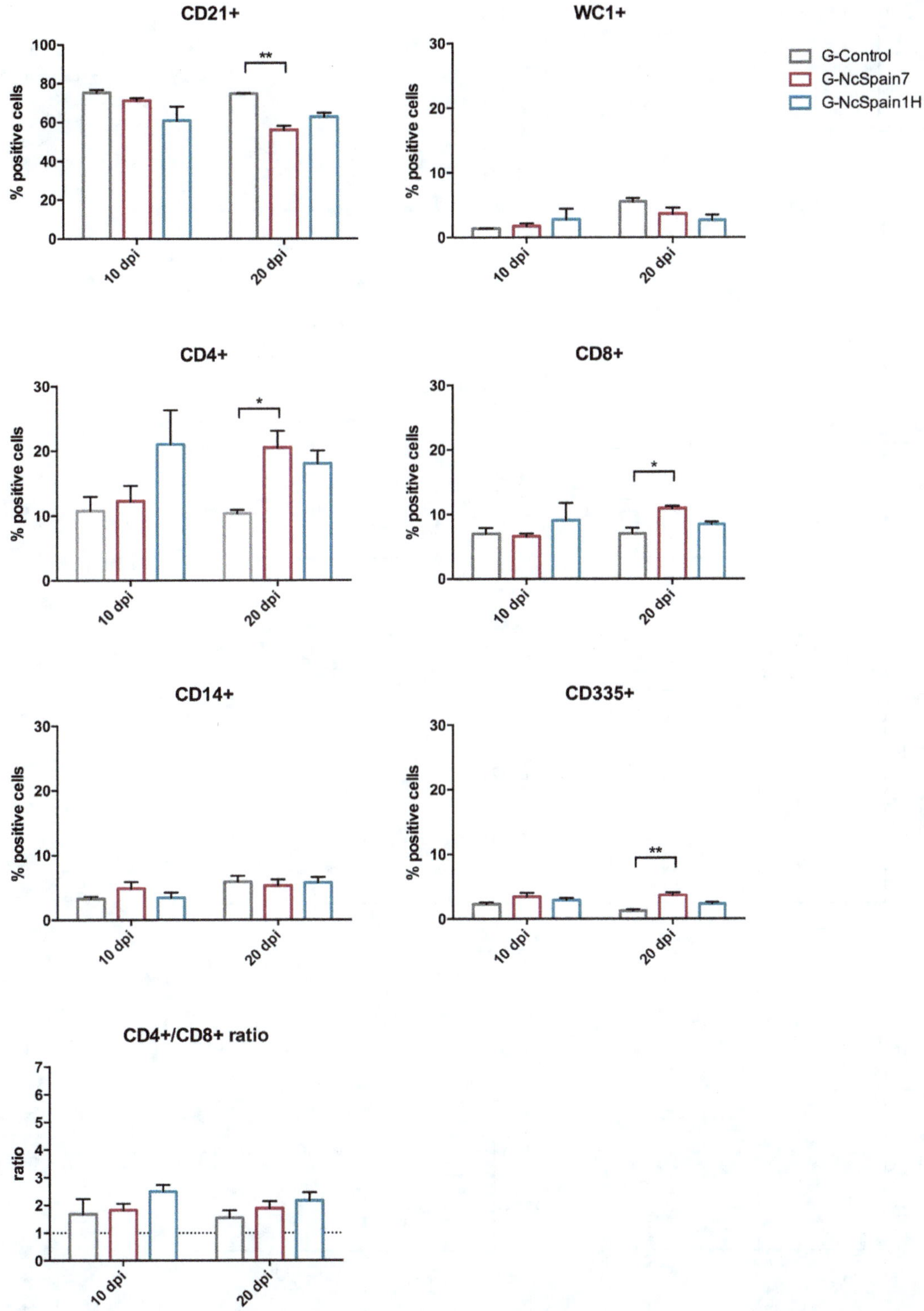

FIGURE 3 | Relative percentage of immune cells in iliofemoral lymph nodes from Nc-Spain7- and Nc-Spain1H-infected heifers. Graphs indicate the relative percentage of cells positive for CD21, WC1, CD4, CD8, CD14 and CD335 surface markers, and CD4+/CD8+ ratio surface markers in the population of immune cells obtained from the iliofemoral lymph node of uninfected heifers (G-Control) and heifers challenged with Nc-Spain7 (G-NcSpain7) and Nc-Spain1H (G-NcSpain1H) tachyzoites culled at 10 or 20 dpi. The results are represented as the mean + SD. Asterisks indicate significant differences. $^{**}P < 0.01$, $^{*}P < 0.05$.

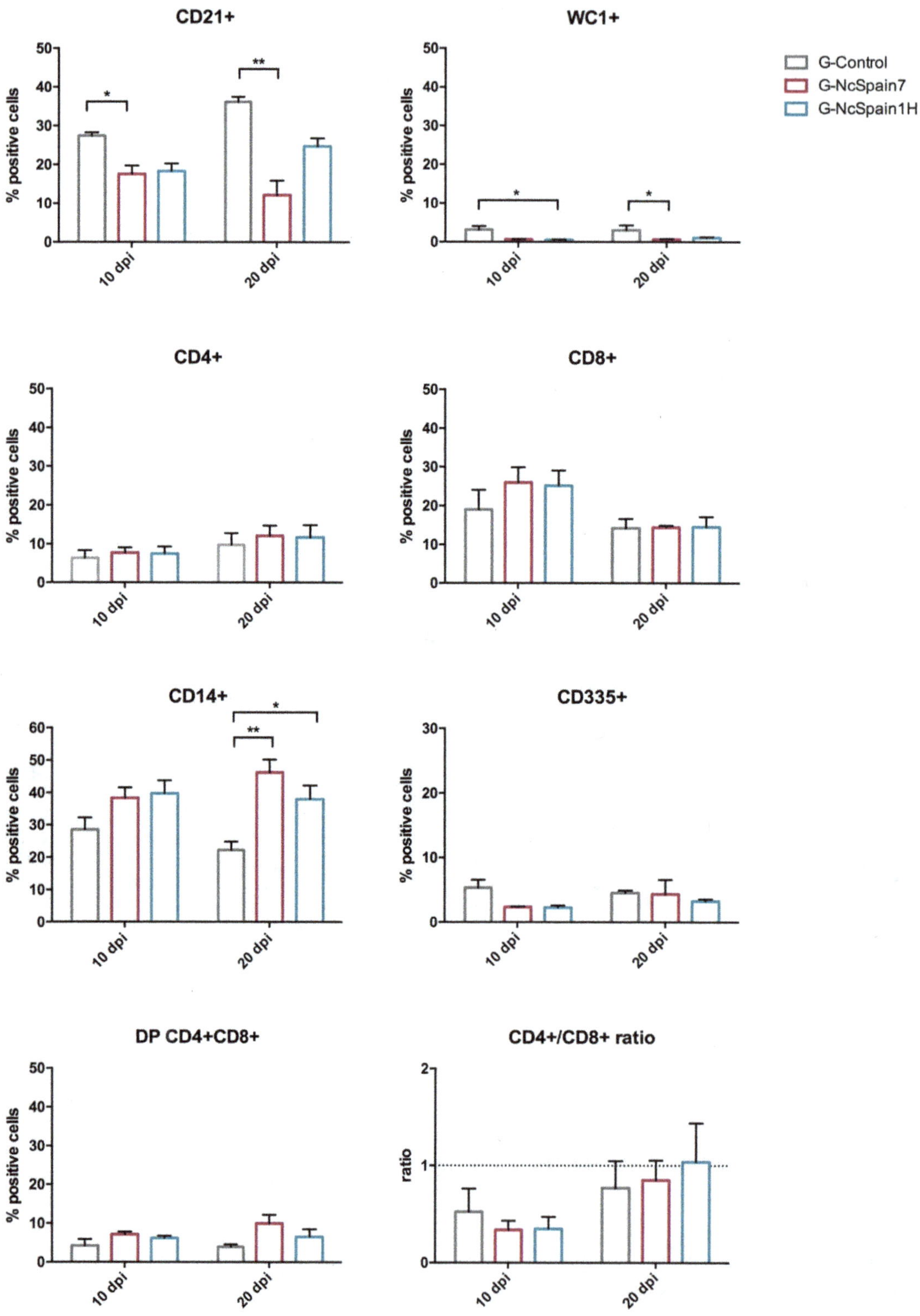

FIGURE 4 | Immune cell populations in the spleen of foetuses from Nc-Spain7 and Nc-Spain1H infected heifers at 10 and 20 dpi. Graphs indicate the relative percentage of cells positive for CD21, WC1, CD4, CD8, CD14 and CD335 surface markers, double positive (DP) CD4+CD8+ cells and CD4+/CD8+ ratio, in the population of immune cells obtained from the spleen of foetuses from uninfected heifers (G-Control) and heifers challenged with Nc-Spain7 (G-NcSpain7) and Nc-Spain1H (G-NcSpain1H) tachyzoites culled at 10 or 20 dpi. The results are represented as the mean + SD. Asterisks indicate significant differences. $^{**}P < 0.01$, $^{*}P < 0.05$.

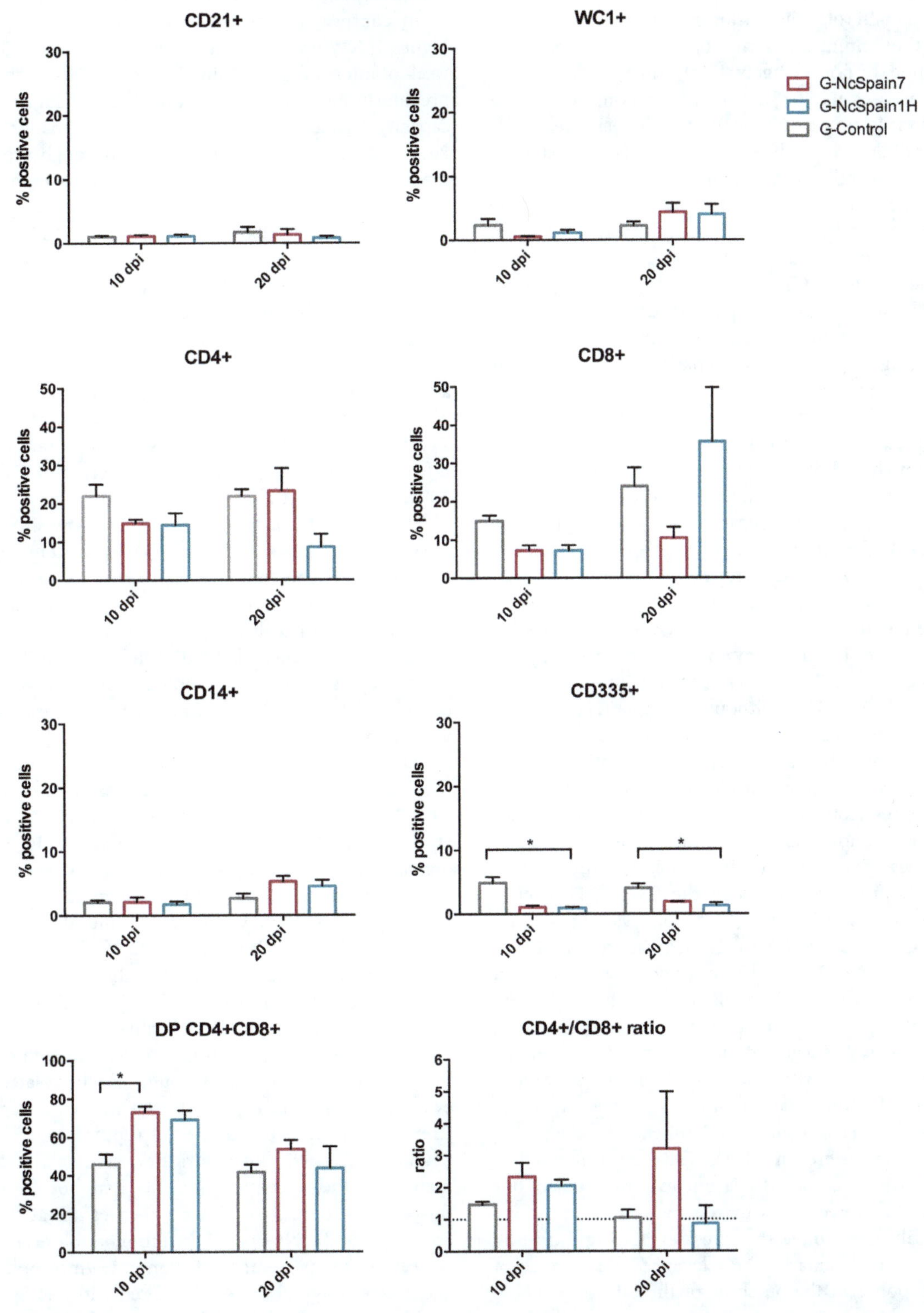

FIGURE 5 | Immune cell populations in the thymus of foetuses from Nc-Spain7 and Nc-Spain1H infected heifers at 10 and 20 dpi. Graphs indicate the relative percentage of cells positive for CD21, WC1, CD4, CD8, CD14 and CD335 surface markers, double positive (DP) CD4+CD8+ cells and CD4+/CD8+ ratio, in the population of immune cells obtained from the thymus of foetuses from uninfected heifers (G-Control) and heifers challenged with Nc-Spain7 (G-NcSpain7) and Nc-Spain1H (G-NcSpain1H) tachyzoites culled at 10 or 20 dpi. The results are represented as the mean + SD. Asterisks indicate significant differences. $^*P < 0.05$.

early increase in circulating CD14+ cells. Although individual differences were found, this result could be remarkable, since these cells play a main role in initiating early immune responses and priming the immune system for the development of adaptive immune responses against infection (Werling and Jungi, 2003; Jensen et al., 2018). A higher response of bovine macrophages to infection by Nc-Spain1H has been previously reported *in vitro* (García-Sánchez et al., 2019b; García-Sánchez et al., 2020) and was related to a higher expression of surface antigens (García-Sánchez et al., 2019a). Moreover, during the early response to an initial infection, mononuclear phagocytes are expected to encounter circulating parasites triggering an innate immune response (Goff et al., 2010). Consequently, phagocytic cells would reduce parasitaemia in the first multiplication cycles of the parasite, thereby possibly negatively affecting to parasite dissemination and the number of tachyzoites reaching the placenta. Second, an early CD4+ T cell increase was also induced by Nc-Spain1H infection in blood. CD4+ T cells could contribute to enhanced control of Nc-Spain1H growth and dissemination by releasing cytokines, activating mononuclear phagocytes, killing *N. caninum*-infected cells and affecting long-term disease progression. Consequently, a higher proportion of CD4+ lymphocytes is likely to be favourable. Previous reports have indicated that CD4+ T cells from experimentally infected cattle proliferate when stimulated with *N. caninum* antigen (Andrianarivo et al., 2001) and are able to inhibit tachyzoite multiplication by the resulting production of IFN-γ (Innes et al., 1995; Lundén et al., 1998; Rocchi et al., 2011). Here, although Nc-Spain1H infection induced lower IFN-γ levels than Nc-Spain7, the production was more maintained over time, and higher levels of IL-4 were induced by the infection with the low-virulent isolate. The ratio between helper and cytotoxic T cells was calculated as a marker of the immune regulation balance. This ratio could be used as a predictor of disease outcome. Various research studies have also described temporary changes in the CD4+/CD8+ ratio during some disease states in cattle (Ellis et al., 1990; Bassey and Collins, 1997; Chang et al., 2005). It is of interest that Nc-Spain1H triggered a shift in blood T lymphocyte subsets with a predominance of the CD4+ subpopulation, thereby raising the CD4+/CD8+ ratio. The role in pregnancy maintenance of a high CD4+/CD8+ was suggested previously (Hecker et al., 2013) and was associated with fewer foetal lesions, as we also observed in placental infiltration of animals infected with Nc-Spain1H (Jiménez-Pelayo et al., 2019; Jiménez-Pelayo et al., 2020). However, how a greater CD4+/CD8+ ratio may aid in protection in bovine neosporosis is unclear. Altogether, our results suggest that infection with the low-virulence isolate could be readily controlled by the developing immune response of dams and remarks the relevance of a balance of the immune response in the outcome of the infection. These results agree with our previous studies, in which the Nc-Spain1H isolate triggered early innate immune recognition in the bovine placenta, characterized by upregulation of genes involved in pathogen recognition inducing a solid Th1 response, which was counterbalanced by a higher expression of anti-inflammatory and regulatory cytokines, minimizing placental pathology and abortion (Jiménez-Pelayo et al., 2020).

In contrast, the highly virulent isolate Nc-Spain7 induced higher IFN-γ production by stimulated blood cells at the first week of infection, predominating over IL-4, which was observed previously and may be attributed to its higher proliferation capacity (Regidor-Cerrillo et al., 2014; Jiménez-Pelayo et al., 2017; García-Sánchez et al., 2019b). Although proinflammatory mediators may be beneficial to eliminate a high parasite load, overexpression may also cause immunopathology (Quin et al., 2002; Innes et al., 2007; Almería et al., 2017) compromising gestation, as we observed in the placentomes from these animals (Jiménez-Pelayo et al., 2020). High IFN-γ levels have been also associated with a failure in protection in different vaccine assays against neosporosis (Vemulapalli et al., 2007; Aguado-Martínez et al., 2009). Thus, a Th1 immune response is not always associated with protection against the progression of *N. caninum* infection (but rather the contrary) and even significant levels of Th2 cytokines are important for controlling infection, especially during acute infection (Nishikawa et al., 2001; Haldorson et al., 2005).

However, the largest differences between isolates were observed in CD8+ cells in PBMC, which appeared in a significantly higher proportion from 9 dpi onwards. CD8 is a marker for cytotoxic T cells, which are largely involved in the recognition and killing of cells infected with intracellular pathogens. Staska et al. (2003) showed that CD8+ cytotoxic lymphocytes from cattle could kill *N. caninum*-infected autologous target cells *in vitro*. The CD8+ increase would be an attempt by the dam to reduce parasite multiplication mediated directly by lysis of infected cells as a consequence of the higher invasion and replication rates of Nc-Spain7 (Regidor-Cerrillo et al., 2011; Jiménez-Pelayo et al., 2017; García-Sánchez et al., 2019b). However, CD8+ increases could enhance tissue damage *in vivo* due to cytotoxic effects (Correia et al., 2015). Previously, we described that CD8 + lymphocytes predominated in placentomes from G-Nc-Spain7 and that severe placental damage and foetal death were found (Jiménez-Pelayo et al., 2020). In this respect, Cantón et al. (2014) also suggested a positive association between a high number of CD8+ T lymphocytes in the placental infiltrate and the occurrence of abortion. Although speculative, an alternative interpretation for this increase in CD8+ cells could also be related to immune evasion mechanisms triggered by the high-virulence isolate, since CD8+ lymphocytes can also exert suppressor effector functions (Inoue et al., 1993; Rocamora-Reverte et al., 2020). Thus, an increase in the percentage of CD8+ lymphocytes may suppress the activity of CD4+ T lymphocytes (Shafer-Weaver and Sordillo, 1997). Nc-Spain7 infection also induced a delayed increase in the percentage of monocytes/macrophages in blood and CD4+ T lymphocytes compared with Nc-Spain1H, which could contribute to delayed host immune responsiveness during the early stages of pathogenesis. In line with these results, we have more evidence supporting that Nc-Spain7 elicits mechanisms to circumvent the immune response that could allow survival during early infection (García-Sánchez et al., 2019a;

García-Sánchez et al., 2019b; García-Sánchez et al., 2020; Jiménez-Pelayo et al., 2020). In addition, only Nc-Spain7 induced changes in the immune cell population at 20 dpi from the maternal iliofemoral lymph node, in which the uterus drains. This result could be clinically correlated with the presence of parasites in the placenta and foetus of Nc-Spain7-infected groups and the occurrence of abortion (Jiménez-Pelayo et al., 2019).

CONCLUSIONS

This study shows that isolates of different virulence may have an inherent ability to trigger different host cellular immune responses in a pregnant cow that these abilities vary in the initial recognition of the pathogen, and the character and duration of the subsequent response. Our results support the hypothesis put forward in previous *in vivo* and *in vitro* studies suggesting that the high-virulence isolate Nc-Spain7 may induce a delayed activation of CD14+ cells. This would favour its survival and arrival at the placenta, where due to its greater proliferative capacity, it would cause tissue damage enhanced by a predominant Th1 immune response. In contrast, early recognition of the low-virulence isolate Nc-Spain1H and the induction of robust responses with a better immunoregulatory balance, although not eliminating the infection, would reduce parasitemia and thus the number of parasites reaching the placenta, allowing foetal survival. We also suggested that some potential immune traits, such as IFN-γ and IL-4 levels, as well as the CD4+/CD8+ ratio and could be correlated with protection against abortion (higher IL-4 levels and CD4+/CD8+ ratio) or with poor prognosis or inflammatory conditions (higher IFN-γ production and increase of CD8+ lymphocytes).

AUTHOR CONTRIBUTIONS

JR-C, PH, KO, LO-M, and EC-F conceived the study and participated in its design. MG-S and EC-F wrote the manuscript, with interpretation of results and discussion inputs from JR-C, PH, and LO-M. PH prepared the parasite inocula. MG-S, LJ-P, PV, and AJ-M performed the collection of the samples. MG-S and LJ-P analysed the samples by flow cytometry and ELISA, carried out statistical analyses and interpreted the results. All authors contributed to the article and approved the submitted version.

REFERENCES

1. Aguado-Martınez, A., Alvarez-Garcıa, G., Fernandez-Garcıa, A., Risco-Castillo, V., Marugan-Hernandez, V., and Ortega-Mora, L. M. (2009). Failure of a Vaccine Using Immunogenic Recombinant Proteins rNcSAG4 and rNcGRA7 Against Neosporosis in Mice. *Vaccine.* 27, 7331–7338. doi: 10.1016/j.vaccine.2009. 09.050
2. Almeria, S., De Marez, T., Dawson, H., Araujo, R., Dubey, J. P., and Gasbarre, L. C. (2003). Cytokine Gene Expression in Dams and Foetuses After Experimental *Neospora Caninum* Infection of Heifers At 110 Days of Gestation. *Parasite Immunol.* 25, 383–392. doi: 10.1046/j.1365-3024.2003.00645.x
3. Almeria, S., Serrano-Perez, B., Darwich, L., Mur-Novales, R., Garcia-Ispierto, I., Cabezon, O., et al. (2016). Cytokine Gene Expression in Aborting and non-Aborting Dams and in Their Foetuses After Experimental Infection With *Neospora Caninum* At 110 Days of Gestation. *Vet. Parasitol* 227, 138–142. doi: 10.1016/j.vetpar.2016.08.006
4. Almerıa, S., Serrano-Perez, B., and Lopez-Gatius, F. (2017). Immune Response in Bovine Neosporosis: Protection or Contribution to the Pathogenesis of Abortion. *Microb. Pathog.* 109, 177–182. doi: 10.1016/j.micpath.2017.05.042
5. Alvarez-Garcia, G., Collantes-Fernandez, E., Costas, E., Rebordosa, X., and Ortega-Mora, L. M. (2003). Influence of Age and Purpose for Testing on the Cut-Off Selection of Serological Methods in Bovine Neosporosis. *Vet. Res.* 34, 341–352. doi: 10.1051/vetres:2003009
6. Andrianarivo, A. G., Barr, B. C., Anderson, M. L., Rowe, J. D., Packham, A. E., Sverlow, K. W., et al. (2001). Immune Responses in Pregnant Cattle and Bovine Fetuses Following Experimental Infection With *Neospora Caninum*. *Parasitol Res.* 87, 817–825. doi: 10.1007/s004360100442
7. Bartley, P. M., Katzer, F., Rocchi, M. S., Maley, S. W., Benavides, J., Nath, M., et al. (2013). Development of Maternal and Foetal Immune Responses in Cattle Following Experimental Challenge With *Neospora Caninum* At Day 210 of Gestation. *Vet. Res.* 44, 91. doi: 10.1186/1297-9716-44-91
8. Bartley, P. M., Wright, S. E., Maley, S. W., Macaldowie, C. N., Nath, M., Hamilton,, et al. (2012). Maternal and Foetal Immune Responses of Cattle Following an Experimental Challenge With *Neospora Caninum* At Day 70 of Gestation. *Vet. Res.* 43, 38. doi: 10.1186/1297-9716-43-38
9. Bassey, E. O., and Collins, M. T. (1997). Study of T-lymphocyte Subsets of Healthy and Mycobacterium Avium Subsp. Paratuberculosis-Infected Cattle. *Infect. Immun.* 65, 4869–4872. doi: 10.1128/IAI.65.11.4869-4872.1997
10. Benavides, J., Collantes-Fernandez, E., Ferre, I., Perez, V., Campero, C., Mota, R., et al. (2014). Experimental Ruminant Models for Bovine Neosporosis: What is Known and What is Needed. *Parasitology* 141, 1471–1488. doi: 10.1017/ S0031182014000638
11. Canton, G. J., Katzer, F., Maley, S. W., Bartley, P. M., Benavides-Silvan, J., Palarea- Albaladejo, J., et al. (2014). Inflammatory Infiltration Into Placentas of *Neospora Caninum* Challenged Cattle Correlates With Clinical Outcome of Pregnancy. *Vet. Res.* 45, 11. doi: 10.1186/1297-9716-45-11
12. Caspe, S. G., Moore, D. P., Leunda, M. R., Cano, D. B., Lischinsky, L., Regidor-Cerrillo, J., et al. (2012). The *Neospora caninum*-Spain 7 Isolate Induces Placental Damage, Fetal Death and Abortion in Cattle When Inoculated in Early Gestation. *Vet. Parasitol* 189, 171–181. doi: 10.1016/j.vetpar.2012.04.034
13. Chang, B. S., Bohach, G. A., Lee, S. U., Davis, W. C., Fox, L. K., Ferens, W. A., et al. (2005). Immunosuppression by T Regulatory Cells in Cows Infected With Staphylococcal Superantigen. *J. Vet. Sci.* 6, 247–250. doi: 10.4142/ jvs.2005.6.3.247
14. Correia, A., Ferreirinha, P., Botelho, S., Belinha, A., Leitão, C., Caramalho, I., et al. (2015). Predominant Role of Interferon-g in the Host Protective Effect of CD8(+) T Cells Against *Neospora Caninum* Infection. *Sci. Rep.* 5, 14913. doi: 10.1038/srep14913
15. Ellis, J. A., Luedke, A. J., Davis, W. C., Wechsler, S. J., Mecham, J. O., Pratt, D. L., et al. (1990). T Lymphocyte Subset Alterations Following Bluetongue Virus Infection in Sheep and Cattle. *Vet. Immunol. Immunopathol.* 24, 49–67. doi: 10.1016/0165-2427(90)90077-6
16. Garcıa-Sanchez, M., Jimenez-Pelayo, L., Horcajo, P., Collantes-Fernandez, E., Ortega-Mora, L. M., and Regidor-Cerrillo, J. (2020). *Neospora Caninum* Infection Induces an Isolate Virulence-Dependent Pro-Inflammatory Gene Expression Profile in Bovine Monocyte-Derived Macrophages. *Parasit Vectors* 13, 374. doi: 10.1186/s13071-020-04239-3
17. Garcıa-Sanchez, M., Jimenez-Pelayo, L., Horcajo, P., Regidor-Cerrillo, J., Collantes-Fernandez, E., and Ortega-Mora, L. M. (2019a). Gene Expression Profiling of *Neospora Caninum* in Bovine Macrophages Reveals Differences Between Isolates Associated With Key Parasite Functions. *Front. Cell Infect. Microbiol.* 9, 354. doi: 10.3389/fcimb.2019.00354
18. Garcıa-Sanchez, M., Jimenez-Pelayo, L., Horcajo, P., Regidor-Cerrillo, J., O lafsson, E. B., Bhandage,, et al. (2019b). Differential Responses of Bovine

Monocyte-Derived Macrophages to Infection by *Neospora Caninum* Isolates of High and Low Virulence. *Front. Immunol.* 10, 915. doi: 10.3389/fimmu.2019.00915

19. Goff, W. L., Bastos, R. G., Brown, W. C., Johnson, W. C., and Schneider, D. A. (2010). The Bovine Spleen: Interactions Among Splenic Cell Populations in the Innate Immunologic Control of Hemoparasitic Infections. *Vet. Immunol. Immunopathol.* 138, 1–14. doi: 10.1016/j.vetimm.2010.07.006
20. Goodswen, S. J., Kennedy, P. J., and Ellis, J. T. (2013). A Review of the Infection, Genetics, and Evolution of *Neospora Caninum*: From the Past to the Present. *Infect. Genet. Evol.* 13, 133–150. doi: 10.1016/j.meegid.2012.08.012
21. Haldorson, G. J., Mathison, B. A., Wenberg, K., Conrad, P. A., Dubey, J. P., Trees, A. J., et al. (2005). Immunization With Native Surface Protein NcSRS2 Induces a Th2 Immune Response and Reduces Congenital *Neospora Caninum* Transmission in Mice. *Int. J. Parasitol* 35, 1407–j.ijpara.2005.05.013 1415. doi: 10.1016/
22. Hecker, Y. P., Canton, G., Regidor-Cerrillo, J., Chianini, F., Morrell, E., Lischinsky, L., et al. (2015). Cell Mediated Immune Responses in the Placenta Following Challenge of Vaccinated Pregnant Heifers With *Neospora Caninum*. *Vet. Parasitol* 214, 247–254. doi: 10.1016/j.vetpar.2015.10.015
23. Hecker, Y. P., Moore, D. P., Quattrocchi, V., Regidor-Cerrillo, J., Verna, A., Leunda, M. R., et al. (2013). Immune Response and Protection Provided by Live Tachyzoites and Native Antigens From the NC-6 Argentina Strain of *Neospora Caninum* in Pregnant Heifers. *Vet. Parasitol* 197, 436–446. doi: 10.1016/j.vetpar.2013.07.027
24. Innes, E. A. (2007). The host-parasite relationship in pregnant cattle infected with Neospora caninum. *Parasitology* 134, 1903–1910.
25. Innes, E. A., Andrianarivo, A. G., Björkman, C., Williams, D. J., and Conrad, P. A. (2002). Immune Responses to *Neospora Caninum* and Prospects for Vaccination. *Trends Parasitol* 18, 497–504. doi: 10.1016/S1471-4922(02) 02372-3
26. Innes, E. A., Panton, W. R., Marks, J., Trees, A. J., Holmdahl, J., and Buxton, D. (1995). Interferon Gamma Inhibits the Intracellular Multiplication of *Neospora Caninum*, as Shown by Incorporation of 3H Uracil. *J. Comp. Pathol.* 113, 95– 100. doi: 10.1016/S0021-9975(05)80075-1
27. Innes, E. A., Wright, S., Bartley, P., Maley, S., Macaldowie, C., Esteban-Redondo, I., et al. (2005). The Host-Parasite Relationship in Bovine Neosporosis. *Vet. Immunol. Immunopathol.* 108, 29–36. doi: 10.1016/j.vetimm.2005.07.004
28. Inoue, T., Asano, Y., Matsuoka, S., Furutani-Seiki, M., Aizawa, S., Nishimura, H., et al. (1993). Distinction of Mouse CD8+ Suppressor Effector T Cell Clones From Cytotoxic T Cell Clones by Cytokine Production and CD45 Isoforms. *J. Immunol.* 150, 2121–2128.
29. Jensen, K., Gallagher, I. J., Johnston, N., Welsh, M., Skuce, R., Williams, J. L., et al. (2018). Variation in the Early Host-Pathogen Interaction of Bovine Macrophages With Divergent Mycobacterium Bovis Strains in the United Kingdom. *Infect. Immun.* 86, e00385-17. doi: 10.1128/IAI.00385-17
30. Jimenez-Pelayo, L., Garcıa-Sanchez, M., Collantes-Fernandez, E., Regidor-Cerrillo, J., Horcajo, P., Gutierrez-Exposito, D., et al. (2020). Crosstalk Between *Neospora Caninum* and the Bovine Host At the Maternal-Foetal Interface Determines the Outcome of Infection. *Vet. Res.* 51, 83. doi: 10.1186/ s13567-020-00803-y
31. Jimenez-Pelayo, L., Garcıa-Sanchez, M., Regidor-Cerrillo, J., Horcajo, P., Collantes-Fernandez, E., Gomez-Bautista,, et al. (2017). Differential Susceptibility of Bovine Caruncular and Trophoblast Cell Lines to Infection With High and Low Virulence Isolates of *Neospora Caninum*. *Parasit Vectors* 10, 463. doi: 10.1186/s13071-017-2409-9
32. Jimenez-Pelayo, L., Garcıa-Sanchez, M., Vazquez, P., Regidor-Cerrillo, J., Horcajo, P., Collantes-Fernandez, E., et al. (2019). Early *Neospora Caninum* Infection Dynamics in Cattle After Inoculation At Mid-Gestation With High (Nc- Spain7)- or Low (Nc-Spain1H)-virulence Isolates. *Vet. Res.* 50, 72. doi: 10.1186/s13567-019-0691-6
33. Klevar, S., Kulberg, S., Boysen, P., Storset, A. K., Moldal, T., Björkman, C., et al. (2007). Natural Killer Cells Act as Early Responders in an Experimental Infection With *Neospora Caninum* in Calves. *Int. J. Parasitol* 37, 329–339. doi: 10.1016/j.ijpara.2006.11.002
34. Lunden, A., Marks, J., Maley, S. W., and Innes, E. A. (1998). Cellular Immune Responses in Cattle Experimentally Infected With *Neospora Caninum*. *Parasite Immunol.* 20, 519–526. doi: 10.1046/j.1365-3024.1998.00184.x
35. Nishikawa, Y., Inoue, N., Xuan, X., Nagasawa, H., Igarashi, I., Fujisaki, K., et al. (2001). Protective Efficacy of Vaccination by Recombinant Vaccinia Virus Against *Neospora Caninum* Infection. *Vaccine* 19, 1381–1390. doi: 10.1016/ S0264-410X(00)00389-3
36. Quinn, H. E., Ellis, J. T., and Smith, N. C. (2002). Neospora caninum: a cause of immune-mediated failure of pregnancy? *Trends Parasitol.* 18, 391–394.
37. Peckham, R. K., Brill, R., Foster, D. S., Bowen, A. L., Leigh, J. A., Coffey, T. J., et al. (2014). Two Distinct Populations of Bovine IL-17 T-Cells can be Induced and WC1IL-17gd T-cells are Effective Killers of Protozoan Parasites. *Sci. Rep.* 4, 5431. doi: 10.1038/srep05431
38. Regidor-Cerrillo, J., Arranz-Solıs, D., Benavides, J., Gomez-Bautista, M., Castro- Hermida, J. A., Mezo, M., et al. (2014). *Neospora Caninum*
39. Regidor-Cerrillo, J., Gómez-Bautista, M., Pereira-Bueno, J., Adúriz, G., Navarro- Lozano, V., Risco-Castillo, V., et al. (2008). Isolation and genetic characterization of Neospora caninum from asymptomatic calves in Spain. *Parasitology* 135, 1651–9.
40. Regidor-Cerrillo, J., Gomez-Bautista, M., Sodupe, I., Aduriz, G., A lvarez-Garcıa, G., Del Pozo, I., et al. (2011). *In Vitro* Invasion Efficiency and Intracellular Proliferation Rate Comprise Virulence-Related Phenotypic Traits of *Neospora Caninum*. *Vet. Res.* 42, 41. doi: 10.1186/1297-9716-42-41
41. Rocamora-Reverte, L., Melzer, F. L., Würzner, R., and Weinberger, B. (2020). The Complex Role of Regulatory T Cells in Immunity and Aging. *Front. Immunol.* 11, 616949. doi: 10.3389/fimmu.2020.616949
42. Rocchi, M. S., Bartley, P. M., Inglis, N. F., Collantes-Fernandez, E., Entrican, G., Katzer, F., et al. (2011). Selection of *Neospora Caninum* Antigens Stimulating Bovine CD4+Ve T Cell Responses Through Immuno-Potency Screening and Proteomic Approaches. *Vet. Res.* 42, 91. doi: 10.1186/1297-9716-42-91
43. Rojo-Montejo, S., Collantes-Fernandez, E., Blanco-Murcia, J., Rodrıguez-Bertos, A., Risco-Castillo, V., and Ortega-Mora, L. M. (2009). Experimental Infection With a Low Virulence Isolate of *Neospora Caninum* At 70 Days Gestation in Cattle did Not Result in Foetopathy. *Vet. Res.* 40, 49. doi: 10.1051/vetres/ 2009032
44. Rosbottom, A., Guy, C. S., Gibney, E. H., Smith, R. F., Valarcher, J. F., Taylor, G., et al. (2007). Peripheral Immune Responses in Pregnant Cattle Following *Neospora Caninum* Infection. *Parasite Immunol.* 29, 219–228. doi: 10.1111/ j.1365-3024.2007.00936.x
45. Shafer-Weaver, K. A., and Sordillo, L. M. (1997). Bovine CD8+ Suppressor Lymphocytes Alter Immune Responsiveness During the Postpartum Period. *Vet. Immunol. Immunopathol.* 56, 53–64. doi: 10.1016/S0165-2427(96) 05725-X
46. Staska, L. M, McGuire, T. C., Davies, C. J., Lewin, H. A., and Baszler, T. V. (2003). Neospora caninum-infected cattle develop parasite-specific CD4+ cytotoxic T lymphocytes. *Infect Immun.* 71 (6), 3272–3279. doi: 10.1128/iai.71.6.3272-3279.2003
47. Vazquez, P., Osoro, K., Fernandez, M., Roman-Trufero, A., Regidor-Cerrillo, J., Jimenez-Pelayo, L., et al. (2019). Effects of Challenge Dose and Inoculation Route of the Virulent *Neospora Caninum* Nc-Spain7 Isolate in Pregnant Cattle At Mid-Gestation. *Vet. Res.* 50, 68. doi: 10.1186/s13567-019-0686-3
48. Vemulapalli, R., Sanakkayala, N., Gulani, J., Schurig, G. G., Boyle, S. M., Lindsay, D. S., et al. (2007). Reduced Cerebral Infection of *Neospora Caninum* in BALB/c Mice Vaccinated With Recombinant *Brucella Abortus* RB51 Strains Expressing N. Caninum SRS2 and GRA7 Proteins. *Vet. Parasitol.* 148, 219–230. doi: 10.1016/j.vetpar.2007.06.029
49. Werling, D., and Jungi, T. W. (2003). TOLL-Like Receptors Linking Innate and Adaptive Immune Response. *Vet. Immunol. Immunopathol.* 91, 1–12. doi: 10.1016/S0165-2427(02)00228-3
50. Williams, D. J., Guy, C. S., Smith, R. F., Ellis, J., Björkman, C., Reichel, M. P., et al. (2007). Immunization of Cattle With Live Tachyzoites of *Neospora Caninum* Confers Protection Against Fetal Death. *Infect. Immun.* 75, 1343–1348. doi: 10.1128/IAI.00777-06

High Antibodies to VAR2CSA in Response to Malaria Infection are Associated with Improved Birthweight in a Longitudinal Study of Pregnant Women

Alistair R. D. McLean[1,2†], *D. Herbert Opi*[1,3,4†], *Danielle I. Stanisic*[5,6], *Julia C. Cutts*[1,4], *Gaoqian Feng*[1,4], *Alice Ura*[5], *Ivo Mueller*[5,7,8], *Stephen J. Rogerson*[4], *James G. Beeson*[1,4,9*] *and Freya J. I. Fowkes*[1,10,11,12*]

[1] *Burnet Institute, Melbourne, VIC, Australia,* [2] *Centre for Tropical Medicine and Global Health, Nuffield Department of Medicine, University of Oxford, Oxford, United Kingdom,* [3] *Department of Immunology and Pathology, Monash University, Melbourne, VIC, Australia,* [4] *Department of Medicine at the Doherty Institute, University of Melbourne, Melbourne, VIC, Australia,* [5] *Papua New Guinea Institute of Medical Research, Madang, Papua New Guinea,* [6] *Institute for Glycomics, Griffith University, Southport, QLD, Australia,* [7] *Population, Health and Immunity Division, Walter and Eliza Hall Institute of Medical Research, Parkville, VIC, Australia,* [8] *Département Parasites et Insectes Vecteurs, Institute Pasteur, Paris, France,* [9] *Department of Microbiology, Monash University, Clayton, VIC, Australia,* [10] *Department of Infectious Diseases, Central Clinical School, Monash University, Melbourne, VIC, Australia,* [11] *Centre for Epidemiology and Biostatistics, University of Melbourne, Melbourne, VIC, Australia,* [12] *Department of Epidemiology and Preventive Medicine, Monash University, Melbourne, VIC, Australia*

***Correspondence:**
Freya J. I. Fowkes
freya.fowkes@burnet.edu.au
James G. Beeson
beeson@burnet.edu.au

†*These authors have contributed equally to this work*

Introduction: Pregnant women have an increased risk of *P. falciparum* infection, which is associated with low birth weight and preterm delivery. VAR2CSA, a variant surface antigen expressed on the parasitized erythrocyte surface, enables sequestration in the placenta. Few studies have prospectively examined relationships between antibody responses during pregnancy and subsequent adverse birth outcomes, and there are limited data outside Africa.

Methods: Levels of IgG against VAR2CSA domains (DBL3; DBL5) and a VAR2CSA-expressing placental-binding *P. falciparum* isolate (PfCS2-IE) were measured in 301 women enrolled at their first visit to antenatal care which occurred mid-pregnancy (median = 26 weeks, lower and upper quartiles = 22, 28). Associations between antibody levels at enrolment and placental infection, birthweight and estimated gestational age at delivery were assessed by linear and logistic regression with adjustment for confounders. For all outcomes, effect modification by gravidity and peripheral blood *P. falciparum* infection at enrolment was assessed.

Results: Among women who had acquired *P. falciparum* infection at enrolment, those with higher levels of VAR2CSA antibodies (75th percentile) had infants with higher mean birthweight (estimates varied from +35g to +149g depending on antibody response) and reduced adjusted odds of placental infection (aOR estimates varied from 0.17 to 0.80), relative to women with lower levels (25th percentile) of VAR2CSA antibodies. However, among women who had not acquired an infection at enrolment, higher VAR2CSA antibodies were associated with increased odds of placental infection (aOR estimates varied from 1.10 to 2.24).

Conclusions: When infected by mid-pregnancy, a better immune response to VAR2CSA-expressing parasites may contribute to protecting against adverse pregnancy outcomes.

Keywords: VAR2CSA antibodies, birthweight, placental infection, Papua New Guinea, malaria in pregnancy (MiP), *Plasmodium falciparum*

INTRODUCTION

Plasmodium falciparum infections during pregnancy are associated with low birth weight and preterm delivery (1). Pregnant women are at an increased risk of detected *P. falciparum* infection relative to non-pregnant women and are at greatest risk during their first pregnancy (2). The variant surface antigen VAR2CSA, expressed on the infected erythrocyte (IE) surface (3–5), mediates adhesion to chondroitin sulfate A (CSA) (6) and thus enables sequestration of IEs in the placenta (7). VAR2CSA is a specific variant of *P. falciparum* erythrocyte membrane protein 1 (PfEMP1). Primigravid women and men in malaria endemic settings generally have low levels of antibodies specific for VAR2CSA but levels increase among women with increasing gravidity (8–12). It has been suggested that the reduced risk of malaria infection in multigravid women relative to primigravid women can be partly explained by the acquisition of naturally acquired antibodies to VAR2CSA with each pregnancy, providing protection against placental *P. falciparum* infection and its adverse consequences (11). On this basis, efforts are underway to design a vaccine to induce immunity against VAR2CSA to protect against placental infection (13, 14). However, there is very limited evidence from population studies to indicate that VAR2CSA antibodies are protective against adverse maternal and birth outcomes (15), especially in Asia-Pacific where a large population is at risk of malaria.

Most cross-sectional studies investigating antibodies in women at delivery have not found significant protective associations between levels of VAR2CSA antibodies and birthweight (15–18) or gestational age at delivery (15, 16) and a limited number of studies have noted protective associations in subsets of women according to clinical outcome or gravidity (3, 19–22). As VAR2CSA antibodies arise in response to placental infection but are also putatively protective against placental infection and its adverse outcomes, cross-sectional studies are limited in their ability to determine the protective effect of VAR2CSA immune responses.

The majority of longitudinal studies have been undertaken in Africa and have not observed significant associations between VAR2CSA antibodies measured mid-pregnancy and birthweight (23–26) or gestational age at delivery (26, 27). However, the presence of malaria infection can confound these associations as they are associated with both VAR2CSA antibodies and birth outcomes. Indeed, one African study demonstrated a positive association between VAR2CSA antibodies and birthweight, but only in women who had peripheral blood *P. falciparum* infection at enrolment; no association was observed in *P. falciparum* negative women (27). The probability of malaria infection is heterogeneous across individuals and in populations of varying malaria transmission. Investigating the potential modification of *P. falciparum* infection on associations between VAR2CSA and birth outcomes is needed. In addition, investigations in other regions that experience a high burden of malaria in pregnancy but may differ from Africa with respect to parasite and host genetics and human behaviour, such as the Asia-Pacific (28), are required.

In this study, we investigated whether antibodies measured at the first visit to ANC were associated with protection against adverse pregnancy outcomes in a longitudinal study in a malaria-endemic region of Papua New Guinea. We evaluated antibodies to VAR2CSA expressed on the surface of IEs and to specific domains expressed as recombinant proteins. We hypothesized that women who have higher magnitude antibody responses when infected during pregnancy will have better pregnancy outcomes than those with lower responses. Because of the heterogeneity of exposure to malaria in populations, we investigated how infection status at enrolment in mid-pregnancy influenced protective associations.

MATERIALS AND METHODS

Study Population and Sample Collection

The study was carried out in the malaria endemic province of Madang in Papua New Guinea (PNG) as described in detail previously (29). Between September 2005 and October 2007, 470 pregnant women >16 years of age attending their first antenatal care visit at Alexishafen Health Centre were recruited following written informed voluntary consent. Women were followed up at 30-34 weeks gestation, at delivery and 6-8 weeks postpartum. Gestational age was estimated from fundal height measurements. At enrolment, women received chloroquine (9 or 12 tablets, 150 mg base) and (when available) sulphadoxine pyrimethamine (500/25 mg, three tablets), followed by weekly chloroquine prophylaxis (two 150 mg tablets weekly), and ferrous sulphate 270 mg and folic acid 0.3 mg daily, according to local policy. Prophylaxis was not monitored. Inclusion criteria included no history of multiple births (e.g. past delivery of twins) and delivery complications, intention to deliver at the Alexishafen Health Centre, haemoglobin (Hb) >5g/dl and evidence of foetal movement. This study included 301 women who had delivery data and peripheral blood samples available at the enrolment visit for antibody analysis. Peripheral blood samples were collected at each visit and plasma and serum samples were separated and frozen. Placental blood and placental biopsy samples were collected at delivery if the delivery occurred at the clinic (n = 233). At each visit peripheral parasitemia was determined by microscopy on thick and thin blood films and *Plasmodium spp* confirmed by PCR. The presence of placental infection was determined by placental histology of fixed Giemsa-stained placental biopsies by light microscopy and samples were classified as no infection (no malaria parasites present) or active infection (presence of malaria parasites) as previously described (30, 31). Data on human genetic polymorphisms of South-East Asian Ovalocytosis (SAO), Complement Receptor 1 (CR1) and α+thalassaemia were available as described (29). Samples from malaria-naive residents of Melbourne, Australia were used as malaria naive controls in all assays. Male Madang samples were collected between 2001 and 2002 from Modilon Hospital, the Madang town clinic, and the Yagaum immunization service (32).

This study received ethical approval from the PNG Medical Research Advisory Council, the Melbourne Health Human Research Ethics Committee and Alfred Health Human Research Ethics Committee.

Parasite Culture and Selection

The CS2 *P. falciparum* parasite line that binds to CSA and predominantly express the *var2csa* transcript (33–35) was used in this study. *P. falciparum* CS2 parasites were cultured in O+ human red blood cells (RBCs) in RPMI-HEPES culture medium supplemented with 5% pooled non-exposed human serum and 0.1% Albumax (32). Parasites were routinely selected for knob expression by gelatin floatation (36).

Measurement of Antibody Levels to Recombinant Proteins

Antibody levels were determined for 3 VAR2CSA recombinant proteins representing 2 allelic variants; DBL5 (3D7), DBL5 (7G8) and DBL3 (7G8) by standard ELISA assays (37). All recombinant proteins were cloned and produced in *Pichia pastoris* (38). DBL5 and DBL3 recombinant proteins were selected because compared to other VAR2CSA domains they are highly immunogenic in natural infections and elicit some degree of cross-reactive and adhesion-blocking antibodies (25, 39–43), and also promote opsonic phagocytosis by monocytes (44). Antibodies to apical membrane antigen 1 were assessed as a broad measure of blood-stage immunity (45). Recombinant proteins were coated onto plates overnight at concentrations of 0.5 μg/ml followed by 2 hour incubation with sera samples (1/500) and 1 hour incubation with goat anti-human IgG conjugated to horseradish peroxidase (HRP) (Millipore) (1/2500). Reactivity was determined by measuring the optical density (OD) at 405 nm following the addition of ABTS [2,2'-azino-bis(3-ethylbenzothiazoline-6-sulphonic acid)] (Thermo Fisher Scientific) for fifteen minutes and the reaction stopped with the addition of 1% sodium dodecyl sulfate in PBS. Results are presented as ODs standardized to five positive control samples (individuals from the study identified as having high IgG reactivity to VAR2CSA during assay optimisation) run on each assay plate to account for inter-plate variability.

Measurement of Antibody Levels to VAR2CSA on the Surface of IEs

We used the CS2 parasite line to measure antibody levels to VAR2CSA expressed on the surface of IEs. The CS2 parasite line predominantly expresses the *var2csa* transcript (32, 33), binds to CSA and is recognized by serum from malaria exposed pregnant women (46, 47). Total IgG reactivity to the surface of CS2 IEs was assessed by flow cytometry as previously described (36, 48). Total IgG binding for each sample was determined by subtracting the geometric Mean Fluorescence Intensity (MFI) of uninfected erythrocytes from that of IEs. Geometric MFI were then expressed as a percentage of the mean geometric MFI (Arbitrary Units) of pooled serum from five positive high responders.

Statistical Analysis

Statistical analyses were performed using Stata Version 16.1 (StataCorp, College Station, TX, USA).

Descriptive statistics were used to describe the included women, categorical variables were summarised with proportions and frequencies; continuous variables were summarised with quartiles. Linear regression was used to assess the associations between the exposures (antibody levels) and outcomes [birth weight (grams) and estimated gestational age at delivery (weeks)]. Logistic regression was used to assess associations between antibody levels and odds of placental infection (defined as presence of *P. falciparum* parasites in placental histology). Potential confounders for all analyses were selected *a priori* using causal diagrams (49). All analyses were adjusted for the following confounders: *P. falciparum* infection at enrolment (from peripheral blood sample, diagnosis by light microscopy of blood smears with confirmation by PCR), gravidity (primigravid/multigravid), haemoglobin at enrolment (g/dl; determined using Hemocue), middle upper arm circumference (cm), SAO (yes/no; by PCR), alpha thalassaemia (yes/no; by PCR). In the birth weight regression model, sex of baby (male/female) was included as a covariate known to be independently predictive of the outcome.

For all models, the assumption of a linear association between antibody levels and outcome was assessed both visually and by testing regression models with categorical (groups cut at quartiles) and pseudo-continuous antibody variables by likelihood ratio tests. As there was no evidence of non-linearity of associations between antibodies and outcomes in all models, antibody measures were fitted as continuous exposures. To aid interpretation, coefficients were presented representing the difference in outcome of a high responder (75th percentile) to a low responder (25th percentile). To assess whether the relationship between antibody levels and the outcome of interest was modified by gravidity (primigravid/multigravid) or *P. falciparum* infection at enrolment detected by light microscopy (yes/no), likelihood ratio tests were performed comparing the model with and without interaction terms. Where evidence supporting an interaction was present ($p < 0.1$ for at least two pregnancy-specific antibody exposures) this model was presented in the main text; results from all models are reported in **Supplementary Material**.

RESULTS

The median age of women was 24 years (lower, upper quartiles = 21, 28); 115 (38%) women were primigravid (**Table 1**). Median estimated gestational age at enrolment was 26 (22, 28) weeks. Primigravid women were more likely to present with peripheral blood *P. falciparum* infection [49/115 (43%); by light microscopy) than multigravid women [54/186 (29%)]. There were 103 (34%) women who had *P. falciparum* infection. Women infected at enrolment were more likely to experience adverse birth outcomes than women uninfected at enrolment with a higher percentage of low birth weight births (20% *vs* 15%) and preterm deliveries (30% *vs* 18%) and were more likely to experience placental *P. falciparum* infection (65% *vs* 53%).

Antibodies to VAR2CSA Were Associated With Gravidity and Exposure

Antibodies to VAR2CSA were assessed by quantifying IgG to recombinant DBL3 and DBL5 domains, and antibodies to the surface of CS2-IEs expressing VAR2CSA. VAR2CSA antibody levels were higher in multigravid women than primigravid women ($p = 0.03$), and higher in pregnant women compared to malaria-exposed men from the same population ($p < 0.001$) or malaria non-exposed adults ($p < 0.001$, **Figure 1A**). Women who were infected at enrolment had higher levels of VAR2CSA antibodies than women who were uninfected at enrolment ($p < 0.001$, **Figure 1B**).

VAR2CSA IgG at Enrolment Was Differentially Associated With Placental Infection Among Women Infected Versus Non-Infected at Enrolment

There was evidence of effect modification of the association between VAR2CSA antibodies and odds of placental infection

TABLE 1 | Study population characteristics in women with and without microscopic peripheral *P. falciparum* infection at enrolment.

	Total (N=301)	Uninfected at enrolment (N=198)	Infected at enrolment (N=103)
Enrolment demographics			
Age (years)	24 (21, 28)	25 (21, 30)	23 (20, 27)
Gravidity			
Primigravid	115/301 (38%)	66/198 (33%)	49/103 (48%)
Multigravid	186/301 (62%)	132/198 (67%)	54/103 (52%)
Gestational age (weeks)	26 (22, 28)	26 (22, 28)	26 (22, 29)
Middle Upper Arm Circumference (cm)	22 (21, 24)	23 (21, 24)	22 (22, 23)
Smokes	60/300 (20%)	40/198 (20%)	20/102 (20%)
Maternal genetics			
South East Asian Ovalocytosis	41/301 (14%)	23/198 (12%)	18/103 (17%)
α+thalassaemia			
Normal	59/301 (20%)	40/198 (20%)	19/103 (18%)
Heterozygous	112/301 (37%)	72/198 (36%)	40/103 (39%)
Homozygous	130/301 (43%)	86/198 (43%)	44/103 (43%)
Complement Receptor 1 (exon 22)			
AA	30/301 (10%)	21/198 (11%)	9/103 (8.7%)
AG	120/301 (40%)	84/198 (42%)	36/103 (35%)
GG	151/301 (50%)	93/198 (47%)	58/103 (56%)
Haemoglobin at enrolment			
Haemoglobin (g/dl)	8.4 (7.6, 9.4)	8.7 (7.9, 9.7)	8.1 (7.2, 9.0)
Severe anaemia (<8g/dl)	111/301 (37%)	60/198 (30%)	51/103 (50%)
Infections at enrolment			
Peripheral *P. falciparum*[a]	103/301 (34%)	0/198 (0%)	103/103 (100%)
Infections at delivery			
Peripheral *P. falciparum*[a]	33/288 (11%)	22/190 (12%)	11/98 (11%)
Placental *P. falciparum*[b]	132/233 (57%)	81/154 (53%)	51/79 (65%)
Haemoglobin at delivery			
Haemoglobin (g/dl)	9.4 (8.2, 10.3)	9.4 (8.1, 10.4)	9.2 (8.2, 10.2)
Severe anaemia (<8g/dl)	68/285 (24%)	45/188 (24%)	23/97 (24%)
Birth Outcomes			
Birth weight (kg)	2.9 (2.6, 3.2)	3.0 (2.6, 3.2)	2.8 (2.5, 3.0)
Low birth weight (<2500g)	50/299 (17%)	30/197 (15%)	20/102 (20%)
Gestational age	38 (37, 40)	38 (37, 40)	38 (36, 40)
Preterm delivery	63/285 (22%)	35/191 (18%)	28/94 (30%)

Data are presented as median (25th percentile, 75th percentile) and n/total (%) for categorical variables. [a]Parasite positive by light microscopy, confirmed by PCR. [b]Parasite positive by placental histology. Smoker missing for 1 participant, Middle Upper Arm Circumference at enrolment missing for 12 participants, Age missing for 10 participants.

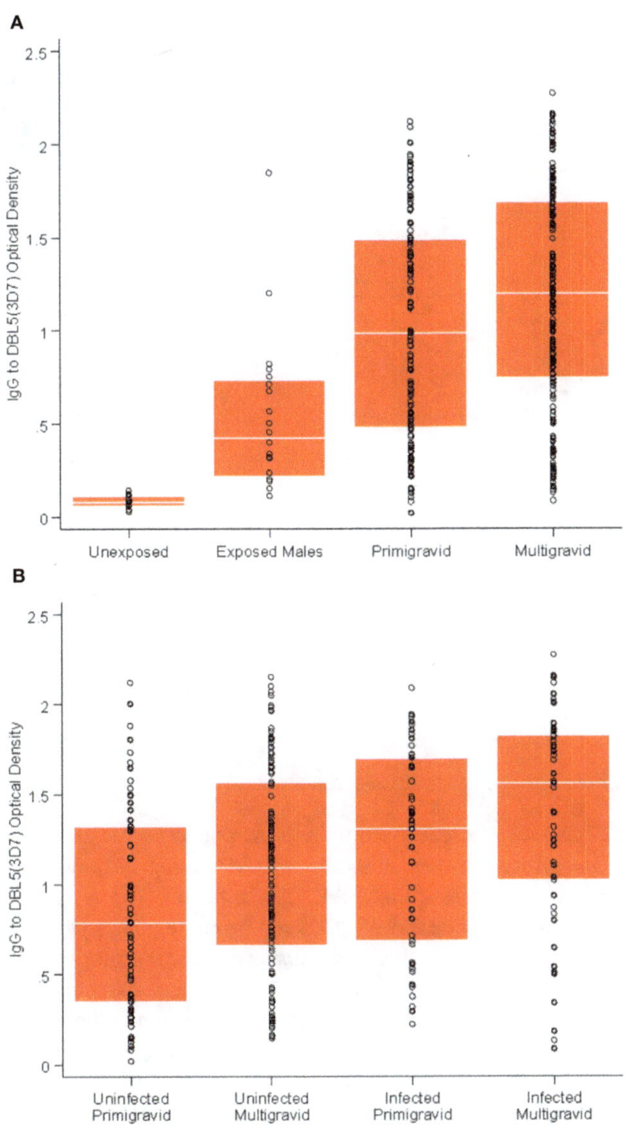

FIGURE 1 | VAR2CSA-specific antibodies are associated with gravidity and exposure. **(A)** Total IgG to DBL5 (3D7) in unexposed Melbourne controls (n = 30); exposed males from Papua New Guinea (n = 20); primigravid women (n = 115); and multigravid (n = 186) women. p = 0.03 for multigravid versus primigravid; p < 0.01 for all other comparisons. **(B)** Total IgG to DBL5 (3D7) in primigravid uninfected at enrolment (n = 66); primigravid infected at enrolment (n = 49); multigravid uninfected at enrolment (n = 132); and multigravid infected at enrolment (n = 54). p = 0.02 and p = 0.08 for multigravid versus primigravid (uninfected and infected respectively); p < 0.01 for infected versus uninfected (primigravid and multigravid respectively).

by *P. falciparum* infection at enrolment (**Supplementary Table S1**, likelihood ratio tests, p < 0.02 for DBL3 and DBL5; p = 0.11 for CS2-IE). Among women with infection detected at enrolment, women with higher levels of antibodies to VAR2CSA had lower adjusted odds of placental infection at delivery [**Figure 2**, Odds Ratio (OR) [95% confidence interval (CI)] = 0.6 (0.2,1.4); 0.2 (0.1,0.5); 0.6 (0.3,1.2); 0.8 (0.6,1.2) for DBL3 (7G8), DBL5 (3D7) and DBL5 (7G8) and CS2-IE respectively]. However, 95% CIs were wide and associations were generally not statistically significant [with the exception of DBL5 (3D7)]. In contrast, among women who were not infected at enrolment, higher levels of VAR2CSA antibodies were associated with an increased adjusted odds of placental infection (**Figure 2**, OR = 2.2 (1.2,4.3); 2.0 (1.0,3.8); 1.7 (1.0,3.1); 1.1 (0.8,1.5) for DBL3 (7G8), DBL5 (3D7) and DBL5 (7G8) and CS2-IE respectively). Levels of AMA1 antibodies (not specific to malaria in pregnancy), were not associated with odds of placental infection among infected women or uninfected women [OR = 0.9 (0.5,1.9) and 1.0 (0.6,1.7) respectively].

VAR2CSA IgG Levels Associated With Increased Birth Weight in Women Infected During Pregnancy

Moderate evidence for effect modification by infection at enrolment was observed for some VAR2CSA antibodies.

Among women infected at enrolment, higher levels of IgG to CS2-IEs, which represents IgG to full-length VAR2CSA (50), were associated with higher birth weight [+90g (20g-150g)] relative to women with lower antibody levels (**Figure 3** and **Supplementary Table S4**). Higher antibodies to VAR2CSA domains DBL5 (3D7 and 7G8) were also associated with higher birth weight [+150g (95% CI: 0g, +300g); +120g (-10g, +240g), respectively]. There was no clear association for DBL3 antibodies (+40g (-110g, + 180g)). The estimated association between levels of antibodies to AMA1 was not significant (-60g (95% CI: -180g, +60g). Among women without infection detected at enrolment, the estimated associations between higher levels of VAR2CSA antibodies and birth weight were close to zero (estimates -10g to +0g). There was very little evidence to support effect modification by gravidity (**Supplementary Table S5**, likelihood ratio tests, p >0.3). Estimates of the associations between VAR2CSA antibodies and gestational age at delivery were of small magnitude and were not significant (**Supplementary Tables S7-9**).

DISCUSSION

In this study, we investigated the association between anti-VAR2CSA antibody responses and pregnancy outcomes, examining the influence of infection with *P. falciparum* at enrolment as well as gravidity on these associations. Women infected at enrolment and women who had been pregnant before had higher levels of anti-VAR2CSA antibodies at enrolment compared to women who were uninfected at enrolment, and women in their first pregnancy, respectively. Among women who were infected with *P. falciparum* at enrolment, those with higher VAR2CSA antibody levels had higher birthweight babies and lower odds of odds of LBW relative to those with low levels. These findings suggest that when women experience *P. falciparum* infection during pregnancy, the ability to generate higher levels of VAR2CSA antibodies may lead to better pregnancy outcomes.

Findings from previous studies investigating the associations between anti-VAR2CSA antibody responses and improved birth outcomes have been inconsistent and contradictory (3, 16–27, 51). Most of the literature reporting positive associations

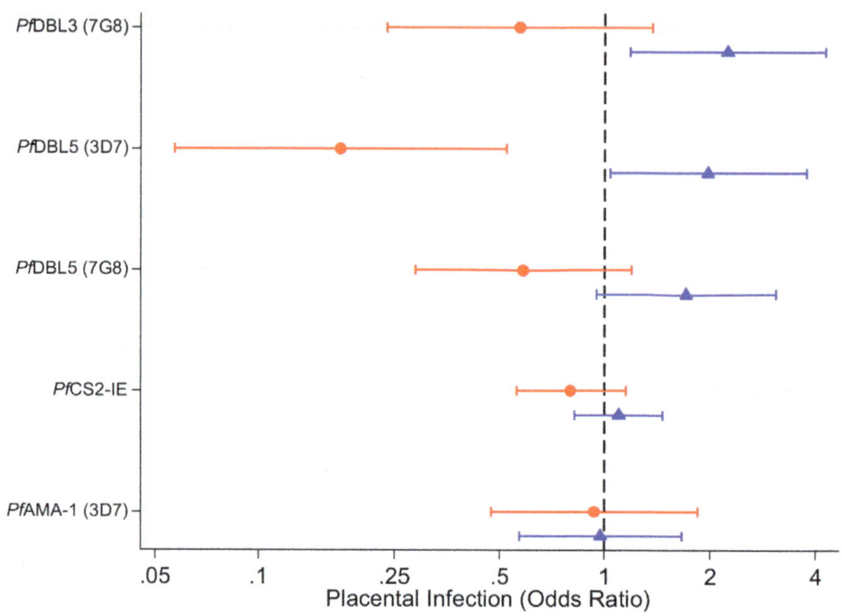

FIGURE 2 | Adjusted odds ratios for placental *P. falciparum* infection in individuals with high antibody levels (75th percentile) relative to individuals with low antibody levels (25th percentile) in women infected at enrolment (red circles) and uninfected at enrolment (blue triangles). Capped bars indicate 95% confidence intervals. See **Supplementary Table 1** for a table with p values. See **Supplementary Tables 2** and **3** for estimates from models fitted with an interaction between antibodies and gravidity; and for estimates from models fitted without an interaction term.

between anti-VAR2CSA antibodies and better birth outcomes have concentrated on particular subsets of infected women (3, 20–22, 27) or in particular strata of gravidity (19, 21), and often analyses were conducted as a cross-sectional study at delivery (15). Importantly, our analysis examined a cohort of pregnant women prospectively and formally tested for effect modification by *P. falciparum* infection and gravidity. This study supports the hypothesis that antibody responses to VAR2CSA are protective against lower birth weight, and possibly placental *P. falciparum* infection, but this protective association is only observed in women with evidence of *P. falciparum* infection at enrolment. Therefore, our findings suggest that women who generate higher antibody responses when infected in pregnancy have a reduced risk of low birthweight. That antibody levels in women with no peripheral blood *P. falciparum* infection at enrolment were instead associated with poor outcomes suggests that in this subset of women, antibodies are likely correlated with unmeasured recent infection, confounding any underlying protective association. Alternatively, it may be important to quantify antibodies during an active infection to better assess the nature and potential beneficial effects of antibody responses.

The strength of associations between antibody response to VAR2CSA and birth outcomes were broadly comparable across each measure of antibody response to VAR2CSA. It is beyond the scope of our immune-epidemiological study to be able to distinguish antibodies that have a truly protective role from antibodies that do not play a protective role but are associated with protection. However, a plausible role for antibodies to VAR2CSA in protective immunity is supported by the absence of any association between antibodies to AMA-1 and birth outcomes as well as observations that VAR2CSA antibodies can function to inhibit placental adhesion of PfIEs and promote phagocytosis (23, 52, 53). There may be other mechanisms that are not yet defined. A stronger association of antibodies specific for one domain relative to another domain may not indicate that these antibodies play a stronger direct role in protection. Strong associations with protection may indicate that these antibodies may be useful biomarkers for protective immunity. Further studies in multiple populations are needed to estimate the causal effect of single antibody responses and determine the importance of a repertoire of antibodies for maximal immunity. This knowledge will be valuable for informing vaccine approaches. Further assessment of functional mechanisms of protection (54, 55) for different epitopes or targets is warranted to clarify their role in the immune system in mediating protection. In this study, we only assessed antibodies to two VAR2CSA domains, DBL3 and DBL5. While these both are targets of acquired immunity and functionally-relevant antibodies (25, 39–44) and served the purpose of providing an assessment of responses to VAR2CSA in our study population, other domains have also been identified as targets of acquired immunity (25, 27). Detailed studies including an evaluation of all VAR2CSA domains and sub-domain could be valuable in future studies.

The longitudinal nature of this study allowed us to investigate a temporal relationship between the presence of antibodies mid-pregnancy at enrolment and subsequent adverse pregnancy outcomes, measured at delivery. Given that antibodies arise in

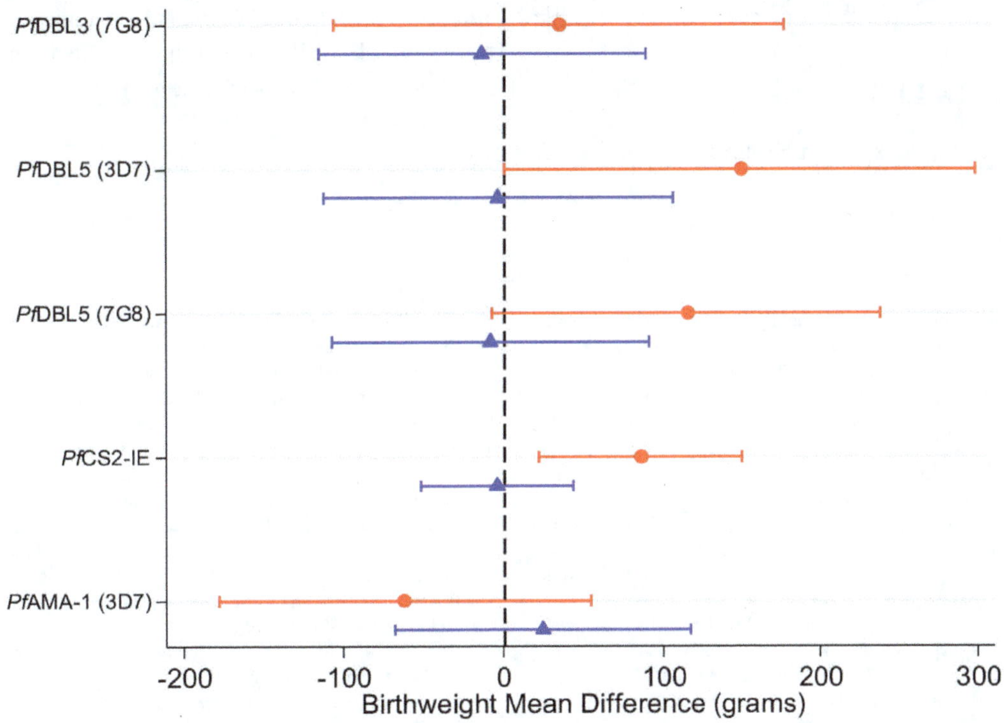

FIGURE 3 | Adjusted mean difference in birthweight (grams) in individuals with high antibody levels (75th percentile) relative to individuals with low antibody levels (25th percentile) in women infected at enrolment (red circles) and uninfected at enrolment (blue triangles). Capped bars indicate 95% confidence intervals. See **Supplementary Table 4** for a table with p values. See **Supplementary Tables 5** and **6** for estimates from models fitted with an interaction between antibodies and gravidity; and for estimates from models fitted without an interaction term.

response to exposure but may also serve a protective role against clinical malaria and adverse outcomes, it is difficult for cross-sectional studies (3, 16–22) to distinguish between women who have high antibody levels that reflect a recent infection and women who have high antibody levels that have successfully kept them infection free. In the absence of detailed exposure history, these studies will likely be subject to residual confounding by unmeasured exposure. A limitation of our study was measurement of *P. falciparum* exposure during, and prior to, the study; *P. falciparum* infection was only measured once using light microscopy and more frequent measurement of infection may have provided more accurate exposure data. Although these *P. falciparum* infections were observed during pregnancy, the acquisition of the infection will predate the moment it was detected, and some infections may have been present prior to conception. It is also possible that some women experienced undetected infections between recruitment and delivery and/or experienced and cleared infection prior to recruitment. This study was conducted in a setting where women received prophylaxis as part of their antenatal care which likely reduced *P. falciparum* infection and its negative effects during pregnancy. As such the magnitudes of protective effects of VAR2CSA immunity we observed may not be generalisable to other populations where malaria prophylaxis is not routinely given to pregnant women or in areas of different malaria endemicity.

In summary, we found that associations between VAR2CSA specific antibodies and birth outcomes varied across groups experiencing different levels of exposure. Among women who had already acquired infection by mid-pregnancy at enrolment, higher levels of antibodies to VAR2CSA were associated with a reduced risk of adverse outcomes. In contrast, among women uninfected at enrolment, anti-VAR2CSA antibodies may indicate women at increased risk of *P. falciparum* exposure and the adverse outcomes that follow. These differences in antibody associations due to exposure history might explain some of the conflicting reports in the published literature. Given the close relationship between exposure, antibodies and protection, ignoring heterogeneous exposure may obscure relevant protective associations. Future population studies should ensure the design and analysis accounts for the possibility of heterogeneous exposure.

AUTHOR CONTRIBUTIONS

JB, FF, SR, and IM designed the research. AM, HO, DS, GF, and AU performed the research, AM and HO analysed the data, and AM, HO, JC, JB, and FF wrote the manuscript with input from all authors. All authors contributed to the article and approved the submitted version. JC are members of the NHMRC-funded Australian Centre for Research Excellence in Malaria Elimination.

ACKNOWLEDGMENTS

We thank the staff of the Alexishafen Health Centre and PNG Institute of Medical Research for their assistance with the study particularly Francesca Baiwog (now deceased), Prof Peter Siba and Prof Willie Pomat. We thank Joe Smith and Marion Avril for provision of VAR2CSA antigens. We thank all the study participants for their participation.

REFERENCES

1. McLean AR, Ataide R, Simpson JA, Beeson JG, Fowkes FJ. Malaria and Immunity During Pregnancy and Postpartum: A Tale of Two Species. *Parasitology* (2015) 142:999–1015. doi: 10.1017/S0031182015000074
2. McGregor IA, Wilson ME, Billewicz WZ. Malaria Infection of the Placenta in The Gambia, West Africa; Its Incidence and Relationship to Stillbirth, Birthweight and Placental Weight. *Trans R Soc Trop Med Hyg* (1983) 77:232–44. doi: 10.1016/0035-9203(83)90081-0
3. Salanti A, Staalsoe T, Lavstsen T, Jensen AT, Sowa MP, Arnot DE, et al. Selective Upregulation of a Single Distinctly Structured Var Gene in Chondroitin Sulphate A-Adhering *Plasmodium falciparum* Involved in Pregnancy-Associated Malaria. *Mol Microbiol* (2003) 49:179–91. doi: 10.1046/j.1365-2958.2003.03570.x
4. Duffy MF, Caragounis A, Noviyanti R, Kyriacou HM, Choong EK, Boysen K, et al. Transcribed Var Genes Associated With Placental Malaria in Malawian Women. *Infect Immun* (2006) 74:4875–83. doi: 10.1128/IAI.01978-05
5. Tuikue Ndam NG, Salanti A, Bertin G, Dahlback M, Fievet N, Turner L, et al. High Level of var2csa Transcription by *Plasmodium falciparum* Isolated From the Placenta. *J Infect Dis* (2005) 192:331–5. doi: 10.1086/430933
6. Fried M, Duffy PE. Adherence of *Plasmodium falciparum* to Chondroitin Sulfate A in the Human Placenta. *Science* (1996) 272:1502–4. doi: 10.1126/science.272.5267.1502
7. Walter PR, Garin Y, Blot P. Placental Pathologic Changes in Malaria. A Histologic and Ultrastructural Study. *Am J Pathol* (1982) 109:330–42. doi: 10.1097/00006254-198308000-00008
8. Ataide R, Mayor A, Rogerson SJ. Malaria, Primigravidae, and Antibodies: Knowledge Gained and Future Perspectives. *Trends Parasitol* (2014) 30:85–94. doi: 10.1016/j.pt.2013.12.007
9. Oleinikov AV, Rossnagle E, Francis S, Mutabingwa TK, Fried M, Duffy PE. Effects of Sex, Parity, and Sequence Variation on Seroreactivity to Candidate Pregnancy Malaria Vaccine Antigens. *J Infect Dis* (2007) 196:155–64. doi: 10.1086/518513
10. Ricke CH, Staalsoe T, Koram K, Akanmori BD, Riley EM, Theander TG, et al. Plasma Antibodies From Malaria-Exposed Pregnant Women Recognize Variant Surface Antigens on *Plasmodium falciparum*-Infected Erythrocytes in a Parity-Dependent Manner and Block Parasite Adhesion to Chondroitin Sulfate a. *J Immunol* (2000) 165:3309–16. doi: 10.4049/jimmunol.165.6.3309
11. Fried M, Duffy PE. Maternal Malaria and Parasite Adhesion. *J Mol Med (Berlin Germany)* (1998) 76:162–71. doi: 10.1007/s001090050205
12. Beeson JG, Ndungu F, Persson KE, Chesson JM, Kelly GL, Uyoga S, et al. Antibodies Among Men and Children to Placental-Binding *Plasmodium falciparum*-Infected Erythrocytes That Express var2csa. *Am J Trop Med Hyg* (2007) 77:22–8. doi: 10.4269/ajtmh.2007.77.22
13. Chene A, Gangnard S, Guadall A, Ginisty H, Leroy O, Havelange N, et al. Preclinical Immunogenicity and Safety of the cGMP-Grade Placental Malaria Vaccine PRIMVAC. *EBioMedicine* (2019) 42:145–56. doi: 10.1016/j.ebiom.2019.03.010
14. Mordmuller B, Sulyok M, Egger-Adam D, Resende M, de Jongh WA, Jensen MH, et al. First-in-Human, Randomized, Double-Blind Clinical Trial of Differentially Adjuvanted PAMVAC, A Vaccine Candidate to Prevent Pregnancy-Associated Malaria. *Clin Infect Dis* (2019) 69:1509–16. doi: 10.1093/cid/ciy1140
15. Cutts JC, Agius PA, Zaw L, Powell R, Moore K, Draper B, et al. Pregnancy-Specific Malarial Immunity and Risk of Malaria in Pregnancy and Adverse Birth Outcomes: A Systematic Review. *BMC Med* (2020) 18:14. doi: 10.1186/s12916-019-1467-6
16. Serra-Casas E, Menendez C, Bardaji A, Quinto L, Dobano C, Sigauque B, et al. The Effect of Intermittent Preventive Treatment During Pregnancy on Malarial Antibodies Depends on HIV Status and Is Not Associated With Poor Delivery Outcomes. *J Infect Dis* (2010) 201:123–31. doi: 10.1086/648595
17. Ataide R, Hasang W, Wilson DW, Beeson JG, Mwapasa V, Molyneux ME, et al. Using an Improved Phagocytosis Assay to Evaluate the Effect of HIV on Specific Antibodies to Pregnancy-Associated Malaria. *PloS One* (2010) 5: e10807. doi: 10.1371/journal.pone.0010807
18. Beeson JG, Mann EJ, Elliott SR, Lema VM, Tadesse E, Molyneux ME, et al. Antibodies to Variant Surface Antigens of *Plasmodium falciparum*-Infected Erythrocytes and Adhesion Inhibitory Antibodies Are Associated With Placental Malaria and Have Overlapping and Distinct Targets. *J Infect Dis* (2004) 189:540–51. doi: 10.1086/381186
19. Duffy PE, Fried M. Antibodies That Inhibit Plasmodium falciparum Adhesion to Chondroitin Sulfate A Are Associated With Increased Birth Weight and the Gestational Age of Newborns. *Infect Immun* (2003) 71:6620–3. doi: 10.1128/IAI.71.11.6620-6623.2003
20. Staalsoe T, Shulman CE, Bulmer JN, Kawuondo K, Marsh K, Hviid L. Variant Surface Antigen-Specific IgG and Protection Against Clinical Consequences of Pregnancy-Associated *Plasmodium falciparum* Malaria. *Lancet* (2004) 363:283–9. doi: 10.1016/S0140-6736(03)15386-X
21. Ataide R, Mwapasa V, Molyneux ME, Meshnick SR, Rogerson SJ. Antibodies That Induce Phagocytosis of Malaria Infected Erythrocytes: Effect of HIV Infection and Correlation With Clinical Outcomes. *PloS One* (2011) 6:e22491. doi: 10.1371/journal.pone.0022491
22. Mayor A, Kumar U, Bardaji A, Gupta P, Jimenez A, Hamad A, et al. Improved Pregnancy Outcomes in Women Exposed to Malaria With High Antibody Levels Against *Plasmodium falciparum*. *J Infect Dis* (2013) 207:1664–74. doi: 10.1093/infdis/jit083
23. Feng G, Aitken E, Yosaatmadja F, Kalilani L, Meshnick SR, Jaworowski A, et al. Antibodies to Variant Surface Antigens of *Plasmodium falciparum*-Infected Erythrocytes are Associated With Protection From Treatment Failure and the Development of Anemia in Pregnancy. *J Infect Dis* (2009) 200:299–306. doi: 10.1086/599841
24. Chandrasiri UP, Fowkes FJ, Beeson JG, Richards JS, Kamiza S, Maleta K, et al. Association Between Malaria Immunity and Pregnancy Outcomes Among Malawian Pregnant Women Receiving Nutrient Supplementation. *Malar J* (2016) 15:547. doi: 10.1186/s12936-016-1597-7
25. Tuikue Ndam NG, Salanti A, Le-Hesran JY, Cottrell G, Fievet N, Turner L, et al. Dynamics of Anti-VAR2CSA Immunoglobulin G Response in a Cohort of Senegalese Pregnant Women. *J Infect Dis* (2006) 193:713–20. doi: 10.1086/500146
26. Aitken EH, Mbewe B, Luntamo M, Maleta K, Kulmala T, Friso MJ, et al. Antibodies to Chondroitin Sulfate A-Binding Infected Erythrocytes: Dynamics and Protection During Pregnancy in Women Receiving Intermittent Preventive Treatment. *J Infect Dis* (2010) 201:1316–25. doi: 10.1086/651578
27. Ndam NT, Denoeud-Ndam L, Doritchamou J, Viwami F, Salanti A, Nielsen MA, et al. Protective Antibodies Against Placental Malaria and Poor Outcomes During Pregnancy, Benin. *Emerg Infect Dis* (2015) 21:813–23. doi: 10.3201/eid2105.141626
28. Rijken MJ, McGready R, Boel ME, Poespoprodjo R, Singh N, Syafruddin D, et al. Malaria in Pregnancy in the Asia-Pacific Region. *Lancet Infect Dis* (2012) 12:75–88. doi: 10.1016/S1473-3099(11)70315-2
29. Stanisic DI, Moore KA, Baiwog F, Ura A, Clapham C, King CL, et al. Risk Factors

for Malaria and Adverse Birth Outcomes in a Prospective Cohort of Pregnant Women Resident in a High Malaria Transmission Area of Papua New Guinea. *Trans R Soc Trop Med Hyg* (2015) 109:313–24. doi: 10.1093/trstmh/trv019

30. Bulmer JN, Rasheed FN, Francis N, Morrison L, Greenwood BM. Placental malaria. I. Pathological Classification. *Histopathology* (1993) 22:211–8. doi: 10.1111/j.1365-2559.1993.tb00110.x
31. Bulmer JN, Rasheed FN, Morrison L, Francis N, Greenwood BM. Placental Malaria. II. A Semi-Quantitative Investigation of the Pathological Features. *Histopathology* (1993) 22:219–25. doi: 10.1111/j.1365-2559.1993.tb00111.x
32. Hommel M, Elliott SR, Soma V, Kelly G, Fowkes FJ, Chesson JM, et al. Evaluation of the Antigenic Diversity of Placenta-Binding Plasmodium falciparum Variants and the Antibody Repertoire Among Pregnant Women. *Infect Immun* (2010) 78:1963–78. doi: 10.1128/IAI.01365-09
33. Duffy MF, Byrne TJ, Elliott SR, Wilson DW, Rogerson SJ, Beeson JG, et al. Broad Analysis Reveals a Consistent Pattern of Var Gene Transcription in *Plasmodium falciparum* Repeatedly Selected for a Defined Adhesion Phenotype. *Mol Microbiol* (2005) 56:774–88. doi: 10.1111/j.1365-2958.2005.04577.x
34. Beeson JG, Mann EJ, Byrne TJ, Caragounis A, Elliott SR, Brown GV, et al. Antigenic Differences and Conservation Among Placental *Plasmodium falciparum*-Infected Erythrocytes and Acquisition of Variant-Specific and Cross-Reactive Antibodies. *J Infect Dis* (2006) 193:721–30. doi: 10.1086/500145
35. Elliott SR, Brennan AK, Beeson JG, Tadesse E, Molyneux ME, Brown GV, et al. Placental Malaria Induces Variant-Specific Antibodies of the Cytophilic Subtypes Immunoglobulin G1 (IgG1) and IgG3 That Correlate With Adhesion Inhibitory Activity. *Infect Immun* (2005) 73:5903–7. doi: 10.1128/IAI.73.9.5903-5907.2005
36. Chan JA, Howell KB, Reiling L, Ataide R, Mackintosh CL, Fowkes FJ, et al. Targets of Antibodies Against *Plasmodium falciparum*-Infected Erythrocytes in Malaria Immunity. *J Clin Invest* (2012) 122:3227–38. doi: 10.1172/JCI62182
37. Persson KE, McCallum FJ, Reiling L, Lister NA, Stubbs J, Cowman AF, et al. Variation in Use of Erythrocyte Invasion Pathways by *Plasmodium falciparum* Mediates Evasion of Human Inhibitory Antibodies. *J Clin Invest* (2008) 118:342–51. doi: 10.1172/JCI32138
38. Avril M, Hathaway MJ, Cartwright MM, Gose SO, Narum DL, Smith JD. Optimizing Expression of the Pregnancy Malaria Vaccine Candidate, VAR2CSA in *Pichia pastoris*. *Malar J* (2009) 8:143. doi: 10.1186/1475-2875-8-143
39. Tutterrow YL, Avril M, Singh K, Long CA, Leke RJ, Sama G, et al. High Levels of Antibodies to Multiple Domains and Strains of VAR2CSA Correlate With the Absence of Placental Malaria in Cameroonian Women Living in an Area of High *Plasmodium falciparum* Transmission. *Infect Immun* (2012) 80:1479–90. doi: 10.1128/IAI.00071-12
40. Salanti A, Dahlback M, Turner L, Nielsen MA, Barfod L, Magistrado P, et al. Evidence for the Involvement of VAR2CSA in Pregnancy-Associated Malaria. *J Exp Med* (2004) 200:1197–203. doi: 10.1084/jem.20041579
41. Fernandez P, Petres S, Mecheri S, Gysin J, Scherf A. Strain-Transcendent Immune Response to Recombinant Var2CSA DBL5-Epsilon Domain Block *P. falciparum* Adhesion to Placenta-Derived BeWo Cells Under Flow Conditions. *PloS One* (2010) 5:e12558. doi: 10.1371/journal.pone.0012558
42. Oleinikov AV, Francis SE, Dorfman JR, Rossnagle E, Balcaitis S, Getz T, et al. VAR2CSA Domains Expressed in *Escherichia coli* Induce Cross-Reactive Antibodies to Native Protein. *J Infect Dis* (2008) 197:1119–23. doi: 10.1086/529526
43. Andersen P, Nielsen MA, Resende M, Rask TS, Dahlback M, Theander T, et al. Structural Insight Into Epitopes in the Pregnancy-Associated Malaria Protein VAR2CSA. *PloS Pathog* (2008) 4:e42. doi: 10.1371/journal.ppat.0040042
44. Hommel M, Chan JA, Umbers AJ, Langer C, Rogerson SJ, Smith JD, et al. Evaluating Antibody Functional Activity and Strain-Specificity of Vaccine Candidates for Malaria in Pregnancy Using *In Vitro* Phagocytosis Assays. *Parasites Vectors* (2018) 11:69. doi: 10.1186/s13071-018-2653-7
45. Stanisic DI, Richards JS, McCallum FJ, Michon P, King CL, Schoepflin S, et al. Immunoglobulin G Subclass-Specific Responses Against *Plasmodium falciparum* Merozoite Antigens Are Associated With Control of Parasitemia and Protection From Symptomatic Illness. *Infect Immun* (2009) 77:1165–74. doi: 10.1128/IAI.01129-08
46. Beeson JG, Brown GV. *Plasmodium falciparum*-Infected Erythrocytes Demonstrate Dual Specificity for Adhesion to Hyaluronic Acid and Chondroitin Sulfate A and Have Distinct Adhesive Properties. *J Infect Dis* (2004) 189:169–79. doi: 10.1086/380975
47. Rogerson SJ, Chaiyaroj SC, Ng K, Reeder JC, Brown GV. Chondroitin Sulfate A Is a Cell Surface Receptor for *Plasmodium falciparum*-Infected Erythrocytes. *J Exp Med* (1995) 182:15–20. doi: 10.1084/jem.182.1.15
48. Kinyanjui SM, Howard T, Williams TN, Bull PC, Newbold CI, Marsh K. The Use of Cryopreserved Mature Trophozoites in Assessing Antibody Recognition of Variant Surface Antigens of *Plasmodium falciparum*-Infected Erythrocytes. *J Immunol Methods* (2004) 288:9–18. doi: 10.1016/j.jim.2004.01.022
49. Williamson EJ, Aitken Z, Lawrie J, Dharmage SC, Burgess JA, Forbes AB. Introduction to Causal Diagrams for Confounder Selection. *Respirology* (2014) 19:303–11. doi: 10.1111/resp.12238
50. Chan JA, Fowkes FJ, Beeson JG. Surface Antigens of *Plasmodium falciparum*-Infected Erythrocytes as Immune Targets and Malaria Vaccine Candidates. *Cell Mol Life Sci CMLS* (2014) 71:3633–57. doi: 10.1007/s00018-014-1614-3
51. Requena P, Arevalo-Herrera M, Menegon M, Martinez-Espinosa FE, Padilla N, Botto-Menezes C, et al. Naturally Acquired Binding-Inhibitory Antibodies to *Plasmodium vivax* Duffy Binding Protein in Pregnant Women Are Associated With Higher Birth Weight in a Multicenter Study. *Front Immunol* (2017) 8:163. doi: 10.3389/fimmu.2017.00163
52. Barfod L, Dobrilovic T, Magistrado P, Khunrae P, Viwami F, Bruun J, et al. Chondroitin Sulfate A-Adhering *Plasmodium falciparum*-Infected Erythrocytes Express Functionally Important Antibody Epitopes Shared by Multiple Variants. *J Immunol* (2010) 185:7553–61. doi: 10.4049/jimmunol.1002390
53. Fried M, Nosten F, Brockman A, Brabin BJ, Duffy PE. Maternal Antibodies Block Malaria. *Nature* (1998) 395:851–2. doi: 10.1038/27570
54. Boyle MJ, Reiling L, Feng G, Langer C, Osier FH, Aspeling-Jones H, et al. Human Antibodies Fix Complement to Inhibit *Plasmodium falciparum* Invasion of Erythrocytes and Are Associated With Protection Against Malaria. *Immunity* (2015) 42:580–90. doi: 10.1016/j.immuni.2015.02.012
55. Irani V, Ramsland PA, Guy AJ, Siba PM, Mueller I, Richards JS, et al. Acquisition of Functional Antibodies That Block the Binding of Erythrocyte-Binding Antigen 175 and Protection Against *Plasmodium falciparum* Malaria in Children. *Clin Infect Dis* (2015) 61:1244–52. doi: 10.1093/cid/civ525

14

Vaccines in Congenital Toxoplasmosis: Advances and Perspectives

*Mariana Barros [1], Daniela Teixeira [1], Manuel Vilanova [2,3,4], Alexandra Correia [2,3,4], Natercia Teixeira [5] and Margarida Borges [5]**

[1] Departamento de Ciências Biológicas, Faculdade de Farmácia, Universidade do Porto, Porto, Portugal, [2] Immunobiology Group, Instituto de Investigação e Inovação em Saúde (i3S), Universidade do Porto, Porto, Portugal, [3] Instituto de Biologia Molecular e Celular (IBMC), Universidade do Porto, Porto, Portugal, [4] Departamento de Imuno-Fisiologia e Farmacologia, Instituto de Ciências Biomédicas Abel Salazar (ICBAS), Universidade do Porto, Porto, Portugal, [5] Applied Molecular Biosciences Unit/Rede de Química e Tecnologia (UCIBIO/REQUIMTE), Departamento de Ciências Biológicas, Faculdade de Farmácia, Universidade do Porto, Porto, Portugal

***Correspondence:**
Margarida Borges
mborges@ff.up.pt

Congenital toxoplasmosis has a high impact on human disease worldwide, inducing serious consequences from fetus to adulthood. Despite this, there are currently no human vaccines available to prevent this infection. Most vaccination studies against *Toxoplasma gondii* infection used animal models in which the infection was established by exogenous inoculation. Here, we review recent research on potential *T. gondii* vaccines using animal models in which infection was congenitally established. Endeavors in this field have so far revealed that live or subunit vaccines previously found to confer protection against extrinsically established infections can also protect, at least partially, from vertically transmitted infection. Nevertheless, there is no consensus on the more adequate immune response to protect the host and the fetus in congenital infection. Most of the vaccination studies rely on the assessment of maternal systemic immune responses, quantification of parasitic loads in the fetuses, and survival indexes and/or brain parasitic burden in the neonates. More research must be carried out not only to explore new vaccines but also to further study the nature of the elicited immune protection at the maternal-fetal interface. Particularly, the cellular and molecular effector mechanisms at the maternal-fetal interface induced by immunization remain poorly characterized. Deeper knowledge on the immune response at this specific location will certainly help to refine the vaccine-induced immunity and, consequently, to provide the most effective and safest protection against *T. gondii* vertical infection.

Keywords: pregnancy, toxoplasmosis, congenital, vaccination, maternal-fetal

INTRODUCTION

Toxoplasma gondii is an obligate intracellular protozoan parasite and the etiologic agent of congenital toxoplasmosis. *T. gondii* is considered one of the most successful parasites worldwide, infecting over 30% of the human population, with high associated disease burden (1, 2). Seroprevalence varies greatly from region to region, ranging from approximately 30% in the American, European, and Asiatic regions, to more than 60% in the African continent (3, 4). The disease is potentially dangerous in women who become infected during pregnancy, as it can lead to transplacental transmission of the parasite upon primary infection or re-infection with highly virulent strains (5, 6). The incidence of congenital toxoplasmosis varies according to the timing of infection during pregnancy. The transmission rate is greater in the final stages of pregnancy, but the severity of infection is greater in early gestation (7). In the more severe cases, hydrocephalus, chorioretinitis, and cerebral calcification may occur, according to the parasite's brain and ocular tropism (5). An association between congenital infection and the development of neurological and psychiatric disorders later in life, including schizophrenia, Alzheimer's disease, bipolar disease, and even suicidal tendencies has also been suggested (8, 9).

Innate and adaptive immunity determines protection against *T. gondii* infection. An effective immune response must control parasite growth while avoiding immunopathology. In both mice and humans, the IL-12- IFN-γ axis is the main immune mechanism responsible for parasite control. Protection mediated by IFN-γ produced by NK and Th1 cells induces the expression of immunity-related GTPase and/or guanylate-binding proteins, indoleamine-2,3-dioxygenase, and NO production. TNF-α has also been associated with host protection, as highlighted in patients with defective IFN-γ signaling (10). TGF-β, IL-6, and IL-23 promote the production of IL-17 that may also play a host protective role in toxoplasmosis by avoiding excessive IFN-γ-dependent inflammation (11). T cells producing IL-10, which include T regulatory cells and Foxp3$^-$T-bet$^+$ Th1 cells, can limit excessive inflammation driven by *T. gondii* (12). A regulatory role for IL-4, and IL-27 in minimizing host tissue injury due to exacerbated inflammation has also been shown (10, 13). A good vaccine candidate would thus induce not only IL-12 and IFN-γ, but also counterbalancing cytokines such as IL-4, IL-10, and IL-27 (14).

It is important to note that there are no licensed human vaccines able to prevent toxoplasmosis (15). The lack of effective treatment makes the development of a vaccine against congenital toxoplasmosis one of the main objectives in the management of this disease. Here, recent findings in vaccination approaches to congenital toxoplasmosis using animal models of vertical *T. gondii* infection will be reviewed and the possible implications in the quest for a vaccine protecting from congenital toxoplasmosis will be discussed.

IN VIVO MODELS TO STUDY CONGENITAL INFECTION

In the study of toxoplasmosis, animal models are used to better understand the disease pathology and the immunological mechanisms induced by infection, as well as to assess the effectiveness of experimental vaccination. However, no single animal model has, so far, been able to mimic all clinical symptoms and signs developed by humans in response to *T. gondii* infection (16). For congenital toxoplasmosis, the murine model is commonly used as it allows a short pregnancy period and mimics features of human congenital toxoplasmosis, namely the co-localization of inflammatory cells and necrosis at the maternal-fetal interface after primo-infection during pregnancy (17). Further, primo-infection confers resistance to maternal fetal transmission throughout later infections (16). However, the immune response to *T. gondii* in mice and humans presents distinct features and this should be adequately considered (18, 19).

Most vaccination studies in congenital infection reviewed here used Kunming, BALB/c, Swiss OF1, and CBA/J mice. No study was found using the C57BL/6 mouse strain. This might be due to excessive susceptibility to disease exhibited by *T. gondii* infected C57BL/6 mice. In contrast, BALB/c mice present higher resistance to infection, more closely resembling humans, rendering this strain more suitable for vaccination studies in congenital infection models (20–22). In murine congenital toxoplasmosis, C57BL/6 mice exhibited higher abortion rate compared to BALB/c due to exacerbated proinflammatory cytokines such as TNF-α (23). Mouse strain differences in major histocompatibility complex haplotypes (*e.g.*, H-2^b, H-2^d, H-2^k for C57BL/6, BALB/c, and CBA/J, respectively), and therefore, antigenic presentation, could explain different susceptibility to *T. gondii* infection and induced immunopathology (20).

Other animal models can be used such as sheep, rats, guinea pig, or hamster (24–28). Rats and sheep are widely used in studies addressing drug effectiveness to *T. gondii* (18). Rats have placental development and hemochorial placentation identical to humans (29). In sheep, congenital toxoplasmosis is very similar to what occurs in humans (15). Thus, sheep is an adequate animal model to study congenital toxoplasmosis, not only because it shares important aspects with the human infection, but also because it directly contributes to the study of new disease control measures in livestock, also severely affected by *T. gondii* (15). There are well established models of toxoplasmosis in pregnant sheep that provide a starting point for the preparation and testing of new vaccines (15).

VACCINES IN VERTICAL INFECTION

This section aims to describe the vaccines already tested in congenital infection models, and to reveal the gap of analysis concerning immune cells and related mechanisms induced by immunization at the level of maternal-fetal interface as wells as in the neonates. Literature research was performed through a PubMed search, using the query "[(*Toxoplasma gondii*) AND (vaccine)] AND (congenital toxoplasmosis [title/abstract])". The results presented pertain to studies using pregnant mice where protection and immune responses of pregnant mice and their offspring was evaluated.

Live-Attenuated Vaccines

Live-attenuated vaccines have been the most studied in the context of congenital transmission (**Table 1**). These vaccines consist of parasites with reduced virulence but are nevertheless capable of inducing an immune response (36). Alternatively,

TABLE 1 | Live-attenuated vaccines tested in vertical *Toxoplasma gondii* infection models.

Strain/animal	Immunogen/strain/ delivery	Day of mating post-immunization	ChallengePregnancy day/route/#parasite form/Strain	Dam sacrifice	Maternal parameters	Progeny parameters	Highlighted results	References
Swiss OF1/ mice*	20 tachyzoites Δ*mic1-3*/ RH/ ip	Day 60	Day 11/oral/ 45 cysts/ 76K strain	-Day 17 of pregnancy (exp#1) -1 month after delivery (exp#2)	-Toxoplasma specific IgG levels -*Ex-vivo* splenocyte specific cytokine production (exp#1) -Brain cyst load (exp#2)	-Fetus parasite load (exp#1) -Survival of neonates and mean weight of pups at day 11 after birth -Brain cyst load at day 35 after birth (exp#2).	-Potent maternal humoral and Th1 responses. -Decreased fetus parasite load and, maternal and neonate brain parasite load. -100% Neonate survival and higher pups weight.	(30)
Bizet, Romanov, and Solognot/ ewes**	10^5(exp#1), $2x10^6$ (exp#2), and 10^5 (exp#3) tachyzoites Δ*mic1-3*/ RH/ sc (exp#1, #2) and ip (exp#3)	Day 60	~ Day 75 (mid gestation)/ oral/ 400 sporulated oocysts (exp#1, #2), 100 sporulated oocysts (exp#3)/ PRU strain	~ Day 135 of pregnancy (exp#1, #3)	-Seroconversion after immunization and before pregnancy (exp#1, #2, #3) -Evaluation of infection clinical signs (febrile response) (exp#1, #2, #3) -Brain cyst load (exp#1, 3)	-Number of non-viable and viable lambs. -Evaluation of abortion. -Mean weights of viable lambs. -Brain cyst load in lambs.	-Maternal seroconversion and lower febrile response. -Protection against *T. gondii* abortion and higher rate of viable lambs. -Decreased brain parasite load in vaccinated ewes and in the lambs.	(31)
Kunming/mice	$5x10^4$ tachyzoites Δ*gra17*/ RH/ ip	Day 70	-Day 12/oral/ 10 Cysts/Pru strain (exp#1) -Day 18/ip/ 200 tachyzoites/ RH strain (exp#2)	-Day 18 of pregnancy (exp#1) -Day 30 after delivery (exp#2)	-*Ex-vivo* splenocyte specific cytokine production (exp#1) -Brain cyst load (exp#2)	-Litter size and survival of delivered pups at birth and 5 days after birth (exp#2). -Body weight 35 days after birth (exp#1) and 5 days after birth (exp#2). -Brain cyst burden in pups at 35 days after birth.	-Higher maternal IFN-γ, IL-12, and IL-10 productions. -Decreased maternal brain parasite load and no clinical signs in immunized dams. -Protection against *T. gondii* abortion. -Higher litter sizes of viable neonates, survival rate and body weight. -Decreased pup brain parasite load.	(32)
Kunming/mice	10^6 tachyzoites Δ*gra17*Δ*npt1*/ RH/ ip	Day 60	Day 5/oral/ 10 cysts/ Pru strain	Day 30 after delivery	Brain cyst load.	-Litter size and survival rates of delivered pups at birth and 30 days after birth - Body weight 30 days after birth. -Brain cysts burden in pups at 30 after birth.	-Decreased maternal brain parasite load. -No abortions in immunized mice. -Increased litter size, pups survival rate, and body weight.	(33)
Kunming/mice	500 tachyzoites Δ*cdpk2*/ Pru/ ip	Day 70	Day 12/oral/ 10 cysts /Pru strain	-Day 18 of pregnancy (exp#1) -Day 5 after delivery (exp#2)	-*Ex-vivo* splenocyte specific cytokine (exp#1). -Brain cyst load (exp#2).	-Litter size and survival of delivered pups at birth and 35 after birth. - Body weight 35 days after birth. - Brain cysts burden in pups at 35 after birth.	-Higher maternal IFN-γ, IL-2, IL-12, and IL-10 production. - Decreased maternal brain parasite load. - Higher litter sizes of viable neonates, survival rate, and body weight. -Decreased pup brain parasite load.	(34)

(Continued)

TABLE 1 | Continued

Strain/animal	Immunogen/strain/delivery	Day of mating post-immunization	ChallengePregnancy day/route/#parasite form/Strain	Dam sacrifice	Maternal parameters	Progeny parameters	Highlighted results	References
Kunming/mice	10^6 tachyzoites Δ*tkl1*/ RH/ ip	Day 60	Day 5/oral/ 10 oocysts/ Pru strain	Day 30 after delivery	Brain cyst load	Evaluation of abortion.	-Healthy dams and decreased maternal brain parasite load. - Protection against *T. gondii* abortion. - Higher litter sizes of viable neonates.	(35)

**Mice: pregnancy length of 21 days; ** ewes: pregnancy length of 152 days. MIC1-3KO: micronemal protein 1 and 3 double deletion mutant; ΔGRA17: dense granule protein 17 deletion mutant; Δgra17Δnpt1/: dense granule protein 17 (gra17) and novel putative transporter (npt1) double deletion mutant; ΔCDPK2: calcium-dependent protein kinase 2 (cdpk2) deletion mutant; Δtkl1: tyrosine kinase-like 1 (tkl1) deletion mutant. RH strain (type I); 76K and PRU strains: type II: ip: intraperitoneal; sc: subcutaneous. exp#1: experimental design 1; exp#2: experimental design 2.*

attenuated virulent strains can also be used, albeit, in this case, the attenuation must be complete to ensure that the vaccine will not cause the disease (37). These vaccines present several advantages, such as using whole parasites, meaning that multiple antigens are available simultaneously. Live vaccines also do not usually require repeated immunizations or the use of adjuvants. However, a concern in using this type of vaccination is the possibility of reversing the parasite to a virulent state causing infection (36). Moreover, live vaccines are not recommended to be used in immunocompromised hosts. Toxovax®, the only licensed vaccine for toxoplasmosis, administered to avoid abortion in sheep, is a live-attenuated vaccine, using the strain S48 tachyzoites, originally isolated from an aborted lamb in New Zealand (14). This vaccine is not licensed for humans due to the possibility of parasite reversion to its virulent form (38). Moreover, it has a short shelf life and does not lead to full parasite elimination (14).

Live-attenuated vaccines may be produced by gene targeted approaches. Such is the case of a modified RH strain lacking two genes, respectively encoding micronemal protein 1 (MIC1), which associates to MICs 4 and 6, rendering them active, and MIC3, a micronemal protein necessary for host cell invasion and MIC8 function. The double deletion of these genes (Δ*mic1-3*) resulted in the loss of function of these five proteins. Female Swiss OF1 mice immunized with Δ*mic1-3* strain exhibited higher levels of IFN-γ and IL-2 and a smaller number of brain cysts compared to non-immunized mice when infected with *T. gondii*. Also, all pups born from immunized animals survived compared to 64% of non-immunized mice. Moreover, 55% of the pups born from immunized mice did not present brain cysts and those with brain cysts exhibited a 91% reduction of cyst burden (30). This vaccine was also tested in Bizet, Romanov, and Solognot ewes, using the same experimental design but adapted to the ewes' pregnancy length. It showed to be effective by both subcutaneous (sc) and intraperitoneal (ip) routes, inducing protection against abortion, a higher rate of viable lambs and a decrease of brain parasite cysts in the lambs born from vaccinated ewes (31). Wang *et al.* attempted immunization before pregnancy with a live attenuated vaccine, using tachyzoites of the RH strain with a deletion of the dense granule protein 17 (*GRA17*) gene (Δ*gra17*) that had previously shown to protect mice from lethal infection (32). The deletion entailed a defective parasitophorous vacuole (PV) and decreased intravacuolar tachyzoite proliferation, due to interference with protein transport across the PV membrane. Ip immunization with Δ*gra17* strain elicited the production of Th1-type response cytokines, IL-12, and IFN-γ, as well as of IL-10 in Kunming mice (32). Thereafter, the same authors have tested this vaccine against vertical transmission using both acute and chronic infection models. No maternal clinical signs of infection and abortion were found and the litter sizes of viable neonates in immunized and RH inoculated dams were higher. In both models of infection, pups presented a higher survival rate. Maternal spleen *T. gondii*-induced cytokine production was evaluated at day 18 of pregnancy, 6 days after infection with Pru strain. Higher levels of Th1-type cytokines IFN-γ, IL-12, and IL-2, and of IL-10 were detected. Significantly lower parasite burden was found in the brain of immunized dams. Further, partial protection was observed, concerning brain parasite load in the progeny of these animals (32). Recently, a live-attenuated vaccine of the RH strain was engineered to harbor a deletion of *Gra17* and of novel putative transporter 1 (*NPT1*) gene, encoding a selective arginine transporter (33). The virulence of this strain (RHΔ*gra17*Δ*npt1*) was completely attenuated *in vivo*. The brain cyst burden of immunized dams was significantly lower and no abortions were observed compared with non-immunized infected mice. All pups born from immunized infected mice had about 15 times fewer brain cysts than non-immunized infected mice pups (33).

A live-attenuated vaccine using tachyzoites of the Pru strain with a deletion of the calcium-dependent protein kinase 2 (*CDPK2*) gene (Δ*cdpk2*) was also developed by Wang *et al.* (34). CDPKs harbored by *T. gondii* are required for cell invasion and gliding motility and are important virulence factors. Specifically, CDPK2 prevents accumulation of amylopectin to toxic levels in the cell, that would cause the parasite to be morphologically defective and unable to form cysts. Therefore, these parasites were incapable of establishing chronic infection since they were not able to form tissue cysts. Dam brain cyst burden was, in average, 43 times lower than that of non-immunized challenged dams. Splenocytes from immunized dams produced higher levels of IFN-γ, IL-2, IL-12, and IL-10 compared with non-immunized mice when stimulated *in vitro* with soluble tachyzoite antigen. These results indicated that this vaccination approach led to a balanced pro- and counter-inflammatory maternal response, useful to control infection but also to avoid potentially harmful excessive inflammation. Pups from non-immunized infected mice harbored in average 919 ± 339 brain cysts, whereas only 41.4% of the pups from immunized infected mice harbored cysts, averaging 60 ± 33 cyst per brain (34). Recently, Wang *et al.* created a live-attenuated vaccine from the *T. gondii* RH strain with a deletion of the tyrosine kinase-like 1 (*TKL1*) gene (RHΔ*tkl1*) (35). Vaccinated Kunming mice remained without clinical signs of infection and showed significant decrease in brain cyst burden 30 days after delivery. No abortions occurred and litter size was unaltered in immunized mice when infected, while all non-immunized infected mice suffered abortions. A decreased brain cyst load was observed in the pups from immunized infected dams indicating reduced vertical transmission (35).

Recombinant Protein Vaccines

Recombinant *T. gondii* surface antigen 1 (rSAG1) protein (39) was assessed in two models of congenital infection (**Table 2**). Haumont *et al.* immunized Dunkin-Hartley guinea pigs subcutaneously (sc) with rSAG1 three times at 3-week intervals and intradermally challenged 3 weeks after breeding (25). Vaccination induced protection against maternal-fetal transmission as assessed by the brain parasite load in the live pups. However, the SAG1-specific IgG levels in newborn pups did not correlate with protection, while cellular responses were not evaluated (25). In another study, BALB/c and CBA/J mice (*H2*^{d} and *H2*^{k} background, respectively) were sc immunized twice with rSAG1 (40). A reduction of 50% of maternal-fetal transmission in BALB/c, but not in CBA/J mice, was observed. Protection found in immunized BALB/c mice correlated with a maternal increase in rSAG1-specific IgG1 and a decrease in rSAG1-specific IgG2a. IFN-γ and IL-10 levels were increased in serum and in supernatants of *T. gondii* lysate antigen (TLA)-stimulated splenocytes obtained from vaccinated animals. In contrast, the immunized CBA/J mice showed no protection and significantly increased serum IL-10 and IL-4 levels. Further, no differences were observed concerning serum IFN-γ or IFN-γ levels in the supernatants of TLA *ex-vivo* stimulated spleen cells from both rSAG1-vaccinated or control CBA/J animals. These observations suggest that the Th1-/Th2-type responses induced by the immunization used were affected by the host genetic background, such as the major histocompatibility complex, leading to the different outcomes after immunization (40).

DNA Vaccines

DNA vaccines are among the most promising in *T. gondii* research. These vaccines have numerous advantages such as ease of development, low-cost production, stable storage, and shipping. More than 50 vaccine variants have been experimentally produced and tested and have shown positive results in their protective capacity using exogenous infection models (36, 37). Vaccination with a DNA plasmid encoding SAG1, which previously showed to protect BALB/c mice against infection with the avirulent Beverly type-2 strain, upon intra-muscular immunization with PltPASAG1 plasmid, was tested in a congenital infection model. However, maternal-fetal transmission was not reduced as compared to sham-immunized control mice (41)

This observation led to the conclusion that different immune mechanisms could mediate protection in adult-acquired infection and congenital parasite transmission (41). Another approach was performed by Mevelec *et al.* combining DNA plasmids encoding SAG1, *T. gondii* dense granule antigen 4 (GRA4) and murine granulocyte-macrophage colony-stimulating factor (GM-CSF) (42). The survival rates of pups from immunized infected dams was significantly higher compared to non-immunized infected dams. These results indicate that DNA plasmid multiantigen vaccine works better than a single antigen vaccine (42). Further studies are however necessary to highlight the suitability and efficacy of this type of vaccines in vertical infection.

Exosome Vaccines

Exosomes are nano-sized vesicles released by most eukaryotic cells (14). These vesicles can contain a wide variety of molecules, such as proteins, lipids, and nucleic acids, able to activate cellular and humoral responses altering the outcome of parasite infections (45).They can transfer mRNA, miRNA, and proteins between cells, representing a communication path between cells, necessary for immune homeostasis (14, 45). Studies showed that immunization with exosomes released from *T. gondii*-pulsed dendritic cells (DCs) induced protection against congenital toxoplasmosis, associated with IFN-γ and IL-10 responses in

TABLE 2 | Non-live vaccines in vertical *Toxoplasma gondii* infection models.

Strain/ animal	Immunogen/delivery	Day of mating post-immunization	ChallengePregnancy day/route/#parasite form/strain	Dam sacrifice	Maternal parameters	Progeny parameters	Highlighted results	References
Dunkin-Hartley/ guinea pigs*	Recombinant SAG1/ sc	Day 21	21 Days after mating/ id/ $5x10^5$ tachyzoites/ C56 strain	NS	-Specific IgG antibodies at the time of delivery	-Number of litters negative, partially positive, and positive. -Number of stillborn and viable pups and *T. gondii* positive. -Pups brain infectious status 2 days after birth. -Specific neonate IgG antibodies.	-Protection against maternal-fetal transmission (66–86%) -No correlation with specific IgG levels in the newborn pups.	(25)
BALB/c and CBA/J/mice	Recombinant SAG1/ sc	Day 60	Day 12 of pregnancy/ oral/ 10 cysts/ Me49 strain	Day 19 of pregnancy	-Maternal SAG1 IgG1 and IgG2a -*Ex-vivo* splenocyte specific cytokine production	-Fetus parasite load	-Protection against maternal-fetal transmission in BALB/c mice (50%) -Increased maternal IFN-γ and IL-10 production. Higher maternal rSAG1 specific IgG1 levels in BALB/c mice. - No protection in CBA/J mice associated with a Th2 response.	(40)
BALB/c/mice	SAG1-DNA plasmid/ im	Day 14	Day 12 of pregnancy/ oral/ 10 cystes/ Beverley strain	NS	Uterus examination (resorptions) or still births (at delivery)	-Survival and specific IgG in pups 12 weeks after birth -Number of survival pups at day 12 after birth	-No protection against maternal fetal transmission (no differences in pups's survival and specific IgG levels).	(41)
Swiss OF1/ mice	pSAG1mut+pGRA4+ pGMCSF DNA plasmids/ im	Day 15	Day 7-10 of pregnancy/oral/ 70 cysts/ 76K strain	NS	NE	-Survival (days 1–30 after birth) - Weight evaluation (days 8, 15, and 30 after birth). - Brain cyst burden (day 30 after birth)	-Higher survival rates but no differences in pups's body weight. -No protection against parasite vertical transmission (equal brain cyst burden).	(42)
CBA/J/mice	Exosomes derived from DC pulsed with *T. gondii* total antigen sc	Day 14	Day13 of pregnancy/ oral/ 25 cysts/ 76K strain	2 months after infection	Brain cyst load	-Survival (days 1–42 after birth) -Weight evaluation every 4 days for 42 days. -Brain cyst burden (6 weeks after birth) -Specific IgG isotypes and IgA response and *ex-vivo* spleen and lymph node specific cytokine production (6 weeks after birth).	- Decreased maternal brain parasite load. - Higher survival rate and pups body weight. - IgG2a, IgG2b, IL-2, IFN-γ, IL-4, and IL-10 responses in the pups. - Decreased pup brain parasite load.	(43)

(Continued)

TABLE 2 | Continued

Strain/ animal	Immunogen/delivery	Day of mating post-immunization	ChallengePregnancy day/route/#parasite form/strain	Dam sacrifice	Maternal parameters	Progeny parameters	Highlighted results	References
CBA/J/mice	Di-palmityol phosphatidyl glycerol-loaded nanoparticles (DGNP) containing total *T. gondii* extract/ in	Day 60	Day 11 of pregnancy/ oral/ 15 cysts/ 76K strain	Day 17 of pregnancy (exp#1) Day 60 after delivery (exp#2) (6 days post-infection the dams were sacrificed and fetus were collected for parasite load quantification)	- *Ex-vivo* cytokine secretion in placentas (Th1H1: IFN-γ and TNF-α, Th2 (IL4), Treg: TGF-β and IL-10, Th17: IL17A, and anti-inflammatory: IL6) (exo#1). -Brain cyst load evaluated 60 days after delivery (chronic infection) (exp#2).	- Parasites load n fetal tissues by real-time PCR (exp#1). - Evaluation of fetal resorption (exp#1). -Litter size and pups weight (exp#2). -Evaluation of protection in offspring against chronic infection (exp#2). -Average weight of each litter at 7, 14, and 21 days—after birth (exp#2). Ophthalmologic clinical signs (exp#2).	-Decreased maternal brain cyst load. -Reduction of IFN-γ and increase IL-6 and IL-10 placental cytokine levels favoring pregnancy maintenance -Protection against vertical transmission (fetus parasite load) or offspring (brain cyst load) - Higher mean weight and protection against ocular toxoplasmosis in the offspring.	(44)

Guinea pigs: pregnancy length of 9 weeks. C56 strain: type III; Me49 and 76K strain: type II. sc, subcutaneous; im, intramuscular; in, intranasal; NS, no sacrifice; NE, not evaluated. exp#1: experimental design 1; exp#2: experimental design 2.

the pups (43). This vaccine, when administered before pregnancy, provided strong fetus protection against infection. Low cyst burden was observed in both immunized dams and pups delivered from immunized dams (43). This was the first description, so far, studying immune responses in the offspring from vaccinated females.

Nanoparticle-Based Vaccines

Advances in research have revealed the use of nanoparticles (NP) as antigen delivery systems, thus setting the basis for a new type of vaccines. This antigen delivery system avoids antigen degradation and increases bloodstream life span, internalization, and presentation by antigen-presenting cells, such as DCs (14). Di-palmitoyl phosphatidyl glycerol-loaded nanoparticles (DGNP) loaded with *T. gondii* total antigen extract were shown to deliver parasitic antigens to mucosa after intranasal immunization, inducing a specific Th1/Th17 response *in vivo* (46). Further work has tested the safety and efficiency of DGNP in congenital toxoplasmosis (44). Placental levels of cytokine production were analyzed, which revealed no signs of inflammation exacerbation in immunized mice, even though, there was an increase in IFN-γ concentration. IL-10 and IL-6 levels were significantly raised. Survival of offspring and dams was 100% and mean litter size and pup weight was not diminished in infected immunized mice. The parasite burden on the fetus was 86% reduced from females immunized with DGNT/TE compared to controls (44).

CONCLUSION

Most of the research work that addresses vaccination using vertical *T. gondii* infection models assessed the immune response to vaccination, determining the IgG isotypes and cytokines produced in response to parasite antigen stimulation. Typically, production of IFN-γ, IL-2, IL-12, IL-10, and, occasionally, IL-4 was found elevated in response to vaccination in non-pregnant mice until 60–70 days post-vaccination. This might explain why this time-point has been referred in the achievement of pregnant animals, since the balance between these cytokines is essential in successful pregnancy as reported in almost all the studies referred here.

Most reports gather data from acute, chronic, and congenital infection experiments. However, the immune status during pregnancy is altered (7), therefore, the data from non-pregnant mice must be carefully discussed and not directly extrapolated to pregnancy due its specific immune status.

In two studies using live attenuated vaccines, mixed maternal Th1-/Th2-type responses were induced, being discussed as Th1 crucial against *T. gondii* congenital infection and Th2 essential for pregnancy maintenance (32, 34). Currently, a balance between several subsets of T cells must be considered such as Th1, Th2, Th9, Th17, Th22, and follicular Th cells (Tfh) for a successful human pregnancy (47). Indeed, these T cell subsets contribute to the immune response occurring at the maternal-fetal interface, known to be important not only in protecting against infection and controlling inflammatory response, but also contributing to immune homeostasis, implantation, decidualization, maternal immune tolerance and acceptance of the fetus, and parturition (47).

A heterogeneity in the experimental designs was found in the studies reported. The difficulty of performing research work with congenital infection models is very high and may explain the scarcity of research in this area. It would be useful to choose a standard experimental design in the study of vaccines, using congenital models able to get valid and robust results. Murine models are the most chosen because they offer simplified logistics, including the facility to monitor physiologic parameters and the short length of pregnancy. Further, mice allow experiments with higher animal numbers, availability of immunological reagents and genetically modified hosts. Mice were largely validated as an adequate model to study congenital toxoplasmosis, by reproducing many features of human infection (21).

None of the vaccines described so far managed to fully protect against *T. gondii* vertical transmission, even if providing multi-antigenic stimulus. The lack of more effective vaccination approaches may be a consequence of the scarce knowledge on the host protective immune molecular and cellular mechanisms operating at the maternal-fetal interface, specifically at decidua and placenta. Indeed, only one work testing nanoparticles containing *T. gondii* total extracts, analyzed the cytokine profile in placentas from vaccinated dams (44). This study found that a reduction in IFN-γ and an increase in IL-6 and IL-10 production was associated with protection against vertical transmission and ocular toxoplasmosis in the offspring (44). Determining the type of immune response at maternal-fetal interface that can correlate with protection will be useful to refine vaccination approaches, by selecting adjuvants that could adequately polarize T cell responses, thereby leading to protection against congenital infection. On the other hand, it would be also important to understand the immune response developed in the pups born from vaccinated dams and infected during pregnancy. To our knowledge, only one study analyzed the immune response in surviving pups born from vaccinated dams, having found a mixed Th1- and Th2-type response associated with a high survival rate, high weight mean, and low cyst brain burden (43). The development of adaptive fetal immune responses are observed in neonates exposed to an infection environment *in uterus* but not necessarily infected themselves (48). Thus, it will be worthy to get new insights into how T cell responses and related mediators operate in fetuses and in neonates. Novel vaccine design formulations and delivery systems can also be improved, concerning parasite antigen determinants and elicited immune mechanisms involved in protection against *T. gondii* vertical infection (36).

AUTHOR CONTRIBUTIONS

MBa, DT, and MBo wrote the initial manuscript. All authors contributed to the article and approved the submitted version.

REFERENCES

1. Torgerson PR, Devleesschauwer B, Praet N, Speybroeck N, Willingham AL, Kasuga F, et al. World Health Organization Estimates of the Global and Regional Disease Burden of 11 Foodborne Parasitic Diseases, 2010: A Data Synthesis. *PLoS Med* (2015) 12(12):e1001920. doi: 10.1371/journal.pmed.1001920
2. Torgerson PR, Mastroiacovo P. The global burden of congenital toxoplasmosis: a systematic review. *Bull World Health Organ* (2013) 91 (7):501–8. doi: 10.2471/blt.12.111732
3. Nayeri T, Sarvi S, Moosazadeh M, Amouei A, Hosseininejad Z, Daryani A. The global seroprevalence of anti-Toxoplasma gondii antibodies in women who had spontaneous abortion: A systematic review and meta-analysis. *PLoS Negl Trop Dis* (2020) 14(3):e0008103. doi: 10.1371/journal.pntd.0008103
4. Pittman KJ, Knoll LJ. Long-Term Relationships: the Complicated Interplay between the Host and the Developmental Stages of Toxoplasma gondii during Acute and Chronic Infections. *Microbiol Mol Biol Rev* (2015) 79(4):387–401. doi: 10.1128/mmbr.00027-15
5. McAuley JB. Congenital Toxoplasmosis. *J Pediatr Infect Dis Soc* (2014) 3 Suppl 1(Suppl 1):S30–5. doi: 10.1093/jpids/piu077
6. Elbez-Rubinstein A, Ajzenberg D, Darde ML, Cohen R, Dumetre A, Yera H, et al. Congenital toxoplasmosis and reinfection during pregnancy: case report, strain characterization, experimental model of reinfection, and review. *J Infect Dis* (2009) 199(2):280–5. doi: 10.1086/595793
7. Borges M, Magalhaes Silva T, Brito C, Teixeira N, Roberts CW. How does toxoplasmosis affect the maternal-foetal immune interface and pregnancy? *Parasite Immunol* (2019) 41(3):e12606. doi: 10.1111/pim.12606
8. Flegr J, Escudero DQ. Impaired health status and increased incidence of diseases in Toxoplasma-seropositive subjects - an explorative cross-sectional study. *Parasitology* (2016) 143(14):1974–89. doi: 10.1017/s0031182016001785
9. Sutterland AL, Fond G, Kuin A, Koeter MW, Lutter R, van Gool T, et al. Beyond the association. Toxoplasma gondii in schizophrenia, bipolar disorder, and addiction: systematic review and meta-analysis. *Acta Psychiatr Scand* (2015) 132(3):161–79. doi: 10.1111/acps.12423
10. Sasai M, Pradipta A, Yamamoto M. Host immune responses to Toxoplasma gondii. *Int Immunol* (2018) 30(3):113–9. doi: 10.1093/intimm/dxy004
11. Moroda M, Takamoto M, Iwakura Y, Nakayama J, Aosai F. Interleukin-17A-Deficient Mice Are Highly Susceptible to Toxoplasma gondii Infection Due to Excessively Induced T. gondii HSP70 and Interferon Gamma Production. *Infect Immun* (2017) 85(12):e00399-17. doi: 10.1128/iai.00399-17
12. Melchor SJ, Ewald SE. Disease Tolerance in Toxoplasma Infection. *Front Cell Infect Microbiol* (2019) 9:185. doi: 10.3389/fcimb.2019.00185
13. Sasai M, Yamamoto M. Innate, adaptive, and cell-autonomous immunity against Toxoplasma gondii infection. *Exp Mol Med* (2019) 51(12):1–10. doi: 10.1038/s12276-019-0353-9
14. Wang JL, Zhang NZ, Li TT, He JJ, Elsheikha HM, Zhu XQ. Advances in the Development of Anti-Toxoplasma gondii Vaccines: Challenges, Opportunities, and Perspectives. *Trends Parasitol* (2019) 35(3):239–53. doi: 10.1016/j.pt.2019.01.005
15. Innes EA, Hamilton C, Garcia JL, Chryssafidis A, Smith D. A one health approach to vaccines against Toxoplasma gondii. *Food Waterborne Parasitol* (2019) 15:e00053. doi: 10.1016/j.fawpar.2019.e00053
16. Munoz M, Liesenfeld O, Heimesaat MM. Immunology of Toxoplasma gondii. *Immunol Rev* (2011) 240(1):269–85. doi: 10.1111/j.1600-065X.2010.00992.x
17. Brito C, MS T, MC M, Wyrwas W, Oliveira B, MF B, et al. Toxoplasma gondii infection reduces serum progesterone levels and adverse effects at the maternal-foetal interface. *Parasite Immunol* (2020) 42(2):e12690. doi: 10.1111/pim.12690
18. Dunay IR, Gajurel K, Dhakal R, Liesenfeld O, Montoya JG. Treatment of Toxoplasmosis: Historical Perspective, Animal Models, and Current Clinical Practice. *Clin Microbiol Rev* (2018) 31(4):e00057-17. doi: 10.1128/cmr.00057-17

19. Fisch D, Clough B, Frickel EM. Human immunity to Toxoplasma gondii. *PLoS Pathog* (2019) 15(12):e1008097. doi: 10.1371/journal.ppat.1008097
20. Suzuki Y, Yang Q, Remington JS. Genetic resistance against acute toxoplasmosis depends on the strain of Toxoplasma gondii. *J Parasitol* (1995) 81(6):1032–4. doi: 10.2307/3284069
21. Roberts CW, Brewer JM, Alexander J. Congenital toxoplasmosis in the Balb/c mouse: prevention of vertical disease transmission and fetal death by vaccination. *Vaccine* (1994) 12(15):1389–94. doi: 10.1016/0264-410X(94)90147-3
22. Menzies FM, Henriquez FL, Roberts CW. Immunological control of congenital toxoplasmosis in the murine model. *Immunol Lett* (2008) 115 (2):83–9. doi: 10.1016/j.imlet.2007.10.009
23. Coutinho LB, Gomes AO, Araújo EC, Barenco PV, Santos JL, Caixeta DR, et al. The impaired pregnancy outcome in murine congenital toxoplasmosis is associated with a pro-inflammatory immune response, but not correlated with decidual inducible nitric oxide synthase expression. *Int J Parasitol* (2012) 42 (4):341–52. doi: 10.1016/j.ijpara.2012.01.006
24. Dos Santos TR, Faria GD, Guerreiro BM, Dal Pietro NH, Lopes WD, da Silva HM, et al. Congenital Toxoplasmosis in Chronically Infected and Subsequently Challenged Ewes. *PLoS One* (2016) 11(10):e0165124. doi: 10.1371/journal.pone.0165124
25. Haumont M, Delhaye L, Garcia L, Jurado M, Mazzu P, Daminet V, et al. Protective immunity against congenital toxoplasmosis with recombinant SAG1 protein in a guinea pig model. *Infect Immun* (2000) 68(9):4948–53. doi: 10.1128/iai.68.9.4948-4953.2000
26. Freyre A, Falcón J, Méndez J, González M. Toxoplasma gondii: an improved rat model of congenital infection. *Exp Parasitol* (2008) 120(2):142–6. doi: 10.1016/j.exppara.2008.06.007
27. Freyre A, Falcón J, Méndez J, Rodriguez A, Correa L, Gonzalez M. Toxoplasma gondii: Partial cross-protection among several strains of the parasite against congenital transmission in a rat model. *Exp Parasitol* (2006) 112(1):8–12. doi: 10.1016/j.exppara.2005.08.009
28. Freyre A, Araujo FA, Fialho CG, Bigatti LE, Falcón JD. Protection in a hamster model of congenital toxoplasmosis. *Vet Parasitol* (2012) 183(3-4):359–63. doi: 10.1016/j.vetpar.2011.07.039
29. Fonseca BM, Correia-da-Silva G, Teixeira NA. The rat as an animal model for fetoplacental development: a reappraisal of the post-implantation period. *Reprod Biol* (2012) 12(2):97–118. doi: 10.1016/s1642-431x(12)60080-1
30. Ismael AB, Dimier-Poisson I, Lebrun M, Dubremetz JF, Bout D, Mevelec MN. Mic1-3 knockout of Toxoplasma gondii is a successful vaccine against chronic and congenital toxoplasmosis in mice. *J Infect Dis* (2006) 194(8):1176–83. doi: 10.1086/507706
31. Mevelec MN, Ducournau C, Bassuny Ismael A, Olivier M, Seche E, Lebrun M, et al. Mic1-3 Knockout Toxoplasma gondii is a good candidate for a vaccine against T. gondii-induced abortion in sheep. *Vet Res* (2010) 41(4):49. doi: 10.1051/vetres/2010021
32. Wang JL, Elsheikha HM, Zhu WN, Chen K, Li TT, Yue DM, et al. Immunization with Toxoplasma gondii GRA17 Deletion Mutant Induces Partial Protection and Survival in Challenged Mice. *Front Immunol* (2017) 8:730. doi: 10.3389/fimmu.2017.00730
33. Liang QL, Sun LX, Elsheikha HM, Cao XZ, Nie LB, Li TT, et al. RHDeltagra17Deltanpt1 Strain of Toxoplasma gondii Elicits Protective Immunity Against Acute, Chronic and Congenital Toxoplasmosis in Mice. *Microorganisms* (2020) 8(3):352. doi: 10.3390/microorganisms8030352
34. Wang JL, Li TT, Elsheikha HM, Chen K, Cong W, Yang WB, et al. Live Attenuated Pru:Deltacdpk2 Strain of Toxoplasma gondii Protects Against Acute, Chronic, and Congenital Toxoplasmosis. *J Infect Dis* (2018) 218 (5):768–77. doi: 10.1093/infdis/jiy211
35. Wang JL, Liang QL, Li TT, He JJ, Bai MJ, Cao XZ, et al. Toxoplasma gondii tkl1 Deletion Mutant Is a Promising Vaccine against Acute, Chronic, and Congenital Toxoplasmosis in Mice. *J Immunol (Baltimore Md 1950)* (2020) 204(6):1562–70. doi: 10.4049/jimmunol.1900410
36. Loh FK, Nathan S, Chow SC, Fang CM. Vaccination challenges and strategies against long-lived Toxoplasma gondii. *Vaccine* (2019) 37(30):3989–4000. doi: 10.1016/j.vaccine.2019.05.083
37. Li Y, Zhou H. Moving towards improved vaccines for Toxoplasma gondii. *Expert Opin Biol Ther* (2018) 18(3):273–80. doi: 10.1080/14712598.2018.1413086
38. Zhang NZ, Chen J, Wang M, Petersen E, Zhu XQ. Vaccines against Toxoplasma gondii: new developments and perspectives. *Expert Rev Vaccines* (2013) 12(11):1287–99. doi: 10.1586/14760584.2013.844652
39. Biemans R, Grégoire D, Haumont M, Bosseloir A, Garcia L, Jacquet A, et al. The conformation of purified Toxoplasma gondii SAG1 antigen, secreted from engineered Pichia pastoris, is adequate for serorecognition and cell proliferation. *J Biotechnol* (1998) 66(2):137–46. doi: 10.1016/S0168-1656(98) 00143-6
40. Letscher-Bru V, Pfaff AW, Abou-Bacar A, Filisetti D, Antoni E, Villard O, et al. Vaccination with Toxoplasma gondii SAG-1 protein is protective against congenital toxoplasmosis in BALB/c mice but not in CBA/J mice. *Infect Immun* (2003) 71(11):6615–9. doi: 10.1128/iai.71.11.6615-6619.2003
41. Couper KN, Nielsen HV, Petersen E, Roberts F, Roberts CW, Alexander J. DNA vaccination with the immunodominant tachyzoite surface antigen (SAG-1) protects against adult acquired Toxoplasma gondii infection but does not prevent maternofoetal transmission. *Vaccine* (2003) 21(21):2813–20. doi: 10.1016/S0264-410X(03)00163-4
42. Mevelec MN, Bout D, Desolme B, Marchand H, Magne R, Bruneel O, et al. Evaluation of protective effect of DNA vaccination with genes encoding antigens GRA4 and SAG1 associated with GM-CSF plasmid, against acute, chronical and congenital toxoplasmosis in mice. *Vaccine* (2005) 23(36):4489–99. doi: 10.1016/j.vaccine.2005.04.025
43. Beauvillain C, Juste MO, Dion S, Pierre J, Dimier-Poisson I. Exosomes are an effective vaccine against congenital toxoplasmosis in mice. *Vaccine* (2009) 27 (11):1750–7. doi: 10.1016/j.vaccine.2009.01.022
44. Ducournau C, Nguyen TT, Carpentier R, Lantier I, Germon S, Precausta F, et al. Synthetic parasites: a successful mucosal nanoparticle vaccine against Toxoplasma congenital infection in mice. *Future Microbiol* (2017) 12:393–405. doi: 10.2217/fmb-2016-0146
45. Coakley G, Maizels RM, Buck AH. Exosomes and Other Extracellular Vesicles: The New Communicators in Parasite Infections. *Trends Parasitol* (2015) 31(10):477–89. doi: 10.1016/j.pt.2015.06.009
46. Dimier-Poisson I, Carpentier R, N'Guyen TT, Dahmani F, Ducournau C, Betbeder D. Porous nanoparticles as delivery system of complex antigens for an effective vaccine against acute and chronic Toxoplasma gondii infection. *Biomaterials* (2015) 50:164–75. doi: 10.1016/j.biomaterials.2015.01.056
47. Wang W, Sung N, Gilman-Sachs A, Kwak-Kim J. T Helper (Th) Cell Profiles in Pregnancy and Recurrent Pregnancy Losses: Th1/Th2/Th9/Th17/Th22/Tfh Cells. *Front Immunol* (2020) 11:2025. doi: 10.3389/fimmu.2020.02025
48. Dauby N, Goetghebuer T, Kollmann TR, Levy J, Marchant A. Uninfected but not unaffected: chronic maternal infections during pregnancy, fetal immunity, and susceptibility to postnatal infections. *Lancet Infect Dis* (2012) 12(4):330–40. doi: 10.1016/s1473-3099(11)70341-3

15

Toxoplasma GRA Peptide-Specific Serologic Fingerprints Discriminate among Major Strains Causing Toxoplasmosis

David Arranz-Solís[1]*, Cristina G. Carvalheiro*[2,3]*, Elizabeth R. Zhang*[2]*, Michael E. Grigg*[2] *and Jeroen P. J. Saeij*[1*]

[1] *Pathology, Microbiology and Immunology Department, Veterinary Medicine School 3A, University of California Davis, Davis, CA, United States,* [2] *Laboratory of Parasitic Diseases, Molecular Parasitology Section, National Institute of Allergy and Infectious Diseases, National Institutes of Health, Bethesda, MD, United States,* [3] *Department of Pediatrics, Ribeirão Preto Medical School, University of São Paulo, Ribeirão Preto, Brazil*

Correspondence:
Jeroen P. J. Saeij
jsaeij@ucdavis.edu

The severity of toxoplasmosis depends on a combination of host and parasite factors. Among them, the *Toxoplasma* strain causing the infection is an important determinant of the disease outcome. Type 2 strains dominate in Europe, whereas in North America type 2, followed by type 3 and 12 strains are commonly isolated from wildlife and patients. To identify the strain type a person is infected with, serological typing provides a promising alternative to the often risky and not always possible biopsy-based DNA methods of genotyping. However, despite recent advances in serotyping, improvements in the sensitivity and specificity are still needed, and it does not yet discriminate among the major *Toxoplasma* lineages infecting people. Moreover, since infections caused by non-1/2/3 strains have been associated with more severe disease, the ability to identify these is critical. In the present study we investigated the diagnostic potential of an ELISA-based assay using 28 immunogenic *Toxoplasma* peptides derived from a recent large-scale peptide array screen. Our results show that a discrete number of peptides, derived from *Toxoplasma* dense granule proteins (GRA3, GRA5, GRA6, and GRA7) was sufficient to discriminate among archetypal strains that infect mice and humans. The assay specifically relies on ratios that compare individual serum reactivities against GRA-specific polymorphic peptide variants in order to determine a "reactivity fingerprint" for each of the major strains. Importantly, nonarchetypal strains that possess a unique combination of alleles, different from types 1/2/3, showed either a non-reactive, or different combinatorial, mixed serum reactivity signature that was diagnostic in its own right, and that can be used to identify these strains. Of note, we identified a distinct "HG11/12" reactivity pattern using the GRA6 peptides that is able to distinguish HG11/12 from archetypal North American/European strain infections.

Keywords: *Toxoplasma*, serotyping, peptide, ELISA, dense granule, rhoptry

INTRODUCTION

The intracellular protozoan parasite *Toxoplasma gondii* is the causative agent of toxoplasmosis in humans and animals. Infection usually occurs after ingestion of tissue cysts present in undercooked meat or by ingestion of soil, water or food contaminated with oocysts shed in feline feces (Robert-Gangneux and Dardé, 2012). In humans, the worldwide seroprevalence is estimated to be approximately 30%, although it can vary widely (10–80%) between countries (Robert-Gangneux and Dardé, 2012; Dard et al., 2016). Although infection is usually benign with occasional flu-like symptoms in immunocompetent individuals, it can also cause severe disease such as ocular toxoplasmosis or encephalitis, especially in immunocompromised patients, as well as abortion or birth defects in pregnant women infected for the first time (Furtado et al., 2011). Hence, progression and severity of toxoplasmosis depends on a combination of host and parasite factors, with the infecting *Toxoplasma* strain type playing a pivotal role in the outcome of disease (Boothroyd and Grigg, 2002; Ajzenberg et al., 2010; Fekkar et al., 2011).

Toxoplasma has a markedly clonal population structure in North America and Europe, with four distinct clonotypes commonly isolated from animals and humans (types 1, 2, 3 and 12), although type 2 strains predominate, especially in Europe (Dubey et al., 2011; Herrmann et al., 2012; Su et al., 2012). By contrast, the majority of characterized isolates from South America are genetically distinct from the North-American/European strains and have been referred to as non-canonical, non-archetypal, non-clonal or atypical strains or lineages (Grigg and Sundar, 2009; Su et al., 2012). Some of these have been associated with severe systemic toxoplasmosis in immunocompetent people (Carme et al., 2009; Hamilton et al., 2019). Conversely, type 2 strains are less often associated with severe clinical disease. In fact, type 1 and non-type 2 strains are more likely to be found infecting immunocompetent individuals suffering from ocular toxoplasmosis and are disproportionately associated with severe congenital toxoplasmosis in the USA and Europe (Howe et al., 1997; Fuentes et al., 2001; Grigg et al., 2001; Carme et al., 2002; Nowakowska et al., 2006; Carme et al., 2009; McLeod et al., 2012; Shobab et al., 2013; Hutson et al., 2015). In addition, the “Cougar” strain, which was isolated from oocysts shed by mountain lions (*Puma concolor*) and belongs to haplogroup 11 (HG11) (Su et al., 2012; Lorenzi et al., 2016), has been epidemiologically linked to a major waterborne toxoplasmosis outbreak in Victoria, British Columbia, Canada (Aramini et al., 1998; Aramini et al., 1999). Similarly, a recent outbreak in Wisconsin, USA, was reported to be caused by consumption of undercooked venison contaminated with cysts from a HG12 strain (Schumacher et al., 2020). It is worth mentioning that in both of these outbreaks, infected patients experienced systemic disease, suggesting that either the number of cysts/oocysts ingested was exceptionally high or that a virulent strain was involved.

Recent advances in genotyping *Toxoplasma* isolates from different continents have identified extensive genetic diversity; however, genotyping has substantial limitations: it is both time consuming and costly, and it often requires parasite isolation by invasive and risky biopsies, which is normally only achieved in severe clinical cases (Robert-Gangneux and Dardé, 2012; Su et al., 2012; Shobab et al., 2013; Lorenzi et al., 2016). In contrast to DNA-dependent techniques, serological typing allows for the inclusion of clinical, as well as subclinical, cases, and represents a rapid, sensitive, and relatively non-invasive alternative (Kong et al., 2003). Serotyping takes advantage of the fact that *Toxoplasma* stimulates a strong and persistent humoral immune response, eliciting the production of antibodies against parasite proteins that are often highly polymorphic among distinct strains. By using polymorphic peptides as antigens and monitoring the reactivity of the serum, a prediction of the infecting strain type can be made. Indeed, several studies employed synthetic peptides or recombinant polypeptides derived from polymorphic regions of *Toxoplasma* secreted/excreted proteins to serologically distinguish type 2 from non-type 2 infections in a variety of hosts (Kong et al., 2003; Peyron et al., 2006; Morisset et al., 2008; Xiao et al., 2009; Sousa et al., 2009; Sousa et al., 2010; Vaudaux et al., 2010; Maksimov et al., 2012b; Maksimov et al., 2012a; McLeod et al., 2012; Shobab et al., 2013; Hutson et al., 2015; Maksimov et al., 2018). Other studies have attempted to develop peptides capable of differentiating type 1 *vs.* 3 and type 2 *vs.* 3 infections, but with only partial success (Xiao et al., 2009; Maksimov et al., 2012a; Maksimov et al., 2018). We recently developed a discrete set of *Toxoplasma* polymorphic peptides capable of discriminating infections caused by type 1, 2 and 3 strains (Arranz-Solís et al., 2019), but these have not yet been widely applied, nor have they been systematically tested against serum collected from patients infected with non-archetypal strains.

Although the serotyping approach lacks the exquisite sensitivity and specificity of DNA genotyping, the recent availability of whole genome sequences from 64 different *Toxoplasma* strains, including atypical ones (Lorenzi et al., 2016), makes it possible to test whether serologic reactivity is determined by the epitope present, and not the underlying genotype of the parasite strain. Based on our previous work, we observed that many atypical strains either possess a type 1/2/3 epitope within the GRA peptides, even though the allele present is not type 1/2/3, or they share the sequence of one of the type 1, 2 and/or 3 strains but in different admixture combinations (Lorenzi et al., 2016). Since arrays are not always readily available and entail a great cost, the aim of the present study was to test a small selection of promising peptides using a larger collection of murine and human serum samples by ELISA, which represents an easier, more accessible and affordable assay platform that is available in most laboratories. To this end, a total of 28 *Toxoplasma* allele-specific peptides were designed and synthesized for screening. By using a ratio that compares the reaction of different variants within the same polymorphic regions, an approach taken by McLeod et al. (2012), we demonstrate that peptides derived from the GRA proteins GRA3, GRA5, GRA6, GRA7 and GRA15 differentiate between types 1, 2, 3, as well as other strain infections produced by non-archetypal strains. These peptides should enable further research to assess whether the genotype of the infecting strain is associated with specific disease phenotypes among different populations, allowing for a better understanding of the molecular epidemiology of toxoplasmosis.

METHODS

Toxoplasma In Vitro Culture

Toxoplasma strains used for animal infections and lysate production (see below) were routinely maintained on Human Foreskin Fibroblast (HFF) monolayers as previously described (Jensen et al., 2015).

Ethics Statement and Mice Infection

All animal experiments were performed in strict accordance with the recommendations in the Guide for the Care and Use of Laboratory Animals of the National Institutes of Health. The MIT Committee on Animal Care (assurance number A-3125-01), the Institutional Animal Care and Use Committee (IACUC) at the University of California, Davis (assurance number A-3433-01), and the Animal Care and Use Committee (ACUC) of the Intramural Research Program of NIAID (Animal study protocol; LPD22E) approved all protocols, and all efforts were made to minimize unnecessary distress to the animals. The animal study protocol LPD22E was reviewed and approved by the Animal Care and Use Committee of the Intramural Research Program of the National Institute of Allergy and Infectious Diseases (NIAID) at the National Institutes of Health.

Mouse Serum Samples

A summary of the mouse breed, parasite, dose, route, treatment and time of collection of sera is presented in **Supplemental File 1A**. Serum samples from mice infected with RH (type 1); M4, ME49 and PRU (type 2); CEP and CL14 (type 3); MAS (type 4), BOF (type 6), CAST (type 7), P89 (type 9), GUY-DOS (type 10), and Cougar (type 11) were used (Jensen et al., 2015; Mukhopadhyay et al., 2020, This study). In addition, samples from mice infected orally with cysts from the type 2 PRU and type 3 CEP strains, as well as intraperitoneally with oocysts of the type 2 M4 strain, were also included. Finally, the most reactive peptides were tested with a set of sera from mice infected with the strains S22, S26, CL13, and STE10, which are F1 progeny from a cross between type 2 (ME49) and 3 (CEP) strains in cats (Sibley et al., 1992). Animals were checked every day to detect signs of illness, such as rough hair coat, apathy or weight loss. Depending on the strain, sulfadiazine, alone or in combination with pyrimethamine, was added to the drinking water (0.4 mg/ml and 0.2 mg/ml, respectively), either at the time of infection or upon detection of clinical signs, to control the acute stage. The sera of infected mice were collected at different time points according to the severity of infection caused by specific strains. Serum samples from individual mice were pooled for each group of infection and used for the ELISAs.

Human Serum Samples

Thirty-four serum samples from infected patients from France, Brazil or the United States were used in the present study (de-la-Torre et al., 2013; Arranz-Solís et al., 2019; This study) (**Supplemental File 1B**). The strain causing the infection was previously assessed by genotyping or serotyping employing GRA6 and GRA7 peptides (6I/III, d6I/III, 6II and 7II) originally described by Kong et al. (2003). Samples included infections caused by type 1, 2, 3, 1/3 and SA (aka atypical) strains. In addition, a number of samples were defined as non-reactive, or NR (i.e., positive serum reactivity against either *Toxoplasma* lysate or rSAG1 antigen with no reaction to the Kong panel of peptides). These patient samples are thought to represent infection by atypical strains (de-la-Torre et al., 2013; Shobab et al., 2013). Human samples were used according to the Committee on the Use of Humans as Experimental Subjects (COUHES) application No. 0808002869.

Toxoplasma Lysate Production

A *Toxoplasma* soluble lysate extract was prepared to be used in the ELISA experiments. To achieve a homogeneous representation of the type 1, 2, and 3 strains, which generally encompass most peptide polymorphisms, *Toxoplasma* tachyzoites of RH and GT1 (type 1); PRU, ME49, and M4 (type 2); and VEG and CEP (type 3) strains were grown as described above. When parasites started to lyse out, flasks were scraped and tachyzoites recovered and syringe lysed (27×G and 30×G). Pellets were collected by centrifugation at 700×g for 7 min and washed twice with 1×PBS to remove residual culture media. Washed pellets were then resuspended in 5 ml 1×PBS and filtered to remove cells and debris by passing the suspensions through PD-10 desalting columns (GE Healthcare). Tachyzoites were counted using a Neubauer chamber and pellets collected by centrifugation and stored at −80 °C until processing. A total of 5×10^9 tachyzoites were used for the soluble antigen production. For this, pellets were thawed on ice and resuspended thoroughly in a lysate solution containing 10mM Tris, 57 mM phenylmethylsulphonyl fluoride (PMSF), and 1× protease inhibitor + phosphatase cocktail (ThermoFisher) in 1×PBS. All lysates were then mixed and subjected to 3 cycles of 3 min sonication (50% amp 15 s pulse + 10 s pause) (EpiShear Q120AM probe sonicator, Active Motif). To avoid overheating of the samples, tubes were placed on a freeze-cold cooler throughout the process. Finally, sonicated lysates were centrifuged at 14,000×g for 30 min at 4 °C and supernatants containing the soluble antigen transferred to new tubes. Protein concentration was determined by the Bradford method (Bradford, 1976) and aliquots were stored at −80 °C until used.

Selection, Design and Production of Peptides

In a recent work from our group, we tested 950 peptides from 62 *Toxoplasma* genes by peptide array (Arranz-Solís et al., 2019). A number of promising peptides were found to be immunogenic and strain-specific; however, arrays are not readily available and are often cost prohibitive. Hence, we prioritized a small selection of promising peptides from the array work to develop an ELISA format assay to test against a broader panel of murine and human serum samples. Only antigenic peptides that consistently discriminated the strain of infection were re-synthesized for the ELISA assay. Some selected peptides were shortened from the originally described peptide (Arranz-Solís et al., 2019) to evaluate their capacity to maintain reactivity and the importance of specific amino acids. Altogether, a total of 28 allele-specific peptides from *Toxoplasma* dense granule (GRA3, GRA5, GRA6, GRA7 and GRA15) and rhoptry (ROP8 and ROP20) proteins, as well as one histidine acid phosphatase superfamily protein (TGME_308950) and a PA14 domain-containing protein (TGME49_258400, only expressed in oocysts) were designed (**Table 1**). When not present, cysteine residues were added to the N or C terminus of the peptide for coupling purposes. Peptides were synthesized with a purity of >95% and coupled to Keyhole-Limpet Hemocyanin (KLH) carrier protein (Biomatik USA, Wilmington, DE). In addition, a KLH-coupled control peptide derived from a randomly generated sequence of GRA6 (Kong et al., 2003) was used to rule out nonspecific reactions against KLH. Lyophilized peptides were resuspended in MilliQ water or in low concentrations (0.1–1%) of glacial acetic acid, depending on their hydrophilic properties, to a final concentration of 1 µg/µl, aliquoted and stored at -80 °C until use. All but one peptide were successfully resuspended; unfortunately, all attempts to resuspend the peptide GRA5-III-38 failed, even with increasing concentrations of Dimethyl Sulfoxide (DMSO), acetonitrile or acetic acid. Therefore, this peptide was subsequently excluded from the study.

Mouse ELISA

An indirect enzyme-linked immunosorbent assay (ELISA) was used to determine the reactivity level shown by different serum samples from mice infected with several *Toxoplasma* strains (**Supplemental File 1A**). Peptides (**Table 1**) were used to coat 96-well microtiter plates (CLS3590, Corning, Sigma). For this, 100 µl/well of peptides at 10 µg/ml (1 µg/well) diluted in carbonate buffer (100 mM, pH 9.6) were incubated overnight at 4 °C. For each sample, the *Toxoplasma* lysate (0.25 µg/well) and the KLH-coupled control peptide were used as positive and negative controls, respectively. Subsequently, non-specific binding was blocked by adding 200 µl of bovine serum albumin diluted to 3% in PBS (pH 7.4) containing 0.05% Tween 20 (PBS-T). After 2 h incubation at room temperature (RT), plates were washed four times with PBS-T. Subsequently, 100 µl of 1/100 sera dilution in block solution was added to each well and incubated for 1 h at 37 °C. In each plate, samples of the same positive and negative control sera were included. These corresponded to a pool of mice infected with the M4 strain and

TABLE 1 | List of peptides used in the ELISA test.

Gene ID	Name[a]	Sequence[b]	type	Reference
TGME49_227280	GRA3-I/III-43	ADQP**E**NHQALAEC	1/3	Arranz-Solís et al., 2019[c]
TGME49_227280	GRA3-II-43	ADQP**G**NHQALAEC	2	Arranz-Solís et al., 2019[c]
TGME49_286450	GRA5-I-38	CSEGA**R**G**R**EQ	1	Arranz-Solís et al., 2019
TGME49_286450	GRA5-II-38	CSEGA**W**G**G**EQ	2	Arranz-Solís et al., 2019
TGME49_286450	GRA5-III-38*	CSEGA**G**G**R**E**R**	3	Arranz-Solís et al., 2019
TGME49_275440	GRA6-I-44	ADS**G**GV**K**QTPC	1	Arranz-Solís et al., 2019[c]
TGME49_275440	GRA6-II-44	ADS**G**GV**R**QTPC	2	Arranz-Solís et al., 2019[c]
TGME49_275440	GRA6-III-44	ADS**D**GV**K**QTPC	3	Arranz-Solís et al., 2019[c]
TGME49_275440	GRA6-II-200	C**N**EGRG**E**GG**EDD**	2	Arranz-Solís et al., 2019
TGME49_275440	GRA6-III-201	CEGRG**Y**GG**RGE**	3	Arranz-Solís et al., 2019[c]
TGME49_275440	GRA6-I/III-213	CLHP**ER**VN**V**FD**Y**	1/2	Kong et al., 2003 [6-I/III]
TGME49_275440	GRA6-II-214	CLHP**GS**VN**E**FD**F**	2	Kong et al., 2003 [6-II]
TGME49_275440	GRA6-II-215	CHP**GS**VN**E**FD	2	Kong et al., 2003[c]
TGME49_203310	GRA7-I-164	CLTE**E**QQ**R**GDEP	1	Arranz-Solís et al., 2019[c]
TGME49_203310	GRA7-III-164	CLTE**Q**QQ**T**GDEP	3	Arranz-Solís et al., 2019[c]
TGME49_203310	GRA7-II-224	CVPESG**K**D**G**EDARQ	2	Kong et al., 2003 [7-II]
TGME49_203310	GRA7-III-224	CVPESG**E**D**R**EDA	3	Kong et al., 2003 [(d)7-III]
TGME49_203310	GRA7-II-226	CESG**K**D**G**EDAR	2	Arranz-Solís et al., 2019
TGME49_203310	GRA7-III-226	CESG**E**D**R**EDA	3	Arranz-Solís et al., 2019[c]
TGME49_275470	GRA15-II-477	CSPHTLLSRS	2	Arranz-Solís et al., 2019
TGME49_215775	ROP8-I/III-61	CPGGASPRHFHS	1/3	Arranz-Solís et al., 2019
TGME49_215775	ROP8-I/III-305	CSN**T**IKQMK**Q**EV	1/3	Arranz-Solís et al., 2019[c]
TGME49_215775	ROP8-II-305	CSN**A**IKQMK**E**EV	2	Arranz-Solís et al., 2019
TGME49_258230	ROP20-I-331	CLRKQG**GN**SLLN	1	Arranz-Solís et al., 2019
TGME49_258230	ROP20-II/III-331	CLRKQG**DT**SLLN	2/3	Arranz-Solís et al., 2019
TGME49_308950	hp-I/II-47	S**IW**RPQGTPEC	1/2	Arranz-Solís et al., 2019[c]
TGME49_308950	hp-III-47	S**TL**RPQGTPEC	3	Arranz-Solís et al., 2019[c]
TGME49_258400	PA14-I/II/III-35	EFRQQHRKTIDGRLC	1/2/3	This study
CONTROL	KLH1	CEVVHDYRLFNP		Kong et al., 2003

All attempts to dissolve GRA5-III-38 were unsuccessful.

[a]*I, II, and III refer to the archetypal strain that includes the peptide sequence, and the numbers following these indicate position in the coding sequence of the first amino acid of each peptide. The cysteine (C) at the N or C terminus was added for coupling purposes and was not present in the protein. Hp stands for hypothetical protein. TGME49_308950 is annotated as histidine acid phosphatase superfamily protein.*

[b]*Bold type indicates polymorphic sites.*

[c]*Modified version of a peptide described in Arranz-Solís et al., 2019 or Kong et al., 2003.*

uninfected mice, respectively. After four washes in PBS-T, 100 µl of horseradish peroxidase (HRP) conjugate-labeled goat α-mice IgG antibody (16-078, Thermo-Fisher Scientific) diluted 1:2,000 in PBS-T was added and incubated for 1 h at 37 °C. Plates were washed as above before the addition of 100 µl per well of ABTS substrate (11684302001, Sigma) and incubated at room temperate in the dark. The reaction was stopped by the addition of 100 µl per well of a solution of 0.3 M oxalic acid, and the optical density (OD) was read at 405 nm (OD_{405}) in a plate reader machine (Molecular Device Spectramax M2e). Plates were stopped when the positive control (lysate) reached OD values of 1.5–1.8, usually within 15–30 min. To normalize the obtained OD values, for each sample and peptide a relative index percent (RIPC) was calculated using the following formula RIPC = (peptide OD_{405} sample – peptide OD_{405} negative control)/(lysate OD_{405} sample – lysate OD_{405} negative control) × 100 (**Supplemental File 2**). To use a more stringent normalization, we decided to employ constant values for both the peptides and lysate OD negative controls. These values were calculated as two times the average of the ODs obtained with the negative control for each peptide and the lysate in all the plates used (0.39 and 0.25, respectively). Since each peptide showed a different level of reactivity, we decided to calculate a ratio between those homologous peptides from the different strain types (for example, GRA3-I/III-43 *vs.* GRA3-II-43). To further normalize the results, before calculating the ratios, RIPC values below 1 (including negative values) were converted to 1, and those higher than 100 were converted to 100.

Human ELISA

Human ELISA assays were performed at the Laboratory of Parasitic Diseases, Bethesda, MD, USA, as described above for mice with the following modifications: 50 µl per well were used in all steps using a different set of 96-well plates (353912, BD Falcon). Peptides were provided by the Saeij lab and labelled with letter codes to ensure that all ELISAs were performed blinded and an unbiased interpretation of results was carried out. To validate the reproducibility of our test and the status of the serum samples, three control peptides, 6I/III, 6II and 7II (Kong et al., 2003), well-known to be able to differentiate type 2 *vs.* non-type 2 infections, were included. These peptides shared the same sequence as our GRA6-I/III-213, GRA6-II-214 and GRA7-II-224 (**Table 1**), although they were manufactured by a different provider and manually coupled with the KLH carrier protein (Shobab et al., 2013). In addition, for each sample a positive control consisting of a universal and highly reactive recombinant SAG1 (rSAG1) antigen was included (Shobab et al., 2013). As a blocking buffer, a 2% casein (C5890, Sigma) solution in PBS was used, whereas several sample dilutions (1/40-1/160) were done for each patient and incubated at room temperature for 1 h. All coupled peptides were reacted with a cohort of 30 negative sera and each serum was tested against an irrelevant peptide-KLH coupled control. As a secondary antibody, a 1/1,000 dilution of the HRP Anti-Human IgG HRP (555788, BD Pharmingen) was used. Finally, after addition of the ABTS reagent, OD_{405} values were obtained for each sample by reading the plate at different time points ranging from 20–40 min for the rSAG1 antigen to 2–4 h for the peptides. Data were presented as an OD index, normalized as described previously (Kong et al., 2003; Shobab et al., 2013). Briefly, the OD_{405} value for each serotyping peptide was divided by the OD_{405} reading for the irrelevant peptide-KLH control and the results expressed as arbitrary units. Serum samples from individuals infected with *T. gondii* for whom the genotype is known served as positive controls for each experiment. Thus, it is expected that samples unreactive to specific peptides have a normalized value close to 1. Threshold values above which each sample-peptide reaction is considered positive were determined by adding 2 standard deviations (SDs) to the average of the normalized OD ratio derived from the 30 seronegative samples. Values were normalized by dividing homologous peptides from the different strain types as described above for the mice ELISA.

RESULTS

Peptide ELISA Using Sera From *Toxoplasma* Infected Mice

Sera from mice infected with different *Toxoplasma* strains were used to test the antigenicity of the peptides described in **Table 1**. Namely, sera from mice infected with one type 1 (RH) strain, three type 2 (M4, ME49, PRU), two type 3 (CEP, CL14), one MAS (type 4), BOF (type 6), CAST (7), P89 (9), GUY-DOS (10) and Cougar (11) strains were assessed to detect specific reactivity. As expected, all these sera showed a strong reactivity against the *Toxoplasma* lysate (soluble antigen), whereas the uninfected negative serum sample did not react against any of the peptides nor the lysate (**Supplemental File 2**). In addition, none but two showed reactivity against the KLH-control peptide (RIPC of 4 and 7 for one ME49 and one M4 sample, respectively), confirming the absence of (or very low) nonspecific reactivity of the samples to the KLH carrier protein. From the final 27 peptides that were tested by ELISA, 14 (GRA3-I/III-43, GRA3-II-43, GRA5-I-38, GRA5-II-38, GRA6-III-201, GRA6-I/III-213, GRA6-II-214, GRA6-II-215, GRA7-I-164, GRA7-II-224, GRA7-III-224, GRA7-II-226, GRA7-III-226 and GRA15-II-477) showed reactivity with at least one of the examined serum (**Figure 1**). None of the other 13 peptides showed reactivity with any of the samples and were therefore not further studied.

The reactivity of different serum samples obtained from mice infected with the same strain but that differed in mouse breed, infection dose, treatment, route of infection or day of collection (**Supplemental File 1A**) was investigated with these 14 peptides. Although a clear pattern was not found when comparing samples from the strains ME49 (type 2, 2 samples), PRU (type 2, 7 samples) and CEP (type 3, 6 samples), this allowed us to confirm the reproducibility of our assay. To simplify the results, an average of the different samples tested for each of the type 2 and 3 strains was calculated (**Figure 1**). The individual values for each sample, as well as the standard deviation of type 2 and 3 strains is shown in **Supplemental File 3**.

Peptide \ Haplogroup	1	2	2	2	3	3	4	6	7	9	10	11
	RH	M4	ME49[a]	PRU[b]	CEP[c]	CL14	MAS	BOF	CAST	P89	GUY-DOS	Cougar
GRA3-I/III-43	46	1	1	3	74	40	1	1	100	1	1	1
GRA3-II-43	40	1	1	5	16	1	1	1	1	1	1	1
GRA5-I-38	58	12	1	28	1	1	1	1	6	1	1	1
GRA5-II-38	1	62	16	66	1	7	1	1	1	1	1	1
GRA6-I-44	1	1	1	1	1	1	1	1	1	1	1	1
GRA6-II-44	1	1	1	1	1	1	1	1	1	1	1	1
GRA6-III-44	1	1	1	1	1	1	1	1	1	1	1	1
GRA6-II-200	1	1	1	1	1	1	1	1	1	1	1	1
GRA6-III-201	1	1	1	1	1	1	1	1	23	1	6	1
GRA6-I/III-213	84	8	3	2	62	24	1	10	64	44	67	56
GRA6-II-214	6	59	73	49	3	1	30	1	1	1	1	12
GRA6-II-215	1	4	25	7	1	1	4	11	1	1	1	1
GRA7-I-164	8	1	1	1	1	1	1	1	1	1	1	1
GRA7-III-164	1	1	1	1	1	1	1	1	1	1	1	1
GRA7-II-224	1	42	20	44	1	1	1	1	1	1	1	1
GRA7-III-224	1	1	1	1	6	1	1	1	1	1	1	1
GRA7-II-226	1	7	7	9	1	1	1	1	1	1	1	1
GRA7-III-226	1	1	1	1	6	1	1	1	1	1	1	1
GRA15-II-477	1	8	1	24	1	1	1	1	1	1	1	1
ROP8-I/III-61	1	1	1	1	1	1	1	1	1	1	1	1
ROP8-I/III-305	1	1	1	1	1	1	1	1	1	1	1	1
ROP8-II-305	1	1	1	1	1	1	1	1	1	1	1	1
ROP20-I-331	1	1	1	1	1	1	1	1	1	1	1	1
ROP20-II/III-331	1	1	1	1	1	1	1	1	1	1	1	1
HP-I/II-47	1	1	1	1	1	1	1	1	1	1	1	1
HP-III-47	1	1	1	1	1	1	1	1	1	1	1	1
PA14-I/II/III-35	1	1	1	1	1	1	1	1	1	1	1	1
KLH-control	1	4	2	1	1	1	1	1	1	1	1	1

FIGURE 1 | Relative index percentage (RIPC) values for ELISAs using *Toxoplasma* peptides and murine sera. OD values for each sample and peptide were normalized by calculating a relative index percentage (RIPC) with the following formula RIPC = (peptide OD_{405} sample – peptide OD_{405} negative control)/(lysate OD_{405} sample – lysate OD_{405} negative control) × 100. To use a more stringent normalization, constant OD values corresponding to two times the average of the ODs obtained with the negative sample for all peptides and the lysate (0.39 and 0.25, respectively) were used. In addition, RIPC values below 1 (including negative values) were converted to 1, and those higher than 100 were converted to 100. [a] average of 2 ME49 samples; [b] average of 7 PRU samples; [c] average of 6 CEP samples.

Sera of Mice Infected With Different *Toxoplasma* Strains React to GRA Peptides in an Epitope-Specific Manner

Peptides that showed good reactivity were derived from GRA proteins: GRA3, 5, 6, 7 and 15. Among these, GRA3-I/III-43, GRA5-II-38, GRA6-I/III-213, GRA6-II-214 and GRA7-II-224 showed a strong and specific reactivity against their respective type. On the other hand, although GRA6-II-215, GRA7-I-164, GRA7-III-224, GRA7-III-226 and GRA15-II-477 were also very strain specific, their response was weak and not always present in all samples from their respective type (**Figure 1**, **Supplemental File 3**). Nevertheless, while an absence of reactivity is the most likely scenario for these latter peptides, provided a reaction is detected, they are capable of predicting the strain causing the infection (potentially for all three type 1, 2 and 3 strains) in a very specific way. The C-terminal part of GRA6 is a very antigenic region that has been previously shown to represent an excellent epitope for serotyping (e.g. Kong et al., 2003; Arranz-Solís et al., 2019). In this work, we observed that GRA6-II-214 (LHPGSVNEFDF) shows a high and specific reactivity against type 2 serum samples, while it dramatically decreases to almost basal levels in GRA6-II-215 (HPGSVNEFD), which lacks the first and last amino acids compared to GRA6-II-214. Moreover, the type 1/3 version of GRA6-II-214 (GRA6-I/III-213) showed an interesting pattern in which all non-type 2 sera reacted to a certain degree to this peptide (except the type 4 MAS, which has the type II sequence), with the lowest reactivity being observed in few type 2 strains and type 6 BOF (**Figure 1** and **Supplemental File 3**). Except for the latter, the constant amino acid in all the strains reacting to this peptide is the last one (F/Y). Only those sharing the type 1/3 (Y) showed reactivity, even when they possess one or two different amino acids in the rest of the peptide (**Figure 2**). However, the amino acid in position 221 (E/V) also seems to influence the reactivity, as apart from the type 2 strains and type 4 MAS (that share the same sequence), only Cougar has reactivity against the type 2 version of this peptide (GRA6-II-214). Remarkably, while all the samples reacted strongly to either one of the two versions of this portion of GRA6 (GRA6-I/III-213 or GRA6-II-214), type 11 Cougar reacted to both, although with a stronger response to the type 1/3 version. The importance that single amino acid substitutions can have on peptide recognition was also observed in GRA7-224/226 and GRA3-43 peptides (K/E and G/E, respectively).

A Ratio Between the Seroreactivity Against Different Strain Versions of the Same Peptide Provides a Strain-Specific Signature

Although most sera reacted better to peptide versions corresponding to the infecting strain, they also did to a lesser extent to other versions of the peptide. Hence, we decided to further analyze the RIPC values for each group of related peptides by calculating a ratio of reactivity against different versions of the peptide (**Figure 2** and **Supplemental File 3**). From these ratios it was clear that a distinction between type 1, 2

Strain \ Peptide		GRA3-I/III-43 ÷ GRA3-II-43	GRA5-I-38 ÷ GRA5-II-38	GRA6-I/III-213 ÷ GRA6-II-214	GRA7-II-224 ÷ GRA7-III-224	GRA7-II-226 ÷ GRA7-III-226
Type 1		1.2 (46÷40)	58.3 (58.3÷1)	15.0 (84.0÷5.6)	NR	NR
Type 2[b]		0.9 (±0.3)	0.3 (±0.2)	0.05 (±0.04)	39.4 (±35.1)	8.0 (±10.8)
Type 3[c]		44.0 (±41.1)	0.9 (±0.3)	43.6 (±31.5)	0.9 (±0.4)	0.9 (±0.4)
4	MAS	NR	NR	0.03 (1÷30.4)	NR	NR
6	BOF	NR	NR	10.3 (10.3÷1)	NR	NR
7	CAST	100 (100÷1)	5.6 (5.6÷1)	63.8 (63.8÷1)	NR	NR
9	P89	NR	NR	43.6 (43.6÷1)	NR	NR
10	GUY-DOS	NR	NR	66.6 (66.6÷1)	NR	NR
11	Cougar	NR	NR	4.6 (56.5÷12.2)	NR	NR

1-RH	ADQPENHQALAE	....R.R..	LHPERVNVFDY	.....E.......	...E.......
2-ME49	....G.......	SEGAWGGEQ	...GS..E..F	VPESGKDGEDARQ	ESGKDGEDARQ
3-VEG	....	....G.R.R	....	.....E.R.....	...E.R.....
4-MAS	....	F...G.R.R	...GS..E..F	.....E.R.....	...E.R.....
6-BOF	....	....R.R..	....	.....E.......	...E.......
7-CAST	....	....R.R..	....	.....E.R.....	...E.R.....
9-p89	....	....G.R.R	...GS......	.....E.R.....	...E.R.....
10-GUY-DOS	....	....G.R.R	....	.....E.......	...E.......
11-COUG	....G.......	D...G...R	.......E...	.....E.......	...E.......
12-ARI	....G.......	....G.R.R	.......E...	.....E.......	...E.......

Strain \ Peptide	GRA3-I/III-43 ÷ GRA3-II-43	GRA5-I-38 ÷ GRA5-II-38	GRA6-I/III-213 ÷ GRA6-II-214	GRA7-II-224 ÷ GRA7-III-224	GRA7-II-226 ÷ GRA7-III-226
RH*	≥1 (S/S)	>1 (S/NR)	>1 (S/W)	NR	NR
M4*, ME49, Pru	NR or ≤1 (W/W)	<1 (W/S)	<1 (W/S)	>1 (S/NR)	>1 (W/NR) or NR
CEP, CL14*	>1 (S/W)	NR or ≤1 (NR/W)	>1 (S/W)	NR or <1 (NR/W)	NR or <1 (NR/W)
MAS*	NR	NR	<1 (NR/S)	NR	NR
BOF*	NR	NR	>1 (W/NR)	NR	NR
CAST*	>1 (S/NR)	>1 (W/NR)	>1 (S/NR)	NR	NR
P89*	NR	NR	>1 (S/NR)	NR	NR
GUY-DOS*	NR	NR	>1 (S/NR)	NR	NR
Cougar*	NR	NR	>1 (S/S)	NR	NR

FIGURE 2 | Different *Toxoplasma* strains show a unique profile of seroreactivity against specific GRA peptides. Ratio values from strain-specific peptides assayed with serum samples from mice infected with different *Toxoplasma* strains. Ratios were calculated by dividing the RIPC values of specific peptides with the homologous version from the different strain types (in parenthesis). Ratios greater than 1 were highlighted with an increasing brown color (being 100 the most intense), whereas values between 1 and 0 were highlighted in an increasing green color (being 0 the most intense). NR, non-reactive, designates ratios of 1 derived from samples that did not react to any of the two peptides. As a reference, type 1 RH, as well as the average ratio for individual M4, ME49 and PRU type 2 ([b]) and CEP and CL14 type 3 ([c]) samples are shown. Readers are referred to **Supplemental File 3** for details on individual values and standard deviation. The specific peptide amino acid sequence for each of the strains is displayed in the middle of the figure, where dots represent identical residues. Type 12 Ari strain has been added for comparative purposes. At the bottom, predictions were made based on the ratio obtained for each infection type. Ratios were classified as non-reactive (NR, when both peptides in the division had an RIPC value of 1), lower than 1 (<1), lower but close or almost equal to 1 (≤1), higher but close or almost equal to 1 (≥1) or higher than 1 (>1). The strength (S, strong; W, weak) of each peptide is indicated in parenthesis and separated by a division mark (/). * indicates a single strain result.

and 3 strains is possible by using the aforementioned GRA peptides in combination. For example, RIPC values from GRA3 and GRA5 peptides showed a high, often nonspecific, reactivity. However, when RIPC values for GRA3-I/III-43 *vs.* GRA3-II-43 and GRA5-I-38 *vs.* GRA5-II-38 were analyzed, a clear specific ratio was detected for their respective type (**Supplemental File 3**). Moreover, the GRA3-I/III-43 *vs.* GRA3-II-43 ratio proved better for differentiating type 3 *vs.* non-type 3 strains (>1 *vs.* ~1 or non-reactive), whereas the GRA5-I-38 *vs.* GRA5-II-38 ratio was more useful to differentiate type 1 *vs.* non-type 1 strains (>1 *vs.* ≤1 or non-reactive). Apart from the GRA6-I/III-213 *vs.* GRA6-II-214 combination that has already been described to distinguish type 2 *vs.* non-type 2 strains and that we have confirmed here, ratio values from the GRA7 peptides also proved useful to discriminate between type 2 and non-type 2, and occasionally type 3, strains. Nevertheless, although all 4 peptides were very specific, the GRA7-II-224 and GRA7-III-224 showed a stronger reactivity compared to their shorter versions (GRA7-II-226 and GRA7-III-226).

Furthermore, the non-archetypal strains tested in the present study behaved in a way compatible with a mixture of types 1, 2, and/or 3 "standard" profiles. For example, CAST (type 7) reacted as a type 3 strain for the GRA3, GRA6 and GRA7 peptides, while it induced a type 1-like reaction against the GRA5 peptides. In all these cases CAST shares the respective type 3 and 1 sequences (**Figure 2**). On the other hand, Cougar (type 11) showed a unique mixed pattern of type 2 and 1/3 reactivity against only two peptides (GRA6-I/III-213 and GRA6-II-214). The Cougar type 11 strain has a distinct GRA6 allele that shares both type I/III and type II characteristics, likely explaining its low GRA6-I/III-213 *vs.* GRA6-II-214 ratio (4.6) when compared to the other strains with ratios >1 that usually were higher than 10 (**Figure 2**). This represents a unique pattern for these GRA6 peptides that is not observed for any other strain tested here (**Supplemental File 3**). Therefore, this pattern observed with Cougar, in which among all peptides it only reacted against this GRA6 pair, could be diagnostic of this strain. Previously, a similar mixed reactivity against these two peptides was observed for other non-type 1/2/3 strains belonging to the haplogroup (HG)12, such as Ari or Ray (McLeod et al., 2012). Since these strains share with Cougar the same peptide sequence (LHPERVNEFDY) for this portion of GRA6 (**Figure 2**), this pattern could potentially be used to differentiate type 11/12 strains from other strains (see below).

Interestingly, apart from CAST, all the other non-archetypal strains tested in the present work only reacted to some of the GRA6 peptides. BOF (type 6) showed a similar low reactivity against GRA6-I/III-213 and GRA6-II-215, but did not react against GRA6-II-214, as opposed to the other strains which showed a stronger reactivity for GRA6-II-214 compared to GRA6-II-215. On the other hand, P89 (type 9) only reacted to GRA6-I/III-213. Taken together, this combination of peptide ratios revealed a unique profile for each of the strains tested that can be potentially used to define a fingerprint for identification, except for GUY-DOS and P89 that showed a very similar signature (**Figure 2**).

Recombinant and Non-Archetypal Strains Display Different Patterns

Since a low reactivity against few peptides was the pattern observed in most of the non-archetypal strains, but not in any of the type 1, 2 or 3 strains, we next investigated whether non-archetypal strains could be differentiated from recombinant strains derived from type 2×3 crosses. To this end, the GRA3, GRA5, GRA6 and GRA7 peptides were tested in combination for their ability to determine the allele type by using sera from mice infected with four different strains derived from a 2×3 cross (Sibley et al., 1992): S22, S26, STE10 and CL13. A prediction of the type for each of these proteins at the GRA3, GRA5 and GRA6 loci was made based on the RIPC ratios (**Figure 3**), which was further confirmed with the genotype of these F1 progeny at those loci (available at http://toxomap.wustl.edu/IIxIII_Typing_Table.html). This result shows that the low reactivity found in some non-archetypal strains that were predicted to react based on the epitope present may instead be explained by the existence of other unique immunodominant epitopes that have yet to be pinpointed.

Human Sera Peptide ELISA

Although the mouse ELISA results provided promising results, the final objective of *Toxoplasma* serotyping is arguably aimed to assist in human toxoplasmosis. Hence, a total of 34 human serum samples (**Supplemental File 1B**) were used to test the 27 final peptides by ELISA, except the GRA7-II-226 peptide that could not be used in this assay due to insufficient amounts. All the samples reacted to the rSAG1 control antigen, indicating that, although titers varied, antibody levels were high enough to be able to compare reactivity against different polymorphic peptides (**Supplemental File 4**). In addition, all samples from France (FR-X) (de-la-Torre et al., 2013) showed a rSAG1 reactivity matching that from the IgG titers reported based on the ARCHITECT IgG assay (**Supplemental File 1B, Supplemental File 4**). The "duplicated" 6I/III, 6II and 7II control peptides (Kong et al., 2003) proved to be reactive against most of their respective serum type samples in our analysis, confirming the validity of our results. Nevertheless, when compared to our GRA6-I/III-213, GRA6-II-214 and GR7-II-214 peptides (which share the same sequence), although values were in general very close to each other, some samples only reacted above the cut-off for one of the duplicates. This indicates that individual variation occurs within each sample and peptide, including peptides from different batches, which highlights the importance of using a large number of peptides to minimize this effect. To make our results more uniform, only our recent batch of peptides was considered for further analysis. All the peptides except GRA5-II-38 elicited a response above the

Strain \ Peptide	GRA3-I/III-43 ÷ GRA3-II-43	GRA5-I-38 ÷ GRA5-II-38	GRA6-I/III-213 ÷ GRA6-II-214	GRA7-II-224 ÷ GRA7-III-224
Type 2	NR or ≤1 (W/W)	<1 (W/S)	<1 (W/S)	>1
Type 3	>1 (S/W)	NR or ≤1 (W/W)	>1 (S/W)	NR or <1
S22	12 (12÷1)	0.2 (11÷65)	46 (46÷1)	NR (1÷1)
S26	68 (68÷1)	0.2 (6÷30)	<0.1 (1÷34)	NR (1÷1)
STE10	69 (69÷1)	0.3 (8÷33)	<0.1 (1÷22)	NR (1÷1)
CL13	NR (1÷1)	0.1 (1÷14)	37 (37÷1)	NR (1÷1)

Alleles	GRA3	GRA5	GRA6	GRA7
S22	3	2	3	3
S26	3	2	2	3
STE10	3	2	2	3
CL13	2	2	3	3

FIGURE 3 | Strains derived from a 2×3 cross can be identified by seroreactivity against a combination of different GRA peptides. Ratio values of reactivity from strain-specific peptides assayed with serum samples from mice infected with *Toxoplasma* S22, S26, STE10 and CL13 strains from a 2×3 cross (Sibley et al., 1992). Ratios were calculated by dividing the RIPC values (in parenthesis) of specific peptides with their homologous peptide from the different strain types. Numbers above 1 were rounded to decrease decimals (readers are referred to **Supplemental File 3** for the exact values). NR, non-reactive, designates ratios of 1 derived from samples that did not react to any of the two peptides. At the top, the observed behavior of type 2 (M4, ME49 and PRU) and 3 (CEP and CL14) samples are shown as a reference (**Figure 2**), where the strength (S, strong; W, weak) of each peptide is indicated in parenthesis and separated by a division mark (/). Predictions were made based on this and highlighted in green and blue for type 2 and 3 alleles, respectively. At the bottom, the actual alleles for each strain that can be found at http://toxomap.wustl.edu/IIxIII_Typing_Table.html are shown.

cut-off for at least one of the serum samples. The most reactive peptides were GRA7-II-224, GRA6-I/III-213 and GRA6-II-214, which produced a response above the cut-off limit in 19/34, 15/34 and 12/34 serum samples, respectively. On the other hand, a number of peptides reacted to only a few of the samples: GRA5-I-38, GRA6-II-215 and GRA15-II-477 to only 4/34 samples, and GRA3-II-43, ROP8-I/III-61, ROP8-I/III-305, ROP20-I-331 and hp-I/II-47 to 5/34 samples (**Supplemental File 4**).

From the 34 human serum samples, all but 7 (FR-96, FR-25, FR-27, FR-30, FR-54, FR-58 and JOS1) reacted to at least one of the peptides. It is worth mentioning that some of the samples considered non-reactive (NR) by previous analysis did react, although weakly, to some of the peptides tested in this study: FR-10, FR-19, FR-31, FR-46, FR-48 and FR-49. On the other hand, FR-96 that reacted weakly to the Kong panel of GRA6 and GRA7 peptides did not react to any of the peptides tested in our study (**Supplemental File 4**). Since all these values were very close to their respective threshold, it is possible that slight variations in reactivity between assays may render them positive or negative to specific peptides. Therefore, low values should be carefully interpreted and not be considered individually. Regardless, samples with a strong positive reaction to *Toxoplasma* lysate or rSAG1 antigen but very low, or absent, reaction against multiple strain-specific peptides have been considered in the past as an "atypical" (i.e. non-type 1, 2 or 3) profile (Shobab et al., 2013). Furthermore, 5 samples reacted above the cut-off limit against the majority of the peptides: FR84 (23/26), JOBE (22/26), 9M (21/26), FR72 (20/26) and 279 (19/26). Because they reacted against peptides from different strain types, it is possible that the strain causing the infection was different from the archetypal 1, 2, or 3 strains, or that these patients had a mixed infection. Moreover, these 5 samples, together with NZJ, were the only ones reacting to the PA-14 peptide derived from the TGME49_258400 protein (CCp5A, sporozoite-specific), which was described to be able to distinguish oocyst *vs.* cyst derived infections (Santana et al., 2015).

A Prediction of the Infecting Strain Can Be Made by Using Peptide Ratios

As described above for mice, a ratio was calculated by dividing individual values from the most reactive peptides by their homologous counterpart versions. While the GRA5-I-38 *vs.* GRA5-II-38 ratio proved useful with murine samples, that was not the case with human sera: GRA5-II-38 did not react to any of the samples and GRA5-I-38 only reacted weakly to very few sera (**Supplemental File 4**). On the other hand, two new ratios were

Sample	Type[a]	GRA3-I/III-43 ÷ GRA3-II-43	GRA6-II-200 ÷ GRA6-III-201	GRA6-I/III-213 ÷ GRA6-II-214	GRA7-I-164 ÷ GRA7-III-164	GRA7-II-224 ÷ GRA7-III-226	GRA3-I/III-43 ÷ GRA3-II-43	GRA6-II-200 ÷ GRA6-III-201	GRA6-I/III-213 ÷ GRA6-II-214	GRA7-I-164 ÷ GRA7-III-164	GRA7-II-224 ÷ GRA7-III-226	PRED.
RO2	fRH	1.4 (1.5÷1.1)	NR (1.4÷1.3)	1.2 (1.5÷1.3)	NR (1.4÷1.3)	1.5 (2.0÷1.3)	1/3	IC (NR)	IC (W/NR)	IC (NR)	2	ATYP
NZJ	G-1	1.6 (2.3÷1.4)	NR (1.3÷1.3)	9.3 (11.0÷1.2)	1.9 (1.9÷1.0)	NR (0.3÷1.1)	1/3	IC (NR)	1/3	1	IC (NR)	1
FON	G-2	NR (1.3÷1.3)	NR (1.3÷1.3)	NR (1.4÷1.4)	NR (1.2÷1.3)	1.5 (2.0÷1.3)	IC (NR)	IC (NR)	IC (NR)	IC (NR)	2	2?
NS	G-2	NR (1.5÷1.5)	0.9 (1.4÷1.5)	0.7 (1.1÷1.6)	NR (1.0÷1.1)	3.9 (3.9÷1.0)	IC (NR)	IC (W/W)	2	IC (NR)	2	2
FR-57	S-2	NR (0.9÷1.3)	NR (1.0÷0.9)	0.3 (1.0÷3.0)	NR (0.9÷1.0)	1.8 (1.6÷0.9)	IC (NR)	IC (NR)	2	IC (NR)	2	2
FR-65	S-2	NR (0.9÷1.1)	NR (1.0÷1.4)	0.5 (1.2÷2.3)	NR (1.1÷1.4)	1.5 (1.7÷1.1)	IC (NR)	IC (NR)	2	IC (NR)	2	2
FR-80	S-2	0.4 (1.0÷2.2)	NR (1.1÷1.2)	0.5 (1.1÷2.1)	NR (1.2÷1.4)	1.4 (2.1÷1.5)	2	IC (NR)	2	IC (NR)	2	2
FR-92	S-2	NR (1.0÷1.2)	NR (1.2÷1.2)	NR (1.3÷1.4)	NR (1.4÷1.2)	1.6 (1.8÷1.1)	IC (NR)	IC (NR)	IC (NR)	IC (NR)	2	2?
FR-96	S-2	NR (0.9÷1.0)	NR (0.9÷1.0)	NR (1.0÷1.1)	NR (0.9÷0.9)	NR (1.3÷1.0)	IC (NR)	IC (NR)	IC (NR)	IC (NR)	IC (NR)	NR
TIL	G-3	NR (1.3÷1.1)	NR (1.1÷1.1)	3.8 (4.4÷1.2)	NR (1.0÷1.3)	NR (1.1÷1.0)	IC (NR)	IC (NR)	1/3	IC (NR)	IC (NR)	1/3
9M	G-ATYP	1.7 (4.4÷2.6)	1.0 (2.6÷2.5)	4.4 (8.5÷1.9)	0.5 (1.3÷2.4)	0.6 (1.9÷3.2)	1/3	IC (S/S)	1/3	3	3	3
JOBE	G-ATYP	1.0 (2.9÷2.8)	3.2 (2.9÷0.9)	2.7 (7.5÷2.7)	0.8 (2.5÷3.1)	0.9 (2.8÷3.2)	1?	2	1/3*	3?	IC (S/S)	ATYP
JOS1	G-ATYP	NR (1.0÷1.2)	NR (1.1÷1.3)	NR (1.5÷1.1)	NR (1.1÷0.8)	NR (1.3÷0.9)	IC (NR)	IC (NR)	IC (NR)	IC (NR)	IC (NR)	NR
258	G-ATYP	NR (1.1÷0.8)	NR (1.2÷1.3)	10.2 (10.1÷1.0)	7.9 (10.1÷1.3)	2.3 (4.4÷1.9)	IC (NR)	IC (NR)	1/3	1	2	ATYP
279	G-ATYP	1.4 (2.1÷1.5)	1.0 (2.1÷2.0)	5.1 (8.5÷1.7)	3.0 (6.6÷2.2)	0.3 (1.9÷6.2)	1/3	IC (W/W)	1/3	1	3	ATYP
FR-100	S-ATYP	NR (1.2÷1.1)	NR (1.2÷1.2)	3.8 (4.3÷1.1)	1.0 (8.6÷8.5)	2 (2.2÷1.1)	IC (NR)	IC (NR)	1/3	IC (S/S)	2	ATYP
FR-36	S-ATYP	NR (1.4÷1.2)	1.5 (1.8÷1.2)	1.6 (2.3÷1.4)	0.7 (1.2÷1.7)	0.9 (2.3÷2.6)	IC (NR)	2	1/3	3	IC (S/S)	ATYP
FR-72	S-ATYP	1.0 (1.6÷1.5)	1.3 (2.3÷1.8)	2.3 (3.4÷1.5)	1.0 (1.6÷1.6)	1.1 (1.9÷1.7)	IC (W/W)	2	1/3	IC (W/W)	IC (W/W)	ATYP
FR-67	S-ATYP	NR (1.3÷1.2)	1.0 (1.5÷1.5)	0.8 (1.5÷2.1)	1.3 (1.9÷1.5)	2.5 (3.7÷1.5)	IC (NR)	IC (W/W)	2	1	2	ATYP
FR-69	S-ATYP	1.5 (1.5÷1.0)	NR 1.2÷1.2)	1.0 (12.6÷12.6)	11.9 (12.6÷1.1)	1.7 (1.9÷1.1)	1/3	IC (NR)	IC (S/S)*	1	2	ATYP
FR-97	S-ATYP	NR (1.5÷0.9)	NR (1.0÷1.0)	1.1 (9.3÷8.6)	9.3 (9.3÷1.0)	NR (1.5÷1.0)	IC (NR)	IC (NR)	IC (S/S)*	1	IC (NR)	11/12-like?
FR-16	S-ATYP	2.2 (1.9÷0.9)	NR (1.5÷1.1)	2.3 (16.6÷7.2)	0.8 (1.3÷1.6)	NR (1.4÷1.3)	3	IC (NR)	1/3*	3?	IC (NR)	3?
FR-84	S-ATYP	1.0 (2.9÷2.9)	1.0 (4.2÷4.0)	2.2 (6.0÷2.8)	0.6 (2.3÷3.6)	0.8 (3.8÷4.5)	1?	IC (S/S)	1/3*	3?	IC (S/S)	ATYP
FR-10	S-NR	NR (1.1÷1.2)	NR (1.2÷1.1)	NR (1.1÷1.1)	NR (1.2÷1.3)	1.5 (1.9÷1.3)	IC (NR)	IC (NR)	IC (NR)	IC (NR)	2	NR-2?
FR-19	S-NR	NR (1.2÷1.1)	NR (1.4÷1.2)	NR (1.2÷1.1)	1.0 (1.5÷1.6)	1.0 (1.7÷1.7)	IC (NR)	IC (NR)	IC (NR)	IC (W/W)	IC (W/W)	NR?
FR-25	S-NR	NR (1.0÷0.8)	NR (1.1÷1.0)	NR (1.0÷1.1)	NR (1.0÷1.0)	NR (1.2÷1.0)	IC (NR)	IC (NR)	IC (NR)	IC (NR)	IC (NR)	NR
FR-27	S-NR	NR (1.0÷0.9)	NR (1.0÷1.0)	NR (1.0÷1.2)	NR (1.1÷1.2)	NR (1.1÷1.3)	IC (NR)	IC (NR)	IC (NR)	IC (NR)	IC (NR)	NR
FR-30	S-NR	NR (1.0÷1.0)	NR (1.1÷1.1)	NR (1.1÷1.0)	NR (1.1÷1.2)	NR (1.1÷1.0)	IC (NR)	IC (NR)	IC (NR)	IC (NR)	IC (NR)	NR
FR-31	S-NR	NR (1.0÷0.9)	NR (1.0÷1.1)	NR (1.0÷1.0)	NR (1.0÷1.2)	0.3 (1.3÷4.0)	IC (NR)	IC (NR)	IC (NR)	IC (NR)	3	NR-3?
FR-46	S-NR	NR (1.2÷1.0)	NR (1.3÷1.1)	NR 1.1÷1.5)	0.7 (1.4÷1.8)	NR (1.3÷1.2)	IC (NR)	IC (NR)	IC (NR)	3	IC (NR)	3-NR?
FR-48	S-NR	NR (0.7÷0.7)	NR (0.8÷0.8)	NR (0.9÷1.0)	NR (0.7÷0.7)	0.3 (0.8÷2.7)	IC (NR)	IC (NR)	IC (NR)	IC (NR)	3	NR-3?
FR-49	S-NR	NR (1.2÷1.2)	1.2 (1.6÷1.3)	NR (1.2÷1.1)	NR (1.2÷1.2)	NR (1.3÷1.2)	IC (NR)	2	IC (NR)	IC (NR)	IC (NR)	2-NR?
FR-54	S-NR	NR (0.8÷0.9)	NR (1.0÷0.7)	NR (0.8÷1.0)	NR (1.1÷1.0)	NR (0.8÷0.8)	IC (NR)	IC (NR)	IC (NR)	IC (NR)	IC (NR)	NR
FR-58	S-NR	NR (1.1÷1.0)	NR (1.0÷0.9)	NR (0.9÷1.0)	NR (0.9÷1.0)	NR (1.3÷0.9)	IC (NR)	IC (NR)	IC (NR)	IC (NR)	IC (NR)	NR

FIGURE 4 | Strain type prediction using human sera reactivity against a panel of *Toxoplasma* polymorphic peptides. On the left, ratios were calculated by dividing individual values from each peptide (in parenthesis). Readers are referred to **Supplemental File 4** for further details on individual values. [a] G and S indicate the type of analysis (genotyping and serotyping, respectively) used to detect the strain type. ATYP: Atypical, non-archetypal (non-type 1, 2 or 3). NR: non-reactive. On the right, a prediction was made based on the ratio for each specific peptide couple and the strain causing the infection inferred considering all individual predictions. IC stands for inconclusive. For IC samples, the strength of the reactivity against each peptide is shown in parenthesis as NR (non-reactive), W/W (weak/weak) or S/S (strong/strong). * denotes an unusual strong reactivity to both peptides in the GRA6-I/III-213 *vs.* GRA6-II-214 ratio.

used here compared to mice samples: GRA6-II-200 *vs.* GRA6-III-201 and GRA7-I-164 *vs.* GRA7-III-164. In addition, the GRA7-II-224 peptide was compared to GRA7-III-226 instead of GRA7-III-224 on account of its stronger reactivity. Despite these differences and considering each one of the peptide combinations as a whole, a prediction of the strain that caused the infection for each sample was performed (**Figure 4**). Predictions from all but 2 samples matched the information gathered in the past by genotyping or serotyping techniques. Of note, the strains causing the infection in the human patients included in this study were in most cases not isolated and thus the actual initially suspected strain may not be accurate or even a mixture of strains be present, which renders the analysis more difficult.

R02 sera was derived from a patient known to be accidentally infected with the mouse virulent fRH (f=French) strain, which is not RH nor a type 1 strain. Its reactivity pattern with the diagnostic peptides (only reacted weakly to some peptides from different types) supports that designation, that it is atypical, neither type 1, 2 or 3. Another sample, 279, is non-archetypal, but possesses the GRA6 I/III-213 epitope, and reacted positively with that peptide, despite the fact that it possesses a novel GRA6 allele. Further, it has a type 1 allele at GRA7, and as expected, did not react with either the GRA7 II-224 or GRA7 III-226 peptide. Finally, sera from JOS1 also failed to react with the GRA6 (I/III and II) and GRA7 (II and III) peptides, an expected result since it possesses a novel epitope at GRA6 and a type 1 epitope at GRA7. These data support the notion that the reactivity profile at the GRA6 and GRA7 antigens is epitope specific.

We also included in our study several samples previously serotyped as NR (all French samples) to test if an expanded set of peptides would be able to identify their type. Although some NR samples showed a weak reactivity against few peptides, most of them failed to react to any peptide, confirming previous results (de-la-Torre et al., 2013). The reason underlying this lack of reactivity to different peptides despite keeping a strong reactivity against rSAG1 is currently unknown. Finally, 5 samples (JOBE, FR-16, FR-69, FR-84 and FR-97) reacted strongly to both GRA6-I/III-213 and GRA6-II-214, although being higher with the former in all but FR-69, which showed similar reactivity with both peptides (**Figure 4**, **Supplemental File 4**). Although this unusual pattern is similar to the one described above for the Cougar (HG11) mouse sample, these human samples reacted strongly to several other peptides (including PA14 for JOBE and FR-84), which indicates the infection was likely produced by an atypical strain or that the patients had a mixed infection. Nevertheless, among these samples, FR-97 displayed a profile that is similar to that observed for the Cougar-infected mice. As opposed to the other four samples, besides the strong reaction against both GRA6 peptides it only reacted to the GRA7-I-164 peptide (which shares the amino acid sequence with Cougar and HG12 Ari and Ray strains), while failing to react to the GRA7-224 and 226 peptides (**Supplemental File 4**). To the best of our knowledge, the Cougar and HG12 strains have not been isolated in France; however, it is possible that this patient acquired the infection abroad or that the spectrum of strains present in France and other European countries are not yet fully characterized.

HG11/12 Strains Can Be Resolved by Their Distinct Reactivity Against GRA6-I/III-213 and GRA6-II-214

Because the C-terminal GRA6 amino acid sequence is identical in the HG11 Cougar and HG12 Ari and Ray strains (**Figure 2**), we further sought to investigate whether the unique GRA6-I/III-213 *vs.* GRA6-II-214 pattern observed both for the Cougar infected mice sample and some human samples could be a signature of HG11/12 infections. For this, we tested the two GRA6 peptides (I/III-213 and II-214) against a new panel of sera from CD1 mice infected with different HG12 isolates (**Table 2**). Mouse sera were collected at 1 month post-infection, and since these strains are highly virulent to outbred CD1 mice, animals needed to be treated with sulfadiazine (0.4 mg/ml in drinking water) at the time of infection or upon detection of clinical signs to survive acute infection. All HG12 infected mice developed a strong mixed reactivity against GRA6-I/III-213 and GRA6-II-214, but with a predominant GRA6-I/III-213 response, which correlates with the results described above for the Cougar strain. Moreover, all these samples also failed to react to the GRA7-II-224 peptide, which is in accordance with the type 1 sequence for

TABLE 2 | HG12 mouse serum samples react distinctively against GRA6 peptides.

Mouse ID	Dose[a]	Strain[b]	Genotype	Sulf.[c]	rSAG1	GRA6-I/III-213÷GRA6-II-214	GRA7-II-224
4338	NA	UI		Y	0.7		
4336	NA	UI		Y	0.7		
4334	1,000	3045	HG12	Y	14.4	1.0 (2.0÷2.1)	0.9
4328	1,000	3133	HG12	Y	16.3	4 (7.2÷1.8)	1.1
4329	1,000	3133	HG12	Y	17.4	1.9 (5.9÷3.1)	1.1
4332	1,000	3133	HG12	Y	11.5	2.2 (8.4÷3.8)	1.4
4331	1,000	3142	HG12	Y	18.6	3.3 (15.7÷4.8)	1
3916	50	3429	HG12	N	24.0	1.6 (5.8÷3.6)	0.7
3917	50	3429	HG12	N	23.5	1.4 (13.5÷9.4)	1.2
BC-3	50	3675	TYPE II	N	23.7	0.1 (1.1÷13.7)	12.2

Mouse sera were collected at 1 month post-infection. GRA6-I/III-213 vs. GRA6-II-214 ratio was calculated by dividing individual normalized values from each peptide (in parenthesis). Threshold values below which each sample-peptide reaction is considered negative are greyed out. Green highlighting represents positive rSAG1 values, while orange and blue colors represent GRA6-I/III-213 vs. GRA6-II-214 ratios above (or close to) and below 1, respectively. (a) Number of tachyzoites unless otherwise stated. NA: not available. (b) UI: uninfected. (c) Sulf.: sulfadiazine treatment (0.4 mg/ml in drinking water) was applied at the time of or early after infection to avoid mortality in the acute phase.

this peptide in Cougar, Ari and Ray strains (**Figure 2** and **Table 2**). Taken together, these results support the notion that HG11/12 strain samples elicit a unique strong reaction against both GRA6-I/III-213 and GRA6-II-214 peptides combined with the absence of reactivity against GRA7-II-224.

Different Allele Combinations Are Formed When Comparing the Amino Acid Sequence of GRA3, GRA5, GRA6, and GRA7 Peptides

When we aligned the amino acid sequences of the GRA peptides used in the ratio analysis and compared the 64 strains available on ToxoDB, we observed that the possible combinations give rise to different allele groups. Namely, 2, 5, 5, 6, 5, and 3 different combinations were observed for GRA3-43, GRA5-38, GRA6-44, GRA6-213, GRA7-164, and GRA7-224 peptides, respectively (**Supplemental File 5**). Furthermore, 30 different allele groups were detected when all these peptides were compared together (**Figure 5**). Among these, all the 6 type 1 strains, together with the type 7 TgCkBr141 strain, had the same peptide sequence combination. In addition, 4 of the type 6 strains, including BOF and FOU, had an almost identical combination compared to the type 1 strains, except one amino acid in the GRA6-44 peptide. On the other hand, the type 2 and 3 strains showed different allele combinations and were distributed in 3 and 5 different groups, respectively. Besides the type 1 group, the next larger group was formed by 5 strains from the types 3, 8, 9 and 16, such as G662M, P89 or CASTELLS. By contrast, most of the groups were only composed of one or two strains. Despite this, it is worth mentioning that numerous combinations were very similar except for one of the peptides and sometimes differing in only one amino acid; therefore, they could be considered virtually identical in practice (**Figure 5, Supplemental File 5**). Taken together, these results show that different strains can react in a similar way to these peptides on account of their sequence similarity, although it is possible that the presence of particular immunodominant regions may differ within strains. Therefore, although epitope is predictive in archetypal strains and some non-archetypal strains, it is the reactivity pattern across multiple peptide pairs that should be used to define a specific signature or fingerprint for each strain.

DISCUSSION

Serological typing relies on the identification of long-lasting antibodies produced against parasite proteins that are polymorphic among distinct strains (Kong et al., 2003; Garcia-Ispierto et al., 2010; Vaudaux et al., 2010; Herrmann et al., 2012; McLeod et al., 2012; Hutson et al., 2015). Through a large-scale peptide array assay we recently identified a large number of novel *Toxoplasma* antigenic peptides able to discriminate between infections caused by different strain types (Arranz-Solís et al., 2019). However, arrays are expensive and not always available or transferable. Hence, in the present work we sought to further

```
                          GRA3-43         GRA5-48      GRA6-44         GRA6-213         GRA7-164         GRA7-224
RH                        ADQPENHQALAE///SEGARGREQ///ADSGGVKQTP///LHPERVNVFDY///LTEEQQRGDEP///VPESGEDGEDARQ
B73                       ....G.......///....G...R///......R...///...GS..E..F///...Q..T....///.......R.....
ME49                      ....G.......///....W.G..///......R...///...GS..E..F///...Q..T.E..///.....K.......
SOU                       ............///....G...R///...D......///...........///...Q..T.E..///.....K.......
p89                       ............///....G...R///...D......///...GS......///...Q..T....///.......R.....
M7741                     ............///....G...R///..........///...........///...Q..T....///.......R.....
VEG                       ............///....G...R///...D......///...........///...Q..T....///.......R.....
TgCkGy2                   ............///....G...R///...D......///...GS......///...........///.............
GUY-2003-MEL              ............///....G...R///..........///...........///...........///.............
MAS                       ............///F...G...R///..........///...GS..E..F///...Q..T....///.......R.....
TgCatBr1                  ............///F...G...R///..........///....H......///...Q..T....///.......R.....
TgCatBr18                 ............///F...G...R///......R...///...GS..E..F///...Q..T....///.......R.....
TgCatBr10                 ............///F...G...R///...D......///...GS......///...Q..T....///.......R.....
VAND                      ............///.........///..........///...........///...Q..A.E..///.............
GUY-2004-ABE              ............///.........///...D......///...GS......///...Q..A.E..///.............
RUB                       ............///....G...R///..........///..L....A...///...Q..A.E..///.............
BOF                       ............///.........///......Q...///...........///...........///.............
TgCATBr9                  ............///.........///......Q...///...........///...Q..T....///.......R.....
TgCatBr72                 ............///F...G...R///......Q...///...........///...Q..T....///.......R.....
CAST                      ............///.........///..........///...........///...Q..A....///.......R.....
TgCatBr3                  ............///....G...R///..........///....H......///...Q..T....///.......R.....
BRC_TgH_18001_GUY-DOS     ............///....G...R///..........///...........///...Q..A.E..///.............
BRC_TgH_18009             ............///....G...R///..........///....H......///...Q..A.E..///.............
COUG                      ....G.......///D...G.G.R///......R...///.......E...///...Q..T.E..///.............
ARI                       ....G.......///....G...R///......R...///.......E...///...Q..T.E..///.............
B41                       ....G.......///....G...R///......R...///...GS..E..F///...Q..T.E..///.............
GAB1-2007-GAL-DOM10       ............///....G...R///......R...///...GS..E..F///...........///.............
TgCkCr10                  ............///....G...R///..........///...........///...Q..A....///.......R.....
TgRsCr1                   ............///.........///...D......///...........///...Q..T....///.......R.....
BRC_TgH_21016             ............///F...G...R///.....FR...///.......E...///...Q..T....///.......R.....
```

FIGURE 5 | Allele combinations in GRA peptide amino acid sequences among 64 *Toxoplasma* strains. Amino acid sequence alignment from GRA3-43, GRA5-38, GRA6-44, GRA6-213, GRA7-164 and GRA7-224 peptides (from left to right, respectively) in the 64 strains available on ToxoDB shows the possible combinations that give rise to different allele groups. The different possible combinations are aligned and a representative strain from each group is given, where dots indicate identical amino acids. For further details and individual sequences for each strain we refer readers to **Supplemental File 5**.

investigate the potential diagnostic properties of the most promising peptides by means of a more accessible and affordable ELISA test with a larger collection of murine and human serum samples. To that end, a total of 28 *Toxoplasma* allele-specific peptides mainly from dense granule (GRA3, GRA5, GRA6, GRA7 and GRA15) and rhoptry (ROP8 and ROP20) proteins were designed and synthetized.

Our results show a number of peptides that discriminate between mice infected with different type 1, 2 and 3 strains. Among these, GRA6-I/III-213, GRA6-II-214, GRA7-II-224 and GRA7-III-224 were already described (Kong et al., 2003), whereas GRA3-I-38, GRA3-II-38, GRA5-I/III-43, GRA5-II-43, GRA7-II-226, GRA7-III-226 and GRA15-II-477 are novel peptides. In accordance with earlier studies, we detected a high degree of individual variability for each peptide and sample (Sousa et al., 2008; Maksimov et al., 2012b). In an attempt to significantly improve *Toxoplasma* serotyping, we calculated a ratio between RIPC values of different strain versions of the same peptides. A similar comparison between GRA6 and GRA7 I/III and II peptides was previously made by McLeod et al. (2012). In that work, when a sample reacted strongly to both peptides, different designations were given depending on the predominance to one of the two peptides. Similarly, we have used a numeric ratio with GRA3, GRA5, GRA6 and GRA7 peptide pairs to determine which one is predominant and hence predict the strain type regardless of the reactions that happen in low-specific or low-sensitive peptides. A clear example of this is the combination of GRA5-I-38 and GRA5-II-38: if considered individually, some samples are difficult to allocate into one group, as they react weakly to only one of them or strongly to both. However, when the ratio is used, type 1 (>1) and type 2 (<1) strains can readily be differentiated. Unfortunately, all our attempts to resuspend the GRA5-III-38 peptide were unsuccessful. Had it worked, this peptide would have also allowed us to individually differentiate type 3 from 1 and 2 strains. Peptides able to distinguish type 2 *vs.* non-type 2 (Kong et al., 2003), type 1 *vs.* type 3 (Xiao et al., 2009) and type 2 *vs.* type 3 infections (Maksimov et al., 2012a) have been previously described. In addition to these, we show peptide combinations able to differentiate type 3 *vs.* non-type 3 (GRA3), 1 *vs.* 2 (GRA5) and 2 *vs.* 3 (GRA7) strains. Nevertheless, it is worth mentioning that only one type 1 mouse infection was available in our study, and given the individual variability shown by other samples, further investigation is needed with a larger number of type 1 serum samples to confirm these results. Be that as it may, we confirmed the utility of these GRA peptides by means of a proof of concept where we accurately determined the allele type for each gene using serum samples from mice infected with F1 progeny derived from a type 2×3 cross (Sibley et al., 1992).

In addition to the variability in the peptide recognition among individuals infected with the same strain, a recent report showed that chickens and turkeys experimentally infected had a peptide recognition pattern that changed over time (Maksimov et al., 2018). Herein, we compared samples from mice infected with the type 2 PRU and type 3 CEP strains under a wide variety of experimental conditions: inoculum dose, parasite stage, route of infection, post-infection treatment, time after infection and mouse breed. As expected, differences in the peptide recognition were observed within the same strain. However, since there was a high number of different possible combinations of parameters and few individual samples, comparison between animals could not be made. Regardless, this adds further evidence as to the high individual variability even in the same group of animals reported previously by others (Sousa et al., 2009; Maksimov et al., 2013; Maksimov et al., 2018). In our study, however, a number of peptides showed a constant strain-specific reactivity irrespective of the experimental variables: GRA3-I/III-43 and GRA6-I/III-213 in type 3 and GRA5-II-38, GRA6-II-214 and GRA7-II-224 in type 2 strains reacted in all cases in a frequently strong manner.

When we tested the peptides with our panel of human samples, we observed different levels of reactivity compared to that of murine samples. While some peptides that reacted strongly in mice were very weak in human samples, other peptides that did not elicit any response with any mouse serum were able to react to some human samples. Nonetheless, it is important to remark that in our study most of the human samples were either genotyped or serotyped as type 2 or atypical (non-type 1/2/3) strains, while only one type 3 sample was included. Despite this shortcoming, with the current panel of peptides we were able to correctly predict the *Toxoplasma* type in the great majority of human samples. This further supports the notion that even though some peptides may react differently depending on the host and individuals, a prediction can be made if a large number of peptides is used (Arranz-Solís et al., 2019).

Although we and others have shown that a distinction between the archetypal strains (type 1, 2 and 3) is possible by serological typing, non-archetypal strains are harder to investigate due to the lack of specific peptides. Maksimov and colleagues attempted to distinguish cats infected with non-type 1/2/3 strains, but they observed a high reactivity against type 2 and, specially, type 1/3 peptides (Maksimov et al., 2013). The current availability in ToxoDB of the whole genome sequences of 64 different *Toxoplasma* strains, including non-archetypal ones (Lorenzi et al., 2016), makes it possible to start investigating specific allelic variations between these and 1/2/3 strains. Unsurprisingly, non-archetypal strains share, in most cases, the sequence of one of 1, 2 or 3 types in different combinations. For example, type 7 CAST shares the sequence of type 1/3 in GRA3-43 peptides, type 1 in GRA5-38, type 1/3 in GRA6-213/214 and type 3 in GRA7-224/226. Another important hindrance in the advancement of non-archetypal strains serotyping is the scarcity of validated serum samples from animals or patients infected with these strains. Herein, we used sera from mice experimentally infected with a number of different atypical strains (type 4 MAS, type 6 BOF, type 7 CAST, type 9 P89, type 10 GUY-DOS and type 11 Cougar). In agreement with what was reported by Maksimov et al. (2013) and the performed alignments, we observed a high reactivity of these samples to few peptides from type 1/3 (GRA3-I/III-43 and GRA6-I/III-213) and/or type 2 (GRA6-II-214 and 215) strains, which correlated in most cases with the specific sequence shared with their respective type. Similarly, Kong and colleagues observed a type 1/3 profile with the GRA6-I/III-213 peptide in mice and human CAST samples that were believed to belong to the type 1 group (Kong et al., 2003), and which is currently classified as type 7 (Lorenzi et al., 2016). As suggested by others and confirmed here, non-archetypal strains contain unique combinations of alleles at any given genetic locus, highlighting the need for the inclusion of a considerably larger number of peptides from different genes to avoid a misprediction of the strain type. This feature should be further exploited in future experiments by employing new peptides from polymorphic antigens that have dissimilar allele segregation not only compared to the archetypal types but also within non-archetypal strains.

In our study, when the ratio between the GRA6-I/III-213 and GRA6-II-214 peptides was analyzed for the type 11 Cougar mouse serum sample, a distinct pattern was observed: while this ratio showed a clear predominance of the respective type-specific peptide in type 1, 2, and 3 strains, it reacted against both 2 and 1/3 peptides, but stronger to the latter, in the Cougar strain. Likewise, a similar pattern with these two GRA6 peptides was observed in mice infected with different recombinant type 12 strains. Considering that the amino acid sequence in the C-terminal epitope of GRA6 is identical in the type 11 Cougar and type 12 Ari and Ray strains, this could be considered as a "HG11/12" profile. Together with the aforementioned mixed GRA6 reactivity, a further trait of this profile would be an absence of reactivity to the GRA7-II-224 peptide, as Cougar, Ari and Ray have the type 1 version for this peptide. In line with this, a mixed reactivity against GRA6 type 1/3 and 2 peptides but not GRA7 type 2 peptides has been already reported and shown to be a characteristic feature of the type 12 Ari and Ray strains (McLeod et al., 2012). Indeed, McLeod et al. described a similar reactivity of type 12 samples to both GRA6 peptides and defined a "II=I/III" profile. Although in our study some non-archetypal human samples showed a similar pattern, most of them had a close but stronger reactivity against GRA6-I/III-213 compared to GRA6-II-214, a profile designated by McLeod as "I/IIIa". Whether this is something specific of the Ari or Ray strains compared to other type 11 or 12 strains deserves further investigation. In fact, the B41 strain, currently classified within haplogroup 12 together with Ari and Ray (Lorenzi et al., 2016), does not share the same sequence in that epitope of GRA6, but rather it has a type 2 sequence. This correlates with the fact that B41 has been described to be an F1 progeny from a type 2 and Ray/WTD3 (belonging to haplogroup 12) cross (Minot et al., 2012). Thus, although serum samples from patients or animals infected with this B41 strain were not tested, it is tempting to hypothesize that the reactivity against the GRA6 peptides could be different from the "HG11/12" of Cougar, Ari or Ray, but similar to PRU or ME49 strains. Nevertheless, it is also possible that other non-archetypal strains may elicit this GRA6 reactivity or that this particular pattern may be observed when a mixed infection is present, as most of the patients showing this HG11/12 profile for GRA6 in our study did also react strongly to several other peptides. Hence, further samples from animals and patients infected with different strains need to be tested to investigate whether this strong and near equal (or slightly higher) reactivity against GRA6-I/III-213 compared GRA6-II-214 is a specific signature of HG11/12 strains. This might prove extremely useful in North America, where type 2, 12 and 3 account for most of strains isolated from wild-life, with the type 12 commonly being found in severe cases of ocular and congenital toxoplasmosis (Grigg et al., 2001; Khan et al., 2011; Minot et al., 2012; Schumacher et al., 2020). In addition, the Cougar strain has been epidemiologically linked to a major waterborne outbreak occurred in Victoria, British Columbia, Canada (Aramini et al., 1998; Aramini et al., 1999), and recently an outbreak in Wisconsin, USA, was reported to be caused by type 12 strains from contaminated venison (Schumacher et al., 2020).

Apart from the "HG11/12" profile, we observed two other characteristic patterns in the non-archetypal serum samples. Firstly, despite having similar high reactivity to the *Toxoplasma* lysate or rSAG1 antigen, some samples reacted to none, or weakly to few, of the peptides. This was apparent in both mouse and human samples, although only few of the human samples failed to react to any of the peptides. This profile, termed non-reactive, has been previously described even after using a high number of peptides, and has been associated with infections by atypical strains, especially in ocular toxoplasmosis patients (Kong et al., 2003; Maksimov et al., 2012a; Maksimov et al., 2012b; Shobab et al., 2013). In these studies, the lack of reactivity against type 1, 2 and 3 strain-specific peptides by samples from non-archetypal strain infections was attributed to possible differences in the amino acid sequence. However, with the current availability of the whole genome sequences of several non-type 1/2/3 strains (Lorenzi et al., 2016), we have observed that the absence of reactivity often does not correlate with differences in amino acid sequence, as even strains sharing the sequence with type 1, 2 and/or 3 strains do not react to their respective peptide. Instead, this non-reactive profile may be explained by the presence of other immunogenic epitopes in the proteins of those strains that are dominant and prevent other epitopes, such as the ones from the peptides, from reacting (Arranz-Solís et al., 2019). Alternatively, it could be possible that this lack of reactivity against short strain-specific peptides may be caused by the Hoskins paradox, aka original antigenic sin. This term was coined more than 60 years ago after observations made in patients that showed a reduced vaccine effectiveness against influenza virus (Thomas Francis, 1960; Monto et al., 2017). The prior exposure to a particular strain of the virus produced a diversion of the antibody response against a second infecting strain to focus on cross-reactive immunodominant epitopes. Although this phenomenon has not been described in *Toxoplasma* and is out of the scope of the present work, superinfection with a different strain than the original strain could provide a plausible explanation for the lack of reactivity which is only observed in human serum samples.

Regardless, the second pattern frequently observed in non-1/2/3 type serum samples was a strong reaction against the majority of the peptides, which was observed exclusively in human samples. This could represent a specific pattern for certain non-archetypal strains, although since we did not observe this pattern in mice experimentally infected with several of them, the possibility that this pattern may just have been caused by mixed natural infections cannot be ruled out (Aspinall et al., 2003; Nowakowska et al., 2006; Vaudaux et al., 2010). Interestingly, together with NZJ, these samples were the only ones reacting to the PA-14 peptide derived from the sporozoite-specific protein CCp5A. This protein has been shown to be able to differentiate infections caused by oocysts (Santana et al., 2015). Therefore, although the origin of infection in the patients included in our study is unknown, it is possible that the reactivity against PA-14 was either the result of infection by ingestion of oocysts, or caused by the high levels of antibodies found in these patients.

Finally, apart from the low type-specificity of particular peptides that may be explained by a strong immunoreactivity in the non-polymorphic parts of these peptides, identical sequences in the peptides employed did not always match with the observed reactivity in different strains. For instance, although several strain types share the same amino acid sequence, only serum samples from mice infected with type 3 strains and type 7 CAST were recognized by GRA3-I/III-43 (ADQPENHQALAE). Similar to the non-reactive pattern discussed above, this effect may be accounted for by the presence of other immunogenic epitopes in the protein for certain strains that prevent short peptides from reacting. On the other hand, we have confirmed the importance that single amino acid substitutions may have on the peptide recognition. For example in the GRA6 C-terminal epitope the GS/ER polymorphisms are not important, while the EFDF/VFDY portion is much more relevant (Kong et al., 2003; Arranz-Solís et al., 2019). Similarly, the K/E in position 229 in GRA7-224 and 226 peptides proved to be the most important amino acid. These results, together with the lower reactivity of shorter peptides (for example GRA6-II-214 *vs.* GRA6-II-215) are in accordance with the notion that the polymorphic site and length of peptides play a pivotal role in serological typing (Kong et al., 2003; Arranz-Solís et al., 2019).

In summary, we present novel antigenic peptides able to differentiate type 1, 2 and 3, as well as some non-archetypal strains, by comparing the reaction to different variants of polymorphic regions rather than relying on individual peptides. As a proof of concept, we show that GRA3, GRA5, GRA6, and GRA7 peptides are able to correctly predict the type for each locus in mice infected with strains derived from a type 2×3 cross. This same principle could be applied in future studies to investigate the strain an animal or a patient is infected with. In addition, we also observed reaction patterns that were exclusive of some atypical strains, especially in human samples. This allowed us not only to clearly differentiate them from the three canonical lineages, but also to identify specific profiles from certain groups of strains, such as the HG11/12, which may spur further investigations on these strains and their frequent association with severe toxoplasmosis cases. In order to advance in *Toxoplasma* serotyping, a wider panel of well characterized samples would prove critical to better characterize their reaction against a large pool of polymorphic peptides from different loci described by us and others. This can further advance in the definition of a clear signature for each host and strain, with a particular growing interest in the understudied non-archetypal strains.

ETHICS STATEMENT

The studies involving human participants were reviewed and approved by Human samples were used according to the Committee on the Use of Humans as Experimental Subjects (COUHES) application No. 0808002869. Written informed consent for participation was not required for this study in accordance with the national legislation and the institutional requirements. The animal study was reviewed and approved by The MIT Committee on Animal Care (assurance number A-3125-01), the Institutional Animal Care and Use Committee (IACUC) at the University of California, Davis (assurance number A-3433-01), and the Animal Care and Use Committee (ACUC) of the Intramural Research Program of NIAID (Animal study protocol; LPD22E) approved all protocols, and all efforts were made to minimize unnecessary distress to the animals. The animal study protocol LPD22E was reviewed and approved by the Animal Care and Use Committee of the Intramural Research Program of the National Institute of Allergy and Infectious Diseases (NIAID) at the National Institutes of Health.

AUTHOR CONTRIBUTIONS

Conceptualization, methodology, validation, and formal analysis: DA-S, MG, and JS. Investigation: DA-S, CC, EZ, and MG. Resources: MG and JS. Data curation: DA-S and MG. Writing original draft: DA-S. Writing review and editing: DA-S, MG, and JS. Supervision, project administration, and funding acquisition: JS. All authors contributed to the article and approved the submitted version.

ACKNOWLEDGMENTS

We would like to thank Hafiz Muhammad Rizwan and Carolina Gómez for their technical contribution.

SUPPLEMENTARY MATERIAL

Supplemental File 1 | Mouse **(A)** and human **(B)** serum samples used for ELISAs.

Supplemental File 2 | Raw mouse ELISA OD values and normalization process.

Supplemental File 3 | Individual RIPC and ratio values of antigenic peptides tested with mouse sera by ELISA.

Supplemental File 4 | Normalized values of human peptide ELISA.

Supplemental File 5 | Amino acid sequence alignment from GRA3-43, GRA5-38, GRA6-44, GRA6-213, GRA7-164 and GRA7-224 peptides in the 64 strains available on ToxoDB shows the possible combinations that give rise to different allele groups.

REFERENCES

1. Ajzenberg, D., Collinet, F., Mercier, A., Vignoles, P., and Darde, M. L. (2010). Genotyping of Toxoplasma gondii isolates with 15 microsatellite markers in a single multiplex PCR assay. *J. Clin. Microbiol.* 48, 4641–4645. doi: 10.1128/JCM.01152-10
2. Aramini, J. J., Stephen, C., and Dubey, J. P. (1998). Toxoplasma gondii in Vancouver Island Cougars (Felis concolor vancouverensis): Serology and Oocyst Shedding. *J. Parasitol.* 84, 438–440. doi: 10.2307/3284508
3. Aramini, J. J., Stephen, C., Dubey, J. P., Engelstoft, C., Schwantje, H., and Ribble, C. S. (1999). Potential contamination of drinking water with Toxoplasma gondii oocysts. *Epidemiol. Infect.* 122, 305–315. doi: 10.1017/S0950268899002113
4. Arranz-Solıs, D., Cordeiro, C., Young, L. H., Darde, M. L., Commodaro, A. G., Grigg, M. E., et al. (2019). Serotyping of toxoplasma gondii infection using peptide membrane arrays. *Front. Cell. Infect. Microbiol.* 9:408. doi: 10.3389/fcimb.2019.00408
5. Aspinall, T. V., Guy, E. C., Roberts, K. E., Joynson, D. H. M., Hyde, J. E., and Sims, P. F. G. (2003). Molecular evidence for multiple Toxoplasma gondii infections in individual patients in England and Wales: Public health implications. *Int. J. Parasitol.* 33, 97–103. doi: 10.1016/S0020-7519(02)00230-8
6. Boothroyd, J. C., and Grigg, M. E. (2002). Population biology of Toxoplasma gondii and its relevance to human infection: do different strains cause different disease? *Curr. Opin. Microbiol.* 5, 438–442. doi: 10.1016/s1369-5274(02)00349-1
7. Bradford, M. M. (1976). A rapid and sensitive method for the quantitation of microgram quantities of protein utilizing the principle of protein-dye binding. *Anal. Biochem.* 72, 248–254. doi: 10.1016/0003-2697(76)90527-3
8. Carme, B., Bissuel, F., Ajzenberg, D., Bouyne, R., Aznar, C., Demar, M., et al. (2002). Severe acquired toxoplasmosis in immunocompetent adult patients in French Guiana. *J. Clin. Microbiol.* 40, 4037–4044. doi: 10.1128/JCM.40.11.4037-4044.2002
9. Carme, B., Demar, M., Ajzenberg, D., Darde, M. L., Darde, M. L., Darde, M. L., et al. (2009). Severe acquired toxoplasmosis caused by wild cycle of Toxoplasma gondii, French Guiana. *Emerg. Infect. Dis.* 15, 656–658. doi: 10.3201/eid1504.081306
10. Dard, C., Fricker-Hidalgo, H., Brenier-Pinchart, M. P., and Pelloux, H. (2016). Relevanceof and new developments in serology for Toxoplasmosis. *Trends Parasitol.* 32, 492–506. doi: 10.1016/j.pt.2016.04.001
11. de-la-Torre, A., Sauer, A., Pfaff, A. W., Bourcier, T., Brunet, J., Speeg-Schatz, C., et al. (2013). Severe South American Ocular Toxoplasmosis Is Associated with Decreased Ifn-g/Il-17a and Increased Il-6/Il-13 Intraocular Levels. *PloS Negl. Trop. Dis.* 7. doi: 10.1371/journal.pntd.0002541
12. Dubey, J. P., Velmurugan, G. V., Rajendran, C., Yabsley, M. J., Thomas, N. J., Beckmen, K. B., et al. (2011). Genetic characterisation of Toxoplasma gondii in wildlife from North America revealed widespread and high prevalence of the fourth clonal type. *Int. J. Parasitol.* 41, 1139–1147. doi: 10.1016/j.ijpara.2011.06.005
13. Fekkar, A., Ajzenberg, D., Bodaghi, B., Touafek, F., Le Hoang, P., Delmas, J., et al. (2011). Direct genotyping of Toxoplasma gondii in ocular fluid samples from 20 patients with ocular toxoplasmosis: predominance of type II in France. *J. Clin. Microbiol.* 49, 1513–1517. doi: 10.1128/JCM.02196-10
14. Fuentes, I., Rubio, J. M., Ramırez, C., and Alvar, J. (2001). Genotypic characterization of Toxoplasma gondii strains associated with human toxoplasmosis in spain: Direct analysis from clinical samples. *J. Clin. Microbiol.* 39, 1566–1570. doi: 10.1128/JCM.39.4.1566-1570.2001
15. Furtado, J. M., Smith, J. R., Belfort, R.Jr, Gattey, D., and Winthrop, K. L. (2011). Toxoplasmosis: a global threat. *J. Glob. Infect. Dis.* 3, 281–284. doi: 10.4103/0974-777X.83536
16. Garcia-Ispierto, I., Nogareda, C., Yaniz, J. L., Almeria, S., Martinez-Bello, D., de Sousa, N. M., et al. (2010). Neospora caninum and coxiella burnetii seropositivity are related to endocrine pattern changes during gestation in lactating dairy cows. *Theriogenology.* 74 (2), 212–220. doi: 10.1016/j.theriogenology.2010.02.004
17. Grigg, M. E., Bonnefoy, S., Hehl, A. B., Suzuki, Y., and Boothroyd, J. C. (2001). Success and virulence in Toxoplasma as the result of sexual recombination between two distinct ancestries. *Science (80-)* 294, 161–165. doi: 10.1126/science.1061888
18. Grigg, M. E., and Sundar, N. (2009). Sexual recombination punctuated by outbreaks and clonal expansions predicts Toxoplasma gondii population genetics. *Int. J. Parasitol.* 39, 925–933. doi: 10.1016/j.ijpara.2009.02.005
19. Hamilton, C. M., Black, L., Oliveira, S., Burrells, A., Bartley, P. M., Melo, R. P. B., et al. (2019). Comparative virulence of Caribbean, Brazilian and European isolates of Toxoplasma gondii. *Parasitol. Vectors* 12, 104. doi: 10.1186/s13071-019-3372-4
20. Herrmann, D. C., Barwald, A., Maksimov, A., Pantchev, N., Vrhovec, M. G., Conraths, F. J., et al. (2012). Toxoplasma gondii sexual cross in a single naturally infected feline host: generation of highly mouse-virulent and avirulent clones, genotypically different from clonal types I, II and III. *Vet. Res.* 43:39. doi: 10.1186/1297-9716-43-39
21. Howe, D. K., Honore, S., Derouin, F., Sibley, L. D., Honore, S., Derouin, F., et al. (1997). Determination of genotypes of Toxoplasma gondii strains isolated from patients with toxoplasmosis. *J. Clin. Microbiol.* 35, 1411–1414.
22. Hutson, S. L., Wheeler, K. M., McLone, D., Frim, D., Penn, R., Swisher, C. N., et al. (2015). Patterns of Hydrocephalus Caused by Congenital Toxoplasma gondii Infection Associate with Parasite Genetics. *Clin. Infect. Dis.* 61, 1831–1834. doi: 10.1093/cid/civ720
23. Jensen, K. D. C. C., Camejo, A., Melo, M. B., Cordeiro, C., Julien, L., Grotenbreg, G. M., et al. (2015). Toxoplasma gondii superinfection and virulence during secondary infection correlate with the exact ROP5/ROP18 allelic combination. *MBio* 6. doi: 10.1128/mBio.02280-14
24. Khan, A., Dubey, J. P., Su, C., Ajioka, J. W., Rosenthal, B. M., and Sibley, L. D. (2011). Genetic analyses of atypical Toxoplasma gondii strains reveal a fourth clonal lineage in North America. *Int. J. Parasitol.* 41, 645–655. doi: 10.1016/j.ijpara.2011.01.005
25. Kong, J., Grigg, M. E., Uyetake, L., Parmley, S., and Boothroyd, J. C. (2003). Serotyping of Toxoplasma gondii infections in Humans Using Synthetic Peptides. *J. Infect. Dis.* 187, 1484–1495. doi: 10.1086/374647
26. Lorenzi, H., Khan, A., Behnke, M. S., Namasivayam, S., Swapna, L. S., Hadjithomas, M., et al. (2016). Local admixture of amplified and diversified secreted pathogenesis determinants shapes mosaic Toxoplasma gondii genomes. *Nat. Commun.* 7. doi: 10.1038/ncomms10147
27. Maksimov, P., Zerweck, J., Maksimov, A., Hotop, A., Groß, U., Pleyer, U., et al. (2012a). Peptide Microarray Analysis of In Silico -Predicted Epitopes for Serological Diagnosis of Toxoplasma gondii Infection in Humans. *Clin. Vaccine Immunol.* 19, 865–874. doi: 10.1128/cvi.00119-12
28. Maksimov, P., Zerweck, J., Maksimov, A., Hotop, A., Groß, U., Spekker, K., et al. (2012b). Analysis of clonal type-specific antibody reactions in toxoplasma gondii seropositive humans from germany by peptide-microarray. *PLoS One* 7, 1–10. doi: 10.1371/journal.pone.0034212
29. Maksimov, P., Zerweck, J., Dubey, J. P., Pantchev, N., Frey, C. F., Maksimov, A., et al. (2013). Serotyping of Toxoplasma gondii in cats (Felis domesticus) reveals predominance of type II infections in Germany. *PLoS One* 8, 1–16. doi: 10.1371/journal.pone.0080213
30. Maksimov, P., Basso, W., Zerweck, J., Schutkowski, M., Reimer, U., Maksimov, A., et al. (2018). Analysis of Toxoplasma gondii clonal type-specific antibody reactions in experimentally infected turkeys and chickens. *Int. J. Parasitol.* 48, 845–856. doi: 10.1016/j.ijpara.2018.04.004
31. McLeod, R., Boyer, K. M., Lee, D., Mui, E., Wroblewski, K., Karrison, T., et al. (2012). Prematurity and severity are associated with toxoplasma gondii alleles (NCCCT-2009). *Clin. Infect. Dis.* 54, 1595–1605. doi: 10.1093/ cid/cis258
32. Minot, S., Melo, M. B., Li, F., Lu, D., Niedelman, W., Levine, S. S., et al. (2012). Admixture and recombination among Toxoplasma gondii lineages explain global genome diversity. *Proc. Natl. Acad. Sci. U. S. A.* 109, 13458–13463. doi: 10.1073/pnas.1117047109
33. Monto, A. S., Malosh, R. E., Petrie, J. G., and Martin, E. T. (2017). The Doctrine of Original Antigenic Sin: Separating Good from Evil. *J. Infect. Dis.* 215, 1782– 1788. doi: 10.1093/infdis/jix173
34. Morisset, S., Peyron, F., Lobry, J. R., Garweg, J., Ferrandiz, J., Musset, K., et al. (2008). Serotyping of Toxoplasma gondii: striking homogeneous pattern between symptomatic and asymptomatic infections within Europe and South America. *Microbes Infect.* 10, 742–747. doi: 10.1016/j.micinf.2008.04.001
35. Nowakowska, D., Colon, I., Remington, J. S., Grigg, M., Golab, E., Wilczynski, J., et al. (2006). Genotyping of Toxoplasma gondii by multiplex PCR and peptide- based serological testing of samples from infants in Poland diagnosed with congenital toxoplasmosis. *J. Clin. Microbiol.* 44, 1382–1389. doi: 10.1128/ JCM.44.4.1382-1389.2006
36. Mukhopadhyay, D., Arranz-Solıs, D., and Saeij, J. P. J. (2020). Toxoplasma GRA15 and GRA24 are important activators of the host innate immune

response in the absence of TLR11. *PLoS Pathog*. 16 (5), e1008586. doi: 10.1371/journal.ppat.1008586

37. Peyron, F., Lobry, J. R., Musset, K., Ferrandiz, J., Gomez-Marin, J. E., Petersen, E., et al. (2006). Serotyping of Toxoplasma gondii in chronically infected pregnant women: predominance of type II in Europe and types I and III in Colombia (South America). *Microbes Infect*. 8, 2333–2340. doi: 10.1016/ J.MICINF.2006.03.023

38. Robert-Gangneux, F., and Darde, M. L. (2012). Epidemiology of and diagnostic strategies for toxoplasmosis. *Clin. Microbiol. Rev*. 25, 264–296. doi: 10.1128/ CMR.05013-11

39. Santana, S. S., Gebrim, L. C., Carvalho, F. R., Barros, H. S., Barros, P. C., Pajuaba, A. C., et al. (2015). CCp5A Protein from Toxoplasma gondii as a Serological Marker of Oocyst-driven Infections in Humans and Domestic Animals. *Front. Microbiol*. 6:1305. doi: 10.3389/fmicb.2015.01305

40. Schumacher, A. C., Elbadawi, L. I., Desalvo, T., Straily, A., Ajzenberg, D., Letzer, D., et al. (2020). Toxoplasmosis outbreak associated with toxoplasma gondii- contaminated venison—high attack rate, unusual clinical presentation, and atypical genotype. *Clin. Infect. Dis*. 30341, 1–9. doi: 10.1093/cid/ciaa285

41. Shobab, L., Pleyer, U., Johnsen, J., Metzner, S., James, E. R., Torun, N., et al. (2013). Toxoplasma Serotype Is Associated With Development of Ocular Toxoplasmosis. *J. Infect. Dis*. 208, 1520–1528. doi: 10.1093/infdis/jit313

42. Sibley, L. D., LeBlanc, A. J., Pfefferkorn, E. R., and Boothroyd, J. C. (1992). Generation of a restriction fragment length polymorphism linkage map for Toxoplasma gondii. *Genetics* 132, 1003–1015.

43. Sousa, S., Ajzenberg, D., Vilanova, M., Costa, J., and Darde, M. L. (2008). Use of GRA6-derived synthetic polymorphic peptides in an immunoenzymatic assay to serotype Toxoplasma gondii in human serum samples collected from three continents. *Clin. Vaccine Immunol*. 15, 1380–1386. doi: 10.1128/CVI.00186-08

44. Sousa, S., Ajzenberg, D., Marle, M., Aubert, D., Villena, I., Da Costa, J. C., et al. (2009). Selection of polymorphic peptides from GRA6 and GRA7 sequences of Toxoplasma gondii strains to be used in serotyping. *Clin. Vaccine Immunol*. 16, 1158–1169. doi: 10.1128/CVI.00092-09

45. Sousa, S., Canada, N., Correia da Costa, J. M., and Darde, M.-L. L. (2010). Serotyping of naturally Toxoplasma gondii infected meat-producing animals. *Vet. Parasitol*. 169, 24–28. doi: 10.1016/j.vetpar.2009.12.025

46. Su, C., Dubey, J. P., Ajzenberg, D., Khan, A., Ajioka, J. W., Rosenthal, B. M., et al. (2012). Globally diverse Toxoplasma gondii isolates comprise six major clades originating from a small number of distinct ancestral lineages. *Proc. Natl. Acad. Sci*. 109, 5844–5849. doi: 10.1073/pnas.1203190109

47. Thomas Francis, J. (1960). On the Doctrine of Original Antigenic Sin on JSTOR. *Proc. Am. Philos. Soc* 104, 572–578.

48. Vaudaux, J. D., Muccioli, C., James, E. R., Silveira, C., Magargal, S. L., Jung, C., et al. (2010). Identification of an Atypical Strain of Toxoplasma gondii as the Cause of a Waterborne Outbreak of Toxoplasmosis in Santa Isabel do Ivai, Brazil. *J. Infect. Dis*. 202, 1226–1233. doi: 10.1086/656397

49. Xiao, J., Buka, S. L., Cannon, T. D., Suzuki, Y., Viscidi, R. P., Torrey, E. F., et al. (2009). Serological pattern consistent with infection with type I Toxoplasma gondii in mothers and risk of psychosis among adult offspring. *Microbes Infect*. 11, 1011–1018. doi: 10.1016/j.micinf.2009.07.007

16

Plasmodium falciparum VAR2CSA-Specific IgG Subclass Responses Reflect Protection against Low Birth Weight and Pregnancy-Associated Malaria

Bernard Tornyigah[1,2], *Tania d'Almeida*[1,3], *Guillaume Escriou*[1], *Firmine Viwami*[4], *Nadine Fievet*[1,4], *Adrian J. F. Luty*[1,4], *Achille Massougbodji*[4], *Morten A. Nielsen*[5], *Philippe Deloron*[1] and *Nicaise Tuikue Ndam*[1,2*]

[1] *Université de Paris, MERIT, IRD, Paris, France,* [2] *Department of Immunology, Noguchi Memorial Institute for Medical Research, College of Health Sciences, University of Ghana, Legon, Ghana,* [3] *Université Pierre et Marie Curie, Ecole doctorale 393 Pierre Louis de Santé publique, Paris, France,* [4] *Centre d'Etude et de Recherche sur le Paludisme Associé à la Grossesse et à l'Enfance, Cotonou, Benin,* [5] *Centre for Medical Parasitology, University of Copenhagen, Copenhagen, Denmark*

***Correspondence:**
Nicaise Tuikue Ndam
nicaise.ndam@ird.fr

Sequestration of *Plasmodium falciparum*-infected erythrocytes expressing the VAR2CSA antigen in the placenta results in poor pregnancy outcomes, including low birth weight and maternal anemia. Antigen-specific antibody-mediated immunity is acquired during successive pregnancies. Thus, evaluating VAR2CSA-specific IgG profiles among pregnant women will increase knowledge on the immunological mechanisms associated with protection, and help in the development of VAR2CSA-based placental malaria vaccines. Using the PAMVAC candidate vaccine antigen, we assessed anti-VAR2CSA IgG subclass responses of a cohort of pregnant Beninese, and analyzed their relationships with pregnancy outcomes. Cytophilic IgG1 and IgG3 responses were the most frequent, with prevalences ranging from 28% (IgG3) up to 50% (IgG1). Elevated levels of VAR2CSA-specific total IgG and cytophilic IgG3 during pregnancy were consistently associated with higher birth weights, whilst high levels of IgG4 were associated with a reduced risk of placental infections. This suggests that protective anti-VAR2CSA IgG responses are coordinated between both cytophilic and non-cytophilic antibodies.

Keywords: pregnancy, malaria, VAR2CSA, IgG subclasses, IgG3, IgG4

INTRODUCTION

Plasmodium falciparum malaria continues to be a significant human disease burden throughout the tropics. In sub-Saharan Africa, placental malaria (PM) is known to cause low birth weight and maternal anemia (1, 2). The adverse effects associated with PM are due to the sequestration of infected erythrocytes (IEs) in the placental intervillous spaces. The often massive accumulation of IEs is mediated by VAR2CSA, a parasite ligand that promotes adhesion of IEs to placental chondroitin sulfate A (CSA) (3–5). This pathophysiological feature, which led to the recognition of placental malaria as a specific syndrome, is particularly frequent in first pregnancies in areas where *P. falciparum* malaria is highly endemic (6). Women who have had PM develop anti-VAR2CSA IgG antibodies that protect them from the adverse effects of PM during subsequent pregnancies, making this protein an attractive target for vaccine development (4, 7). Anti-VAR2CSA IgGs have been shown to inhibit the binding of VAR2CSA-expressing infected erythrocytes to CSA (8–10). Further studies identified the Id1-DBL2X-Id2 region, in the N-terminal part of VAR2CSA, as being the minimal binding domain mediating binding between VAR2CSA and placental CSA (9), thus making it appropriate for the development of a VAR2CSA-based vaccine with an antigenic construct easier to produce in recombinant form. A Phase 1 clinical trial has recently been completed with such an antigenic construct (10).

Our team has already demonstrated in a longitudinal study that high levels of IgG with specificity for the N-terminal part of VAR2CSA present in women early in pregnancy were associated with better pregnancy outcomes (11). Additionally, a recent systematic review suggests that IgG levels against VAR2CSA antibodies are likely markers of infection rather than correlates of protection (12). However, information is lacking on which of the IgG subclasses targeting the vaccine construct are responsible for protective immunity and also on the dynamics of such protective antibody levels during pregnancy. Here, we used samples from a group of women whose pregnancy outcomes were well characterized in the Strategies to Prevent Pregnancy Associated Malaria (STOPPAM) study in Benin and from whom consecutive blood samples and clinical data were available from the time of inclusion until delivery. Using measurements of naturally acquired antibody targeting the PAMVAC vaccine Id1-Id2a recombinant antigen on consecutive plasma samples, we analyzed the link between IgG subclasses with different pathological outcomes of pregnancy.

METHODS

Study Site and Population

The current study made use of samples collected from a subgroup of women drawn from the STOPPAM project initially designed to characterize the pathology of placental malaria, to determine the factors important for optimal use of intermittent preventive treatment of malaria in pregnancy (IPTp) and for vaccine development against pregnancy-associated malaria. A detailed description of the STOPPAM study design has been reported (13). For the current work, 470 women were included based on their pregnancy outcome as previously reported (14). This subgroup included women who had placental infection at delivery, were anemic, whose infants had low birth weight, in whom intrauterine growth retardation was identified based on fetal growth curves derived from ultrasounds to define children born small-for-gestational-age (SGA), or whose infants were born prematurely. Another group of pregnant women from the same area with no pathological outcome at delivery was also included. Briefly, babies were classified as premature if their gestational age, assessed by ultrasound before 24 weeks of gestation, was <37 weeks at delivery. Fetal growth restriction was approximated by low birth weight for gestational age. A baby was defined as SGA if the birth weight was below the 10th percentile of fetal weight for the gestational age (15). Maternal anemia at delivery was defined as a hemoglobin level below 10 g/dl. Placental malaria was defined as a positive placental blood smear (16). At inclusion and each antenatal or emergency visit, a thick blood smear was processed for malaria diagnosis. Venous blood was collected, and plasma samples were separated and frozen at −80°C for further use. All women diagnosed with *P. falciparum* infection by thick blood smear during the follow up were treated with quinine according to national guidelines applicable at the time of the study.

Ethical Statement

The STOPPAM study obtained ethical approval from two independent institutional ethics committees: the Comité Consultatif de Déontologie et d'Éthique of IRD in France and the Comité d'Éthique de la Faculté des Science de la Santé, Université d'Abomey Calavi, in Benin. All participants provided written consent.

Total IgG and Subclasses Quantification

To measure antibody response against VAR2CSA, we used the PAMVAC vaccine candidate, a recombinant protein representing the ID1-ID2a construct of VAR2CSA from the FCR3 variant of *P. falciparum* (10, 17). Antibody levels with specificity for the ID1-ID2a recombinant protein were determined by a previously described indirect ELISA protocol (7, 10). In brief, antigen-coated (0.5 μg/mL) and bovine serum albumin (BSA)-blocked 96-well ELISA plates (Maxisorp, NUNC, Denmark) were incubated overnight at 4°C with 100 μl/well of test plasma samples in duplicate at dilutions optimized for each subclass (1:200 for total IgG; 1:100 for IgG1 and IgG2 and 1:50 for IgG3 and IgG4) in phosphate-buffered saline (PBS) with 2% BSA. Pools of highly reactive plasma from exposed pregnant Beninese previously characterized on recombinant full-length ectodomain of VAR2CSA (FV2) (11), and non-immune plasma from unexposed French volunteers, were used on each plate as internal controls. Reactions were developed with goat anti-human IgG conjugated to horseradish peroxidase (SIGMA, France) followed by the substrate TMB (SIGMA, France). The color reaction was stopped by the addition of 0.2M H_2SO_4 and optical densities (ODs) were read at 450 nm. In between all incubation steps, plates were washed 3 times with PBS, pH 7.4, containing 0.1% Tween 20, using an automated plate washer.

ELISA for the subclasses followed the same procedure except using mouse anti-human IgG subclasses Fc secondary antibody conjugated to HRP (MH1715, MH1722, MH1732, or MH1742, all from Invitrogen, France). IgG4 antibody levels were also measure against ICAM1 binding DBL-β domain from IT4 VAR13 *Pf*EMP1 (18) donated by Professor Jensen. All reagents were used at predetermined concentrations and optical densities (OD) generated from the antibody measurements were converted to arbitrary units (AUs), as described (19). Briefly,

AUs were calculated as follows:

$$AU = 100 * \frac{\ln(0D\, test\, sample) - \ln(0D\, negative\, sample)}{\ln(0D\, positive\, sample) - \ln(0D\, negative\, sample)}$$

Statistical Analysis

For each measured IgG subtype, the mean ODs from non-immune plasma from each plate were calculated plus 2 standard deviations to define a common cut-off value for each IgG isotype above which samples were deemed antibody-positive. Seroprevalence was calculated as the proportion of samples with OD above this cut-off. The outcome variable was the level of IgG antibodies in peripheral maternal blood. Five principal outcome variables were created: the level of total IgG, the levels of IgG1, IgG2, IgG3, and IgG4. As multiple antibody measurements (inclusion, antenatal visits, and delivery) were available, appropriate hierarchical mixed models were used for univariate and multivariate analyses, performed with Stata® software, Version 12 (StatCorp LP, College Station, TX, USA). The level of antibodies was tested in relation to the following different covariates: maternal age, gravidity, malaria at inclusion, number of peripheral malaria infections identified until the date of plasma collection, parasite density, and at delivery according to pregnancy outcome including anemia and placental infection in mothers; low birth weight, prematurity, intrauterine growth retardation in newborns.

All factors with a *p*-value <0.20 during univariate analyses were included in the multivariate step. A backward stepwise procedure was used to select factors of the final model. Statistical significance was set at $p<0.05$.

TABLE 1 | Characteristics of the population.

Mothers	N=470
Maternal age (years)	26.48± 6.18
Primigravidae	78 (16.6%)
Multigravidae	392 (83.4%)
Malaria infection during the follow-up (BS)	
0	234 (49.8%)
1	132 (28.1%)
2	63 (13.4%)
≥3	41 (8.7%)
Placental malaria	
Yes	63 (13.4%)
No	405 (86.2%)
Unknown	2 (0.4%)
Maternal anemia at delivery	
Yes	82 (17.4%)
No	358 (76.2%)
Unknown	30 (6.4%)
Malaria at inclusion (BS and PCR)	
Negative	265 (56.4%)
Submicroscopic	121 (25.74%)
BS Positive	80 (17.0%)
Newborns	
Birth weight (grams)	2982.22± 434.23
Low birth weight	
Yes	49 (10.1%)
No	418 (88.9%)
Unknown	3 (0.6%)
SGA	
Yes	53 (11.3%)
No	417 (88.7%)
Prematurity	
Yes	24 (5.1%)
No	446 (94.9%)

BS, Blood smear; SGA, small for gestational age.

RESULTS

The STOPPAM cohort subgroup used in this work comprises Beninese pregnant women (mean age, 26 years) followed up during the course of pregnancy. Among the 470 women included in this study, 11 (2.3%) attended 3 antenatal visits (ANV) while 415 (88.3%) attended all the 5 scheduled visits (inclusion, ANV1, ANV2, ANV3, and delivery). Amongst the study cohort 78 (16.6%) were primigravidae, 63 (13.4%) had evidence of placental malaria at delivery, and 82 (17.4%) were anemic at delivery. Forty-nine (10.1%) women gave birth to infants with LBW (<2500g), 53 (11.3%) with SGA, 24 (5.1%) women gave birth prematurely (before 37 gestational weeks), and 272 women had no pathological outcomes. The characteristics of women who had their IgG profiles determined are presented in **Table 1**.

Antibody Profiling and Factors Associated

The distribution of IgG subclass responses shows that cytophilic IgG1 and IgG3 were measured in a higher number of women compared to IgG2 and IgG4 (**Figure 1A**). Analysis of the seroprevalence of the different IgG subclasses shows that IgG1 and IgG3 were the most prevalent with rates ranging from 49.6% to 53.8% for IgG1 and from 27.6% to 27.4% for IgG3 according to the time of pregnancy. IgG2 and IgG4 were less prevalent with rates ranging from 8.3% to 12.1% and from 3.4% to 8.9%, respectively (**Figure 1B**). The ranges were larger for subclass measurements compared to total IgG leading to larger dispersion of values (**Figure 1**). When taking into account repeated measurements made on consecutive samples of the same woman in the analyses, plasma levels of IgG (both total and subclasses) gradually decreased over the course of pregnancy, except for IgG4 which was consistently low throughout. (**Table 2, Figure 1A**).

When comparing levels by gravidity, it was clear that total IgG levels remained consistently higher in multigravid women compared to primigravidae, in both univariate and multivariate analysis. However, this observation was not so clear for individual IgG subclasses. When taking into account infections that were documented during the follow-up in relation to the time of antibody measurement, a high level of all subclasses were consistently observed in infected women, even though this reached significance only for IgG1 and IgG3. A similar observation was made for antibody subclass levels and parasite density of the infections documented during follow-up, but statistical significance in multivariate analysis was reached only for total IgG (**Table 2**) (P = 0.028) and IgG2 (P = 0.03).

Relationship With Pregnancy Outcomes

To compare the level of IgG during pregnancy in women with well-defined pregnancy outcomes, we performed a

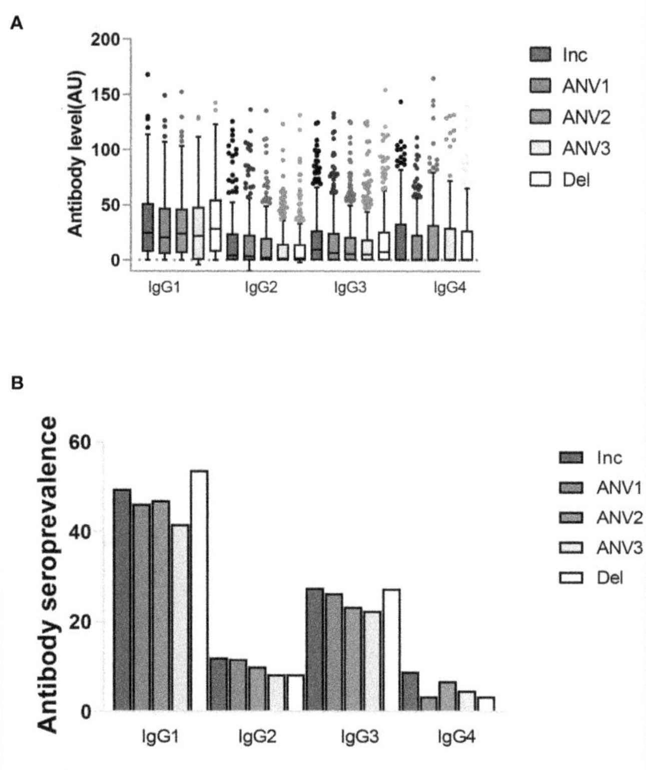

FIGURE 1 | IgG subclass profile to ID1-ID2a recombinant protein from pregnant women followed during the course of pregnancy (inclusion, antenatal visits (ANV) and delivery). **(A)** The distribution of IgG subclasses. Shown are IgG subclasses antibody levels (median and IQR) in arbitrary units. **(B)** IgG subclass seroprevalence. The profile of IgG subclasses clearly shows a cytophilic IgG's (IgG1 and IgG3) are the predominant IgGs while low prevalence of non-cytophilic IgG's (IgG2 and IgG4) were also observed.

hierarchical mixed model analysis and factors with p-value < 0.2 were further incorporated into the final multivariate model (**Table 3**). For total IgG, low levels of antibodies were consistently observed throughout the follow-up in women who delivered babies with low birth weight in univariate analysis (P = 0.014). This observation was further confirmed in the multivariate model (P = 0.004). However, for the other adverse pregnancy outcomes, no significant difference in the antibody levels of total IgG with specificity for the ID1-ID2a PAMVAC antigen was observed. We then tested in a similar way the antibody levels of the IgG subclasses. For IgG1 and IgG2, no significant differences were observed with the different pathological markers at delivery. Levels of IgG3 antibodies were consistently low in women who delivered low birth weight babies compared to those who delivered babies with normal birth weight (multivariate analysis, P = 0.01). Throughout pregnancy, IgG4 antibody levels were low in women presenting with placental infection at delivery compared to women without parasites in their placenta (multivariate analysis, P = 0.03). However, there was no association between IgG4 and placenta infection in data obtained in the same way using a comparable construct from a ICAM1 binding DBL-β domain from IT4 VAR13 *Pf*EMP1 which is not implicated in PM (β=-0.004; p-value = 0.33). Apart from LBW and placental malaria, we did not observe an association between the other pregnancy outcomes and antibody levels measured.

DISCUSSION

In this study of a cohort of pregnant Beninese, we determined the levels of total IgG and of IgG subclasses with specificity for

TABLE 2 | Relationship between antibody levels to ID1-ID2a construct of VAR2CSA and pregnancy outcomes (Total IgG and IgG1).

Covariates	Total IgG						IgG 1					
	Univariate			Multivariate(**)			Univariate			Multivariate(**)		
	β	95% CI	*p*	Adj β	95% CI	*p*	β	95% CI	*p*	Adj β	95% CI	*p*
Primiparity No	–			–			–					
Yes	-9.07	-14,94; -3,21	**0.002**	-9.9	-15,91; -3,90	**0.001**	-3.29	-12,68; 6,10	0.49			
Malaria Infections(*) 0	–			–			–			–		
1	5.18	3,62; 6,75		4.46	2,83; 6,09		6.16	3,24; 9,7	**$<10^{-3}$**	4.92		**$<10^{3}$**
2	7.73	3,75; 11,70	**$<10^{-3}$**	7.93	3,83; 12,02	**$<10^{-3}$**	12.92	4,50; 21,34		12.37		
≥3	13.56	3,13; 23,99		14.30	3,92; 24,68		7.66	-9,20; 24,52		5.44		
Parasite density	0.0002	0,00008; 0,0002	**$<10^{-3}$**	0.0001	0,000016; 0,00027	**0.028**	0.0004	0,0002; 0,0005	**$<10^{-3}$**	0,00002	-0,0003; 0,0003	0,89
Prematurity No	–						–					
Yes	-6.93	-16,93; 3,08	0.17	-4,04	-14,45; 6,38	0,45	0.05	-13,75; 13,84	0.99	-0,84	-18,01; 16;33	0,93
SGA No	–						–			–		
Yes	-4.45	-11,48; 2,58	0.22	-4,04	-12,04; 3,96	0,32	1.47	-9,39; 12,35	0.79	-1,58	-13,65; 10,48	0,80
Placental malaria No	–			–			–			–		
Yes	3.69	-2,77; 10,14	0.26	1,73	-4,70; 8,16	0,59	11.43	-0,88; 23,73	0.07	7,88	-4,65; 20,41	0,22
LBW No	–						–			–		
Yes	-9.04	-16,22; -1,85	**0.014**	-10.74	-18,04; -3,45	**0.004**	-0,59	-11,48; 10,30	0.92	-6,24	-17,33; 4,86	0,27
Maternal anemia No	–						–			–		
Yes	1,74	-3,99; 7,48	0.55	0,44	-5,18; 6,06	0,88	3.31	-5,87; 12,49	0.48	1,65	-7,52; 10,82	0,73

(*) *number of documented blood smear positive during follow-up.*
(**) *Multivariate analysis were adjusted for timepoint.*

TABLE 3 | Relationship between antibody levels to ID1-ID2a construct of VAR2CSA and pregnancy outcomes (IgG2, IgG3 and IgG4).

Covariates	IgG 2						IgG 3						IgG 4					
	Univariate			Multivariate[**]			Univariate			Multivariate[**]			Univariate			Multivariate[**]		
	β	95% CI	*p*	Adj β	95% CI	*p*	β	95% CI	*p*	Adj β	95% CI	*p*	β	95% CI	*p*	Adj β	95% CI	*p*
Primiparity	–						–						–					
No																		
Yes	-7.15	-15,52; 1,23	0.09	-7,32	-15,69; 1,05	0,09	2.17	-4,89; 9,23	0.55				-0.08	-6,32; 6,16	0.98			
Malaria Infections[*]	–						–			–			–					
0																		
1	2.21	0,09; 4,32	0.23				8.12	5,47; 10,77	**$<10^{-3}$**	7.94	5,21; 10,66	**$<10^{-3}$**	-1.81	-6,57; 2,96	0.7			
2	0.93	-4,78; 6,64					10.08	2,46; 17,69		10.12	2,47; 17,76		-1.54	-15,43; 12,36				
≥3	-0.35	-14,35; 13,64					2.97	-12,26; 18,22		2.93	-12,37; 18,22		-13.56	-41,33; 14,20				
Parasite density	0.0001	-0,0001; 0,0002	0.09	0.0001		**0.03**	0.00004	-0,0001; 0,0002	0,59				-0.0001	-0,0004; 0,0001	0.33			
Prematurity	–			–			–			–			–			–		
No																		
Yes	-2.9	-14,13; 8,33	0.61	-3,49	-15,17; 8,19	0,56	-0.46	-10,75; 9,82	0.92	9,29	-3,39; 21,98	0,15	-1.46	-10,54; 7,62	0.75	-0,26	-11,61; 11,09	0,96
SGA	–						–						–					
No																		
Yes	0.25	-9,10; 9,60	0.96	-1,48	-11,73; 8,77	0,78	1.87	-6,36; 10,09	0.66	6,62	-2,38; 15,61	0,15	-4.39	-11,54; 2,76	0,23	-3,33	-10,56; 3,89	0,36
Placental malaria	–			–			–			–			–					
No																		
Yes	8.99	-1,89; 19,88	0.10	10,09	-1,20; 21,39	0,08	-1.06	-10,17; 8,05	0.82	-2,18	-11,47; 7,11	0,65	-8.86	-16,97; -0,75	**0.03**	-8.86	-16,97; -0,75	**0.03**
LBW	–			–			–			–			–			–		
No																		
Yes	-1.01	-10,40; 8,38	0.83	-0,91	-14,75; 12,94	0,89	-5.58	-13,69; 2,52	0,18	-10.79	-19,15; -2,45	**0.01**	-4,15	-11,32; 3,01	0,26	-2,49	-10,23; 5,23	0,53
Maternal anemia	–			–			–			–			–			–		
No																		
Yes	-2.27	-10,03; 5,50	0.56	-2,04	-10,27; 6,18	0,63	1.04	-5,95; 8,03	0.77	-0,64	-7,64; 6,36	0,86	-0.92	-7,09; 5,25	0.77	-0,91	-7,27; 5,44	0,77

[*] *number of documented blood smear positive during follow-up.*

[**] *Multivariate analysis were adjusted for timepoint.*

the PAMVAC vaccine antigen. We focused on the PAMVAC antigen currently undergoing vaccine development to decipher the specific antibody response that women develop when exposed to placental-type parasites. The levels of total IgG with specificity for the PAMVAC antigen were consistently lower in women giving birth to low birth weight babies, unlike other women, regardless of the gestational age at which the plasma sample was taken. These results confirmed our initial observations that low levels of total IgG directed to recombinant DBL1X-Id1-DBL2X of VAR2CSA in early pregnancy were associated with an increased risk of low birth weight (11). The current study emphasizes the fact that this particular association with risk of low birth weight persists throughout pregnancy. Moreover, it should be noted that, as was expected, there were relationships between the antibody levels measured here and the level of exposure to malarial infections or the gravidity status of the women, further supporting the relevance of the observations. Importantly, a recent systematic review by Cutts and his colleagues (12) by analyzing antibody data, most of which was obtained at delivery suggests that IgG levels against VAR2CSA antigen are "likely markers of infection rather than correlates of protection". These observations are in line with those of this work which analyzed antibody levels during pregnancy on a longitudinal angle. This allowed underline the antigenic properties which can differ between different domains or epitopes of an antigen and thus provides additional justification for assessing whether VAR2CSA antibody subclass might better explain the discrepancies between studies.

One noteworthy observation is the association between low levels of cytophilic IgG3 antibody with low birth weight, although IgG1 was the predominant antibody subclass. This finding is similar to that of a study in Senegal (19) and suggests cytophilic IgG3 is the main effector in the prevention of LBW, reflecting the observation with total IgG. From a mechanistic point of view, IgG3 could be acting through either a direct inhibition of infected erythrocyte adhesion to CSA in the placenta, or an ability to mediate opsono-phagocytosis by effector cells, or through sensitization and activation of natural killer cells and the complement system (20–22). As LBW is among the most frequent detrimental outcomes of PM, this is an indication that any vaccine for PM should be demonstrably able to elicit IgG3.

Interestingly, we also observed that higher levels of IgG4 were associated with a reduced risk of placental infection. The IgG4 subclass, unlike IgG3, does not activate complement or act as an opsonin, suggesting that the role of such antibodies in any protective mechanism could only be achieved through the inhibition of infected erythrocyte adhesion to the placental receptor. In helminth infections, antibody isotype patterns are an indicator of the host's immune regulatory status, pointing to the relative level of IgG4 as a corollary of chronic parasite carriage favored by regulatory cytokines. Pathology of chronic helminth infections are characterized by elevated IL-10 and TGFβ that mediate IgG4 production by B cells (23–25). In the context of the STOPPAM study, sub-microscopic parasite carriage revealed by PCR-based diagnosis carried out with samples from this cohort (26) shows that the women who have elevated IgG4 levels are consistently those with low-density (sub-microscopic) parasite carriage at 4 different time points during pregnancy, strongly suggestive of persisting chronic infections. As we have always found, in all our studies, that IL-10 is elevated in the presence of *P. falciparum* infection, whether peripheral (27) or placental (14), we conclude that the conditions therefore likely favored IgG4 production. Further, data obtained using a ICAM-1 binding DBL-β domain protein showed no association with placental infection. This data suggest that our observation with PAMVAC antigen was pregnancy specific and not donor specific. It is also known that the IgG4 titers fall rapidly following curative drug treatment as compared to other subclasses (28). In the context of intermittent preventive treatment administered to pregnant women it is possible that this has contributed to disrupting the association with active infections detected by microscopy in this study. However, the plasma levels of IgG1 and IgG2 subclasses appeared here to represent markers of infection. The observations from this study thus further underline the complex mechanisms underlying antibody responses, the properties of which can both mark the presence of an infection and the success of its control. While this study clearly highlights the importance of the IgG3 subclass in the acquired protection against placental malaria, it also demonstrates for the first time the role that IgG4 could play in this protective mechanism.

One of the limitations of this study is based on the lack of functional data to demonstrate the particular properties of the various purified IgG subclasses. This study opens up on the need for some perspective to confirm the observations. The fact of having used other recombinant antigens reproducing the minimal binding domains of other PfEMP1 (ICAM-1 MBD) and for which we did not observe the same association suggests that the data of this work are of obvious interest. The other limitation is the absence of similar data on the full-length VAR2CSA or other epitopes of the VAR2CSA in this study which would have allowed verify if this association is specific to VAR2CSA in its entirety or just a portion.

In conclusion, the association of IgG3 subclass antibody levels with the risk of low birth weight and that of IgG4 to that of placental infections at delivery, strongly suggest mechanisms of protection mediated by antibody responses against VAR2CSA that rely on different IgG subclasses. This observation further suggests that PM vaccines should ideally target the elicitation of both IgG3 and IgG4 to achieve optimal protection.

AUTHOR CONTRIBUTIONS

NTN, PD and MA contributed to the design of the STOPPAM project. FV and NF collected the samples. BT and GE carried out all the lab experiments. MN provided us with the PAMVAC antigen. Td'A performed the statistical analysis. BT and NTN wrote the MS. AL reviewed the MS. All authors contributed to the article and approved the submitted version.

ACKNOWLEDGMENTS

We are grateful to all the women who participated in the study. Also, we wish to extend our profound thanks to Professor Jessen for the antigen she gave us. This paper describes work undertaken using samples from the STOPPAM project, 'Strategies To Prevent Pregnancy Associated Malaria' supported by the European 7th Framework Programme, contract number: 200889".

REFERENCES

1. Guyatt HL, Snow RW. Impact of Malaria During Pregnancy on Low Birth Weight in Sub-Saharan Africa. *Clin Microbiol Rev* (2004) 17(4):760–9. doi: 10.1128/CMR.17.4.760-769.2004
2. Desai M, ter Kuile FO, Nosten F, McGready R, Asamoa K, Brabin B, et al. Epidemiology and Burden of Malaria in Pregnancy. *Lancet Infect Dis* (2007) 7 (2):93–104. doi: 10.1016/S1473-3099(07)70021-X
3. Tuikue Ndam NG, Salanti A, Bertin G, Dahlbäck M, Fievet N, Turner L, et al. High Level of Var2csa Transcription by *Plasmodium Falciparum* Isolated From the Placenta. *J Infect Dis* (2005) 192(2):331–5. doi: 10.1086/430933
4. Hviid L, Salanti A. VAR2CSA and Protective Immunity Against Pregnancy-Associated *Plasmodium Falciparum* Malaria. *Parasitology* (2007) 134(Pt 13):1871–6. doi: 10.1017/S0031182007000121
5. Salanti A, Dahlbäck M, Turner L, Nielsen MA, Barfod L, Magistrado P, et al. Evidence for the Involvement of VAR2CSA in Pregnancy-Associated Malaria. *J Exp Med* (2004) 200(9):1197–203. doi: 10.1084/jem.20041579
6. Rogerson SJ, Hviid L, Duffy PE, Leke RFG, Taylor DW. Malaria in Pregnancy: Pathogenesis and Immunity. *Lancet Infect Dis* (2007) 7(2):105–17. doi: 10.1016/S1473-3099(07)70022-1
7. Tuikue Ndam NG, Salanti A, Le-Hesran J-Y, Cottrell G, Fievet N, Turner L, et al. Dynamics of Anti-VAR2CSA Immunoglobulin G Response in a Cohort of Senegalese Pregnant Women. *J Infect Dis* (2006) 193(5):713–20. doi: 10.1086/500146
8. O'Neil-Dunne I, Achur RN, Agbor-Enoh ST, Valiyaveettil M, Naik RS, Ockenhouse CF, et al. Gravidity-Dependent Production of Antibodies That Inhibit Binding of *Plasmodium Falciparum*-Infected Erythrocytes to Placental Chondroitin Sulfate Proteoglycan During Pregnancy. *Infect Immun* (2001) 69 (12):7487–92. doi: 10.1128/IAI.69.12.7487-7492.2001
9. Clausen TM, Christoffersen S, Dahlbäck M, Langkilde AE, Jensen KE, Resende M, et al. Structural and Functional Insight Into How the *Plasmodium Falciparum* VAR2CSA Protein Mediates Binding to Chondroitin Sulfate A in Placental Malaria. *J Biol Chem* (2012) 287 (28):23332–45. doi: 10.1074/jbc.M112.348839
10. Mordmüller B, Sulyok M, Egger-Adam D, Resende M, de Jongh WA, Jensen MH, et al. First-In-Human, Randomized, Double-Blind Clinical Trial of Differentially Adjuvanted PAMVAC, A Vaccine Candidate to Prevent Pregnancy-Associated Malaria. *Clin Infect Dis* (2019) 69(9):1509–16. doi: 10.1093/cid/ciy1140
11. Ndam NT, Denoeud-Ndam L, Doritchamou J, Viwami F, Salanti A, Nielsen MA, et al. Protective Antibodies Against Placental Malaria and Poor Outcomes During Pregnancy, Benin. *Emerg Infect Dis* (2015) 21(5):813–23. doi: 10.3201/eid2105.141626
12. Cutts JC, Agius PA, Lin Z, Powell R, Moore K, Draper B, et al. Pregnancy-Specific Malarial Immunity and Risk of Malaria in Pregnancy and Adverse Birth Outcomes: A Systematic Review. *BMC Med* (2020) 18(1):14. doi: 10.1186/s12916-019-1467-6
13. Huynh B-T, Fievet N, Gbaguidi G, Dechavanne S, Borgella S, Guézo-Mévo B, et al. Influence of the Timing of Malaria Infection During Pregnancy on Birth Weight and on Maternal Anemia in Benin. *Am J Trop Med Hyg* (2011) 85 (2):214–20. doi: 10.4269/ajtmh.2011.11-0103
14. Chêne A, Briand V, Ibitokou S, Dechavanne S, Massougbodji A, Deloron P, et al. Placental Cytokine and Chemokine Profiles Reflect Pregnancy Outcomes in Women Exposed to *Plasmodium Falciparum* Infection. *Infect Immun* (2014) 82(9):3783–9. doi: 10.1128/IAI.01922-14
15. Schmiegelow C, Scheike T, Oesterholt M, Minja D, Pehrson C, Magistrado P, et al. Development of a Fetal Weight Chart Using Serial Trans-Abdominal Ultrasound in an East African Population: A Longitudinal Observational Study. *PLoS One* (2012) 7(9):e44773. doi: 10.1371/journal.pone.0044773
16. Jafari-Guemouri S, Ndam NT, Bertin G, Renart E, Sow S, Le Hesran J-Y, et al. Demonstration of a High Level of Parasite Population Homology by Quantification of *Plasmodium Falciparum* Alleles in Matched Peripheral, Placental, and Umbilical Cord Blood Samples. *J Clin Microbiol* (2005) 43 (6):2980–3. doi: 10.1128/JCM.43.6.2980-2983.2005
17. Nielsen MA, Resende M, de Jongh WA, Ditlev SB, Mordmüller B, Houard S, et al. The Influence of Sub-Unit Composition and Expression System on the Functional Antibody Response in the Development of a VAR2CSA Based *Plasmodium Falciparum* Placental Malaria Vaccine. *PLoS One* (2015) 10(9):e0135406. doi: 10.1371/journal.pone.0135406
18. Olsen RW, Ecklu-Mensah G, Bengtsson A, Ofori MF, Kusi KA, Koram KA, et al. Acquisition of IgG to ICAM-1-Binding DBLβ Domains in the *Plasmodium Falciparum* Erythrocyte Membrane Protein 1 Antigen Family Varies Between Groups A, B, and C. *Infect Immun* (2019) 87(10):e00224-19. doi: 10.1128/IAI.00224-19
19. Guitard J, Cottrell G, Magnouha NM, Salanti A, Li T, Sow S, et al. Differential Evolution of Anti-VAR2CSA- IgG3 in Primigravidae and Multigravidae Pregnant Women Infected by *Plasmodium Falciparum*. *Malaria J* (2008) 7 (1):10. doi: 10.1186/1475-2875-7-10
20. Fried M, Nosten F, Brockman A, Brabin BJ, Duffy PE. Maternal Antibodies Block Malaria. *Nature* (1998) 395(6705):851–2. doi: 10.1038/27570
21. Dechavanne S, Srivastava A, Gangnard S, Nunes-Silva S, Dechavanne C, Fievet N, et al. Parity-Dependent Recognition of DBL1X-3X Suggests an Important Role of the VAR2CSA High-Affinity CSA-Binding Region in the Development of the Humoral Response Against Placental Malaria. *Infect Immun* (2015) 83(6):2466–74. doi: 10.1128/IAI.03116-14
22. Khunrae P, Dahlbäck M, Nielsen MA, Andersen G, Ditlev SB, Resende M, et al. Full-Length Recombinant *Plasmodium Falciparum* VAR2CSA Binds Specifically to CSPG and Induces Potent Parasite Adhesion-Blocking Antibodies. *J Mol Biol* (2010) 397(3):826–34. doi: 10.1016/j.jmb. 2010.01.040
23. Hagan P, Blumenthal UJ, Dunn D, Simpson AJ, Wilkins HA. Human IgE, IgG4 and Resistance to Reinfection with Schistosoma Haematobium. *Nature* (1991) 349(6306):243–5. doi: 10.1038/349243a0
24. McSorley HJ, Maizels RM. Helminth Infections and Host Immune Regulation. *Clin Microbiol Rev* (2012) 25(4):585–608. doi: 10.1128/CMR.05040-11
25. Hussain R, Grögl M, Ottesen EA. IgG Antibody Subclasses in Human Filariasis. Differential Subclass Recognition of Parasite Antigens Correlates with Different Clinical Manifestations of Infection. *J Immunol* (1987) 139(8):2794–8.
26. Cottrell G, Moussiliou A, Luty AJF, Cot M, Fievet N, Massougbodji A, et al. Submicroscopic *Plasmodium Falciparum* Infections Are Associated With Maternal Anemia, Premature Births, and Low Birth Weight. *Clin Infect Dis* (2015) 60(10):1481 8. doi: 10.1093/cid/civ122

27. Boström S, Ibitokou S, Oesterholt M, Schmiegelow C, Persson J-O, Minja D, et al. Biomarkers of *Plasmodium Falciparum* Infection During Pregnancy in Women Living in Northeastern Tanzania. *PLoS One* (2012) 7(11):e48763. doi: 10.1371/journal.pone.0048763

28. Atmadja AK, Atkinson R, Sartono E, Partono F, Yazdanbakhsh M, Maizels RM. Differential Decline in Filaria-Specific IgG1, IgG4, and IgE Antibodies in Brugia Malayi-Infected Patients after Diethylcarbamazine Chemotherapy. *J Infect Dis* (1995) 172(6):1567–72. doi: 10.1093/infdis/172.6.1567

17

Trypanosoma cruzi and *Toxoplasma gondii* Induce a Differential MicroRNA Profile in Human Placental Explants

Lisvaneth Medina [1], Christian Castillo [1], Ana Liempi [1], Jesús Guerrero-Muñoz [1], Maura Rojas-Pirela [2], Juan Diego Maya [3], Humberto Prieto [4] and Ulrike Kemmerling [1]*

[1] Programa de Anatomía y Biología del Desarrollo, Facultad de Medicina, Instituto de Ciencias Biomédicas, Universidad de Chile, Santiago, Chile, [2] Instituto de Biología, Pontificia Universidad Católica de Valparaíso, Valparaíso, Chile, [3] Programa de Farmacología Molecular y Clínica, Facultad de Medicina, Instituto de Ciencias Biomédicas, Universidad de Chile, Santiago, Chile, [4] Instituto de Investigaciones Agropecuarias, Ministerio de Agricultura, Santiago, Chile

***Correspondence:**
Ulrike Kemmerling
ukemmerling@uchile.cl*

Trypanosoma cruzi and *Toxoplasma gondii* are two parasites than can be transmitted from mother to child through the placenta. However, congenital transmission rates are low for *T. cruzi* and high for *T. gondii*. Infection success or failure depends on complex parasite-host interactions in which parasites can alter host gene expression by modulating non-coding RNAs such as miRNAs. As of yet, there are no reports on altered miRNA expression in placental tissue in response to either parasite. Therefore, we infected human placental explants *ex vivo* by cultivation with either *T. cruzi* or *T. gondii* for 2 h. We then analyzed the miRNA expression profiles of both types of infected tissue by miRNA sequencing and quantitative PCR, sequence-based miRNA target prediction, pathway functional enrichment, and upstream regulator analysis of differentially expressed genes targeted by differentially expressed miRNAs. Both parasites induced specific miRNA profiles. GO analysis revealed that the *in silico* predicted targets of the differentially expressed miRNAs regulated different cellular processes involved in development and immunity, and most of the identified KEGG pathways were related to chronic diseases and infection. Considering that the differentially expressed miRNAs identified here modulated crucial host cellular targets that participate in determining the success of infection, these miRNAs might explain the differing congenital transmission rates between the two parasites. Molecules of the different pathways that are regulated by miRNAs and modulated during infection, as well as the miRNAs themselves, may be potential targets for the therapeutic control of either congenital Chagas disease or toxoplasmosis.

Keywords: *Trypanosoma cruzi*, *Toxoplasma gondii*, human placental explants, miRNA profile, host gene expression

INTRODUCTION

More than one billion people worldwide are burdened by parasitic diseases (1). Of these, Chagas disease (American trypanosomiasis) and toxoplasmosis are caused by *Trypanosoma cruzi* (*T. cruzi*) and *Toxoplasma gondii* (*T. gondii*), respectively (2–4). Chagas disease is a devastating but neglected health problem in Latin America. Due to the extensive global migration of asymptomatic individuals, this infection has become an emerging disease in non-endemic countries. Congenital transmission is partially responsible for the progressive globalization of Chagas disease (5, 6). *T. gondii* is one of the most successful parasites on earth and is estimated to infect over one billion people worldwide (7). Importantly, both parasites can be congenitally transmitted and cause perinatal morbidity and mortality (2–4) but present different transmission rates. *T. cruzi* has a low transmission rate (1–12%) (6, 8) while *T. gondii* has a high transmission rate (22–72%) (3). Moreover, both parasites elicit a different local placental immune response that might be related to infection susceptibility (9, 10). Thus, *T. cruzi* and *T. gondi* infection is related to the expression and activation of different Toll-like receptors, which in turn mediate the secretion of different cytokines and chemokines in defense against both parasites in the placenta (9, 11).

However, the probability of congenital transmission depends on a variety of complex interactions between the pathogen and the host (4, 12). In particular, parasite factors, placental factors, and maternal and developing fetal immune systems determine infection occurrence (4, 13). In this context, both parasites display sophisticated strategies to avoid host defenses and virulence factors that increase the chance of establishing infection and long-term persistence. One of these strategies is the ability to modulate host cell gene expression (14–16) through small non-coding RNAs such as microRNAs (miRNAs) that repress mRNAs in a sequence-specific manner by either an mRNA degradation process or through mRNA translation inhibition (17–19). MiRNAs play a key role in fine tuning gene expression in multiple physiological and pathological conditions including *T. cruzi* (20) or *T. gondii* (21) infection. Interestingly, the largest miRNA cluster in humans is encoded in chromosome 19 (C19MC; 19q13.41) and is almost exclusively expressed in the placenta (22). Both C19MC-derived and non-C19MC-derived miRNAs have been associated with placental development pathologies such as pre-eclampsia and infection (23, 24). However, there is no report in the literature regarding altered miRNA expression in placental tissue in response to either parasite.

Here, we infected human placental explants (HPE) *ex vivo* by 2 h of incubation with either *T. cruzi* or *T. gondii*, then analyzed both miRNA expression profiles by miRNA sequencing and quantitative PCR of selected miRNAs. In addition, we used sequence-based miRNA target prediction and performed pathway functional enrichment and upstream regulator analysis of differentially expressed genes targeted by differentially expressed miRNAs (DEMs).

MATERIALS AND METHODS

Parasite Culture and Harvesting

For *T. cruzi*, Y strain (*T. cruzi* II) trypomastigotes were obtained from previously infected Vero cells (ATCC® CCL-81) grown in RPMI medium supplemented with 5% fetal bovine serum and 1% antibiotics (penicillin-streptomycin) at 37°C in a humid atmosphere with 5% CO_2. Parasites invaded the cells and replicated intracellularly as amastigotes. After 48–72 h, amastigotes transformed back to trypomastigotes and lysed the host cells. The infective trypomastigotes were separated from cellular debris by low speed centrifugation (500 × *g*) for 10 min. Parasites were isolated from the supernatant by centrifugation at 3500×*g* during 15 min, suspended in RPMI media (without fetal bovine serum, 1% (penicillin-streptomycin) (RPMI 1640®, Biological Industries Ltd.), and quantified in a Neubauer chamber (9).

For *T. gondii*, semi-confluent HFF cells were infected with RH tachyzoites at a multiplicity of infection of 3 to 5 parasites per cell. After 40 h, the infected cells were washed, then monolayers were scraped from the flasks and passed through 20-, 23-, and 25-gauge needles. Tachyzoites were purified from host cell debris with a 3.0 µm Isopore filter (Merck Millipore®) (25).

The laboratory has been certificated as a Biosafety level 2 laboratory by the Biosafety Committee ("Unidad de Prevención de Riesgo") of the "Facultad de Medicina, Universidad de Chile" (approval # 0403/2019).

HPE Infection

Human term placentas were obtained from 3 women with uncomplicated pregnancies with vaginal or caesarean delivery. Informed consent for experimental use of the placenta was given by each patient as stipulated by the Code of Ethics of the "Servicio de Salud Metropolitana Norte" (approval number 0010/2019). Exclusion criteria consisted of the following: major fetal abnormalities, placental tumor, intrauterine infection, obstetric pathology, positive serology for Chagas disease, and any other maternal disease. Donor patients were negative for anti-*T. gondii* IgG/IgM antibodies. The organs were collected in cold, sterile, saline-buffered solution (PBS) and processed no more than 30 min after delivery. The dissected explants (approximately 50 mg of tissue) were washed with sterile PBS to remove the blood and co-cultivated with *T. cruzi* trypomastigotes or *T. gondii* tachyzoites (10^5 parasites/ml) in serum free RPMI media. After 2 h of co-cultivation, explants were collected in RNAlater™ solution (ThermoFisher Scientific®), then stored at 4°C for 24 h and at -80°C for posterior RNA isolation (9). Three independent experiments were carried out in triplicates; HPEs from each placenta were infected with either *T. cruzi* or *T. gondii* parasites. The parasite load in the HPEs was confirmed by real-time PCR as described previously by us (9, 10, 26).

RNA Extraction

Total RNA was extracted from HPE by mechanical disruption in 1.3 ml of RNA-solv® reagent (Omega Bio-tek) and isolated using an E.Z.N.A® total RNA kit I (Omega Bio-tek) according to manufacturer instructions. RNA was stored at -80°C until analysis. The concentration and quality of RNA was determined with a Qubit® RNA HS Assay kit and an IQ Assay kit (Invitrogen), respectively. Only RNA samples with an IQ ≥8 were further analyzed for quality with an Agilent 2100 Bioanalyzer System (Agilent Technologies, USA) using an RNA Nano 6000 Assay Kit. RNA samples with RNA integrity numbers >5.0 were used for miRNA profiling analysis (9).

Library Construction and Sequencing

Small RNA-Seq libraries were constructed with an Illumina TruSeq Small RNA library preparation kit according to manufacturer protocols. To assess the quality of the libraries, a DNA High Sensitivity Chip was used in an Agilent 2100 Bioanalyzer (Agilent Technologies, USA). The libraries were sequenced on an Illumina NextSeq 500 platform. For each condition, three independent biological replicates were sequenced and paired-end reads were generated.

Data Analysis

Raw read quality was evaluated using the FastQC tool (https://www.bioinformatics.babraham.ac.uk/projects/fastqc/). Raw reads were analyzed with Trim Galore Cutadapt software (27) and low-quality reads were removed (phred value < 30) in order to obtain clean reads. Clean reads with a length range of 18–35 nucleotides were chosen to perform all subsequent analyses. The sofware STAR (28) was used to align all reads to the reference human genome sequence (Hg38). The read counts per coding sequence were determined using HTSeq-count (29). To evaluate replicates, we used Principal Component Analysis, Pearson correlation and standardized median correlation analyses and box plots. The program EdgeR was used for differential expression analysis (30). Differentially expressed genes were defined as genes with p-value <0.05. Target gene prediction performed by using miRDB, psRNA target, and TargetScan sofwares.

Enrichment Analyses

miRNA set enrichment analysis was performed using the TAM 2.0 tool (http://www.lirmed.com/tam2/). KEGG pathways and functional annotation of the predicted target genes (https://www.genome.jp/kegg/kegg2.html) were also analyzed to determine the biological processes, molecular functions, cellular components, and associations with disease.

RT-qPCR

RNA enriched in small RNAs was extracted from HPEs (approximately 50 mg of tissue) by mechanical disruption in 1 ml RNAzol® RT (Sigma-Aldrich) according to manufacturer instructions and stored at -80°C until analysis. The concentration of the isolated miRNAs was determined using a Qubit® Quant-iT™ microRNA Assay Kit (Molecular Probes). cDNA of mature miRNAs was synthesized with a MystiCq™ microRNA cDNA Synthesis Mix Kit (Sigma-Aldrich Merck) per manufacturer guidelines. The 25 µl RT-qPCR reaction contained 12.5 µl 2× MystiCq microRNA SYBR Green qPCR Ready Mix, 0.5 µl of 10 µM MystiCq Universal PCR Primer, 0.5 µl of 10 µM of each specific MystiCq microRNA qPCR Assay Primer (**Supplementary Table 1**), 10.5 µl nuclease-free water, and 1 µl cDNA. All RT-qPCR reactions were performed in triplicates. RT-qPCR was performed under the following cycling conditions: initial denaturation at 95°C for 2 min, followed by 40 cycles of 95°C for 5 s and 60°C for 30 s. Gene expressions were calculated using the $2^{-\Delta\Delta CT}$ relative expression method and normalized to snRNA U6 (RNU6-1) expression levels (31).

RESULTS

T. cruzi and *T. gondii* Change the miRNA Expression Profile in HPE

The effects of *T. cruzi* and *T. gondii* on placental tissue were assayed in HPE after a 2 h challenge with 10^5 parasites/ml. Total miRNA extracted from infected and non-infected control HPE was analyzed by miRNA Seq. Key characteristics of the obtained sequencing data are summarized in **Table 1**. A total of 680 and 686 DEMs were identified in *T. cruzi* and *T. gondii* infected HPE, respectively. Only 14 DEMs with a minimum 1.5-fold change in expression and a 95% probability of being differentially expressed (p ≤ 0.05) were identified in *T. cruzi* challenged samples (**Figure 1A**). In *T. gondii* challenged samples, the number of DEMs increased to 42 (**Figure 1B**). Comparison of *T. cruzi* infected HPE with non-infected control samples showed that five

TABLE 1 | Statistics of the small RNA sequences obtained in this study.

	M reads (millions)	M Aligned (millions)	% aligned	Mature microRNA reads	# Mature MicroRNAs	# Mature MicroRNA (single aligned)
S1 Control	12,96	11,68	90,12	3489287	922	732
S2 Control	15,17	13,87	91,43	4855933	938	760
S3 Control	15,58	13,16	84,50	3030989	843	714
S4 *T. cruzi*	14,35	12,60	87,77	3000672	907	712
S5 *T. cruzi*	14,76	12,94	87,69	3910944	907	737
S6 *T. cruzi*	16,13	13,15	81,55	3571933	914	720
S7 *T. gondii*	13,57	11,82	87,07	3160630	916	737
S8 *T. gondii*	14,40	12,79	88,77	4747358	962	757
S9 *T. gondii*	13,51	12,16	89,99	4148647	931	763

M reads, total of sequences in analysis after raw data processing (millions); M aligned, total of mapped sequences to the human genome (millions); % aligned, total of mapped sequences to the human genome (percentage); Mature microRNA reads, mapped reads counted as mature miRNAs; # Mature microRNAs, number of mature miRNAs; # Mature MicroRNA (single aligned), number of mature miRNAs associated to unique miRNA precursors in the reference.

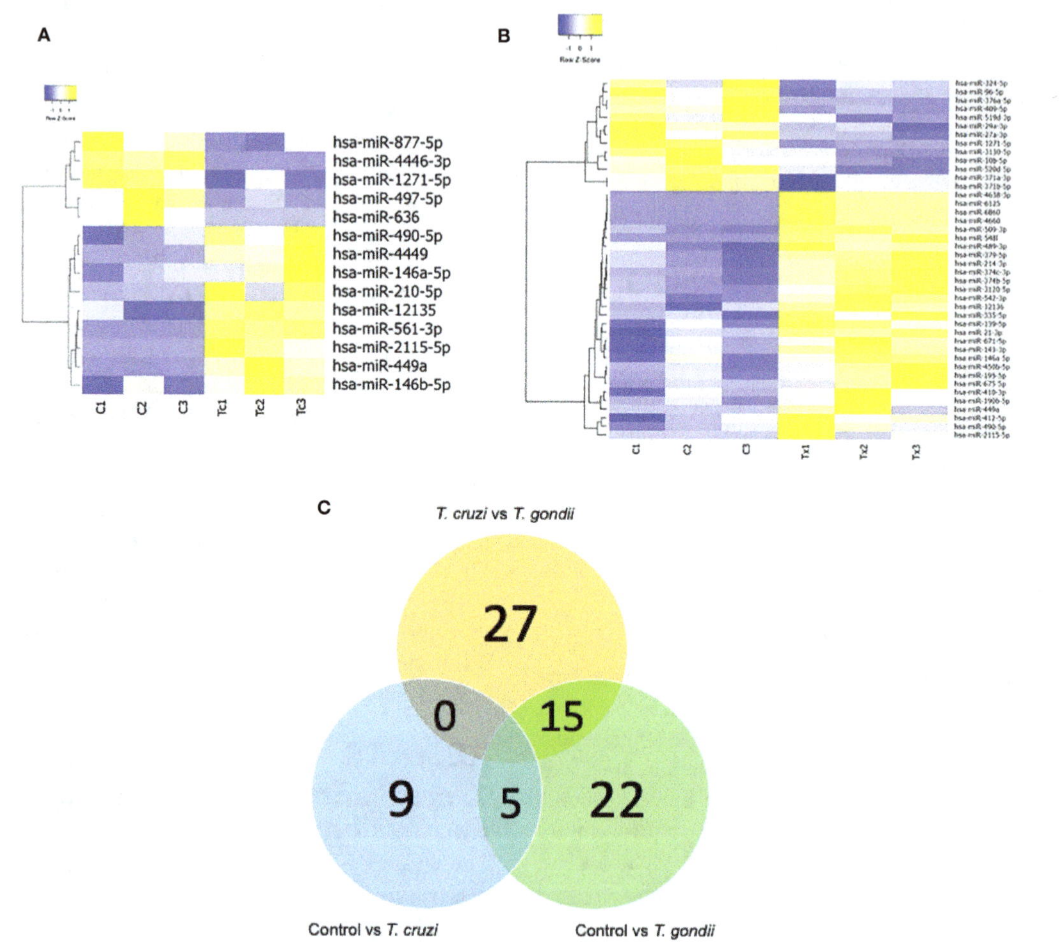

FIGURE 1 | Expression profiling of mature miRNAs in human placental explants (HPEs) following *T. cruzi* or *T. gondii* infection. **(A)** Heat-map of differentially expressed microRNAs (DEMs) in control vs. *T. cruzi* infected HPE and **(B)** control vs. *T. gondii* infected HPE. The filtered miRNA data were subjected to unsupervised hierarchical clustering analysis. The metric was set as the Euclidean distance. Control: C1, C2, C3; *T. cruzi:* Tc1, Tc2, Tc3; *T. gondii:* Tx1, Tx2, Tx3. **(C)** Venn diagram showing the number of commonly expressed and specifically expressed miRNAs between the infected HPE groups. Significant miRNAs for HPE with *T cruzi* infection vs. those with *T. gondii* infection are shown in the yellow circle. The blue circle represents the miRNAs that discriminate between the control (uninfected HPE) and *T. cruzi* infected HPE, while the green circle represents the miRNAs that distinguish the control (uninfected HPE) and *T. gondii* infected HPE.

miRNAs were downregulated and nine were upregulated. In *T. gondii* infected tissues, 13 miRNAs were downregulated and 29 were upregulated. The Venn diagram in **Figure 1C** shows the miRNAs that were differentially expressed in the presence of both parasites compared to non-infected control samples and in HPE infected with either parasite. The complete list of DEMs in response to *ex vivo T. cruzi* and *T. gondii* infection is shown in **Table 2**.

Functional Annotation and KEGG Pathway Enrichment Analysis of miRNA Target Genes

To better understand the roles of the miRNAs identified in HPE in response to *ex vivo* infection with both parasites, the target genes of the miRNAs were identified using miRDB, psRNA target, and TargetScan. GO and KEGG enrichment analyses used to identify the biological functions of the DEMs ($p < 0.05$) during *ex vivo T. cruzi* and *T. gondii* infection revealed 679 best scored target genes of the 14 miRNAs from *T. cruzi* vs. control, 1970 best scored target genes of the 42 miRNAs from *T. gondii* vs. control, and 2011 best scored target genes of the 42 miRNAs from *T. cruzi* vs. *T. gondi*. The target genes of the DEMs are shown in **Supplementary Table 2**. Among the significantly enriched GO terms in *T. cruzi* vs. control samples, DEMs were significantly enriched in regulation of NFκB pathways, chondrocyte development, cell death including apoptosis, peritoneal cavity homeostasis, angiogenesis, cell cycle, megakaryocyte differentiation, Toll-like receptor signaling pathway, and immune response including innate immunity (**Figure 2A**). Among the significantly enriched GO terms in *T. gondii* vs. control samples, DEMs were significantly enriched in cell proliferation, cell migration, osteoblast differentiation, oxidative stress, lipid metabolism, regulation of stem cells including embryonic stem cells, hepatotoxicity, DNA damage response, regulation of NFκB pathways, smooth muscle

TABLE 2 | The top differentially expressed miRNAs (P < 0.05) in HPE challenged with 10^5 *T. cruzi* trypomastigotes or *T. gondii* tachyzoites during 2 h.

	miRNAs	Fold Change	p-value	p-adjustment	Expression
Control vs *T. cruzi*	hsa-miR-490-5p	1,47644601	0,011939305	1	Up-regulated
	hsa-miR-497-5p	-0,95822045	0,021380502	1	Down-regulated
	hsa-miR-146a-5p	0,9111643	0,024398238	1	Up-regulated
	hsa-miR-12135	2,76826832	0,025125553	1	Up-regulated
	hsa-miR-210-5p	1,17471038	0,038576256	1	Up-regulated
	hsa-miR-146b-5p	0,70985057	0,041583753	1	Up-regulated
	hsa-miR-877-5p	-0,71572824	0,049301458	1	Down-regulated
	hsa-miR-1271-5p	-1,48497011	0,049553349	1	Down-regulated
T. cruzi (*treatment exclusive)	hsa-miR-636		0,003652701	1	Up-regulated
	hsa-miR-4449		0,005197851	1	Up-regulated
	hsa-miR-449a		0,009529598	1	Up-regulated
	hsa-miR-2115-5p		0,013101594	1	Up-regulated
	hsa-miR-561-3p		0,023021063	1	Up-regulated
	hsa-miR-4446-3p		0,041796581	1	Up-regulated
Control vs *T. gondii*	hsa-miR-12136	1,79576197	0,00017626	0,120736654	Up-regulated
	hsa-miR-335-5p	1,35817451	0,0007489	0,227732906	Up-regulated
	hsa-miR-10b-5p	-1,51399053	0,00099737	0,227732906	Down-regulated
	hsa-miR-1271-5p	-2,41452099	0,00206894	0,267855922	Down-regulated
	hsa-miR-409-5p	-2,51430487	0,00225422	0,267855922	Down-regulated
	hsa-miR-27a-3p	-0,97356696	0,00234618	0,267855922	Down-regulated
	hsa-miR-29a-3p	-0,92877383	0,00344997	0,337603687	Down-regulated
	hsa-miR-214-3p	0,9642214	0,00435186	0,372627686	Up-regulated
	hsa-miR-379-5p	1,46136088	0,00619518	0,453658878	Up-regulated
	hsa-miR-3120-5p	1,05085403	0,00662276	0,453658878	Up-regulated
	hsa-miR-376a-5p	-1,06317073	0,00928715	0,578335925	Down-regulated
	hsa-miR-542-3p	1,36466429	0,01456701	0,760274481	Up-regulated
	hsa-miR-195-5p	1,29637989	0,01520981	0,760274481	Up-regulated
	hsa-miR-3130-5p	-2,64645685	0,01847345	0,760274481	Down-regulated
	hsa-miR-519d-3p	-0,91993812	0,0188483	0,760274481	Down-regulated
	hsa-miR-490-5p	1,42743639	0,01886813	0,760274481	Up-regulated
	hsa-miR-450b-5p	1,11411811	0,02263153	0,763303449	Up-regulated
	hsa-miR-374b-5p	0,86524386	0,02512358	0,763303449	Up-regulated
	hsa-miR-374c-3p	0,87017312	0,02523843	0,763303449	Up-regulated
	hsa-miR-143-3p	0,78495077	0,02900217	0,763303449	Up-regulated
	hsa-miR-21-3p	0,79317052	0,0291757	0,763303449	Up-regulated
	hsa-miR-675-5p	1,1546043	0,03213608	0,763303449	Up-regulated
	hsa-miR-671-5p	1,76630085	0,03293839	0,763303449	Up-regulated
	hsa-miR-146a-5p	0,86261284	0,03359957	0,763303449	Up-regulated
	hsa-miR-489-3p	1,02467619	0,03372793	0,763303449	Up-regulated
	hsa-miR-96-5p	-2,45982286	0,03878464	0,77095716	Down-regulated
	hsa-miR-509-3p	0,86545472	0,03909277	0,77095716	Up-regulated
	hsa-miR-190b-5p	2,26556495	0,04749263	0,77095716	Up-regulated
	hsa-miR-371b-5p	-0,92943309	0,04875339	0,77095716	Down-regulated
	hsa-miR-520d-5p	-0,6667811	0,04979001	0,77095716	Down-regulated
	hsa-miR-371a-3p	-0,92563764	0,04993063	0,77095716	Down-regulated
	hsa-miR-412-5p	0,86533956	0,0514002	0,77095716	Up-regulated
	hsa-miR-324-5p	-1,01010797	0,05178532	0,77095716	Down-regulated
	hsa-miR-410-3p	0,63475365	0,05378966	0,77095716	Up-regulated
	hsa-miR-139-5p	0,66901369	0,0543406	0,77095716	Up-regulated
T. gondii (*treatment exclusive)	hsa-miR-548l		0,01756271	0,760274481	Up-regulated
	hsa-miR-449a		0,02617767	0,763303449	Up-regulated
	hsa-miR-6125		0,03454366	0,763303449	Up-regulated
	hsa-miR-4638-3p		0,03454366	0,763303449	Up-regulated
	hsa-miR-6860		0,03454366	0,763303449	Up-regulated
	hsa-miR-4660		0,03454366	0,763303449	Up-regulated
	hsa-miR-2115-5p		0,04354449	0,77095716	Up-regulated

Treatment Exclusive: refers to miRNAs sequenced only in the T. cruzi or T. gondii infected condition (treatment), they are not expressed in control explants.

proliferation, T-helper 17 cell differentiation, T-cell activation, and response to estrogen (**Figure 2B**).

In addition, we performed GO and KEGG analyses to identify different pathologies in which the *T. cruzi*- and *T. gondii*-induced DEMs were related. In *T. cruzi* vs. control samples, significantly enriched DEMs were related to metabolic syndrome, IgA-nephropathy, acute childhood lymphoblastic leukemia, atherosclerosis, oral lichen planus, human papilloma virus

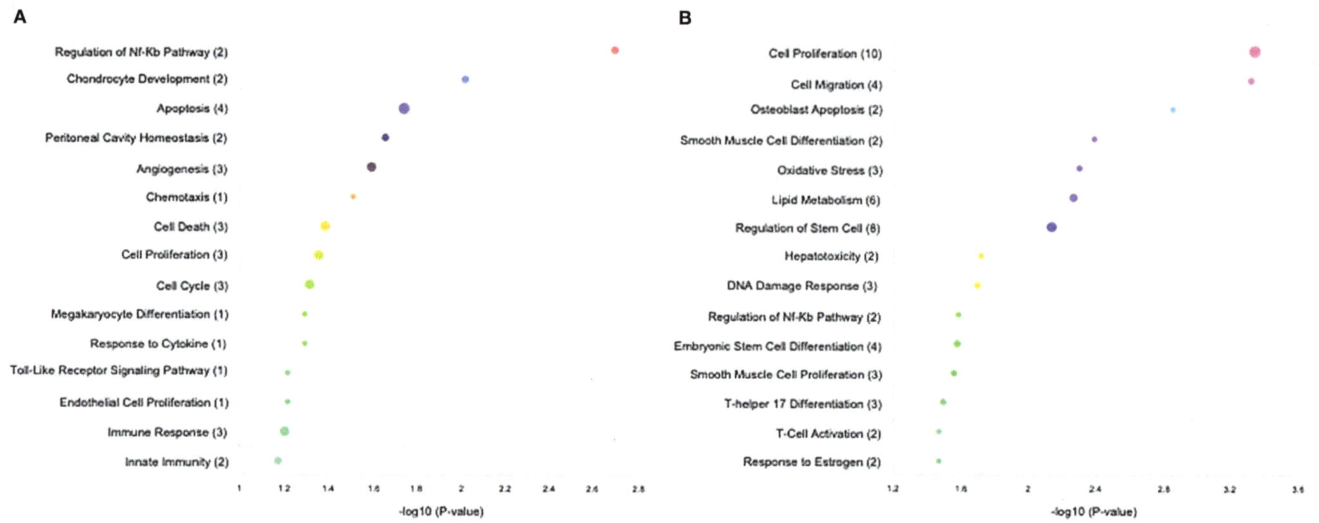

FIGURE 2 | KEGG analysis of the differentially expressed miRNAs ($P < 0.05$) revealed significant enrichment in immune-related and cell cycle pathways. The top 15 enriched pathways of the differentially expressed miRNAs are presented for **(A)** control vs. *T. cruzi* and **(B)** control vs. *T. gondii*. The sizes and colors of the circles represent the number of predicted gene targets of the differentially expressed miRNAs ($P < 0.05$) and the q-value, respectively.

infection, psoriasis, neuropsychiatric disorders, heart diseases, pancreatic carcinoma, Löfgren's syndrome, *Mycobacterium tuberculosis* infection, male infertility, and gastric carcinoma (**Figure 3A**). In *T. gondii* vs. control samples, the significantly enriched DEMs were related to ankylosing spondylitis, type 2 diabetes mellitus, hypertrophic cardiomyopathy, congenital heart disease, fetal alcohol syndrome, pulmonary hypertension, ulcerative colitis, cystic fibrosis, vascular diseases, human cytomegalovirus infection, muscular dystrophy, liver diseases, coxsackievirus infection, and diabetic retinopathy (**Figure 3B**).

Specific GO and KEGG enrichment analyses focused on the functions of DEMs in response to both parasites that were related to parasitic diseases and/or placenta pathology. These DEMs are listed in **Table 3**. In this context, we found that the significantly enriched DEMs were related to the regulation of apoptosis, wound healing, cardiomyocyte apoptosis, heart development, skeletal muscle cell differentiation, Toll-like receptor signaling pathway, innate immunity, epithelial to mesenchymal transition, chromatin remodeling, and nephrotoxicity (**Figure 4**). Moreover, we analyzed the significantly enriched DEMs related

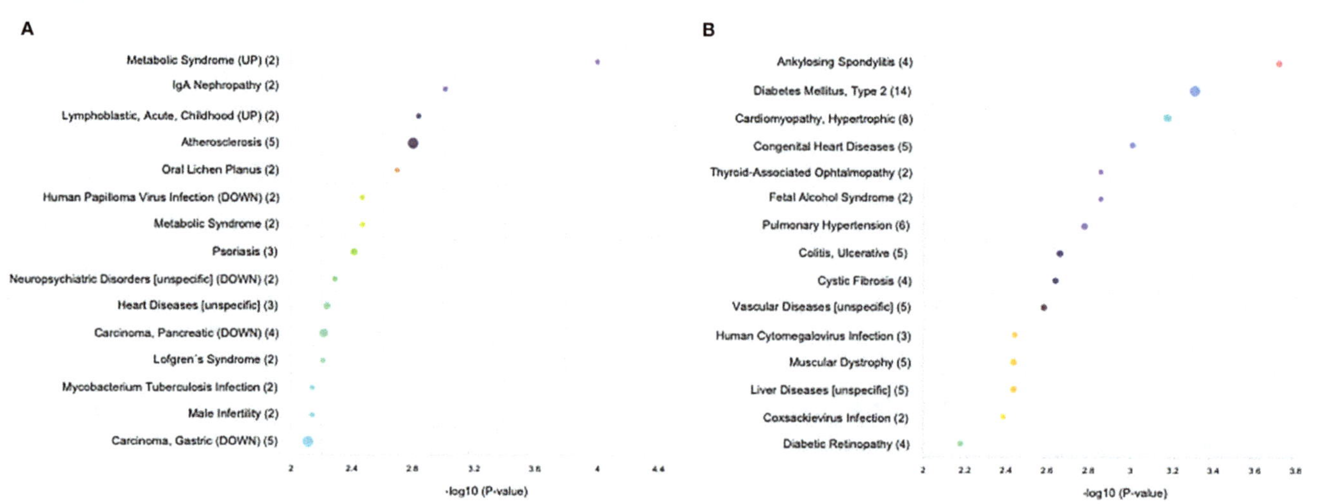

FIGURE 3 | KEGG analysis of the differentially expressed miRNAs ($P < 0.05$) revealed significant enrichment in cancer-related, infections, and inflammatory disease pathways. The top 15 enriched pathways of the differentially expressed miRNAs are presented for **(A)** control vs. *T. cruzi* and **(B)** control vs. *T. gondii*. The sizes and colors of the circles represent the number of predicted gene targets of the differentially expressed miRNAs ($P < 0.05$) and the q-value, respectively.

TABLE 3 | Sequenced miRNA related to placental and/or parasitic diseases in HPE challenged with 10^5 *T. cruzi* trypomastigotes or *T. gondii* tachyzoites during 2 h.

miRNAs	Control vs T. cruzi		Control vs T. gondii	
	Expression	p-value	Expression	p-value
hsa-miR-3074	Up-regulated	0,282778175	Down-regulated	0,906716427
hsa-miR-518e-5p	Down-regulated	0,736493282	Up-regulated	0,655921033
hsa-miR-127-3p	Down-regulated	0,454473692	Up-regulated	0,899001399
hsa-miR-512-3p	Up-regulated	0,893095693	Up-regulated	0,554888541
hsa-miR-516a-5p	Down-regulated	0,573579895	Down-regulated	0,875664943
hsa-miR-376a-3p	Up-regulated	0,26239456	Up-regulated	0,890873441
hsa-miR-523-5p	Down-regulated	0,736493282	Up-regulated	0,655921033
hsa-miR-517-5p	Down-regulated	0,356215385	Down-regulated	0,131367096
hsa-miR-523-3p	Up-regulated	0,558965508	Down-regulated	0,070624754
hsa-miR-519a-5p	Down-regulated	0,902087668	Up-regulated	0,683786458
hsa-miR-526a-5p	Down-regulated	0,878621126	Up-regulated	0,975623088
hsa-miR-519a-3p	Up-regulated	0,855200309	Down-regulated	0,216046946
hsa-miR-518e-3p	Up-regulated	0,878596629	Down-regulated	0,062749763
hsa-miR-520c-5p	Down-regulated	0,878525243	Up-regulated	0,981710662
hsa-miR-526a-3p	Down-regulated	0,648457618	Down-regulated	0,194744348
hsa-miR-29b-3p	Up-regulated	0,688264908	Down-regulated	0,461394462
hsa-miR-520c-3p	Down-regulated	0,492741665	Down-regulated	0,321148465
hsa-miR-133a-3p	Up-regulated	0,800691009	Down-regulated	0,140142195
hsa-miR-525-5p	Down-regulated	0,892625222	Down-regulated	0,624806979
hsa-miR-525-3p	Up-regulated	0,896175408	Down-regulated	0,075998808
hsa-miR-519c-5p	Down-regulated	0,736493282	Up-regulated	0,655921033
hsa-miR-518b	Up-regulated	0,991656949	Down-regulated	0,078353573
hsa-miR-519c-3p	Down-regulated	0,262008953	Down-regulated	0,786169155
hsa-miR-520e-5p	Down-regulated	0,485165729	Up-regulated	0,996288443
hsa-miR-520e-3p	Up-regulated	1	Up-regulated	0,818473073
hsa-miR-21-5p	Up-regulated	0,783933507	Up-regulated	0,129614377
hsa-miR-21-3p	Up-regulated	0,749764521	Up-regulated	0,029175701
hsa-miR-517a-3p	Up-regulated	0,596271375	Down-regulated	0,461347018
hsa-miR-519e-5p	Up-regulated	0,105129034	Up-regulated	0,757374294
hsa-miR-519e-3p	Up-regulated	0,385269175	Up-regulated	0,69099671
hsa-miR-518d-5p	Down-regulated	0,878525243	Up-regulated	0,981710662
hsa-miR-520g-5p	Up-regulated	0,892300156	Up-regulated	0,751979117
hsa-miR-518d-3p	Up-regulated	0,55414416	Down-regulated	0,942071295
hsa-miR-520b-5p	Down-regulated	0,421187791	Down-regulated	0,477328076
hsa-miR-520g-3p	Up-regulated	0,728189158	Down-regulated	0,352658846
hsa-miR-519a-2-5p	Down-regulated	0,421187791	Down-regulated	0,477328076
hsa-miR-520b-3p	Up-regulated	0,530509712	Down-regulated	0,954450249
hsa-miR-517c-3p	Up-regulated	0,760586655	Down-regulated	0,675509383
hsa-miR-524-5p	Down-regulated	0,490615316	Down-regulated	0,115381834
hsa-miR-210-5p	Up-regulated	0,038576256	Up-regulated	0,576691951
hsa-miR-204-5p	Up-regulated	0,62227226	Down-regulated	0,583793777
hsa-miR-524-3p	Down-regulated	0,907890609	Down-regulated	0,099098809
hsa-miR-519b-5p	Down-regulated	0,736493282	Up-regulated	0,655921033
hsa-miR-210-3p	Up-regulated	0,497217414	Down-regulated	0,843820092
hsa-miR-378a-5p	Down-regulated	0,915728534	Down-regulated	0,504825517
hsa-miR-526b-5p	Down-regulated	0,501400731	Down-regulated	0,534886926
hsa-miR-519b-3p	Up-regulated	0,996536077	Up-regulated	0,986254335
hsa-miR-518a-5p	Down-regulated	0,396658878	Down-regulated	0,099042516
hsa-miR-520d-5p	Down-regulated	0,163923317	Down-regulated	0,049790011
hsa-miR-526b-3p	Up-regulated	0,690372369	Down-regulated	0,356016985
hsa-miR-520d-3p	Down-regulated	0,368956264	Down-regulated	0,595399092
hsa-miR-30e-3p	Up-regulated	0,708643074	Down-regulated	0,606142557
hsa-miR-520h	Up-regulated	0,420508027	Down-regulated	0,48103803
hsa-miR-519d-5p	Down-regulated	0,699132481	Down-regulated	0,210250996
hsa-miR-515-5p	Down-regulated	0,451420159	Down-regulated	0,479490879
hsa-miR-519d-3p	Up-regulated	0,795099209	Down-regulated	0,018848296
hsa-miR-515-3p	Down-regulated	0,961837732	Down-regulated	0,056222245
hsa-miR-518c-5p	Down-regulated	0,433629597	Down-regulated	0,461615584
hsa-miR-155-5p	Up-regulated	0,089556012	Up-regulated	0,307144182
hsa-miR-518c-3p	Up-regulated	0,825417746	Down-regulated	0,393062915
hsa-miR-520a-5p	Up-regulated	0,829237058	Down-regulated	0,786085152

(Continued)

TABLE 3 | Continued

miRNAs	Control vs T. cruzi		Control vs T. gondii	
	Expression	**p-value**	**Expression**	**p-value**
hsa-miR-376a-5p	Down-regulated	0,101845272	Down-regulated	0,009287146
hsa-miR-520a-3p	Up-regulated	0,303331111	Down-regulated	0,733502488
hsa-miR-144-5p	Up-regulated	0,979441392	Down-regulated	0,781688613
hsa-miR-204-5p	Up-regulated	0,62227226	Down-regulated	0,583793777
hsa-miR-424-5p	Up-regulated	0,52797867	Down-regulated	0,318765339
hsa-miR-346	Down-regulated	0,996223653	Up-regulated	0,484560011

to transcription activation and found that the following transcription factors or its activators were modulated by them: MYOG, calcineurin, AP-1, TNFSF12, NFκB1, myogenin, MYOD, MYF5, MRF4, and TP53 (**Figure 5**).

Validation of miRNA Expression by RT-qPCR

Validation of miRNAs associated with parasite infection or pregnancy related pathologies was performed by selecting six miRNAs [miR-3074 (26), miR-127-3p (27, 28), miR-30e-3p (29), miR-512-3p (30), miR-515-5p (31), and miR-190b (32)] for confirmation by real time PCR to verify the DEM expression levels. Expression of miR-3074, miR-127-3p, and miR-30e-3p (**Figures 6A–C**) was analyzed in HPE in response to both parasites. miR-512-3p and miR-515-5p (**Figures 6D–E**) expression was determined in response to *T. cruzi* infection and miR-190b expression in response to *T. gondii* infection (**Figure 6F**). All selected miRNAs except for miR-30e-3p (**Figure 6C**) were differentially expressed. Thus, miR-3074 expression (**Figure 6A**) was significantly decreased (*T. cruzi*: 57.03 ± 19.99%, $p \leq 0.01$; *T. gondii*: 69.84 ± 24.67%, $p \leq 0.01$) with respect to the control but not the infected samples. Decreased miR-3074 expression was expected in the *T. gondii* infected samples but not in the *T. cruzi* infected samples. According to the miRNA Seq data, miR-3074 was upregulated in *T. cruzi* challenged samples. Similar results were observed for miR-127-3p (**Figigure 6B**). Expression of miR-127-3p was significantly decreased in HPE infected with either parasite (*T. cruzi*: 68.218 ± 16.41%, $p \leq 0.01$; *T. gondii*: 73.13 ± 22.45%, $p \leq 0.01$) compared to the control but not to infected samples; we expected an increase in miR-127-3p expression in the presence of *T. gondii* since in the miRNA Seq data this particular miRNA was increased (**Table 3**). RT-qPCR validation results for miR-512-3p, miR-515-5p, and miR-190b confirmed the miRNA Seq data. Thus, miR-512-3p expression increased (40.83 ± 22.53%, $p \leq 0.01$) (**Figure 6D**) and miR-515-5p expression decreased (21.44 ± 8.60%, $p \leq 0.01$) (**Figure 6E**) significantly in *T. cruzi* infected samples. In *T. gondii* infected HPE, miR-190b expression was significantly increased (59.02 ± 37.73%, $p \leq 0.01$) (**Figure 6F**).

DISCUSSION

Pathogens have evolved strategies to exploit resources from their hosts to maximize their own survival, replication, and dissemination. Thus, different kinds of pathogens (including

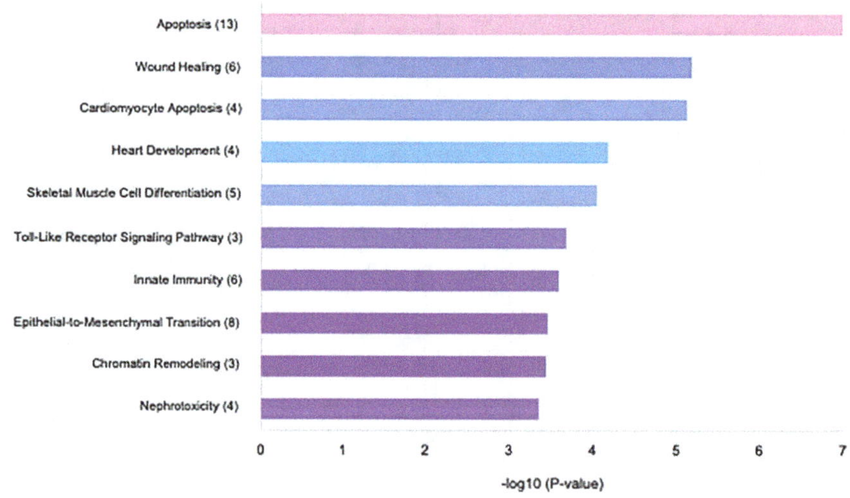

FIGURE 4 | Bar plot illustrating the top 10 significant miRNA-function associations of the sequenced miRNA related to placental and/or parasitic diseases in human placental explants infected with *T. cruzi* or *T. gondii*.

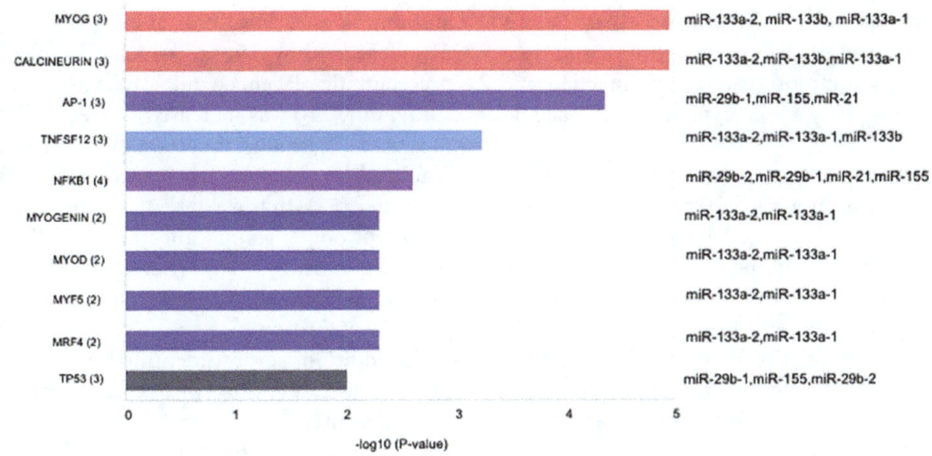

FIGURE 5 | Bar plot illustrating the top 10 significant miRNA transcription factor associations of the sequenced miRNA related to placental and/or parasitic diseases in human placental explants infected with *T. cruzi* or *T. gondii*.

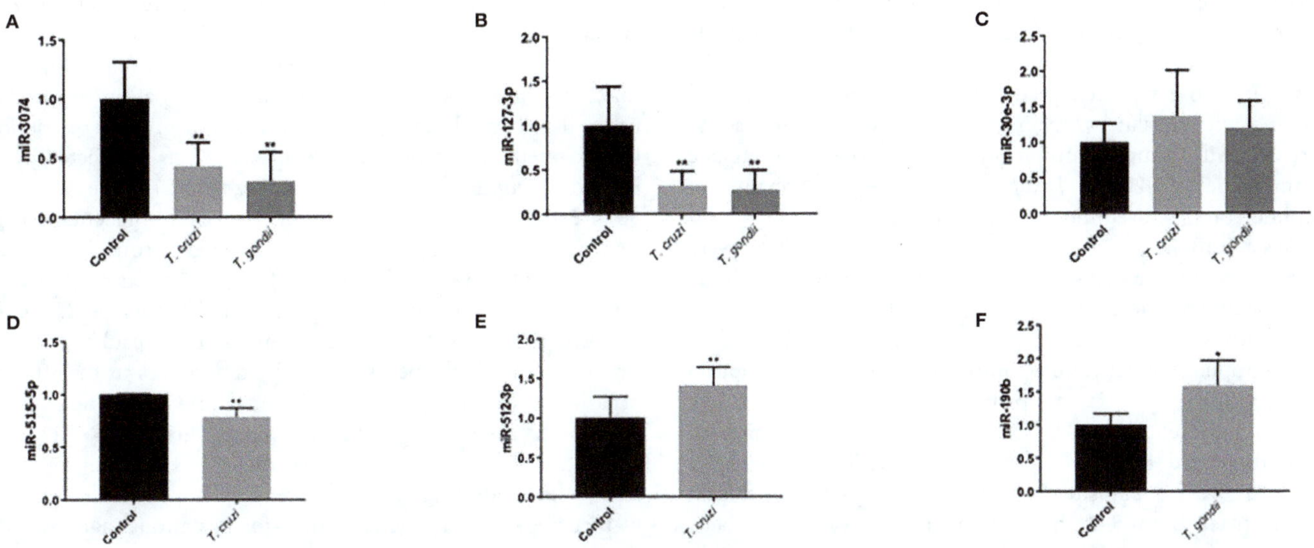

FIGURE 6 | Validation of miRNAs related to placental and/or parasitic diseases using RT-qPCR. Human placental explants were challenged with 10^5 *T. cruzi* trypomastigotes or *T. gondii* tachyzoites for 2 h. The presence of miRNA was determined by real-time PCR. *T. cruzi* and *T. gondii* decreased miR-3074 and miR-127-3p expression, while no change was observed in miR-30e-3p expression **(A–C)**. *T. cruzi* inhibited miR-515-5p expression and induced miR512-3p **(D, E)**. *T. gondii* induced miR-190b-5p **(F)**. All values are the mean ± S.D. and correspond to at least three independent experiments that were performed in triplicate. Data were normalized in terms of the control values and analyzed by Student's t-test or ANOVA. *$p \leq 0.05$; **$p \leq 0.01$.

parasites) have developed sophisticated mechanisms that include hijacking host cellular machinery to modulate host gene expression to inhibit defense responses (16, 32, 33). Both of the parasites studied here are able to manipulate host gene expression. For instance, during *T. cruzi* cell and tissue invasion, cell reprogramming affects cellular stress responses, host metabolism, and a significant number of transcription factors (16, 34). *T. gondii* also reprograms host cells, primarily targeting cell-specific transcription factors that regulate host defenses (i.e., NF-κB, interferon regulatory factor, and JAK/STAT) by regulating their intrinsic activities and expression levels (35). In addition, certain parasites including *T. cruzi* and *T. gondii* can alter host miRNA expression to favor both parasite clearance and infection (18, 19). Moreover, different strains of *T. gondii* can induce specific miRNAs in mice that have been proposed as biomarkers for early infection (19, 36).

Mature miRNAs regulate the expression of over 30% of fundamental genes; these are involved in key biological processes including development, cellular proliferation and differentiation, apoptosis, metabolism, and immune response (18, 19, 37); all of these determine infection success or failure. Moreover, epigenetic and genetic defects in miRNAs and their processing machinery are a common hallmark of infection and diseases that include pregnancy-specific pathologies such as preeclampsia (17, 38).

Most of the transcriptomic studies as well as those analyzing miRNA profiles have focused on a single type of cell response (34) or on tissues or organs in animal models (39, 40); no studies have focused on human tissues. The present study is the first report on the miRNA profile of the human placenta in response to *T. cruzi* or *T. gondii* infection. We identified 680 and 686 DEMs, respectively, in *T. cruzi* and *T. gondii* infected samples. *T. cruzi* modulated only 14 DEMs with a minimum of a 1.5-fold change in expression and a 95% probability of being differentially expressed (**Figure 1A**). In contrast, the number of DEMs increased to 42 in *T. gondii* challenged HPE (**Figure 2B**). Our results showed that the DEMs identified here are related to the regulation of different fundamental cellular processes (**Figure 2**) as well as different pathologies (**Figure 3**). Moreover, fundamental cellular processes related to placenta pathologies and embryonic development are affected by the presence of both parasites (**Figures 4–5**). It is important to point out, that tissue response to infection is relevant during disease progression. The presence of the parasites leads to tissue damage as well as immune and regulatory/repair responses, which can lead to fibrosis and tissue dysfunction as observed in chagasic cardiomyopathy (41) or *Toxoplasma* induced encephalitis in immune-compromised individuals (42).

Three miRNAs, miR-21, miR-146a/b, and miR-210, were overrepresented in most of the ontology terms (**Table 2, Supplementary Tables 3–4**). Previous studies have implicated these miRNAs in immune and inflammatory response regulation *via* macrophage polarization controlled through transcription factor regulation in response to signals from the microenvironment (43, 44). Concordantly, in *T. cruzi*-infected mice, increased miR-21 expression in the heart has been correlated with a parasitemia peak at 30 days post-infection (39). In placenta, miR-21 has been associated with trophoblast differentiation and invasion and miR-21 dysregulation leads to placental pathology (45). MiR-146a is a negative feedback regulator in TLR-4 signaling that acts by repressing TRAF6 to inhibit NFκB transcription factor activation (46, 47). In macrophages, TRAF6 mediates the induction of the pro-inflammatory cytokine IL-12, which is essential to control *T. gondii* infection (48). TRAF6 activation is also required for vacuole-lysosome fusion, a fundamental step during *T. gondii* infection (49). Our results showed that in HPEs, *T. gondii* and *T. cruzi* infection increased miR-146a expression. Our previous studies showed that both parasites modulate placental immune response differentially through TLRs and NFκB pathways in HPEs (9, 10) Interestingly, the inhibition of these pathways increased the DNA loads of both parasites in HPEs (10). Increased *T. gondii* infection in placental tissue is also induced by TLR-4 inhibition (9). In addition, increased levels of miR-146a have been reported in the brains of mice infected with *T. gondii*, moreover, miR-146a ablation affects early parasite burden and improves survival (50). It was previously reported that miR-210 is induced by damage associated molecular patterns (51). In preeclamptic placentas, miR-210 is increased (52); in the present study, miR-210 was increased in HPE infected with *T. cruzi* but not with *T. gondii*. Expression of miR-210 can be directly regulated by the specific binding of NF-κB p50 to its putative promoter (53). In this context, it is important to mention that *T. cruzi*, but not *T. gondii*, infection of HPE activates both NF-κB signaling pathways (10). Therefore, the increased level of miR-210 might be a placental response to signal transduction pathway activation.

In addition, several identified pathways, important, e.g. for chondrocyte development, megakaryocyte smooth and muscle cell differentiation, hepatotoxicity, and DNA damage response, are neither related to infection or with placental tissues (**Figure 3**). This can be explained be the fact, that miRNAs target multiple genes, while individual genes are targeted by multiple miRNAs. Moreover, the same miRNA regulates different genes in different tissues and organs (54, 55). Here, we chose to validate six miRNAs that were associated specifically with parasite infection and/or pregnancy related pathologies (**Figure 6**). Deregulation of miR-30e-3p has been reported in mice that were experimentally infected with *T. gondii* (40). This miRNA is also related to Chagas cardiomyopathy (39) and is upregulated in placentas with intrauterine growth restriction (56). Nonetheless, miR-30e-3p expression was unaffected by *T. cruzi* or *T. gondii* infection in HPE (**Figure 6C**). Increased miR-3074-5p expression has been described in placentas from recurrent miscarriages (57) and in livers from *T. gondii*-infected cats (42). However, miR-3074-5p expression was diminished in HPE infected either with *T. cruzi* or *T. gondii* (**Figure 6A**). The differences between our results and the reported data might be explained by differences in the studied organs (heart and liver *versus* placenta) and the complexity of the above mentioned placental pathologies. MiR-127 is a placenta-specific miRNA codified in the C14MC cluster (58) and its levels are decreased in placenta-related pathologies such as recurrent miscarriage and small-for-gestational age (59, 60); the downregulation of MiR-127 was also detected in babies infected congenitally with either parasite (3, 4). Concordantly, our results showed that HPE infection with either *T. cruzi* or *T. gondii* led to the decrease of this miRNA (**Figure 6B**). Moreover, a decreased expression of miR-127-3p in non-placental tissues has been reported during *T. gondii* infection in mice and cats (40, 42, 61), but there is no report regarding miR-127-3p expression in response to *T. cruzi* infection. Both miR-515-5p and miR-512-3p are placenta-specific miRNAs that are codified in the C19MC cluster (62). Decreased miR-515-5p expression is related to fetal growth restriction (63) and preeclampsia (64). Importantly, this miRNA inhibits human trophoblast differentiation by directly repressing the aromatase P450 (*CYP19A1*), frizzled 5 (*FZD5*), and glial cells missing 1 transcription factor (*GCM1*) genes (65). Trophoblast differentiation is part of the trophoblast epithelial turnover

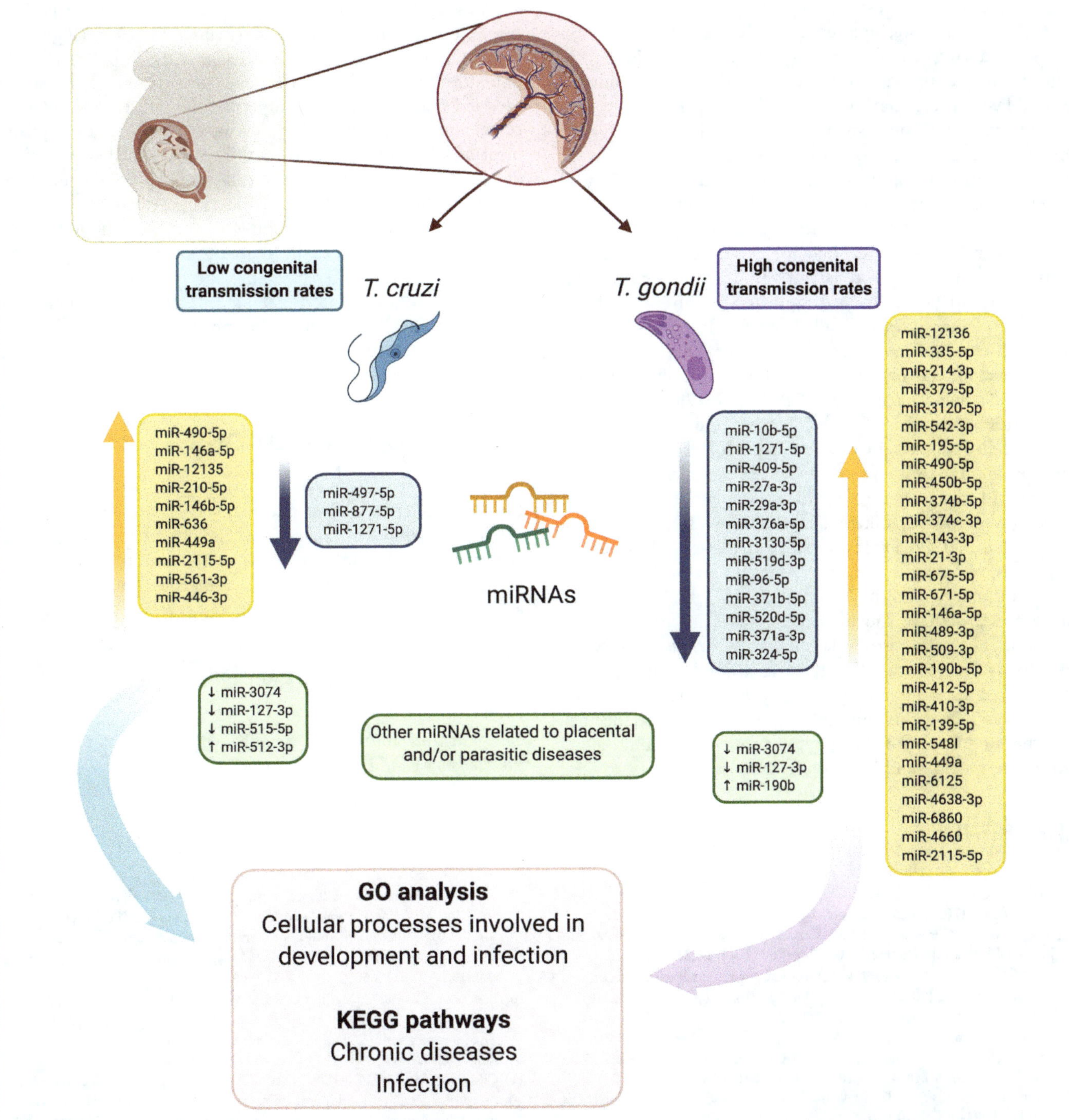

FIGURE 7 | Schematic summary of the comparative analysis of RNA sequencing-based miRNA profiles in HPEs in response to *ex vivo T. cruzi* and *T. gondii* infection. Fourteen, and 42 DEMs were identified in *T. cruzi* and *T. gondii* infected samples. In *T. cruzi* infected HPEs, 5 miRNAs were downregulated and 9 were upregulated. In *T. gondii* infected HPEs, 13 miRNAs were downregulated and 29 were upregulated. In addition, five miRNAs that are associated specifically with parasite infection and/or pregnancy-related pathologies were validated. GO analysis revealed that the predicted targets of the DEMs were different cellular processes involved in development and immunity, and most of the identified KEGG pathways were related to chronic diseases and infection. Considering that the DEMs identified herein modulate crucial host cellular targets potentially determining the success of infection, these miRNAs might explain the differences in the congenital transmission rates of the two parasites. This figure was created using BioRender.com.

and it has been proposed that this mechanism is part of an antiparasitic placental response against *T. cruzi* infection (11, 13, 66, 67). Therefore, our reported decrease of miR-515-5p expression during *ex vivo T. cruzi* infection of HPE (**Figure 6D**) might be at least partially responsible for the parasite-induced trophoblast differentiation. In contrast, miR-512-3p was upregulated in HPE in response to *T. cruzi* infection (**Figure 6E**). Interestingly, miR-512-3p confers resistance to vesicular stomatitis virus in non-placental recipient cells (68) and represses the caspase 8 inhibitor c-FLIP (cellular FLICE-like inhibitory protein); it consequently increases caspase 8 activity (69). Caspase 8 regulates trophoblast differentiation and apoptotic cell death and is activated by *T. cruzi* (66). Therefore, miR-512-3p upregulation might also be a protective placental response to *T. cruzi* infection, as it is to viral infection. The upregulation of miR-190b in HPE during *T. gondii* infection was observed in the RNAseq analysis (**Figure 1B**, **Table 3**), then validated by qPCR (**Figure 6F**). Upregulation of miR-190b promotes cell proliferation and migration and reduces cell apoptosis in different types of cancer (70, 71). Parasites modulate apoptotic responses in infected cells to avoid rapid clearance; *T. gondii* is particularly capable of blocking apoptosis by different mechanisms (33). In neurons, increased miR-190b expression also increases cell viability, suppresses autophagy, and significantly decreases the levels of pro-inflammatory TNF-α, IL-6, and IL-1β cytokines (72). In this context, we have shown that *T. gondii*, in contrast to *T. cruzi*, does not induce pro-inflammatory cytokines in HPE (9). Therefore, it is postulated that the lack of pro-inflammatory cytokine secretion in response to *T. gondii* in HPE might be related to an increase in miR-190b expression and that, together with the modulation of the apoptotic pathway, it could allow parasite persistence and infection in the placenta.

In conclusion, the present study provides a comparative analysis of RNA sequencing-based miRNA profiles in HPE in response to *ex vivo T. cruzi* and *T. gondii* infection (**Figure 7**). Our findings provide new insight into the capacity of both parasites to modulate host gene expression. GO analysis revealed that the predicted targets of the DEMs were different cellular processes involved in development and immunity, and most of the identified KEGG pathways were related to chronic diseases and infection. Considering that the DEMs identified herein modulate crucial host cellular targets that participate in determining the success of infection, these miRNAs might explain the differences in congenital transmission rates. Molecules of the different pathways that are regulated by miRNAs and modulated during infection, as well as the miRNAs themselves, may be potential targets for the therapeutic control of either congenital Chagas disease or toxoplasmosis.

AUTHOR CONTRIBUTIONS

LM and UK conceived of and planned experiments. LM, CC, MR-P, AL, and JG-M carried out experiments. JM and HP contributed to the interpretation of the results. UK and LM wrote the manuscript. All authors contributed to the article and approved the submitted version.

ACKNOWLEDGEMENTS

The authors thank Dr. Sergio Angel for providing the *Toxoplasma gondii* parasites.

REFERENCES

1. Dotters-Katz S, Kuller J, Heine RP. Parasitic infections in pregnancy. *Obstet Gynecol Surv* (2011) 66:515–25. doi: 10.1097/OGX.0b013e3182385fde
2. Błaszkowska J, Góralska K. Parasites and fungi as a threat for prenatal and postnatal human development. *Ann Parasitol* (2014) 60:225–34.
3. Carlier Y, Truyens C, Deloron P, Peyron F. Congenital parasitic infections: a review. *Acta Trop* (2012) 121:55–70. doi: 10.1016/j.actatropica.2011.10.018
4. Kemmerling U, Osuna A, Schijman AG, Truyens C. Congenital Transmission of Trypanosoma cruzi: A Review About the Interactions Between the Parasite, the Placenta, the Maternal and the Fetal/Neonatal Immune Responses. *Front Microbiol* (2019) 10:1854. doi: 10.3389/fmicb.2019.01854
5. Schmuñis G. Status of and cost of Chagas disease worldwide. *Lancet Infect Dis* (2013) 13:283–4. doi: 10.1016/S1473-3099(13)70032-X
6. Pérez-Molina JA, Molina I. Chagas disease. *Lancet (London England)* (2018) 391:82–94. doi: 10.1016/S0140-6736(17)31612-4
7. Melo MB, Jensen KDC, Saeij JPJ. Toxoplasma gondii effectors are master regulators of the inflammatory response. *Trends Parasitol* (2011) 27:487–95. doi: 10.1016/j.pt.2011.08.001
8. Rendell VR, Gilman RH, Valencia E, Galdos-Cardenas G, Verastegui M, Sanchez L, et al. Trypanosoma cruzi-infected pregnant women without vector exposure have higher parasitemia levels: implications for congenital transmission risk. *PloS One* (2015) 10:e0119527. doi: 10.1371/journal.pone.0119527
9. Castillo C, Muñoz L, Carrillo I, Liempi A, Gallardo C, Galanti N, et al. Ex vivo infection of human placental chorionic villi explants with Trypanosoma cruzi and Toxoplasma gondii induces different Toll-like receptor expression and cytokine/chemokine profiles. *Am J Reprod Immunol* (2017) 78:1–8. doi: 10.1111/aji.12660
10. Liempi A, Castillo C, Medina L, Rojas M, Maya JD, Parraguez VH, et al. Ex vivo infection of human placental explants with Trypanosoma cruzi and Toxoplasma gondii: Differential activation of NF kappa B signaling pathways. *Acta Trop* (2019) 199:105153. doi: 10.1016/j.actatropica.2019.105153
11. Castillo C, Muñoz L, Carrillo I, Liempi A, Medina L, Galanti N, et al. Toll-like receptor-2 mediates local innate immune response against Trypanosoma cruzi in ex vivo infected human placental chorionic villi explants. *Placenta* (2017) 60:40–6. doi: 10.1016/j.placenta.2017.10.005
12. Sen R, Nayak L, De RK. A review on host–pathogen interactions: classification and prediction. *Eur J Clin Microbiol Infect Dis* (2016) 35:1581–99. doi: 10.1007/s10096-016-2716-7
13. Liempi A, Castillo C, Carrillo I, Muñoz L, Droguett D, Galanti N, et al. A local innate immune response against Trypanosoma cruzi in the human placenta: The epithelial turnover of the trophoblast. *Microb Pathog* (2016) 99:123–9. doi: 10.1016/j.micpath.2016.08.022

14. De Souza W, Ulisses de Carvalho TM. Active penetration of Trypanosoma cruzi into host cells: Historical considerations and current concepts. *Front Immunol* (2013) 4:2. doi: 10.3389/fimmu.2013.00002
15. Hakimi Ma, Cannella D. Apicomplexan parasites and subversion of the host cell microRNA pathway. *Trends Parasitol* (2011) 27:481–6. doi: 10.1016/j.pt.2011.07.001
16. Castillo C, Carrillo I, Libisch G, Juiz N, Schijman AG, Robello C, et al. Host-parasite interaction: Changes in human placental gene expression induced by Trypanosoma cruzi. *Parasit Vectors* (2018) 11:1–13. doi: 10.1186/s13071-018-2988-0
17. Hayder H, O'Brien J, Nadeem U, Peng C. MicroRNAs: crucial regulators of placental development. *Reproduction* (2018) 155:R259–71. doi: 10.1530/REP-17-0603
18. Zheng Y, Cai X, Bradley JE. MicroRNAs in parasites and parasite infection. *RNA Biol* (2013) 10:377–85. doi: 10.4161/rna.23716
19. Acuña SM, Floeter-Winter LM, Muxel SM. MicroRNAs: Biological Regulators in Pathogen–Host Interactions. *Cells* (2020) 9:113. doi: 10.3390/cells9010113
20. Ferreira LRP, Frade AF, Santos RHB, Teixeira PC, Baron MA, Navarro IC, et al. MicroRNAs miR-1, miR-133a, miR-133b, miR-208a and miR-208b are dysregulated in Chronic Chagas disease Cardiomyopathy. *Int J Cardiol* (2014) 175:409–17. doi: 10.1016/j.ijcard.2014.05.019
21. Cai Y, Shen J. Modulation of host immune responses to Toxoplasma gondii by microRNAs. *Parasite Immunol* (2017) 39:1–6. doi: 10.1111/pim.12417
22. Sadovsky Y, Mouillet JF, Ouyang Y, Bayer A, Coyne CB. The function of trophomirs and other micrornas in the human placenta. *Cold Spring Harb Perspect Med* (2015) 5:1–16. doi: 10.1101/cshperspect.a023036
23. Dumont TMF, Mouillet JF, Bayer A, Gardner CL, Klimstra WB, Wolf DG, et al. The expression level of C19MC miRNAs in early pregnancy and in response to viral infection. *Placenta* (2017) 53:23–9. doi: 10.1016/j.placenta.2017.03.011
24. Delorme-Axford E, Sadovsky Y, Coyne CB. The Placenta as a Barrier to Viral Infections. *Annu Rev Virol* (2014) 1:133–46. doi: 10.1146/annurev-virology-031413-085524
25. Nardelli SC, Che F-Y, Silmon de Monerri NC, Xiao H, Nieves E, Madrid-Aliste C, et al. The histone code of Toxoplasma gondii comprises conserved and unique posttranslational modifications. *MBio* (2013) 4:e00922–13. doi: 10.1128/mBio.00922-13
26. Liempi A, Castillo C, Medina L, Galanti N, Maya JD, Parraguez VH, et al. Comparative ex vivo infection with Trypanosoma cruzi and Toxoplasma gondii of human, canine and ovine placenta: Analysis of tissue damage and infection efficiency. *Parasitol Int* (2020) 76:102065. doi: 10.1016/j.parint.2020.102065
27. Lindgreen S. AdapterRemoval: Easy cleaning of next-generation sequencing reads. *BMC Res Notes* (2012) 5:337. doi: 10.1186/1756-0500-5-337
28. Dobin A, Davis CA, Schlesinger F, Drenkow J, Zaleski C, Jha S, et al. STAR: Ultrafast universal RNA-seq aligner. *Bioinformatics* (2013) 29:15–21. doi: 10.1093/bioinformatics/bts635
29. Anders S, Pyl PT, Huber W. HTSeq-A Python framework to work with high-throughput sequencing data. *Bioinformatics* (2015) 31:166–9. doi: 10.1093/bioinformatics/btu638
30. Robinson MD, McCarthy DJ, Smyth GK. edgeR: A Bioconductor package for differential expression analysis of digital gene expression data. *Bioinformatics* (2009) 26:139–40. doi: 10.1093/bioinformatics/btp616
31. Androvic P, Valihrach L, Elling J, Sjoback R, Kubista M. Two-tailed RT-qPCR: a novel method for highly accurate miRNA quantification. *Nucleic Acids Res* (2017) 45:e144. doi: 10.1093/nar/gkx588
32. Villares M, Berthelet J, Weitzman JB. The clever strategies used by intracellular parasites to hijack host gene expression. *Semin Immunopathol* (2020) 42:215–26. doi: 10.1007/s00281-020-00779-z
33. Mammari N, Halabi MA, Yaacoub S, Chlala H, Dardé M-L, Courtioux B. Toxoplasma gondii Modulates the Host Cell Responses: An Overview of Apoptosis Pathways. *BioMed Res Int* (2019), 2019:6152489. doi: 10.1155/2019/6152489
34. Chiribao ML, Libisch G, Parodi-Talice A, Robello C. Early Trypanosoma cruzi infection reprograms human epithelial cells. *BioMed Res Int* (2014) 2014:439501. doi: 10.1155/2014/439501
35. Hakimi MA, Olias P, Sibley LD. Toxoplasma effectors targeting host signaling and transcription. *Clin Microbiol Rev* (2017) 30:615–44. doi: 10.1128/CMR.00005-17
36. Jia B, Chang Z, Wei X, Lu H, Yin J, Jiang N, et al. Plasma microRNAs are promising novel biomarkers for the early detection of Toxoplasma gondii infection. *Parasit Vectors* (2014) 7:433. doi: 10.1186/1756-3305-7-433
37. Salehi M, Sharifi M. Exosomal miRNAs as novel cancer biomarkers: Challenges and opportunities. *J Cell Physiol* (2018) 233:6370–80. doi: 10.1002/jcp.26481
38. Mouillet JF, Ouyang Y, Coyne CB, Sadovsky Y. MicroRNAs in placental health and disease. *Am J Obstet Gynecol* (2015) 213:S163–72. doi: 10.1016/j.ajog.2015.05.057
39. Navarro IC, Ferreira FM, Nakaya HI, Baron MA, Vilar-Pereira G, Pereira IR, et al. MicroRNA transcriptome profiling in heart of trypanosoma cruzi-infected mice: Parasitological and cardiological Outcomes. *PloS Negl Trop Dis* (2015) 9:1–17. doi: 10.1371/journal.pntd.0003828
40. Hu RS, He JJ, Elsheikha HM, Zhang FK, Zou Y, Zhao GH, et al. Differential brain microRNA expression profiles after acute and chronic infection of mice with toxoplasma gondii oocysts. *Front Microbiol* (2018) 9:2316. doi: 10.3389/fmicb.2018.02316
41. Machado FS, Dutra WO, Esper L, Gollob KJ, Teixeira MM, Factor SM, et al. Current understanding of immunity to Trypanosoma cruzi infection and pathogenesis of Chagas disease. *Semin Immunopathol* (2012) 34:753–70. doi: 10.1007/s00281-012-0351-7
42. Cong W, Zhang XX, He JJ, Li FC, Elsheikha HM, Zhu XQ. Global miRNA expression profiling of domestic cat livers following acute Toxoplasma gondii infection. *Oncotarget* (2017) 8:25599–611. doi: 10.18632/oncotarget.16108
43. Cătană CS, Calin GA, Berindan-Neagoe I. Inflamma-miRs in aging and breast cancer: Are they reliable players? *Front Med (Lausanne)* (2015) 2:85. doi: 10.3389/fmed.2015.00085
44. Li H, Jiang T, Li MQ, Zheng XL, Zhao GJ. Transcriptional regulation of macrophages polarization by microRNAs. *Front Immunol* (2018) 9:1175. doi: 10.3389/fimmu.2018.01175
45. Chaiwangyen W, Ospina-Prieto S, Photini SM, Schleussner E, Markert UR, Morales-Prieto DM. Dissimilar microRNA-21 functions and targets in trophoblastic cell lines of different origin. *Int J Biochem Cell Biol* (2015) 68:187–96. doi: 10.1016/j.biocel.2015.08.018
46. Hou J, Wang P, Lin L, Liu X, Ma F, An H, et al. MicroRNA-146a Feedback Inhibits RIG-I-Dependent Type I IFN Production in Macrophages by Targeting TRAF6, IRAK1, and IRAK2. *J Immunol* (2009) 183:2150–8. doi: 10.4049/jimmunol.0900707
47. Taganov KD, Boldin MP, Chang KJ, Baltimore D. NF-κB-dependent induction of microRNA miR-146, an inhibitor targeted to signaling proteins of innate immune responses. *Proc Natl Acad Sci U S A* (2006) 103:12481–6. doi: 10.1073/pnas.0605298103
48. Mason NJ, Fiore J, Kobayashi T, Masek KS, Choi Y, Hunter CA. TRAF6-dependent mitogen-activated protein kinase activation differentially regulates the production of interleukin-12 by macrophages in response to Toxoplasma gondii. *Infect Immun* (2004) 72:5662–7. doi: 10.1128/IAI.72.10.5662-5667.2004
49. Subauste CS, Andrade RM, Wessendarp M. CD40-TRAF6 and autophagy-dependent anti-microbial activity in macrophages. *Autophagy* (2007) 3:245–8. doi: 10.4161/auto.3717
50. Cannella D, Brenier-Pinchart MP, Braun L, vanRooyen JM, Bougdour A, Bastien O, et al. MiR-146a and miR-155 delineate a microRNA fingerprint associated with toxoplasma persistence in the host brain. *Cell Rep* (2014) 6:928–37. doi: 10.1016/j.celrep.2014.02.002
51. Unlu S, Tang S, Wang E, Martinez I, Tang D, Bianchi ME, et al. Damage associated molecular pattern molecule-induced micrornas (DAMPmiRs) in human peripheral blood mononuclear cells. *PloS One* (2012) 7(6):e38899. doi: 10.1371/journal.pone.0038899
52. Zhu Xm, Han T, Sargent IL, Yin G, Yao Yq. Differential expression profile of microRNAs in human placentas from preeclamptic pregnancies vs normal pregnancies. *Am J Obstet Gynecol* (2009) 7(6):e38899. doi: 10.1016/j.ajog.2008.12.045

53. Zhang Y, Fei M, Xue G, Zhou Q, Jia Y, Li L, et al. Elevated levels of hypoxia-inducible microRNA-210 in pre-eclampsia: New insights into molecular mechanisms for the disease. *J Cell Mol Med* (2012) 16:249–59. doi: 10.1111/j.1582-4934.2011.01291.x
54. Peter ME. Targeting of mRNAs by multiple miRNAs: The next step. *Oncogene* (2010) 29:2161–4. doi: 10.1038/onc.2010.59
55. Cai Y, Yu X, Hu S, Yu J. A Brief Review on the Mechanisms of miRNA Regulation. *Genomics Proteomics Bioinformatics* (2009) 7:147–54. doi: 10.1016/S1672-0229(08)60044-3
56. Wen H, Chen L, He J, Lin J. MicroRNA expression profiles and networks in placentas complicated with selective intrauterine growth restriction. *Mol Med Rep* (2017) 16:6650–73. doi: 10.3892/mmr.2017.7462
57. Gu Y, Zhang X, Yang Q, Wang J, He Y, Sun Z, et al. Aberrant Placental Villus Expression of miR-486-3p and miR-3074-5p in Recurrent Miscarriage Patients and Uterine Expression of These MicroRNAs during Early Pregnancy in Mice. *Gynecol Obstet Invest* (2016) 81:112–7. doi: 10.1159/000435879
58. Williams Z, Ben-Dov IZ, Elias R, Mihailovic A, Brown M, Rosenwaks Z, et al. Comprehensive profiling of circulating microRNA via small RNA sequencing of cDNA libraries reveals biomarker potential and limitations. *Proc Natl Acad Sci U S A* (2013) 110:4255–60. doi: 10.1073/pnas.1214046110
59. Yang Q, Gu WW, Gu Y, Yan NN, Mao YY, Zhen XX, et al. Association of the peripheral blood levels of circulating microRNAs with both recurrent miscarriage and the outcomes of embryo transfer in an in vitro fertilization process. *J Transl Med* (2018) 16(1):186. doi: 10.1186/s12967-018-1556-x
60. Rodosthenous RS, Burris HH, Sanders AP, Just AC, Dereix AE, Svensson K, et al. Second trimester extracellular microRNAs in maternal blood and fetal growth: An exploratory study. *Epigenetics* (2017) 12:804–10. doi: 10.1080/15592294.2017.1358345
61. He JJ, Ma J, Wang JL, Xu MJ, Zhu XQ. Analysis of miRNA expression profiling in mouse spleen affected by acute Toxoplasma gondii infection. *Infect Genet Evol* (2016) 37:137–42. doi: 10.1016/j.meegid.2015.11.005
62. Donker RB, Mouillet JF, Chu T, Hubel CA, Stolz DB, Morelli AE, et al. The expression profile of C19MC microRNAs in primary human trophoblast cells and exosomes. *Mol Hum Reprod* (2012) 18:417–24. doi: 10.1093/molehr/gas013
63. Higashijima A, Miura K, Mishima H, Kinoshita A, Jo O, Abe S, et al. Characterization of placenta-specific microRNAs in fetal growth restriction pregnancy. *Prenat Diagn* (2013) 33:214–22. doi: 10.1002/pd.4045
64. Hromadnikova I, Kotlabova K, Ondrackova M, Pirkova P, Kestlerova A, Novotna V, et al. Expression profile of C19MC microRNAs in placental tissue in pregnancy-related complications. *DNA Cell Biol* (2015) 34:437–57. doi: 10.1089/dna.2014.2687
65. Zhang M, Muralimanoharan S, Wortman AC, Mendelson CR. Primate-specific miR-515 family members inhibit key genes in human trophoblast differentiation and are upregulated in preeclampsia. *Proc Natl Acad Sci* (2016) 113:E7069–76. doi: 10.1073/pnas.1607849113
66. Carrillo I, Droguett D, Castillo C, Liempi A, Muñoz L, Maya JDJDJD, et al. Caspase-8 activity is part of the BeWo trophoblast cell defense mechanisms against Trypanosoma cruzi infection. *Exp Parasitol* (2016) 168:9–15. doi: 10.1016/j.exppara.2016.06.008
67. Liempi A, Castillo C, Duaso J, Droguett D, Sandoval A, Barahona K, et al. Trypanosoma cruzi induces trophoblast differentiation: A potential local antiparasitic mechanism of the human placenta? *Placenta* (2014) 35:1035–42. doi: 10.1016/j.placenta.2014.09.017
68. Delorme-Axford E, Donker RB, Mouillet J-F, Chu T, Bayer A, Ouyang Y, et al. Human placental trophoblasts confer viral resistance to recipient cells. *Proc Natl Acad Sci* (2013) 110:12048–53. doi: 10.1073/pnas.1304718110
69. Chen F, Zhu H-H, Zhou L-F, Wu S-S, Wang J, Chen Z. Inhibition of c-FLIP expression by miR-512-3p contributes to taxol-induced apoptosis in hepatocellular carcinoma cells. *Oncol Rep* (2010) 23:1457–62. doi: 10.3892/or_00000784
70. Dai W, He J, Zheng L, Bi M, Hu F, Chen M, et al. miR-148b-3p, miR-190b, and miR-429 regulate cell progression and act as potential biomarkers for breast cancer. *J Breast Cancer* (2019) 22:219–36. doi: 10.4048/jbc.2019.22.e19
71. Zhao Q, Liu C, Cui Q, Luan X, Wang Q, Zhou C. miR-190b promotes colorectal cancer progression through targeting forkhead box protein P2. *Exp Ther Med* (2019) 19:79. doi: 10.3892/etm.2019.8175
72. Pei X, Li Y, Zhu L, Zhou Z. Astrocyte-derived exosomes transfer miR-190b to inhibit oxygen and glucose deprivation-induced autophagy and neuronal apoptosis. *Cell Cycle* (2020) 19:906–17. doi: 10.1080/15384101.2020.1731649

18

Protective Immunity Induced by TgMIC5 and TgMIC16 DNA Vaccines against Toxoplasmosis

Yu-Chao Zhu[1†], Li-Juan Ma[2†], Ji-Li Zhang[1], Jian-Fa Liu[3], Yong He[1], Ji-Ye Feng[4] and Jia Chen[1,3*]*

[1] Department of Radiology, The Affiliated Hospital of Medical School of Ningbo University, Ningbo University School of Medicine, Ningbo, China, [2] Department of Integrated Chinese and Western Medicine Oncology, The Affiliated People's Hospital of Ningbo University, Ningbo, China, [3] Immunology Innovation Team, Ningbo University School of Medicine, Ningbo, China, [4] Department of Hepatobiliary Surgery, The Affiliated People's Hospital of Ningbo University, Ningbo, China

***Correspondence:**
Jia Chen
chenjia@nbu.edu.cn
Ji-Ye Feng
fengjiye@163.com

[†]These authors have contributed equally to this work

Toxoplasma gondii is an obligate intracellular parasite, which is responsible for a widely distributed zoonosis. Effective vaccines against toxoplasmosis are necessary to protect the public health. The aim of this study is to evaluate the immune efficacy of DNA vaccines encoding TgMIC5 and TgMIC16 genes against *T. gondii* infection. The recombinant plasmid pVAX-MIC5 and pVAX-MIC16 were constructed and injected intramuscularly in mice. The specific immune responses and protection against challenge with *T. gondii* RH tachyzoites were evaluated by measuring the cytokine levels, serum antibody concentrations, lymphocyte proliferation, lymphocyte populations, and the survival time. The protection against challenge with the *T. gondii* RH tchyzoites and PRU cysts was examined by evaluation of the reduction in the brain cyst burden. The results indicated that immunized mice showed significantly increased levels of IgG, IFN-γ, IL-2, IL-12p70, and IL-12p40 and percentages of $CD4^+$ and $CD8^+$ T cells. Additionally, vaccination prolonged the mouse survival time and reduced brain cysts compared with controls. Mouse groups immunized with a two-gene cocktail of pVAX-MIC5 + pVAX-MIC16 were more protected than mouse groups immunized with a single gene of pVAX-MIC5 or pVAX-MIC16. These results demonstrate that TgMIC5 and TgMIC16 induce effective immunity against toxoplasmosis and may serve as a good vaccine candidate against *T. gondii* infection.

Keywords: *Toxoplasma gondii*, DNA vaccine, MIC5, MIC16, parasite

INTRODUCTION

Toxoplasma gondii, an intracellular protozoan parasite, is able to infect almost all warm-blooded animals and humans (Mohamed-Ali et al., 2017; Florence and Marie-Laure, 2012). *T. gondii* is one of the most widespread parasites, with one-third of the world's population estimated to be chronically infected (Dubey, 2009; Pappas et al., 2009). In common, intermediate hosts including humans acquire infection by eating raw meat, and exposure to soil containing oocysts excreted by the only final host of *T. gondii*, cats. Toxoplasmosis is usually characterized as asymptomatic or subclinical infection in immunocompetent individuals, but it can cause serious complications or even a fatal disease in immunocompromised populations (e.g., HIV infected patients, cancer patients, and transplant recipients) (Saki et al., 2013; Wang et al., 2017; Elsheikha et al., 2020). If pregnant women acquire primary infection with *T. gondii*, fetal abortion may occur (Elsheikha, 2008; Flegr et al., 2014; Elsheikha et al., 2020). Also, *T. gondii* infection can lead to abortion and stillbirth in livestock, including goats and sheep, thereafter causing financial losses to the livestock industry (Tenter et al., 2000). Unfortunately, currently available drugs can only target the tachyzoite stage of *T. gondii*, while no effective chemotherapy can eliminate tissue cysts that persist life-long in the infected hosts (Wang et al., 2019). Therefore, immunoprophylaxis is considered to be an alternative approach for the prevention and control of toxoplasmosis (Zhang et al., 2013; Zhang et al., 2015).

The licensed vaccine which has been used for ovine toxoplasmosis (Toxovax) is obtained from the non-cyst forming S48 strain. However, it is unknown whether the vaccination has any effect on the tissue cyst formation and thus it is inapplicable to humans due to safety concerns (Erik et al., 2009; Burrells et al., 2015). Until now, no available vaccine has been used for protection against *T. gondii* infection in other animal species or humans (Wang et al., 2019). Hence, safe and effective vaccines would be extremely valuable for controlling of *T. gondii* infections in animals and humans. There is an urgent need to find a novel, effective, and safe vaccine to combat *T. gondii* infections.

The DNA vaccine is well known as safe, convenient, low cost, and can induce vigorous cellular and humoral immune responses (Margaret, 2011). A number of *T. gondii* excretory secretory antigens have been tested as DNA vaccine candidates (e.g. TgGRA24, TgGRA25, TgROP5, TgROP18, and TgDOC2C, etc.) and they showed effective immunity against *T. gondii* infection, with inductive Th1 type and CD8+ cytotoxic T-lymphocyte responses, and prolonged survival time in mice after infection with *T. gondii* (Zhang et al., 2018; Xu et al., 2019; Zhu et al., 2020)., Some microneme proteins (MICs) have also been shown to have immunogenic capabilities (Dodangeh et al., 2019). TgMIC5 is one of a large member of microneme proteins, which can regulate the activity of proteases and it is related to the proteolytic susceptibility of other microneme protein substrates (Susannah et al., 2006). TgMIC16 is indispensable for binding to aldolase and is also involved in rhomboid cleavage and trafficking signals during *T. gondii* invasion (Lilach et al., 2010). These important features suggest that TgMIC5 and TgMIC16 proteins may be good DNA vaccine candidates, which can elicit protective immunity against infection with *T. gondii*.

The objectives of this study were to assess the potential of TgMIC5 and TgMIC16 as DNA vaccine candidates against infection with *T. gondii*. We constructed the eukaryotic plasmids, pVAX-MIC5 and pVAX-MIC16, and determined the protective immunity elicited by the DNA vaccine based on pVAX-MIC5 and/or pVAX-MIC16 against acute and chronic *T. gondii* infection in Kunming mice.

MATERIALS AND METHODS

Mice and Parasite

Seven-week-old specific-pathogen-free (SPF) Kunming female mice were purchased from Zhejiang Laboratory Animal Center, Hangzhou, China. All mice in this study were handled in strict accordance with the Animal Ethics Procedures and Guidelines of the People's Republic of China. This study was approved by the Animal Ethics Committee of Ningbo University (permission: SYXK(ZHE)2013-0190).

T. gondii tachyzoites of the RH strain (Type I) and cysts of the PRU strain (Type II) were used in this study, which were propagated and harvested according to the methods described in previous studies (Chen et al., 2016). The obtained tachyzoites were used for the preparation of *Toxoplasma* lysate antigen (TLA) and also for total RNA extraction (RNAprep Pure Tissue Kit, TIANGEN, China), as described previously (Chen et al., 2015). In brief, prior to centrifugation, the cellular lysate was prepared by disruption of *T. gondii* RH tachyzoites using three cycles of freezing at –20°C and thawing, followed by sonication on ice at 60 W/s. Then, TLA was obtained from the supernatants, and then pooled and sterile-filtered with 0.2 μm nitrocellulose filters (Sartorius, Germany).

Construction of the Eukaryotic Expression Plasmid

The coding sequences of the TgMIC5 and TgMIC16 gene were amplified by polymerase chain reaction (PCR) from tachyzoite cDNA of *T. gondii* RH strain, using two pairs of oligonucleotide primers: (MIC5F, forward primer: 5′-GGGGTACCATGCTGCG ACCTACTGTT -3′); (MIC5R, reverse primer: 5′-GCCTAGACT ATGCGAGTTTCACCTC -3′); (MIC16F, forward primer: 5′-GG GGTACCATGCTGCGACCTACTGTT -3′); (MIC16R, reverse primer: 5′-GCTCTAGACTATGCGAGTTTCACCTC -3′). The two obtained PCR products were inserted into pMD18-T vector (TaKaRa, China) and sequenced in both directions to ensure fidelity and the construction of pMD-MIC5 and pMD-MIC16. The TgMIC5 and TgMIC16 fragments were cleaved by *Xba* I and *Kpn* I (TaKaRa, China) from pMD-MIC5 and pMD-MIC16 and then subcloned into the pVAX I vector. The recombinant plasmids pVAX-MIC5 and pVAX-MIC16 were transferred into *E. coli* DH5α, and positive clones were selected *via* double restriction enzyme digestion and DNA sequencing. Then, these two plasmids were purified by anion exchange chromatography (EndoFree plasmid giga kit, Qiagen Sciences, Maryland) following the manufacturer's instructions, and were diluted with sterile phosphate buffered saline (PBS) and stored at –20°C until use. The concentration of pVAX-MIC5 and pVAX-MIC16 was determined with spectrophotometer at OD_{260} and OD_{280}.

Expression of pVAX-MIC5 and pVAX-MIC16 Plasmid *In Vitro*

Indirect immunofluorescence assay (IFA) was used to detect the expression of pVAX-MIC5 and pVAX-MIC16 *in vitro*, followed by pVAX-MIC5 and pVAX-MIC16 transfection into 293-T cells using Lipofectamine 2000 reagent (Invitrogen, Carlsbad, CA) according to the manufacturer's instructions as previously described (Chen et al., 2015). In brief, 48 h post-transfection with pVAX-MIC5 or pVAX-MIC16, cells were fixed with 100% chilled acetone for 30 min. Following washing with PBS-0.1% Triton-X-100 (PBST), anti-*T. gondii* polyclonal antiserum (1:50 dilution in PBS-0.1% Triton-X-100 [PBST]) and fluorescein isothiocyanate (FITC)-labeled donkey-anti-goat IgG (Proteintech Group Inc., Chicago) were added to each well. Finally, the stained monolayers were covered with glycerin and then fluorescence was imaged using a Zeiss Axioplan fluorescence microscope (Carl Zeiss, Germany). 293-T cells transfection with empty pVAX I was used as the negative control.

Immunization and *T. gondii* Challenge in Mice

The experiment groups (25 mice/group) consisting of mice immunized with 100 μL (1 μg/μL) plasmids diluted in PBS, including pVAX-MIC5, pVAX-MIC16, and pVAX-MIC5 + pVAX-MIC16, respectively, which were injected intramuscularly (i.m.) three times at 2-week intervals. Control groups include mice that received 100 μL PBS (negative control group), 100 μg empty pVAX I plasmid (vector control group; 1 μg/μL), and no treatment (blank control). Blood from each group of mice was collected from the tail vein at 0, 2, 4, and 6 weeks prior to immunization. Sera were collected after centrifugation for 5 min at 4000 g and stored at -20°C until further study.

The mice (10 per group) in all groups were intraperitoneally (i.p.) inoculated with 1×10^3 tachyzoites of RH strain 2 weeks after the third immunization, and the survival was recorded daily until 35 days. The mice (another 6 mice per group) were inoculated orally with 20 cysts of the PRU strain at 2 weeks after the third immunization, the mouse brains were removed and homogenized in 1 ml of PBS, and the mean number of brain cysts was determined under a microscope (40 × objective) using three aliquots of 20 μL of brain homogenates. All samples were analyzed in triplicate. Two weeks after the last immunization, a total of 9 mice per group were sacrificed and their splenocytes were used for cytokine measurements (3 mice), lymphocyte proliferation assay (3 mice), and flow cytometric analysis (another 3 mice).

Measurement of Antibody Responses

According to the manufacturer's instruction of SBA Clonotyping System-HRP Kit (Southern Biotech Co., Ltd, Birmingham, United Kingdom) and as described in methods previously (Chen et al., 2015), ELISA was used to determine the levels of IgG, IgG1, and IgG2a in sera samples collected at 0, 2, 4, and 6 weeks. In brief, the microtiter plates were coated with 100 μL (10 μg/mL) TLA diluted in PBS and incubated at 4°C overnight. The plates were then washed three times by PBS containing 0.05% Tween20 (PBST) and blocked by PBS containing 1% BSA for 1 h at 37°C. After washing with PBS, the plates were incubated with the sera diluted by PBS for 1 h at room temperature. The anti-mouse-IgG, IgG1, and IgG2a horseradish peroxidase (HRP)-conjugated antibodies were added to each well for 1 h at 37°C. The efficient binding was visualized by incubation with substrate solution (100 μL; pH 4.0; 1.5% ABTS, 1.05% citrate substrate buffer, 0.03% H_2O_2) for 30 min at room temperature. The absorbance was measured at 405 nm using the ELISA reader (Bio-TekEL×800, U.S.). All samples were analyzed in triplicate.

Lymphoproliferation Assay

Splenocyte suspensions from 3 mice in each group were prepared by pushing the spleens through a wire mesh, and purified through removing the red blood cells by using RBC erythrocyte lysis buffer, and then resuspended in DMEM medium supplemented with 10% fetal bovine serum (FBS; Gibco, Carlsbad, CA). In brief, 3×10^6 cells per well were cultured in 96-well Costar plates stimulated with TLA (10 μg/ml), concanavalin A (ConA; positive control; 5 μg/ml; Sigma, St. Louis, MO), or medium alone (negative control), at 37°C for 72 h with 5% CO_2. Then, 10 ul of 3-(4,5-dimethylthylthiazol-2-yl)-2,5-diphenyltetrazolium bromide (MTT, 5 mg/ml, Sigma, St. Louis, MO) was added to each well and incubated for 4 h. The stimulation index (SI) was calculated as per the following formula: stimulation index (SI) = (OD570 TLA/OD570 Control):(OD570 ConA/OD570 Control). All samples were analyzed in triplicate, which were obtained from 3 different mice.

Flow Cytometry Analysis

The percentages of CD4+ and CD8+ T lymphocytes in the purified splenocytes obtained from the mice after the last immunization were analyzed by flow cytometry. Splenocytes suspensions were prepared as mentioned previously and then stained with fluorochrome-labeled mAbs including PE-CD3, APC-CD4, and FITC-CD8 (eBioscience, United States) at 4°C for 30 min in the dark. After washing with 2 ml PBS, the cultures were fixed with FACScan buffer (PBS containing 1% FBS and 0.1% sodium azide) and 2% paraformaldehyde. The samples were run in a FACScan flow cytometer (BD Bio-sciences, United States) and then were analyzed for fluorescence by SYSTEM II software (Coulter). All samples were run in triplicate independently, which were obtained from three different mice.

Cytokine Assays

Spleen cells grown in 96-well plates were restimulated with TLA (10 μg/ml) or medium alone (negative control). The commercial ELISA kits (Biolegend, United States) were used to detect the levels of cytokines harvested from cell-free supernatants, which were assayed for IL-2, IL-4, and IL-12p40 levels at 24 h, for IL-10 levels at 72 h, and for gamma interferon (IFN-γ) and IL-12p70 levels.

Statistical Analysis

All statistical analyses were conducted with SPSS17.0 Data Editor (SPSS, Inc., Chicago, IL). The differences (e.g., antibody and percentage of $CD4^+$ and $CD8^+$ T cells) between all the groups were compared by one-way ANOVA. The level of significant difference between groups was considered significantly different if $P<0.05$. The survival time after challenge with RH strain was conducted with Kaplan-Meier.

RESULTS

Expression of pVAX-MIC5 and pVAX-MIC16 Plasmid *In Vitro*

Specific green fluorescence was observed in the 293T cells transfected with pVAX-MIC5 and pVAX-MIC16, while no fluorescence was observed in cells transfected with the empty pVAX I (**Figure 1**).

Antibody Response and Isotype Determination

The levels of total IgG and subclasses IgG1 and IgG2a were detected by ELISA. As shown in **Figure 2A**, a higher IgG titer was detected in the serum of mice vaccinated with single or two genes than that in three control groups. Also, pVAX-MIC5 + pVAX-MIC16 increased the antibody levels induced by DNA immunization than with pVAX-MIC5 or pVAX-MIC16. As shown in **Figure 2B**, the ratios of IgG2a/IgG1 in all immunized groups were higher, especially in pVAX-MIC5 + pVAX-MIC16 group compared with the control groups ($p < 0.05$).

Evaluation of the Proliferative Response in Spleen Cells

The proliferative activity in splenocytes was assayed by MTT. As shown in **Figure 3A**, the SI in mice vaccinated with pVAX-MIC5 + pVAX-MIC16 was higher than that in mice immunized with a single-gene plasmid or the control groups ($P<0.05$). In contrast, mice immunized with pVAX-MIC5 or pVAX-MIC16 induced a higher SI than the control groups. However, no significant difference was observed in the control groups ($P > 0.05$).

The Percentages of CD4$^+$ and CD8$^+$ T Lymphocytes

Similar to the results mentioned previously, the percentages of CD4$^+$ T cells were significantly increased ($P<0.05$) in the immunized mice compared to that in the control groups. The mice immunized with pVAX-MIC5 + pVAX-MIC16 induced higher percentages of CD4$^+$ T cells than that in mice immunized with a single-gene plasmid (pVAX-MIC5 or pVAX-MIC16) (**Figure 3B**). However, there was no significant difference among the three control groups ($P>0.05$). Similar to the results of the percentages of CD4$^+$ T cells, the percentages of CD8$^+$ T cells showed obvious increase in all immunized mice in comparison with that in control groups (**Figure 3C**) ($P < 0.05$).

Cytokine Production

Splenocyte supernatants were obtained at 2 weeks after the last immunization, which were used to assess the levels of IFN-γ, IL-2, IL-12p70, IL-12p40, IL-4, and IL-10 in mice. As shown in **Figure 4**, the higher levels of IL-12p70 and IL-12p40, especially IFN-γ and IL-2 in DNA immunized mice, were detected in comparison to that in the controls ($P<0.05$). The mice immunized with pVAX-MIC5 + pVAX-MIC16 showed higher levels of these cytokines than the groups of mice immunized with a single-gene plasmid (pVAX-MIC5 or pVAX-MIC16). Regarding the production of IL-4 and IL-10, a slight increased production of IL-4 and IL-10 was observed in all the immunized groups compared with that in controls ($P>0.05$).

Protective Efficacy of DNA Vaccination Against Acute and Chronic *T. gondii* Infection

To evaluate the protective efficacy induced by the DNA immunization, the survival curve in immunized mice after challenge of *T. gondii* RH strain as shown in **Figure 5** and this suggested that the three immunized groups had significantly prolonged survival time compared with the control groups, which died within 6 days post challenge ($P<0.05$). As shown in **Figure 6**, a significant reduction of brain cyst was observed in mice immunized with pVAX-MIC5 (28%), pVAX-MIC16 (39.44%), and especially pVAX-MIC5 + pVAX-MIC16 (48.06%) compared to the controls ($P<0.05$). No statistical difference was observed between the three control groups ($P>0.05$).

DISCUSSION

In recent years, DNA vaccines can evoke durable immune responses, which is critical to provide protective immunity against infection with *T. gondii* (Li and Zhou,, 2018). Previous studies have evaluated the immunoprotective efficacy of *T. gondii* MIC antigens, including TgMIC2, TgMIC2, TgMIC11, and

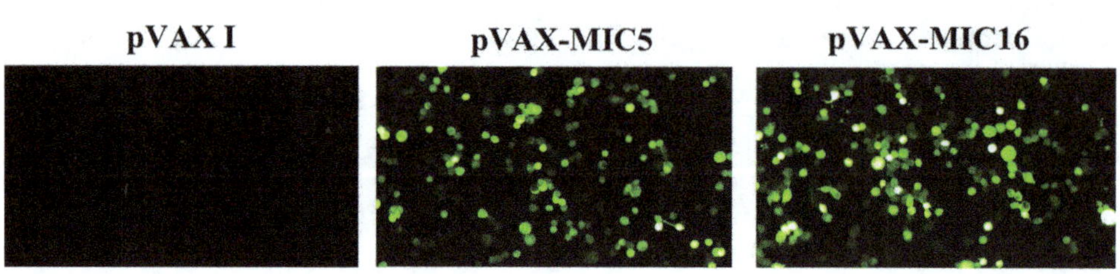

FIGURE 1 | Detection of the recombinant TgMIC5 and TgMIC16 protein expressed in 293T cells. 293T cells were transfected with empty pVAX I, pVAX-MIC5, or pVAX-MIC16.

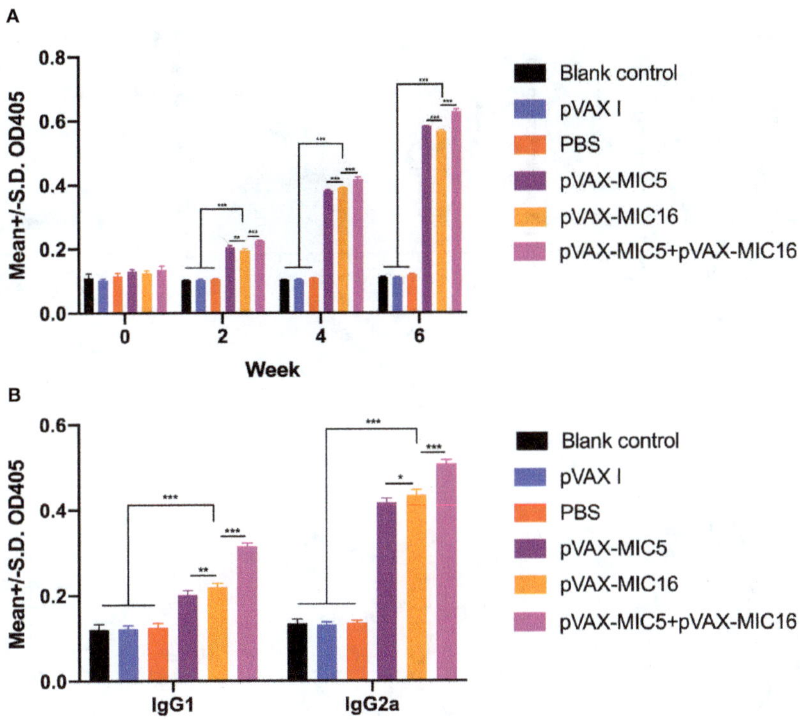

FIGURE 2 | Detection of specific humoral immune responses induced by DNA immunization with single or multiple genes. **(A)** Determination of IgG antibodies in the sera of Kunming mice at 0, 2, 4, and 6 weeks; **(B)** detection of IgG1 and IgG2a antibodies in immunized mice 2 weeks after the last immunization. *$P < 0.05$, **$P < 0.01$, ***$P < 0.001$. Data are presented as the means ± SD.

TgMIC14 (Foroutan et al., 2018). In the present study, DNA immunization with pVAX-MIC5 and/pVAX-MIC16 has activated humoral and Th1-type cellular immune responses, which may contribute to the increased survival of mice challenged with *T. gondii* RH strain and the reduction in the brain cysts post challenge with *T. gondii* PRU strain. Additionally, these two antigen-based cocktail DNA vaccines mounted more protective immunity than a single antigen-based DNA immunization, which is consistent with studies based on vaccination with multiple antigenic peptides (Sun et al., 2014;

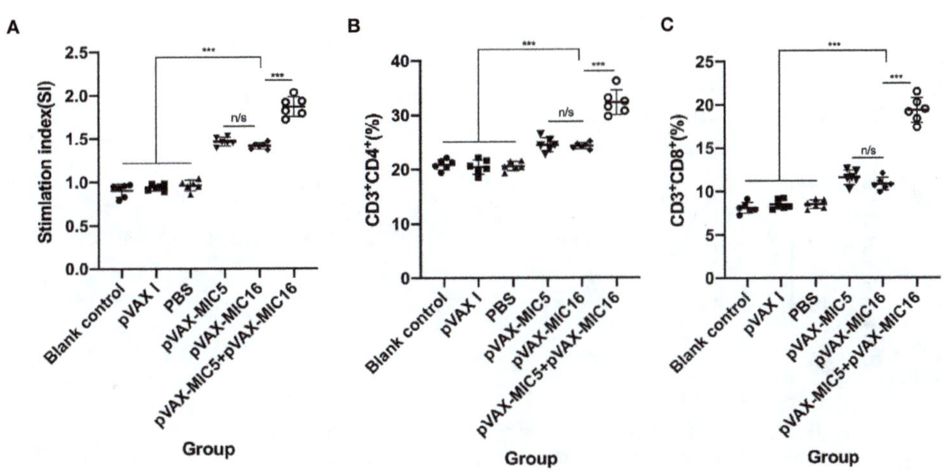

FIGURE 3 | Splenocyte proliferative response and the percentages of $CD4^+$ and $CD8^+$ of T cells in immunized and control mice two weeks after the challenge. **(A)** Lymphocyte proliferation stimulation index (SI). **(B, C)** Determination of the percentages of $CD4^+$ or $CD8^+$ T cells in immunized and control mice. ***$P < 0.001$,"n/s", no significant. Data are presented as the means ± SD.

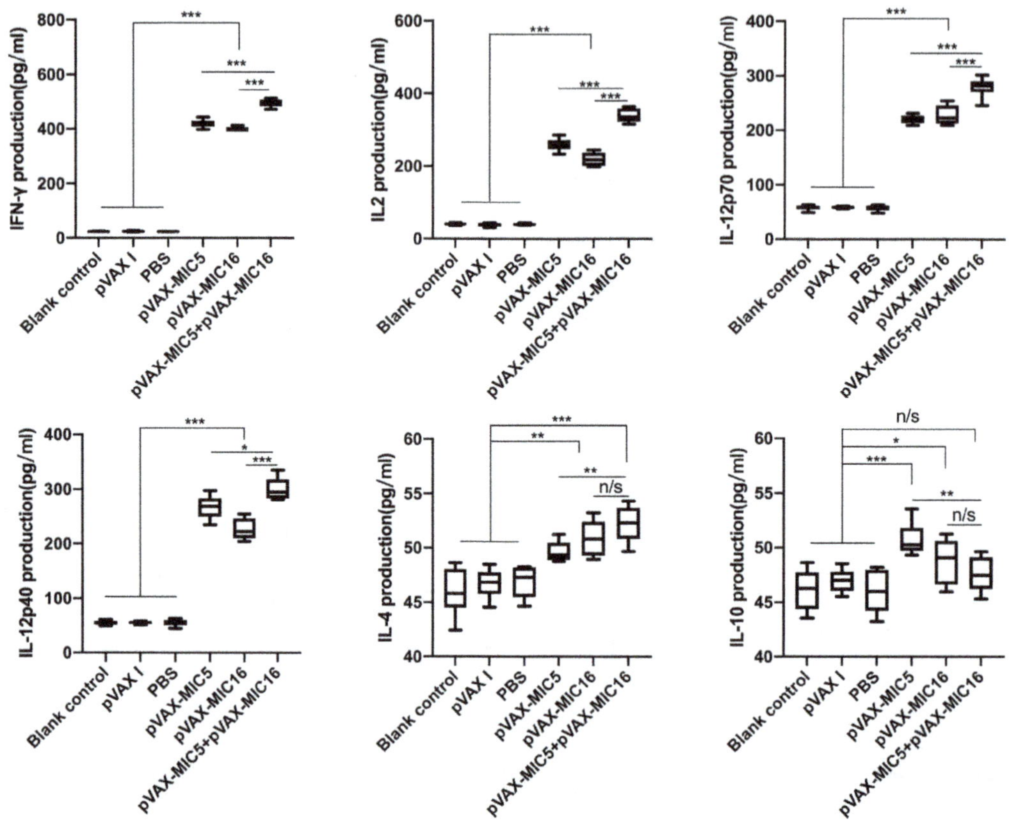

FIGURE 4 | Cytokine production by splenocytes of mice immunized with single or multiple genes. $^{*}P < 0.05$, $^{**}P < 0.01$, $^{***}P < 0.001$. "n/s", no significant. Data are presented as the means ± SD.

Zhou and Wang, 2017). These results suggest that DNA immunization with TgMIC5 and TgMIC6 can induce considerable protection against acute and chronic *T. gondii* infection, demonstrating that a cocktail DNA vaccine can trigger a more potent protective immunity than that induced by single antigen-based DNA vaccine (Foroutan et al., 2018).

Following natural infection with *T. gondii*, B cells are activated and specific antibodies are produced (Sikorski et al., 2021).

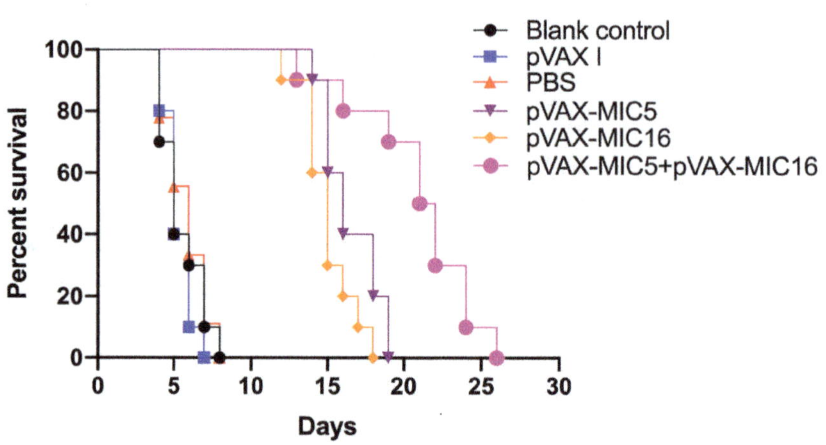

FIGURE 5 | The survival rate of immunized Kunming mice challenged with 1×10^3 tachyzoites 2 weeks after the last immunization.

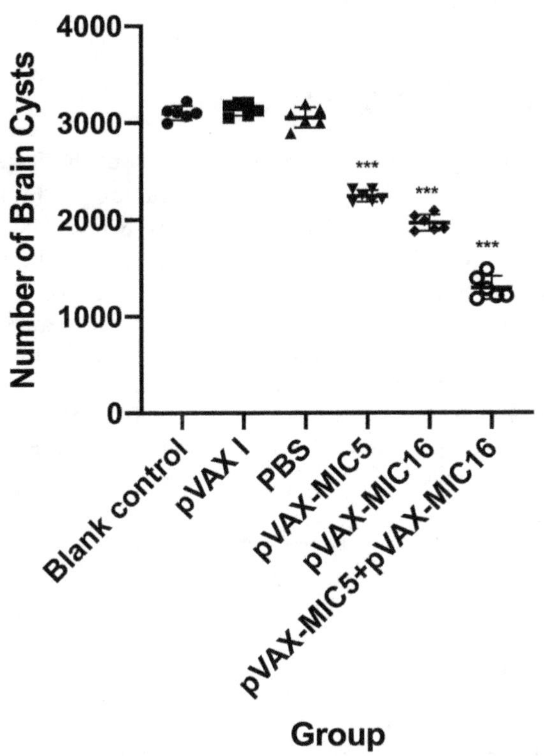

FIGURE 6 | Protection against chronic toxoplasmosis in immunized mice 2 weeks after the final booster immunization. The bars represent the mean cyst burden per mouse brain after oral challenge with 20 cysts of the PRU strain. Cyst load was determined from whole brain homogenates of mice 4 weeks after challenge. Data are means ± SD (representative of three experiments). $^{***}p < 0.001$, compared with the control groups.

Therefore, efficient humoral responses are of great significance in limiting the spread of *T. gondii* tachyzoites (Sayles et al., 2000). In the present study, the significantly increased levels of anti-*T. gondii* IgG in the mice immunized with the cocktail vaccine may have contributed to limiting the infection with *T. gondii* tachyzoites, which was in line with the results from DNA immunization with TgROP18, TgROP5, or TgGRA25, TgGRA25, and TgMIC5 (Chen et al., 2015; Xu et al., 2019). Furthermore, DNA immunization with single gene vaccine, especially two-gene cocktail vaccine, significantly increased the levels of IgG2a and IgG1 compared with that in the control groups. Meanwhile, the higher ratio of IgG2a/IgG1 in immunized groups suggests that Th1-type immune responses were predominant, in accordance with previous DNA vaccination studies (Gigley et al., 2009; Matowicka et al., 2009).

T cell-mediated adaptive immune responses are critical to efficient control of *T. gondii* infection (Silva et al., 2009). In this study, a significant *T. gondii* specific splenocyte proliferation was induced in all immunized mice, suggesting an activated adaptive immune response against *T. gondii* infection, which may contribute to effective cellular immune responses against *T. gondii* infection. Generally, T helper type 1 (Th1) cells are major effectors against intracellular pathogens, including *T. gondii*, mediated by the production of Th1 type cytokines, IFN-γ, IL-12, and IL-2 (LaRosa et al., 2008; Christopher et al., 2012). IFN-γ is more critical for protective immunity than cytotoxicity-based effector functions during *T. gondii* infection (Silva et al., 2009). IL-2 is also indispensable for the development of immunological memory in T cells, depending on the expansion of the number and function in antigen-selected T cell clones (Matowicka et al., 2009). Furthermore, IL-12p40 can facilitate the proliferation of T cells and the production of IFN-γ (Matowicka et al., 2009). Additionally, IL-12p70 plays a key role in the Th1 cells immune response, and also can effectively promote the generation of Th1-biased cytokine, such as IFN-γ (LaRosa et al., 2008). The concomitant IL-10 and IL-4 responses, which are associated with T helper type 2 (Th2) cells and are also required for restraining the production of systemic type-1 cytokine, can prevent lethal immunopathology during acute infection with *T. gondii* (Christopher et al., 2012). Therefore, the significant up-regulated of IFN-γ, IL-2, IL-12p40, IL-12p70, in combination with the slight increased production of IL-4 and IL-10 in all the immunized groups suggest that an appropriate Th1-type and Th2-type cellular response conferred host resistance to *T. gondii* infection. Furthermore, the highest levels of these cytokines induced by the two-gene cocktail DNA immunization in mice indicate that multi-gene DNA vaccine candidate could significantly enhance Th1-type immune responses that areinduced by a single-gene DNA vaccine.

$CD4^+$ T and $CD8^+$ T cells are activated once the intracellular parasite *T. gondii* invades the host cell and play critical roles in adaptive immune responses against *T. gondii* infection (Erik et al., 2010; Zhang et al., 2015). Especially, in synergy with $CD4^+$ T lymphocytes, $CD8^+$ T lymphocytes are key to limit *T. gondii* invasion during acute spreading of *T. gondii* tachyzoites or to limit the formation of brain cysts in the late stage of infection (Gigley et al., 2009; Christopher et al., 2012). In accordance with previous studies on DNA vaccination (Zhang et al., 2018), our results showed that the increased percentage of $CD4^+$ and $CD8^+$ T cells was observed in immunized groups, especially in two-gene immunized groups, suggesting that the DNA immunization with pVAX-MIC5 and or pVAX-MIC16 induces T lymphocytes, which contribute to the inhibition of the formation of tissue cysts in brain and restriction of *T. gondii* dissemination inside the body.

T. gondii strains belong to different genotypes with variable virulence in animals and humans (Sibley and Ajioka, 2008; Gigley et al., 2009). In this study, we used Kunming mice, which are highly susceptible to *T. gondii*, to evaluate the protective efficacy of DNA vaccine including pVAX-MIC5, and/or pVAX-MIC16 against *T. gondii* virulent RH strain (Type I) and avirulent PRU strain (Type II) challenge. As expected, TgMIC5 or TgMIC16 induced cross-protection against infection with different genotypes of *T. gondii*, which is similar to previous studies involving TgMIC13 and TgMIC6 (Yuan et al., 2013), indicating that these two TgMICs are good DNA vaccine candidates against *T. gondii* infection. However, the high levels of Th1-type based immune response and antibody response led to only partial protection against *T. gondii*, which may be ascribed to limited immunity to *T. gondii* induced by DNA vaccine.

In conclusion, the present study demonstrates that the recombinant plasmids encoding TgMIC5 and/or TgMIC16, are good DNA vaccine candidates, which induce immune protection against acute and chronic *T. gondii* infection in mice. Further studies are needed to investigate the protective immunity induced by using a combination with more *T. gondii* antigens.

AUTHOR CONTRIBUTIONS

Y-CZ and JC conceived and designed the study. Y-CZ, L-JM and JC performed the experiments and assisted in the preparation of the manuscript. Y-CZ, J-LZ, J-FL and YH analyzed the data. JC prepared the manuscript. Y-CZ and JC assisted in the design of the experiments, data interpretation, and manuscript preparation. All authors contributed to the article and approved the submitted version.

ACKNOWLEDGMENTS

The project support was provided by funds of the State Key Laboratory of Veterinary Etiological Biology (Grant No. SKLVEB2019KFKT017), the National Natural Science Foundation of China (Grant No. 31402190), and the China Postdoctoral Science Foundation (Grant No. 132764). *T. gondii* strains and 293-T cells were kindly supplied by Professor Xing-Quan Zhu (State Key Laboratory of Veterinary Etiological Biology, Key Laboratory of Veterinary Parasitology of Gansu Province, Lanzhou Veterinary Research Institute, Chinese Academy of Agricultural Sciences, Lanzhou, Gansu Province, People's Republic of China).

REFERENCES

1. Burrells, A., Benavides, J., Canton, G., Garcia, J. L., Bartley, P. M., Nath, M., et al. (2015). Vaccination of Pigs With the S48 Strain of Toxoplasma Gondii–Safer Meat for Human Consumption. *Vet. Res.* 46 (1), 47. doi: 10.1186/s13567-015-0177-0
2. Chen, J., Li, Z. Y., Eskild, P., Huang, S. Y., Zhou, D. H., and Zhu, X. Q. (2015). DNA Vaccination With Genes Encoding Toxoplasma Gondii Antigens ROP5 and GRA15 Induces Protective Immunity Against Toxoplasmosis in Kunming Mice. *Expert Rev. Vaccines* 14, 617–624. doi: 10.1586/14760584.2015.1011133
3. Chen, J., Li, Z. Y., Eskild, P., Liu, W. G., and Zhu, X. Q. (2016). Co-Administration of Interleukins 7 and 15 With DNA Vaccine Improves Protective Immunity Against Toxoplasma Gondii. *Exp. Parasitol.* 162, 18–23. doi: 10.1016/ j.exppara.2015.12.013
4. Christopher, D. D., David, A. C., and Christopher, A. H. (2012). Immune Response and Immunopathology During Toxoplasmosis. *Semin. Immunopathol.* 34, 793–813. doi: 10.1007/s00281-012-0339-3
5. Dodangeh, S., Daryani, A., Sharif, M., Aghayan, S. A., Pagheh, A. S., Sarvi, S., et al. (2019). A Systematic Review on Efficiency of Microneme Proteins to Induce Protective Immunity Against Toxoplasma Gondii. *Eur. J. Clin. Microbiol. Infect. Dis.* 38, 617–629. doi: 10.1007/s10096-018-03442-6
6. Dubey, J. P. (2009). History of the Discovery of the Life Cycle of Toxoplasma Gondii. *Int. J. Parasitol.* 39, 877–882. doi: 10.1016/j.ijpara.2009.01.005
7. Elsheikha, H. M. (2008). Congenital Toxoplasmosis: Priorities for Further Health Promotion Action. *Public Health* 122 (4), 335–353. doi: 10.1016/j.puhe.2007.08.009
8. Elsheikha, H. M., Marra, C. M., and Zhu, X. Q. (2020). Epidemiology, Pathophysiology, Diagnosis, and Management of Cerebral Toxoplasmosis. *Clin. Microbiol. Rev.* 34, e00115–e00119. doi: 10.1128/CMR.00115-19
9. Erik, J., Arnaud, L., Jo, V. G., Stephane, D. C., Kris, H., and Sushila, D. (2010). Functional Characterization of *In Vivo* Effector CD4(+) and CD8(+) T Cell Responses in Acute Toxoplasmosis: An Interplay of IFN-Gamma and Cytolytic T Cells. *Vaccine* 28, 2556–2564. doi: 10.1016/j.vaccine.2010.01.031
10. Erik, J., Craig, W. R., Nicola, G., Elisabeth, F., and Eskild, P. (2009). Vaccines Against Toxoplasma Gondii: Challenges and Opportunities. *Mem Inst Oswaldo Cruz.* 104, 252–266. doi: 10.1590/s0074-02762009000200019
11. Flegr, J., Prandota, J., Sovickova, M., and Israili, Z. H. (2014). Toxoplasmosis–a Global Threat. Correlation of Latent Toxoplasmosis With Specific Disease Burden in a Set of 88 Countries. *PloS One* 9, e90203. doi: 10.1371/journal.pone.0090203
12. Florence, R. G., and Marie-Laure, D. (2012). Epidemiology of and Diagnostic Strategies for Toxoplasmosis. *Clin. Microbiol. Rev.* 25 (2), 264–296. doi: 10.1128/CMR.05013-11
13. Foroutan, M., Zaki, L., and Ghaffarifar, F. (2018). Recent Progress in Microneme- Based Vaccines Development Against Toxoplasma Gondii. *Clin. Exp. Vaccine Res.* 7, 93–103. doi: 10.7774/cevr.2018.7.2.93
14. Gigley, J. P., Fox, B. A., and Bzik, D. J. (2009). Cell-Mediated Immunity to Toxoplasma Gondii Develops Primarily by Local Th1 Host Immune Responses in the Absence of Parasite Replication. *J. Immunol.* 182, 1069–1078. doi: 10.4049/jimmunol.182.2.1069
15. LaRosa, D. F., Stumhofer, J. S., Gelman, A. E., Rahman, A. H., Taylor, D. K., Hunter, C. A., et al. (2008). T Cell Expression of Myd88 Is Required for Resistance to *Toxoplasma Gondii*. *Proc. Natl. Acad. Sci. U.S.A.* 105, 3855–3860. doi: 10.1073/pnas.0706663105
16. Lilach, S., Joana, M. S., Natacha, K., Fabiola, P., Noelle, J., Nikolas, F., et al. (2010). *Toxoplasma Gondii* Transmembrane Microneme Proteins and Their Modular Design. *Mol. Microbiol.* 77, 912–929. doi: 10.1111/j.1365-2958.2010.07255.x
17. Li, Y. W., and Zhou, H. Y. (2018). Moving Towards Improved Vaccines for Toxoplasma Gondii. *Expert Opin. Biol. Ther.* 18, 273–280. doi: 10.1080/14712598.2018.1413086
18. Margaret, A. L. (2011). DNA Vaccines: An Historical Perspective and View to the Future. *Immunol. Rev.* 239 (1), 62–84. doi: 10.1111/j.1600-065X.2010.00980.x
19. Matowicka, K. J., Dymicka, P. V., and Kemona, H. (2009). Does Toxoplasma Gondii Infection Affect the Levels of Ige and Cytokines (IL-5, IL-6, IL-10, IL- 12, and TNF-Alpha)? *Clin. Dev. Immunol.* 2009:374696. doi: 10.1155/2009/374696
20. Mohamed-Ali, H., Philipp, O., and Sibley, L. D. (2017). *Toxoplasma* Effectors Targeting Host Signaling and Transcription. *Clin. Microbiol. Rev.* 30 (3), 615–645. doi: 10.1128/CMR.00005-17
21. Pappas, G., Roussos, N., and Falagas, M. E. (2009). Toxoplasmosis Snapshots: Global Status of Toxoplasma Gondii Seroprevalence and Implications for Pregnancy and Congenital Toxoplasmosis. *Int. J. Parasitol.* 39, 1385–1394. doi: 10.1016/j.ijpara.2009.04.003
22. Saki, J., Khademvatan, S., Soltani, S., and Shahbazian, H. (2013). Detection of Toxoplasmosis in Patients With End-Stage Renal Disease by Enzyme-Linked Immunosorbent Assay and Polymerase Chain Reaction Methods. *Parasitol. Res.* 112, 163–168. doi: 10.1007/s00436-012-3120-6

23. Sayles, P. C., Gibson, G. W., and Johnson, L. L. (2000). B Cells are Essential for Vaccination-Induced Resistance to Virulent Toxoplasma Gondii. *Infect. Immun.* 68 (3), 1026–1033. doi: 10.1128/iai.68.3.1026-1033.2000
24. Sibley, L. D., and Ajioka, J. W. (2008). Population Structure of Toxoplasma Gondii: Clonal Expansion Driven by Infrequent Recombination and Selective Sweeps. *Annu. Rev. Microbiol.* 62, 329–351. doi: 10.1146/annurev.micro.62.081307.162925
25. Sikorski, P. M., Commodaro, A. G., and Grigg, M. E. (2021). A Protective and Pathogenic Role for Complement During Acute Toxoplasma Gondii Infection. *Front. Cell Infect. Microbiol.* 11:634610. doi: 10.3389/fcimb.2021.634610
26. Silva, N. M., Vieira, J. C. M., Carneiro, C. M., and Tafuri, W. L. (2009). *Toxoplasma Gondii: The* Role of IFN-Gamma, Tnfrp55 and Inos in Inflammatory Changes During Infection. *Exp. Parasitol.* 123, 65–72. doi: 10.1016/j.exppara.2009.05.011
27. Sun, X., Mei, M., Zhang, X., Han, F., Jia, B., Wei, X., et al. (2014). The Extracellular Matrix Protein Mindin as a Novel Adjuvant Elicits Stronger Immune Responses for Rbag1, Rsrs4 and Rsrs9 Antigens of Toxoplasma Gondii in BALB/C Mice. *BMC Infect. Dis.* 14:429. doi: 10.1186/1471-2334-14-429
28. Susannah, D. B., Xing, W. Z., My-Hang, H., Jill, M., Jeffrey, M., Koku, D. Z. A., et al. (2006). Targeted Deletion of MIC5 Enhances Trimming Proteolysis of Toxoplasma Invasion Proteins. *Eukaryot Cell.* 5, 2174–2183. doi: 10.1128/ EC.00163-06
29. Tenter, A. M., Heckeroth, A. R., and Weiss, L. M. (2000). *Toxoplasma Gondii*: From Animals to Humans. *Int. J. Parasitol.* 30, 1217–1258. doi: 10.1016/s0020- 7519(00)00124-7
30. Wang, Z. D., Liu, H. H., Ma, Z. X., Ma, H. Y., Li, Z. Y., Yang, Z. B., et al. (2017). *Toxoplasma Gondii* Infection in Immunocompromised Patients: A Systematic Review and Meta-Analysis. *Front. Microbiol.* 8:389. doi: 10.3389/fmicb.2017.00389
31. Wang, J. L., Zhang, N. Z., Li, T. T., He, J. J., Elsheikha, H. M., and Zhu, X. Q. (2019). Advances in the Development of Anti-*Toxoplasma Gondii* Vaccines: Challenges, Opportunities, and Perspectives. *Trends Parasitol.* 35, 239–253. doi: 10.1016/j.pt.2019.01.005
32. Xu, X. P., Liu, W. G., Xu, Q. M., Zhu, X. Q., and Chen, J. (2019). Evaluation of Immune Protection Against Toxoplasma Gondii Infection in Mice Induced by a Multi-Antigenic DNA Vaccine Containing Tggra24, Tggra25 and Tgmic6. *Parasite* 26, 58. doi: 10.1051/parasite/2019050
33. Yuan, Z. G., Ren, D., Zhou, D. H., Zhang, X. X., Petersen, E., Li, X. Z., et al. (2013). Evaluation of Protective Effect of Pvax-Tgmic13 Plasmid Against Acute and Chronic Toxoplasma Gondii Infection in a Murine Model. *Vaccine* 31, 3135– 3139. doi: 10.1016/j.vaccine.2013.05.040
34. Zhang, N. Z., Chen, J., Wang, M., Eskild, P., and Zhu, X. Q. (2013). Vaccines Against Toxoplasma Gondii: New Developments and Perspectives. *Expert Rev. Vaccines* 12, 1287–1299. doi: 10.1586/14760584.2013.844652
35. Zhang, N. Z., Gao, Q., Wang, M., Elsheikha, H. M., Wang, B., Wang, J. L., et al. (2018). Immunization With a DNA Vaccine Cocktail Encoding Tgpf, Tgrop16, Tgrop18, Tgmic6, and Tgcdpk3 Genes Protects Mice Against Chronic Toxoplasmosis. *Front. Immunol.* 29:1505. doi: 10.3389/fimmu.2018.01505
36. Zhang, N. Z., Gao, Q., Wang, M., Hou, J. L., Zhang, F. K., Hu, L. Y., et al. (2018). Protective Efficacy Against Acute and Chronic Toxoplasma Gondii Infection Induced by Immunization With the DNA Vaccine Tgdoc2c. *Front. Microbiol.* 4:2965. doi: 10.3389/fmicb.2018.02965
37. Zhang, N. Z., Wang, M., Xu, Y., Eskild, P., and Zhu, X. Q. (2015). Recent Advances in Developing Vaccines Against Toxoplasma Gondii: An Update. *Expert Rev. Vaccines* 14, 1609–1621. doi: 10.1586/14760584.2015.1098539
38. Zhou, J., and Wang, L. (2017). SAG4 DNA and Peptide Vaccination Provides Partial Protection Against T. Gondii Infection in BALB/C Mice. *Front. Microbiol.* 8:1733. doi: 10.3389/fmicb.2017.01733
39. Zhu, Y. C., He, Y., Liu, J. F., and Chen, J. (2020). Adjuvantic Cytokine IL-33 Improves the Protective Immunity of Cocktailed DNA Vaccine of ROP5 and ROP18 Against Toxoplasma Gondii Infection in Mice. *Parasite* 27, 26. doi: 10.1051/parasite/2020021

19

Innate Immune Response to Viral Infections at the Maternal-Fetal Interface in Human Pregnancy

*Ana Espino [1], Hicham El Costa [1], Julie Tabiasco [1], Reem Al-Daccak [2] and Nabila Jabrane-Ferrat [1]**

[1] Infinity, Université de Toulouse - CNRS – Inserm, CHU Purpan, Toulouse, France, [2] Inserm UMRS976 - Université de Paris - Hôpital Saint-Louis, Paris, France

***Correspondence:**
Nabila Jabrane-Ferrat
nabila.jabrane-ferrat@inserm.fr

The placenta, the first and largest organ to develop after conception, not only nurtures and promotes the development of the conceptus, but, it also functions as a barrier against invading pathogens. Early phases of pregnancy are associated with expansion of specific subsets of Natural Killer cells (dNK) and macrophages (dMφ) at the maternal uterine mucosa, the basal decidua. In concert with cells of fetal origin, dNK cells, and dMφ orchestrate all steps of placenta and fetus development, and provide the first line of defense to limit vertical transmission. However, some pathogens that infect the mother can overcome this protective barrier and jeopardize the fetus health. In this review, we will discuss how members of the classical TORCH family (Toxoplasma, Other, Rubella, Cytomegalovirus, and Herpes simplex virus) and some emerging viruses (Hepatitis E virus, Zika virus, and SARS-CoV2) can afford access to the placental fortress. We will also discuss how changes in the intrauterine environment as a consequence of maternal immune cell activation contribute to placental diseases and devastating pregnancy outcomes.

Keywords: **pregnancy, viral infection, maternal-fetal transmission, innate immunity, Natural Killer cells, macrophages, cytokine environment**

INTRODUCTION

Human pregnancy is associated with tremendous changes of the maternal uterine mucosa (endometrium), called decidua, to promote the implantation, and the development of the blastocyst. The interstitial implantation, in humans and non-human primates, is characterized by complete enclosure of the blastocyst by the decidua (1). A privileged crosstalk between the endometrium and a competent 256-cell blastocyst must be completed in a limited time called the implantation window. The outer surface of the blastocyst also is composed of cytotrophoblasts (CTBs), a unique cell type of the placenta, which will follow two differentiation programs (2). In the first program CTBs fuse to form the multinucleated syncytiotrophoblast (STB) outermost layer surrounding the inner core of the placental villi. The villous core containing mesenchymal/fibroblastic stroma stem cells, immature fetal capillaries and a population of yolk sac-derived macrophages termed Hofbauer cells (HBCs), is surrounded by a bilayer of CTBs.

In the second program, CTBs of the cell column differentiate into interstitial and endovascular invasive cytotrophoblast cells (iCTBs). Subsequently, iCTBs invade the decidua and remodel the maternal spiral arteries through active replacement of smooth muscle and vascular endothelial cells. Completion of vascular remodeling by trophoblast cells which happens by the end of first trimester of pregnancy (10–12 weeks), promotes the switch from high-resistance to low-resistance vessels with enlarged lumen to ensure routing of high blood flow into the intervillous space (3). As the development advances, the highly branched villous trees of the placenta are bathed with maternal blood till parturition. The invasion fetal trophoblast cells and tissue remodeling are under strict control by maternal immune cells to ensure confinement of the placenta to the allocated space within time constraints of pregnancy. Flaws in these developmental steps have been clearly incriminated in many great obstetrical syndromes including pre-eclampsia and fetal growth restriction (FGR), both associated with faulty placental development (3).

Unlike the fetus, the placenta is in direct contact with maternal cells. Intermingling between fetal and maternal cells, which is mandatory for placenta and fetal development, happens within privileged sites (maternal-fetal interface, composed of the basal decidua, and the intervillous space). Hormones are able to prime the decidua-associated remodeling (2), complete "physiological change" requires the presence of trophoblast cells. The extent of trophoblast cell invasion and tissue remodeling, both necessary for efficient and healthy placenta in late pregnancy, are dictated by a finely tuned crosstalk between fetal cells and maternal tissue resident immune cells. Leukocytes represent more than 40% of total cells in the basal decidua (4). While a large fraction of immune cells are tissue resident leukocytes, many factors produced by decidual stromal cells and trophoblast cells could contribute to the recruitment of additional leukocytes from the periphery (5, 6). A high percentage of decidual immune cells are non-cytotoxic CD56 super bright Natural Killer (dNK) cells that lack the expression of the Fc gamma receptor IIIA, CD16, and are endowed with angiogenic and regulatory activities. In the first trimester of pregnancy, dNK cell population represents 70% of leukocytes (7–9). Their rate remains relatively high in the second trimester but declines in the third trimester to reach normal uterine level at parturition (10). Other immune cell populations are also present in first trimester basal decidua, although, at lower levels. Decidual macrophages (dMφ) represent 20–25% of total leukocytes, while dendritic cells and mast cells only represent 1–2% (11). The decidua contains only 5–10% T lymphocytes, including CD8, CD4, and γδT cells, but B cells are barely present. The low level of B cells suggests that it is very unlikely that any eventual antibody response would harm invading trophoblast cells (12). Minor immune cell subsets include innate lymphoid cells (ILCs) (13) and mucosal-associated invariant T cells (MAIT) (14). The interaction of these immune cells with decidual stroma and invading fetal trophoblast cells is crucial for the establishment of an environment rich in soluble mediators including hormones, growth factors cytokines, chemokines and lipids, which are necessary for the development of the placenta and of the fetus. Given their dominance and active contribution to protection against pathogens, this review will mainly discuss the key features of dNK cells and dMφ during healthy pregnancy as well as their functional adaptations during viral invasion, and how viral infections disrupt the maternal-fetal barrier resulting in congenital infections.

DECIDUAL NK CELLS

Natural killer (NK) cells are innate lymphoid cells with documented anti-viral and anti-tumor functions. They are found in the bloodstream (pNK), where they represent up to 15% of circulating lymphocytes, but also in various tissues such as lymphoid organs, liver and uterus. NK cells are classified in two major populations according to the cell surface expression of CD56 (NCAM) and CD16. The majority of pNK cells (~95%) are $CD56^{dim}CD16^{pos}$ and characterized by a highly cytotoxic capacity, the remaining 5% are $CD56^{bright}CD16^{neg}$ (8, 15). At the implantation bed, the majority of dNK cells are CD56 super bright (dNK^{bright}) that share some phenotypic similarities with the minor population of pNK and only a small fraction $CD56^{dim}$ (dNK^{dim}) (8, 15, 16). dNK cells express most of the activating and inhibitory NK cell receptors including the NKp30, NKp46, NKG2C, NKG2E, NKG2D, NKG2A, 2B4, CD85/LILRB1/ILT2 (LILRB1), and Killer-cell immunoglobulin-like family of receptors (KIR) such as KIR2DL1, KIR2DL2/3, KIR2DL4, KIR3DL2 (10, 16–18). However, the function of several NKR is different as compared with pNK cells (15, 19). For example, the inhibitory LILRB1 in the periphery is an activating receptor in the decidua, whist the co-activating 2B4 receptor functions as inhibitory receptors in dNK cells. dNK cells also express many other receptors that are not expressed on resting pNK cells. dNK cells have a constitutive expression of CD69 and CD25, and display differential expression of NKp44/NCR2 and NKp30/NCR3 splice variants implying the involvement of the decidual environment in shaping their cell fate (20). dNK cells also express high levels of integrins (αD, αX, β1, and β5) and other receptors such as CD53, CD63, and CD151 (8) as well as tissue residency markers (CD49a, CD9, and CD103). In addition, several chemokine receptors (CXCR3, CXCR4, CCR1, and CCR9) endow them with high mobility to warrant a fine-tuned dialogue with other cells (21).

dNK cells can be classified under three major subsets dNK1, dNK2, and dNK3. dNK1 is the most abundant subset (>30%), followed by dNK2 and dNK3 (22, 23). While all three subsets express of NKG2A, LILRB1 expression is a major hallmark of dNK1 cells. dNK1 cells also express the regulatory CD39 ATPase, involved in the shift between pro-inflammatory and immunosuppressive environment, large amounts of cytotoxic granules enriched in perforin and granzymes (8), and a combination of KIRs expression that further discriminates four dNK1 subgroups. Similar to dNK1, dNK2 cells express the NKG2C and NKG2E activating receptors as well as the NKG2A inhibitory receptor counterpart that recognize HLA molecules on fetal trophoblast cells. In addition, dNK2 cells express the ANXA1 and ITGB2 receptors. Finally, the third subset expresses CD160, CD161, TIGIT, KLRB1, ITGB2, and CD103 (22, 24).

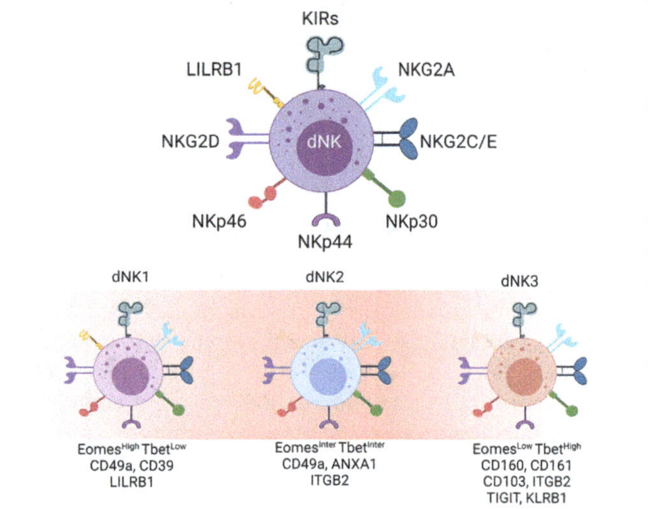

FIGURE 1 | Decidual Natural Killer cells. dNK cells, the main innate immune cell population at the maternal-fetal interface. Inhibitory and activating receptors are presented. Transcription factors (Eomes and Tbet) and cell surface markers (LILRB1, ITGB2, CD160, CD161) defined by single cell RNA sequencing and large scale phenotyping allow the distinction of three dNK cell subsets (dNK1, dNK2, and dNK3).

The differential levels of NKp44 and NKG2A receptors suggest the presence of at least two subgroups of dNK3 cells.

In contrast to other tissues, all three CD49a^{pos} dNK cell subsets express the Eomes and Tbet transcription factors although, at variable levels. Compared to Eomes^{high}Tbet^{low} dNK1 cells, dNK3 cells are Eomes^{low}Tbet^{high} whilst dNK2 cell express intermediate levels of both transcription factors (**Figure 1**).

How these three subsets interact with each other's, with fetal trophoblast cells and decidual stromal cells (DSC), and whether they are all needed to direct the invasion of trophoblast cells, remodeling of the maternal-fetal interface and the development of the placenta are still in debate. Nonetheless, a finely tuned dialogue between different subsets of dNK cells, decidual cells, and invading trophoblast cells seems necessary to promote the complete establishment of the maternal-fetal interface but also the development of the fetus and the placenta (25).

Indeed, through direct interaction with iCTBs and production of a highly diverse secretome rich in cytokines, chemokines metalloproteinases, and growth promoting factors such as VEGF, IGF2, pleiotrophin, osteoglycin, and osteopontin), dNK cells direct the extent of trophoblast invasion, tissue remodeling as well as placental and fetal growth (26, 27). Some of these soluble factors are also important for the establishment of a local pro- and anti-inflammatory cytokine balance that is necessary for fetal tolerance as well as protection against mother-to-child transmission of pathogens.

By contrast to pNK, dNK cells are devoid of cytotoxicity during healthy pregnancies preventing harmful reaction against the semi-allogeneic trophoblast cells (15, 28). Several mechanisms have been suggested for their involvement in restricting dNK cell lytic machinery. These include (i) a defective polarization of the microtubule organizing center (MTOC), resulting in the formation of an immature immunologic synapse with target cells (29); (ii) the lack of SAP adapter molecule expression preventing activating signal from 2B4 (CD244) (19); (iii) the engagement of the NKG2A inhibitory receptor by its natural ligand HLA-E on trophoblast cells (30); and (iv) the expression of inhibitory isoforms of the Natural Cytotoxicity Receptors, NKp44 and NKp30 (16, 17, 20). Finally, the pressure of the local environment maintains cell cytotoxicity under a tight control (24).

Despite these regulatory mechanisms, dNK cell cytotoxic machinery can be unleashed resulting in failure in the harmonious mother-fetus dialogue and adverse pregnancy outcomes. For instance, patients with recurrent spontaneous abortion exhibit a change in the distribution of dNK cell subsets was associated with enhanced production of inflammatory cytokines and lytic granules, but impaired ability to produce growth promoting factors (27, 31). Thus, changes in dNK cell functions and the finely-tuned dialogue at the maternal-fetal interface is probably responsible for fetal trophoblast cells apoptosis and the resulting miscarriage. In addition, genetic studies demonstrated that particular combinations of HLA-C haplotypes and maternal inhibitory KIRs can be linked to defaults in trophoblast invasion and pregnancy disorders including pre-eclampsia pathologies (32, 33).

DECIDUAL MACROPHAGES

Decidual macrophages (dMφ) represent the second largest population of leukocytes. The local environment at the maternal-fetal interface orchestrates dMφ differentiation and functions. In early stages of pregnancy, dMφ have an M1 phenotype, then they switch to a mixed M1/M2 profile during trophoblast cell invasion. Once the placenta is fully developed, they switch toward an M2 phenotype to prevent fetal rejection (34). Consequently, dMφ share features of pro-inflammatory and tolerogenic macrophages, simultaneously expressing M1 (CD64, CD80, CD86) and M2 markers (CD163, CD206, DC-SIGN) (35–39).

Similar to dNK cells, dMφ secrete a large panel of pro-angiogenic factors and pro- and anti-inflammatory cytokines (40, 41). Their localization in the vicinity of spiral arteries and secretion of metalloproteinases allude to their active involvement in vascular remodeling (42). In concert with dNK cells, dMφ promote trophoblast cell invasion and placental development (43, 44) while contributing to defense against threatening pathogens.

VIRAL INFECTIONS DURING PREGNANCY

The maternal-fetal interface constitutes a physical and immune barrier shielding the fetus from pathogens in the maternal circulation. However, some pathogens especially viruses can reach the fetal compartment either through hematogeneous or decidual spread, resulting in congenital syndrome and high case-fatality (**Figure 2**). Even in the absence of maternal-to-fetal transmission, previous epidemics of many emerging viral threats have resulted in poor pregnancy outcomes including maternal and fetal morbidity and mortality and peripartum infections with severe sequelae.

Threatening TORCH Pathogens During Human Pregnancy

The TORCH family [Toxoplasma, Other (syphilis, varicella-zoster, parvovirus B19), Rubella, Cytomegalovirus and Herpes simplex viruses 1 and 2] are well-recognized as pregnancy threating pathogens for human pregnancy.

The Human cytomegalovirus (HCMV), a large DNA virus that belongs to the herpesviridae family, is the most common cause of maternal and fetal morbidity and mortality. Primary maternal infection carries a 30–40% risk of vertical transmission. Congenital infection during the first trimester of pregnancy can result in severe congenital syndrome characterized by irreversible damage including deafness, psychomotor delays, myopathies, chorioretinitis, and devastating microcephaly (45). Even asymptomatic newborns can develop late neuro-developmental damage within the first 3 years of life (46). These congenital disorders could be partially attributed to severe placenta disruption with increased edema, massive inflammation, and avascular villi. HCMV infected placenta are characterized by massive viral-induced cytopathic effects in the villous capillaries and stromal cells and chronic villitis due to maternal inflammatory response.

The highly pathogenic Human immunodeficiency virus 1 (HIV-1) is an RNA virus from the retroviridae family. Histological analyses of first trimester placenta from untreated HIV-infected women revealed the presence of decidual necrosis and chorioamnionitis associated with the presence of HIV-1 in fetal tissues. Syncytin, the envelope glycoprotein of human endogenous retrovirus highly expressed by fetal trophoblast, mediates HIV entry through cell-to-cell fusion contributing to viral dissemination, and establishment of viral reservoir in deep tissues (47). Despite the high permissivity of trophoblast cells and dMφ, intrauterine transmission of HIV-1 is very rare during the first trimester of pregnancy (48) but occurs more frequently during labor and delivery. Although, ART can lower considerably the transmission rate, cesarean delivery is recommended for HIV-infected women with high viral loads.

Emerging Viruses

Lessons from recent outbreaks and the current pandemic crisis, designated genotype 1 of Hepatitis E virus (HEV-1), Zika virus (ZIKV), and SARS-CoV2 as emerging viruses that can threaten human pregnancy.

Hepatitis E virus (HEV), a water-borne pathogen transmitted by the fecal-oral route, belongs to the *Hepeviridae* family. Strains that infect humans are classified in two species, *Orthohepevirus A* (eight genotypes) and *Orthohepevirus C* (49). HEV-1, prevalent in developing countries, is highly pathogenic during pregnancy with high maternal and fetal mortality rate (20%) due to fulminant hepatitis, hemorrhage, preeclampsia like syndrome, and severe placental diseases (50). The transmission rate of HEV-1 ranges from 50 to 100% (51). Trans-placental transmission has been documented by the presence of progeny virions in the fetal placenta and umbilical cord (52). Significant effort has been recently made by our team to understand mechanisms underlying HEV-1-related placental disorders (53). We demonstrate that pathogenic HEV-1 replicates efficiently both in maternal and fetal tissues, produces infectious progeny virions, and induces alteration of the local secretome leading to severe tissue damage.

ZIKV, a mosquito-borne *Flavivirus*, is able to surmount the physical and immunological barrier of the placenta to reach the developing conceptus in ~1 out of 10 infected pregnancies. In the 2015 outbreak in the western hemisphere, ZIKV was declared a serious public health concern, in particular for pregnant women due to surge of devastating microcephaly in newborns and increased frequency of placental pathology including preeclampsia, miscarriage and still birth (54, 55). Histological analysis of term placenta from congenital infected neonates, revealed the presence of immature villi with a large increase in the number of proliferating HBCs. Our group, among others, provided the proof that ZIKV targets a wide range of maternal and fetal cells including dMφ and HBCs, triggers massive inflammation and tissue damage, which may lead to placental insufficiency (56, 57). More recently, we described potential mechanisms for ZIKV-induced pathogenesis during early pregnancy (58). We showed that the virus usurps the placenta lipidome and the mitochondrial network to build replication factories necessary for the production of infectious progeny virions, and to overcome the placental intrinsic defense mechanisms through impairment of the homeostatic equilibrium of pro-/anti-inflammatory environment.

Pregnancy increases the risk of adverse maternal and offspring outcomes from many respiratory viral infections including Influenza virus. In December 2019, Wuhan, China, was faced with the outbreak of the deadliest acute respiratory distress syndrome, COVID-19 disease. On March 11, 2020 COVID-19 was declared a pandemic by the World Health Organization. The etiological agent of COVID-19, SARS-CoV2, is a newly identified member of a zoonotic family of coronaviruses responsible for severe acute respiratory syndrome (SARS). The former two family members SARS-CoV and Middle East respiratory syndrome (MERS)-CoV are the respective etiological agents responsible for the 2002 and 2012 outbreaks (59, 60).

Although, the COVID-19 pandemic has now infected large numbers of pregnant women, the risks and specific effects of SARS–CoV-2 are still largely unknown. Early reports of Chinese pregnancy cohorts did not provide evidence for maternal-fetal transmission in late gestation, but infection was clearly associated with increased risk of admission to intensive care, miscarriage, pre-eclampsia, premature membrane rupture, preterm labor and preterm birth (61–63). Neonates born to infected mothers presented fetal distress with abnormal respiratory gastrointestinal symptoms and refractory shock with multiple organ failure was reported (64). Furthermore, the presence of SARS-CoV-2 was detected either in amniotic fluid, umbilical cord blood or placental sections (65, 66). Vertical

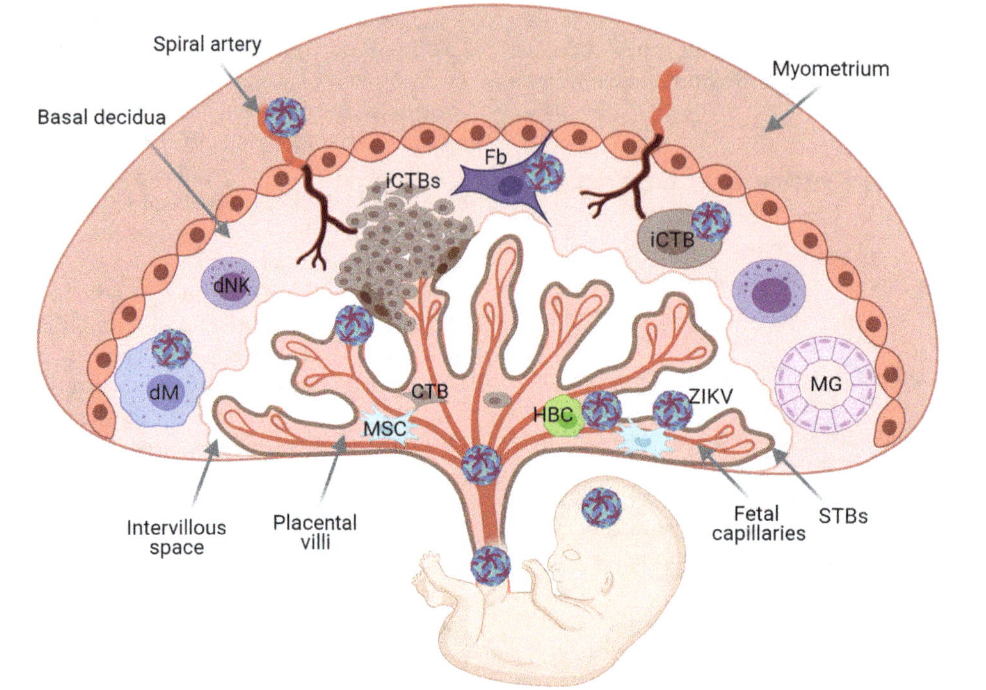

FIGURE 2 | Schematic representation of the human maternal-fetal interface and fetus, and transmission of pathogens. Basal decidua containing decidual Natural Killer cells (dNK), maternal macrophages (dMφ), and stroma cells [mesenchymal (Ms) and fibroblasts (Fb)]. Maternal gland (MG). Extravillous invasive cytotrophoblast cells (iCTBs) invade the maternal decidua. Trophoblast Villous core contains trophoblast cells, mesynchymal cells, Hoffbauer cells (HBC), and fetal capillaries protected with an outermost layer of multinucleacted syncytiotrophoblast cells (STBs). Placental chorionic villi floating bathed by maternal blood within the intervillous space. Viruses can reach the fetus through hematogenous spread or through the basal decidua. Illustration of Zika virus (ZIKV), as model. ZIKV can replicate in the decidua and placental cells before dissemination to the fetus.

transmission of SARS-CoV2 has been suspected in several cases but the mechanisms that allow the virus to breach the placental fortress and reach developing fetus are still lacking. Recent analyses of infected case reports and small cohorts from infected mothers and newborn dyad, revealed the presence of SAR-CoV2 antigens or viral RNA in fetal trophoblast cells and stromal cells (65, 66). The observation of SARS-CoV-2 spike protein in both maternal and fetal side is associated with tissue necrosis and massive recruitment of inflammatory cells to the intervillous space, termed chronic histiocytic intervillositis (67). Thus, placenta from COVID-19 pregnancies are highly likely to develop tissue inflammation and abnormal or injured maternal vessels.

As a cardinal unit for growth and regeneration, fetal trophoblast cells are central for the maintenance and development of the placenta and fetus, and defense against invading pathogens. The trophoblast rich in stem cells is endowed with intrinsic defense mechanisms, which include the production of type III interferons and a set of interferon stimulated genes (ISGs). In addition, a variety of receptors known as pattern recognition receptors (PRRs) including the Toll like receptors (TLRs) are widely expressed in the fetal placenta, but, very little is known about the expression of TLRs at the maternal decidua (68). Both innate immune cells and non-immune cells of the maternal-fetal unit including decidual cells, mesenchymal and trophoblast stem cells, and the amniotic epithelium express TLRs 3, 7, 8, and 9 that can sense viral infection (69). In addition to the intrinsic defense mechanisms and inducible antiviral defenses could lead to beneficial effects by restricting viral replication and dissemination. However, the downstream signaling pathways and induced differential response may determine the final outcome. Our group and others demonstrate the placenta increases the production of a large number of ISGs including IFITM family members, IFI6 and ISG20, and type III IFNs to preempt ZIKV infection (58, 70, 71). Similarly, we reported the involvement of many factors in limiting HEV-1 infection (53). However, trophoblasts function as an active barrier preventing the transmission of certain viral infections to the fetus and sustained inflammatory response may result in disruption of the fine-tuned microenvironment leading to viral dissemination and major pregnancy disorders such as preeclampsia, or UGR.

Immunity to Viral Infection

The "immune privilege" status of the maternal-fetal interface prevents harmful immune response to semi allogeneic embryonic cells. Nevertheless, there is an accumulating body of evidence supporting the active role of decidual immune cells in particular dNK cells and dMφ in controlling infections (72–74).

Our previous studies demonstrated that dNK cells can infiltrate HCMV-infected maternal-fetal tissues and colocalize with infected cells. dNK cells are then able to specifically detect and kill infected cells *via* the activating NKG2C/E and NKG2D receptors. They are also able to acquire specific cytotoxic functions directed against infected decidual fibroblasts (73). Interestingly, HCMV infection is also linked to a change in the secretome of dNK cells. Overall, by modulating the secretory profile of dNK cells toward increased production of cytotoxic factors, HCMV-infection likely constitutes virus-specific immune response (73).

Likewise, the secretion of IFN-γ by dNK cells during HIV-1 infection shapes the polarization of dMφ endowing them with natural resistance to infection (72, 74). This resistance is lost when the dNK cells are no longer in contact with dMφ or when the IFN-γ is neutralized by blocking antibodies, further confirming the role of the local environment in the control of the infection (72). In addition to their role during viral infection, dNK cells are able to balance the contradictory demands of fetal tolerance and protection against bacterial infection. Recent work by the group of Lieberman demonstrated that dNK cells are able to kill intracellular Listeria monocytogenes in trophoblasts and dMφ, through the transfer of granulysin cytotoxic molecules *via* tunneling nanotube (75).

The role of dMφ in the protection against pathogens did not receive much attention. However, dMφ express high levels of Toll-like receptors (TLRs 1–9) and engagement of these receptors *in vitro* enhances the secretion of pro- and anti-inflammatory cytokines that are compatible with maintenance of the fetotolerant immune environment during initiation of immune responses to pathogens (76). Likewise, dMφ antiviral innate immune response to HIV-1 is initiated by activation of TLRs 7 and 8 which in turn would restrict genome replication (74). Activation of TLR pathway induces downstream signaling cascades that ultimately lead to the production interferons (IFNs) and hundreds of IFN-stimulated genes (ISGs) with antiviral activity (77).

Our recent work highlighted the involvement of IFNs and a set of ISGs in placental defense against viral infection (53, 70).

Cytokine Induced Immunopathology

The microenvironment of the uterine mucosa, within first semester of pregnancy, is mandatory not only for embryo implantation but also for the maternal-fetal tolerance (24). Despite the protective effect of immune cells, an overwhelming immune response at the maternal-fetal interface may constitute the other edge of the sword. Viral-induced disequilibrium of pro-inflammatory and anti-inflammatory factors could mediate tissue injury, leading to virus spread, and adverse pregnancy outcomes (78).

In the context of HCMV, modulation of the cytokine environment is considered as a potential initiator and/or exacerbator of placental and fetal injury. Indeed, HCMV infection during pregnancy is associated with a shift toward a proinflammatory cytokine status. Levels of the cytokines, TNFα, IL-1β, IL-12, and IL-17; the chemokines CCL-2 (MCP1), CCL-4 (MIP-1β), and CXCL10; and the growth factors GM-CSF and PDGF-bb were significantly elevated in amniotic fluids from congenital HCMV fetuses (79). In addition, stillborn HCMV-infected placenta have significantly elevated levels of CCL-2 and TNFα levels than uninfected placenta (80). Our team has shown that dNK cells produce high levels of sICAM-1, CXCL-1 (GROα), IL-6, Granzyme B when stimulated with infected autologous decidual cells. On the other hand, dNK cell production of CCL-4, IL-8, CXCL-10 (IP-10), GM-CSF, RANTES, and CCL-3 (MIP-1α) was significantly decreased. These changes in dNK cell secretome are necessary for the recruitment and initiation of anti-viral immune response but reduce trophoblast cell invasion and might be partially responsible for HCMV-associated fetal damages (73).

Increased production of pro-inflammatory cytokines was also associated with pregnancy disorders upon HEV-1 infection. Several pro-inflammatory factors (TNFα, IL-6, IFN-γ, and TGF-β1) were increased in the maternal-fetal interface and peripheral blood from HEV-1 infected women with adverse pregnancy outcomes (81). Our studies revealed that HEV-1 skews the cytokine, chemokine, and growth factor secretory profile in both the decidua and placenta tissues with increased levels of IL-6, sICAM-1, CCL-3, CCL-4, G-CSF, and GM-CSF (53). These alterations in the local secretome were not only correlated with viral load but also promoted tissue apoptosis and necrosis, and may be responsible for HEV-1-associated pregnancy disorders. HEV-1 infection was also associated with decrease of CXCL-10 at the maternal fetal interface that could impair the invasion/migration of the fetal trophoblast and remodeling of maternal spiral arteries, both of which are mandatory for successful placentation.

ZIKV infection has been associated modulation of many factors such as VEGF-A, MMP-2, and MMP-9 that play a role in angiogenesis and ECM degradation. In contrast, the levels of sICAM-1 and IL-8, which could favor transmission of ZIKV, were increased. We found that ZIKV does not interfere type I or type II IFNs, but induces strong increase in the production of type III IFNs (IFN-λ2/3) and a set of interferon stimulated genes (70). We also provided the first evidence that ZIKV infection induces the production of several active lipid mediators which plays can modulate the placenta pro- and anti-inflammatory responses (58). The association between ZIKV-induced pro- and anti-inflammatory lipid metabolites and cytokines/chemokines have been implicated in the physiopathology of several infectious inflammatory disorders.

Modification of the local cytokine profile has also been reported in SARS-CoV-2 infection. SARS-CoV-2 infection is associated with immune cell activation, which may be responsible for a cytokine storm, leading at least to multiple system organ failure (82). The infection is associated with increased levels of pro-inflammatory cytokines IL-6, IL-10, GCSF, CXCL10, MCP-1, MIP-1α, and TNF (83). Taken together, the cytokine storm induced during SARS-CoV-2 infection could impair the migration of trophoblasts cells and the remodeling of the maternal spiral arteries and contribute to placentation defects. The permanent increased pro-inflammatory state could also be likely to impact the fetal brain development of the fetus, thus increasing the risk of autism, mental health disorders, or schizophrenia (84).

CONCLUDING REMARKS

Lessons from the TORCH pathogens and emerging viruses have demonstrated that the infection of the maternal-fetal interface during early pregnancy is often associated with placental diseases and is highly detrimental to fetal development. Viral tropism and efficient replication combined with altered local environment dictate the extent of tissue damage. Significant effort has been made toward understanding the essential role of dNK cells in viral spread. However, why in some cases these cells fail to control the infection or participate to tissue damage need to be further investigated. dNK cell responsiveness to pathogens can be dependent on host factors. Thus, one research axis can focus on KIR and HLA alleles expressed by the host. Indeed, several examples of matched and mismatched KIR and HLA were previously described to be protective or deleterious during viral infections. Metabolic alterations may also underlie the failure of the immune response especially that viral infections are known to deplete and/or enrich the local environment with several metabolites that alters immune cell function. Viral factors may also shape the immune response. For instance, HEV-1 and ZIKV downregulate IFNλ and other ISGs in infected target cells, favoring their own replication and spread at the maternal-fetal interface. Although, similar alterations were previously reported in cell line-based models, the mechanisms that are at play in the decidua and placenta tissue remain elusive. The impact of such mechanisms on dNK cells need also to be further investigated. Another open question is whether dNK cells can expand in response to infected cells and generate a "memory-like" response. Such a memory may generate a natural vaccine against viruses and contribute to the control of viral transmission to the fetus. Finally, a particular attention should be given to dMφ since these cells constitutes the first barrier against different infections in other tissues.

AUTHOR CONTRIBUTIONS

AE and NJ-F wrote and edited the manuscript. All authors contributed to the article and approved the submitted version.

FUNDING

AE holds doctoral-fellowship from the Region Midi-Pyrenées Occitanie. NJ-F was supported by the French National Agency for Research on AIDS and Hepatitis (ANRS, ECTZ103104), JT was supported by the French Association against Endometriosis (EndoFrance).

REFERENCES

1. Bischof P, Campana A. A model for implantation of the human blastocyst and early placentation. *Hum Reprod Update.* (1996) 2:262–70. doi: 10.1093/humupd/2.3.262
2. Pijnenborg R, Vercruysse L, Hanssens M. The uterine spiral arteries in human pregnancy: facts and controversies. *Placenta.* (2006) 27:939–58. doi: 10.1016/j.placenta.2005.12.006
3. Moffett A, Loke C. Immunology of placentation in eutherian mammals. *Nat Rev Immunol.* (2006) 6:584–94. doi: 10.1038/nri1897
4. Trundley A, Moffett A. Human uterine leukocytes and pregnancy. *Tissue Antigens.* (2004) 63:1–12. doi: 10.1111/j.1399-0039.2004.00170.x
5. Carlino C, Stabile H, Morrone S, Bulla R, Soriani A, Agostinis C, et al. Recruitment of circulating NK cells through decidual tissues: a possible mechanism controlling NK cell accumulation in the uterus during early pregnancy. *Blood.* (2008) 111:3108–15. doi: 10.1182/blood-2007-08-105965
6. Huang Y, Zhu X-Y, Du M-R, Li D-J. Human trophoblasts recruited T lymphocytes and monocytes into decidua by secretion of chemokine CXCL16 and interaction with CXCR6 in the first-trimester pregnancy. *J Immunol.* (2008) 180:2367–75. doi: 10.4049/jimmunol.180.4.2367
7. Cooper MA, Fehniger TA, Caligiuri MA. The biology of human natural killer-cell subsets. *Trends Immunol.* (2001) 22:633–40. doi: 10.1016/S1471-4906(01)02060-9
8. Koopman LA, Kopcow HD, Rybalov B, Boyson JE, Orange JS, Schatz F, et al. Human decidual natural killer cells are a unique NK cell subset with immunomodulatory potential. *J Exp Med.* (2003) 198:1201–12. doi: 10.1084/jem.200 30305
9. Moffett-King A. Natural killer cells and pregnancy. *Nat Rev Immunol.* (2002) 2:656–63. doi: 10.1038/nri886
10. Jabrane-Ferrat N, Siewiera J. The up side of decidual natural killer cells: new developments in immunology of pregnancy. *Immunology.* (2014) 141:490–7. doi: 10.1111/imm.12218
11. Gardner L, Moffett A. Dendritic cells in the human decidua. *Biol Reprod.* (2003) 69:1438–46. doi: 10.1095/biolreprod.103.017574
12. Bulmer JN, Longfellow M, Ritson A. Leukocytes and resident blood cells in endometriuma. *Ann N Y Acad Sci.* (1991) 622:57–68. doi: 10.1111/j.1749-6632.1991.tb37850.x
13. Vacca P, Montaldo E, Croxatto D, Loiacono F, Canegallo F, Venturini PL, et al. Identification of diverse innate lymphoid cells in human decidua. *Mucosal Immunol.* (2015) 8:254–64. doi: 10.1038/mi.2014.63
14. Gibbs A, Leeansyah E, Introini A, Paquin-Proulx D, Hasselrot K, Andersson E, et al. MAIT cells reside in the female genital mucosa and are biased towards IL-17 and IL-22 production in response to bacterial stimulation. *Mucosal Immunol.* (2017) 10:35–45. doi: 10.1038/mi.2016.30
15. Hanna J, Goldman-Wohl D, Hamani Y, Avraham I, Greenfield C, Natanson-Yaron S, et al. Decidual NK cells regulate key developmental processes at the human fetal-maternal interface. *Nat Med.* (2006) 12:1065–74. doi: 10.1038/nm1452
16. El Costa H, Casemayou A, Aguerre-Girr M, Rabot M, Berrebi A, Parant O, et al. Critical and differential roles of NKp46- and NKp30-activating receptors expressed by uterine NK cells in early pregnancy. *J Immunol.* (2008) 181:3009–17. doi: 10.4049/jimmunol.181.5.3009
17. El Costa H, Tabiasco J, Berrebi A, Parant O, Aguerre-Girr M, Piccinni M-P, et al. Effector functions of human decidual NK cells in healthy early pregnancy are dependent on the specific engagement of natural cytotoxicity receptors. *J Reprod Immunol.* (2009) 82:142–7. doi: 10.1016/j.jri.2009.06.123
18. Male V, Sharkey A, Masters L, Kennedy PR, Farrell LE, Moffett A. The effect of pregnancy on the uterine NK cell KIR repertoire. *Eur J Immunol.* (2011) 41:3017–27. doi: 10.1002/eji.201141445
19. Vacca P, Pietra G, Falco M, Romeo E, Bottino C, Bellora F, et al. Analysis of natural killer cells isolated from human decidua: evidence that 2B4 (CD244) functions as an inhibitory receptor and blocks NK-cell function. *Blood.* (2006) 108:4078–85. doi: 10.1182/blood-2006-04-017343
20. Siewiera J, Gouilly J, Hocine H-R, Cartron G, Levy C, Al-Daccak R, et al. Natural cytotoxicity receptor splice variants

orchestrate the distinct functions of human natural killer cell subtypes. *Nat Commun.* (2015) 6:10183. doi: 10.1038/ncomms10183

21. Lockwood CJ, Huang SJ, Chen C-P, Huang Y, Xu J, Faramarzi S, et al. Decidual cell regulation of natural killer cell-recruiting chemokines: implications for the pathogenesis and prediction of preeclampsia. *Am J Pathol.* (2013) 183:841–56. doi: 10.1016/j.ajpath.2013.05.029
22. Vento-Tormo R, Efremova M, Botting RA, Turco MY, Vento-Tormo M, Meyer KB, et al. Single-cell reconstruction of the early maternal-fetal interface in humans. *Nature.* (2018) 563:347–53. doi: 10.1038/s41586-018-0698-6
23. Huhn O, Ivarsson MA, Gardner L, Hollinshead M, Stinchcombe JC, Chen P, et al. Distinctive phenotypes and functions of innate lymphoid cells in human decidua during early pregnancy. *Nat Commun.* (2020) 11:381. doi: 10.1038/s41467-019-14123-z
24. Jabrane-Ferrat N. Features of human decidual NK cells in healthy pregnancy and during viral infection. *Front Immunol.* (2019) 10:1397. doi: 10.3389/fimmu.2019.01397
25. Lash GE, Schiessl B, Kirkley M, Innes BA, Cooper A, Searle RF, et al. Expression of angiogenic growth factors by uterine natural killer cells during early pregnancy. *J Leukoc Biol.* (2006) 80:572–580. doi: 10.1189/jlb.0406250
26. Fraser R, Whitley GS, Johnstone AP, Host AJ, Sebire NJ, Thilaganathan B, et al. Impaired decidual natural killer cell regulation of vascular remodelling in early human pregnancies with high uterine artery resistance. *J Pathol.* (2012) 228:322–32. doi: 10.1002/path.4057
27. Fu B, Zhou Y, Ni X, Tong X, Xu X, Dong Z, et al. Natural Killer cells promote fetal development through the secretion of growth-promoting factors. *Immunity.* (2017) 47:1100–13.e6. doi: 10.1016/j.immuni.2017.11.018
28. Kalkunte SS, Mselle TF, Norris WE, Wira CR, Sentman CL, Sharma S. VEGF C facilitates immune tolerance and endovascular activity of human uterine NK cells at the maternal-fetal interface. *J Immunol.* (2009) 182:4085–92. doi: 10.4049/jimmunol.0803769
29. Kopcow HD, Allan DSJ, Chen X, Rybalov B, Andzelm MM, Ge B, et al. Human decidual NK cells form immature activating synapses and are not cytotoxic. *Proc Natl Acad Sci U S A.* (2005) 102:15563–8. doi: 10.1073/pnas.0507835102
30. King A, Allan DS, Bowen M, Powis SJ, Joseph S, Verma S, et al. HLA-E is expressed on trophoblast and interacts with CD94/NKG2 receptors on decidual NK cells. *Eur J Immunol.* (2000) 30:1623–31. doi: 10.1002/1521-4141(200006)30:6<1623::AID-IMMU1623>3.0.CO;2-M
31. Nakashima A, Shiozaki A, Myojo S, Ito M, Tatematsu M, Sakai M, et al. Granulysin produced by uterine natural killer cells induces apoptosis of extravillous trophoblasts in spontaneous abortion. *Am J Pathol.* (2008) 173:653–64. doi: 10.2353/ajpath.2008.071169
32. Hiby SE, Regan L, Lo W, Farrell L, Carrington M, Moffett A. Association of maternal killer-cell immunoglobulin-like receptors and parental HLA-C genotypes with recurrent miscarriage. *Hum Reprod.* (2008) 23:972–6. doi: 10.1093/humrep/den011
33. Hiby SE, Apps R, Sharkey AM, Farrell LE, Gardner L, Mulder A, et al. Maternal activating KIRs protect against human reproductive failure mediated by fetal HLA-C2. *J Clin Invest.* (2010) 120:4102–10. doi: 10.1172/JCI43998
34. Houser BL, Tilburgs T, Hill J, Nicotra ML, Strominger JL. Two unique human decidual macrophage populations. *J Immunol.* (2011) 186:2633–42. doi: 10.4049/jimmunol.1003153
35. Wynn TA, Chawla A, Pollard JW. Macrophage biology in development, homeostasis and disease. *Nature.* (2013) 496:445–55. doi: 10.1038/nature12034
36. Martinez FO, Gordon S, Locati M, Mantovani A. Transcriptional profiling of the human monocyte-to-macrophage differentiation and polarization: new molecules and patterns of gene expression. *J Immunol.* (2006) 177:7303–11. doi: 10.4049/jimmunol.177.10.7303
37. Italiani P, Boraschi D. From monocytes to M1/M2 macrophages: phenotypical vs. functional differentiation. *Front Immunol.* (2014) 5:514. doi: 10.3389/fimmu.2014.00514
38. Repnik U, Tilburgs T, Roelen DL, van der Mast BJ, Kanhai HHH, Scherjon S, et al. Comparison of macrophage phenotype between decidua basalis and decidua parietalis by flow cytometry. *Placenta.* (2008) 29:405–12. doi: 10.1016/j.placenta.2008.02.004
39. Heikkinen J, Möttönen M, Komi J, Alanen A, Lassila O. Phenotypic characterization of human decidual macrophages. *Clin Exp Immunol.* (2003) 131:498–505. doi: 10.1046/j.1365-2249.2003.02092.x
40. Engert S, Rieger L, Kapp M, Becker JC, Dietl J, Kämmerer U. Profiling chemokines, cytokines and growth factors in human early pregnancy decidua by protein array. *Am J Reprod Immunol.* (2007) 58:129–37. doi: 10.1111/j.1600-0897.2007.00498.x
41. Lidström C, Matthiesen L, Berg G, Sharma S, Ernerudh J, Ekerfelt C. Cytokine secretion patterns of NK cells and macrophages in early human pregnancy decidua and blood: implications for suppressor macrophages in decidua. *Am J Reprod Immunol.* (2003) 50:444–52. doi: 10.1046/j.8755-8920.2003.00112.x
42. Lash GE, Pitman H, Morgan HL, Innes BA, Agwu CN, Bulmer JN. Decidual macrophages: key regulators of vascular remodeling in human pregnancy. *J Leukoc Biol.* (2016) 100:315–25. doi: 10.1189/jlb.1A0815-351R
43. Nagamatsu T, Schust DJ. The immunomodulatory roles of macrophages at the maternal—fetal interface. *Reprod Sci.* (2010) 17:209–18. doi: 10.1177/1933719109349962
44. Co EC, Gormley M, Kapidzic M, Rosen DB, Scott MA, Stolp HAR, et al. Maternal decidual macrophages inhibit nk cell killing of invasive cytotrophoblasts during human pregnancy. *Biol Reprod.* (2013) 88:155. doi: 10.1095/biolreprod.112.099465
45. Enders G, Daiminger A, Bäder U, Exler S, Enders M. Intrauterine transmission and clinical outcome of 248 pregnancies with primary cytomegalovirus infection in relation to gestational age. *J Clin Virol.* (2011) 52:244–6. doi: 10.1016/j.jcv.2011.07.005
46. Boppana SB, Fowler KB, Britt WJ, Stagno S, Pass RF. Symptomatic congenital cytomegalovirus infection in infants born to mothers with preexisting immunity to cytomegalovirus. *Pediatrics.* (1999) 104:55–60. doi: 10.1542/peds.104.1.55
47. Tang Y, Woodward BO, Pastor L, George AM, Petrechko O, Nouvet FJ, et al. Endogenous retroviral envelope syncytin induces HIV-1 spreading and establishes HIV reservoirs in placenta. *Cell Rep.* (2020) 30:4528–39.e4. doi: 10.1016/j.celrep.2020.03.016
48. Le Coeur S, Kanshana S, Jourdain G. [HIV-1 transmission from mother to child and its prevention]. *Med Trop.* (2003) 63:381–90.
49. Primadharsini PP, Nagashima S, Okamoto H. Genetic variability and evolution of hepatitis E virus. *Viruses.* (2019) 11:456. doi: 10.3390/v11050456
50. Patra S, Kumar A, Trivedi SS, Puri M, Sarin SK. Maternal and fetal outcomes in pregnant women with acute hepatitis E virus infection. *Ann Intern Med.* (2007) 147:28–33. doi: 10.7326/0003-4819-147-1-200707030-00005
51. Sharma S, Kumar A, Kar P, Agarwal S, Ramji S, Husain SA, et al. Risk factors for vertical transmission of hepatitis E virus infection. *J Viral Hepat.* (2017) 24:1067–75. doi: 10.1111/jvh.12730
52. Bose PD, Das BC, Hazam RK, Kumar A, Medhi S, Kar P. Evidence of extrahepatic replication of hepatitis E virus in human placenta. *J Gen Virol.* (2014) 95:1266–71. doi: 10.1099/vir.0.063602-0
53. Gouilly J, Chen Q, Siewiera J, Cartron G, Levy C, Dubois M, et al. Genotype specific pathogenicity of hepatitis E virus at the human maternal-fetal interface. *Nat Commun.* (2018) 9:4748. doi: 10.1038/s41467-018-07200-2
54. Melo AS de O, Aguiar RS, Amorim MMR, Arruda MB, Melo F de O, Ribeiro STC, et al. Congenital Zika virus infection: beyond neonatal microcephaly. *JAMA Neurol.* (2016) 73:1407–16. doi: 10.1001/jamaneurol.2016.3720
55. Dudley DM, Van Rompay KK, Coffey LL, Ardeshir A, Keesler RI, Grigsby PL, et al. Miscarriage and stillbirth following maternal Zika virus infection in non-human primates. *Nat Med.* (2018) 24:1104–7. doi: 10.1038/s41591-018-0088-5
56. Miner JJ, Cao B, Govero J, Smith AM, Fernandez E, Cabrera OH, et al. Zika virus infection during pregnancy in mice causes placental damage and fetal demise. *Cell.* (2016) 165:1081–91. doi: 10.1016/j.cell.2016.05.008
57. El Costa H, Gouilly J, Mansuy J-M, Chen Q, Levy C, Cartron G, et al. Zika virus reveals broad tissue and cell tropism during the first trimester of pregnancy. *Sci Rep.* (2016) 6:35296. doi: 10.1038/srep35296
58. Chen Q, Gouilly J, Ferrat YJ, Espino A, Glaziou Q, Cartron G, et al. Metabolic reprogramming by Zika virus provokes inflammation in human placenta. *Nat Commun.* (2020) 11:2967. doi: 10.1038/s41467-020-16754-z
59. Zaki AM, van Boheemen S, Bestebroer TM, Osterhaus ADME, Fouchier RAM. Isolation of a novel coronavirus from a man with pneumonia in Saudi Arabia. *N Engl J Med.* (2012) 367:1814–20. doi: 10.1056/NEJMoa1211721

60. Zhong N, Zheng B, Li Y, Poon L, Xie Z, Chan K, et al. Epidemiology and cause of severe acute respiratory syndrome (SARS) in Guangdong, People's Republic of China, in February, 2003. *Lancet.* (2003) 362:1353–8. doi: 10.1016/S0140-6736(03)14630-2
61. Baud D, Greub G, Favre G, Gengler C, Jaton K, Dubruc E, et al. Second-trimester miscarriage in a pregnant woman with SARS-CoV-2 infection. *JAMA.* (2020) 323:2198–200. doi: 10.1001/jama.2020.7233
62. Di Mascio D, Khalil A, Saccone G, Rizzo G, Buca D, Liberati M, et al. Outcome of coronavirus spectrum infections (SARS, MERS, COVID-19) during pregnancy: a systematic review and meta-analysis. *Am J Obstet Gynecol MFM.* (2020) 2:100107. doi: 10.1016/j.ajogmf.2020.100107
63. Zaigham M, Andersson O. Maternal and perinatal outcomes with COVID-19: a systematic review of 108 pregnancies. *Acta Obstet Gynecol Scand.* (2020) 99:823–9. doi: 10.1111/aogs.13867
64. Schwartz DA. An analysis of 38 pregnant women with COVID-19, their newborn infants, and maternal-fetal transmission of SARS-CoV-2: maternal coronavirus infections and pregnancy outcomes. *Arch Pathol Lab Med.* (2020) 144:799–805. doi: 10.5858/arpa.2020-0901-SA
65. Verma S, Joshi CS, Silverstein RB, He M, Carter EB, Mysorekar IU. SARS-CoV-2 colonization of maternal and fetal cells of the human placenta promotes alteration of local renin-angiotensin system. *Med.* (2021) 2:575–90.e5. doi: 10.1016/j.medj.2021.04.009
66. Algarroba GN, Rekawek P, Vahanian SA, Khullar P, Palaia T, Peltier MR, et al. Visualization of severe acute respiratory syndrome coronavirus 2 invading the human placenta using electron microscopy. *Am J Obstet Gynecol.* (2020) 223:275–8. doi: 10.1016/j.ajog.2020.05.023
67. Schwartz DA, Baldewijns M, Benachi A, Bugatti M, Collins RRJ, De Luca D, et al. Chronic histiocytic intervillositis with trophoblast necrosis are risk factors associated with placental infection from coronavirus disease 2019 (COVID-19) and intrauterine maternal-fetal severe acute respiratory syndrome coronavirus 2 (sars-cov-2) transmission in liveborn and stillborn infants. *Arch Pathol Lab Med.* (2020) 145: 517–28. doi: 10.5858/arpa.2020-0771-SA
68. Krikun G, Lockwood CJ, Abrahams VM, Mor G, Paidas M, Guller S. Expression of toll-like receptors in the human decidua. *Histol Histopathol.* (2007) 22:847–54. doi: 10.14670/HH-22.847
69. Koga K, Izumi G, Mor G, Fujii T, Osuga Y. Toll-like receptors at the maternal-fetal interface in normal pregnancy and pregnancy complications. *Am J Reprod Immunol.* (2014) 72:192–205. doi: 10.1111/aji.12258
70. Dukhovny A, Lamkiewicz K, Chen Q, Fricke M, Jabrane-Ferrat N, Marz M, et al. A CRISPR activation screen identifies genes that protect against Zika virus infection. *J Virol.* (2019) 93:e00211-19. doi: 10.1128/JVI.00211-19
71. Buchrieser J, Degrelle SA, Couderc T, Nevers Q, Disson O, Manet C, et al. IFITM proteins inhibit placental syncytiotrophoblast formation and promote fetal demise. *Science.* (2019) 365:176–80. doi: 10.1126/science.aaw7733
72. Quillay H, El Costa H, Duriez M, Marlin R, Cannou C, Madec Y, et al. NK cells control HIV-1 infection of macrophages through soluble factors and cellular contacts in the human decidua. *Retrovirology.* (2016) 13:39. doi: 10.1186/s12977-016-0271-z
73. Siewiera J, El Costa H, Tabiasco J, Berrebi A, Cartron G, Bouteiller P, et al. Human cytomegalovirus infection elicits new decidual natural killer cell effector functions. *PLoS Pathog.* (2013) 9:e1003257. doi: 10.1371/journal.ppat.1003257
74. El Costa H, Quillay H, Marlin R, Cannou C, Duriez M, Benjelloun F, et al. The local environment orchestrates mucosal decidual macrophage differentiation and substantially inhibits HIV-1 replication. *Mucosal Immunol.* (2016) 9:634–46. doi: 10.1038/mi.2015.87
75. Crespo ÂC, Mulik S, Dotiwala F, Ansara JA, Sen Santara S, Ingersoll K, et al. Decidual NK cells transfer granulysin to selectively kill bacteria in trophoblasts. *Cell.* (2020) 182:1125–39.e18. doi: 10.1016/j.cell.2020.07.019
76. Duriez M, Quillay H, Madec Y, El Costa H, Cannou C, Marlin R, et al. Human decidual macrophages and NK cells differentially express toll-like receptors and display distinct cytokine profiles upon TLR stimulation. *Front Microbiol.* (2014) 5:316. doi: 10.3389/fmicb.2014.00316
77. Schneider WM, Chevillotte MD, Rice CM. Interferon-stimulated genes: a complex web of host defenses. *Annu Rev Immunol.* (2014) 32:513–45. doi: 10.1146/annurev-immunol-032713-120231
78. Lash GE, Ernerudh J. Decidual cytokines and pregnancy complications: focus on spontaneous miscarriage. *J Reprod Immunol.* (2015) 108:83–9. doi: 10.1016/j.jri.2015.02.003
79. Scott GM, Chow SSW, Craig ME, Pang CNI, Hall B, Wilkins MR, et al. Cytomegalovirus infection during pregnancy with maternofetal transmission induces a proinflammatory cytokine bias in placenta and amniotic fluid. *J Infect Dis.* (2012) 205:1305–10. doi: 10.1093/infdis/jis186
80. Hamilton ST, Scott G, Naing Z, Iwasenko J, Hall B, Graf N, et al. Human cytomegalovirus-induces cytokine changes in the placenta with implications for adverse pregnancy outcomes. *PLoS ONE.* (2012) 7:e52899. doi: 10.1371/journal.pone.0052899
81. Kumar A, Devi SG, Kar P, Agarwal S, Husain SA, Gupta RK, et al. Association of cytokines in hepatitis E with pregnancy outcome. *Cytokine.* (2014) 65:95–104. doi: 10.1016/j.cyto.2013.09.022
82. Channappanavar R, Perlman S. Pathogenic human coronavirus infections: causes and consequences of cytokine storm and immunopathology. *Semin Immunopathol.* (2017) 39:529–39. doi: 10.1007/s00281-017-0629-x
83. Huang C, Wang Y, Li X, Ren L, Zhao J, Hu Y, et al. Clinical features of patients infected with 2019 novel coronavirus in Wuhan, China. *Lancet.* (2020) 395:497–506. doi: 10.1016/S0140-6736(20)30183-5
84. Chudnovets A, Lei J, Na Q, Dong J, Narasimhan H, Klein SL, et al. Dose-dependent structural and immunological changes in the placenta and fetal brain in response to systemic inflammation during pregnancy. *Am J Reprod Immunol.* (2020) 84:e13248. doi: 10.1111/aji.13248

20

Human Anelloviruses: Prevalence and Clinical Significance during Pregnancy

Chandrashekara Kyathanahalli[1,2], Madeline Snedden[1] and Emmet Hirsch[1,2]*

[1] Department of Obstetrics and Gynecology, NorthShore University HealthSystem, Evanston, IL, United States, [2] Department of Obstetrics and Gynecology, Pritzker School of Medicine, University of Chicago, Chicago, IL, United States

***Correspondence:**
Chandrashekara Kyathanahalli
ckyathanahalli@northshore.org

Although the bacterial microbiota of various compartments (e.g. vagina, amniotic fluid, and placenta) have been studied in pregnancy, there has been far less emphasis on normal and pathological viral communities. Cumulative evidence shows the presence of a number of apathogenic viruses in various tissues of healthy people, including pregnant individuals. What role, if any, these viruses play in human physiology is unknown. Anelloviruses (family *Anelloviridae)* are circular, single-stranded DNA viruses commonly detected with high prevalence in vertebrate hosts, including primates. Humans are nearly always colonized with at least 1 of 3 *anellovirus* subtypes, namely *Alphatorquevirus* (torque teno virus, TTV), *Betatorquevirus* (torque teno midi virus, TTMDV), and *Gammatorquevirus* (torque teno mini virus, TTMV). In healthy pregnant people, the prototype anellovirus, TTV, has been found in maternal and (variably) fetal blood, amniotic fluid, cervical and vaginal secretions, breast milk, and saliva. Nonetheless, the relevance of human anelloviruses in pregnancy and labor is unclear. There is evidence suggesting a link between anellovirus colonization and preterm birth. In this review, we discuss what is known about this family of commensal viruses in health and disease, and specifically the roles they might play during pregnancy and in the timing of delivery.

Keywords: human virome, *Anelloviridae*, anelloviruses, commensal virus, pregnancy, preterm birth

INTRODUCTION

The human body serves as a host to a highly diverse community of microorganisms. These microorganisms may benefit the host (creating a "mutualistic" relationship), harm the host (forming a "pathogenic" relationship), or have no apparent effect (a "commensal" relationship). From time to time, mutualistic or commensal microorganisms may assume a pathogenic character (for example, in the case of vaginal yeast infections). The genomes that constitute the human microbiome include bacteria, archaeans, other eukaryotes, and viruses (1). These microbial communities are highly dynamic and vary based on the individual's age and health status, the biology of the anatomical site, diet, and hygiene (2).

While research on the human microbiome has focused mainly on bacterial populations, much less is known about viral communities residing at different sites in and on the human body and their roles in health. Advances in sequencing have uncovered myriad novel viruses in humans, many of which cause no apparent illness (3). Most humans are colonized in almost every tissue type by members of *Anelloviridae*, a family of diverse, non-enveloped, circular, single-stranded

DNA eukaryotic viruses (4, 5). Thus far, anelloviruses have not been linked definitively to any disease states (6), although there is some evidence suggesting a link to human disease (7). This review discusses this novel class of human viruses, including their prevalence, genome diversity, transmission routes, and potential association with human health and disease. We focus on pregnancy, including a possible role in the timing of delivery. Anelloviruses have been detected in maternal and—to a lesser and highly variable extent, depending on the study—fetal tissues (8–10). We discuss the potential mechanisms by which anelloviruses may interact with and modulate maternal immune responses and influence pregnancy outcomes.

DISCOVERY AND NOMENCLATURE

In 1997, while searching for a viral agent responsible for non-A to E hepatitis, Nishizawa et al. found a novel DNA virus in the serum of a Japanese patient with post-transfusion hepatitis of unknown etiology (11). The viral clone was designated TT virus (TTV) after the patient from whom it was recovered. Subsequent studies revealed TTV as a small, non-enveloped, single-stranded, circular DNA virus (12). After the discovery of the original TTV isolate, smaller variants of TTV were identified and subsequently named torque teno mini virus (TTMV) (13), and torque teno midi virus (TTMDV) (14), derived from the Latin terms *torque* meaning "necklace" and *tenuis* meaning "thin" (15). Recent changes in nomenclature have classified the 3 anellovirus genera found in humans: *Alphatorquevirus* (TTV), *Betatorquevirus* (TTMV), and *Gammatorquevirus* (TTMDV), which together comprise the human *Anelloviridae* family (16).

ANELLOVIRUS AND HUMAN DISEASE

A clear link between anellovirus positivity and human disease has not been established (6). On the one hand, the fact that anelloviruses are rarely detected earlier than 3 months of age and are acquired later in life in healthy individuals (17–19) suggests that anellovirus acquisition over the lifespan is normal. On the other hand, recent studies have suggested that certain anellovirus subtypes are associated with various illness and diseases such as unexplained fever (20), diabetes (7), cirrhosis in liver transplant patients (21), respiratory disease (22–26), cancer (27–30), and autoimmune disorders (31–33). There is some evidence suggesting a high occurrence of anellovirus with *Epstein-Barr virus* (34) and hepatitis B or C (5). Whether this means that anelloviruses have a role in enabling pathological viral infections remains to be elucidated. Given the prevalence of TTV in organ transplant recipients, TTV load has been suggested as a candidate indicator of immune suppression (35–37).

PREVALENCE OF ANELLOVIRUS BY AGE AND GENDER

Anelloviruses are reported at a high prevalence in the general population across the globe (38). TTV, the prototypical anellovirus, is multitropic, i.e., found in nearly every body site, fluid, and tissue tested, as summarized in **Table 1**.

A plethora of evidence suggests that anelloviruses are detected by PCR in all age groups. A study analyzed fecal specimens collected longitudinally from day of life 1–4 (month 0) and at 3, 6, 12, 18, and 24 months of age from 4 healthy twin pairs (18). Anelloviruses were rarely detected earlier than 3 months of age. Thereafter the prevalence increased significantly, peaking at 6–12 months of age, and began to decline at 18 and 24 months of age. Among 8 infants enrolled in the study, 1 infant harbored no less than 47 anellovirus species at 12 months of age. In some infants, the same anelloviruses could be detected from fecal samples collected up to 12 months apart, suggesting persistence and expansion of anellovirus richness in the gut of infants. Another study of 20 twin pairs (0–30 months of age) showed the abundance of anellovirus species increased until 15–18 months of age, after which time abundance diminished (66). A prospective single-center study of 98 clinically healthy breastfeeding infants (1–12 months of age) demonstrated a significant increase in whole blood anellovirus load during the first year of life, reaching a plateau after 6 months of age (17).

A study investigated the epidemiology of anellovirus in blood samples derived from healthy children (1–14 years) and healthy blood donors (18–59 years) (67). Among 208 children, 141 were

TABLE 1 | Tissues tested for anellovirus.

	Citations
Tissues with detectable anellovirus	
Whole blood, plasma, or serum*	(3, 39–48)
Peripheral blood mononuclear cells (PBMCs)	(43, 49–51)
Exosomes-enriched vesicles from plasma	(52)
Bone marrow, lymphoid tissue, thyroid gland, muscle, pancreas, spleen, kidney, lung	(48)
Bronchoalveolar lavage	(53)
Nasal or throat swabs	(24, 53)
Saliva*	(10, 40–42, 54)
Liver	(43, 55)
Bile	(56)
Feces	(41, 42, 46, 49, 56–59)
Urine	(60, 61)
Skin, hair follicle	(62)
Tears	(42)
Semen	(42, 54)
Amniotic fluid*	(9)
Cervix*	(63, 64)
Vaginal secretions*	(65)
Umbilical cord blood*	(9, 10)
Breast milk*	(9, 45, 47)
Tissues without detectable anellovirus	
RBCs	(50, 51)
Platelets	(50, 51)
Sweat	(42)

**Tissues tested in pregnant or post-partum people.*

TTV-positive. TTV prevalence was highest in 1–2-year-olds, lower for 8-year-olds, and higher again in 14-year-old children. Among 196 healthy blood donors representing the normal population, 103 were TTV-positive; there was no difference in the TTV DNA prevalence with age. However, other studies (68–70) with larger sample sizes have consistently demonstrated positive correlations between anellovirus prevalence and age in healthy populations. Phylogenetic analyses did not find associations between anellovirus genotypes and particular age groups (67) or geographic locations (68, 71). One study (68) noted viral loads were highest in blood donors more than 50 years old, but a longitudinal analysis of plasma TTV loads after 2 years showed minimal changes in TTV viremia (70). The findings suggest that although anelloviruses are acquired over the lifetime, healthy aging causes only minimal increases in TTV viremia.

Anellovirus prevalence and viral load may be gender-specific. One study found TTV prevalence was significantly higher in males than in females (70). A separate study found that young women (20–30 years) had lower plasma loads of anellovirus than men in the same age group (19).

Substantial evidence suggests that anellovirus load is governed by the immune system (72). Although the mechanisms by which the immune system reacts to anellovirus colonization are unknown, studies have shown that people receiving a solid organ transplant (73–77), and those with cancer (47), HIV infection (78), and sepsis (79) have higher plasma anellovirus loads than healthy donors. Other studies have shown an inverse correlation between levels of TTV and CD4+ lymphocytes in HIV-positive patients (80) and pediatric lung transplantation patients (81). The latter study findings revealed that patients with low anellovirus genome copies are at risk of transplant rejection or death. There is also evidence of increased anellovirus DNA concentrations after antiviral therapy (6). Thus, it appears that anellovirus load is inversely correlated to and may serve as a marker of general immune status.

ANELLOVIRUS GENOME

Despite their nucleotide sequence diversity, anelloviruses share virion structure and genomic organization (13). Electron microscopy of the prototype anellovirus, TTV, isolated from serum specimens (82) and a TTV-infected HEK293 cell line (83) demonstrate TTV as an unenveloped icosahedral virus with a diameter between 30 and 50 nm. As indicated by their names, the human anelloviruses differ in genome size: 3.9 kb for TTV, 3.2 kb for TTMDV, and 2.8–2.9 kb for TTMV. The TTV genome consists of an untranslated region (UTR) of ~1.2 kb and a potential coding region of ~2.6 kb. The non-coding UTR of the TTV genome contains a GC-rich segment (>60% GC) flanked by a TATA box upstream of the coding region and a poly-A sequence downstream (84), and multiple stem-loop structures that facilitate virus replication (71). The coding region consists of 3–5 overlapping open reading frames (ORF1-5) which encode at least 6 proteins with structural (85), host immune suppression (86, 87), cell cycle regulation, and apoptosis-inducing properties, respectively (88). ORF1 also contains hypervariable regions where mutations occur more frequently than in other regions. These hypervariable regions help the virus evade the immune system (89).

Genetic Heterogeneity

In addition to size, the 3 *Anelloviridae* genera can be grouped according to their degree of genetic similarity in the ORF1 region. TTV, TTMV, and TTMDV have at least 105, 68, and 34 species, respectively. Phylogenetic analysis of TTV isolates recovered from disparate locations have identified 7 major clusters, with genomic sequence differences of up to 35% (90). It has been hypothesized that in a given individual, genetic variability within a viral group is high, and that coinfection by distinct viral strains in blood and other tissues is common (91, 92). A study investigated possible relationships between the number of genogroups carried and the total TTV load present in 239 TTV-positive subjects (93). Individuals with high viral loads tended to possess more TTV genogroups than those with low viral loads. TTV genogroups 1 and 3 were the most prevalent, followed by genogroups 4 and 5, while genogroup 2 was rather infrequent.

DETECTION AND QUANTITATION OF ANELLOVIRUSES

To date, polymerase chain reaction (PCR) is the most prominent method used to detect anellovirus. Because of the extensive heterogeneity among the genomes of anelloviruses, detection of the entire spectrum of the anellovirus variants is impossible using a single set of primers. For genotyping, primer pairs designed either in the ORF1 region or the sequences spanning 5' or 3' UTRs are widely used (93, 94). Taking advantage of these regions, nested and semi-nested PCR assays are developed in which the genomic DNA of all anelloviruses is amplified by first-round PCR with universal primers, and then species-specific DNA are amplified by using a second set of primers (7). In a number of studies, sequences spanning N22-ORF1 regions are utilized for the detection of anellovirus DNA (11, 92). However, this strategy allows detection of only some genotypes of TTV, a genus with more than 30 genotypes (95). For example, N22 primers can efficiently amplify genotypes in group 1, but amplifies certain genotypes in group 2 less efficiently (96) and fails to amplify many genotypes in groups 2, 3, and 4 at all. Over time, studies have increasingly focused on utilizing degenerate primers and highly conserved regions located just downstream of the TATA box to potentially detect all known genetic forms of anelloviruses (97–99). The results are validated across multiple iterations followed by phylogenetic analysis (94, 100, 101). In recent studies 5'UTR primer sets are often used, but these primers differ in their abilities to detect TTV and related genotypes by PCR (95). Therefore, differences in primer selection could explain some of the considerable variation in estimates of anellovirus prevalence between studies. Even within a single healthy cohort, TTV detection ranged from 53% (251/471) to 90% (90/100) depending on which primers were used (68). In addition, measuring prevalence of detectable TTV is highly dependent on the type of specimen analyzed—for example, TTV titer is higher in whole blood than in plasma (70). Therefore, TTV negativity in a sample could be a laboratory artifact due to sub-optimal sensitivity of the detection methods. A study validated the commonly used PCR primer sequences to detect TTV and TTV-like virus in different populations (102). Primer alignment and PCR product characterization consistently indicated that a minimum of five primer sets (NG, TT, TLMV-S, TLMV-L, and a genotype 21-specific set of primers) are required to detect all known genotypes of TTV and TTV-like viruses in healthy individuals.

In addition to the PCR method, antibody-based detection of TTV has also been developed and used for the diagnosis of TTV colonization (103).

SITES OF ANELLOVIRUS REPLICATION

Despite decades of research, the main site of anellovirus replication remains unknown. Studies have indicated the association of TTV with peripheral blood mononuclear cells (PBMCs) and distinct distribution of TTV subtypes between plasma and PBMCs (104, 105). Research has also shown that TTV is abundant in granulocytes compared with other peripheral blood cell types in healthy individuals (51). Given the reported evidence of elevated TTV titers with immunosuppression and transplant-related complications (6, 106), a study investigated TTV levels in plasma samples and potential sites of TTV replication in individual blood cell types derived from pediatric allogeneic hematopoietic stem cell transplant (HSCT) recipients (107). Among 43 HSCT patients enrolled in the study, 34 had detectable TTV in plasma before transplantation, and all patients tested positive for TTV by day+50 post-transplant. TTV copies reached peak titer around day+100, and then gradually declined to pre-transplantation levels over a period of about 2 years. TTV DNA was not present in NK cells, B- and T-cells. On the other hand, granulocytes isolated from peripheral blood or bone marrow were invariably positive in post-transplant samples of all patients. Until day+30 post-transplantation, TTV tested either near or below the detection limit in granulocytes, but dramatically increased between days +30 and +100 days post-transplantation in peripheral blood and bone marrow granulocytes. At the same time, TTV DNA was absent in granulocytes derived from healthy immunocompetent controls throughout the study period. Together, these findings suggest granulocytes as potential TTV replication sites, particularly in immunosuppressed individuals.

Evidence comparing viral titers between different tissues within a single patient suggests anellovirus replication can occur in bone marrow (108), liver (109, 110), lungs (111), lymphoid tissue (112), oropharyngeal and/or salivary glands (40). These findings suggest that viral replication takes place in multiple tissues at distinct levels in infected individuals (48).

Attempts to replicate anellovirus *in vitro* have been unsuccessful thus far. Human cell lines, including Chang liver (109), HEK293TT (113), lymphoma and T-cell leukemia (83), and the Raji cell line (109), have demonstrated TTV infection in initial passages, but the virus did not propagate to later passages (83, 113, 114).

IMMUNOBIOLOGY OF HUMAN ANELLOVIRUSES

Toll-like receptors (TLRs) are members of a family of cell-surface proteins responsible for recognition of a diverse spectrum of pathogens and generation of an innate immune response. TLR9 recognizes intracellular unmethylated heterodimers of guanosine and cytosine (CpGs), which are abundant in the genomes of DNA viruses. Depending on the number of nucleotides flanking CpGs, this may stimulate the production of either pro- or anti-inflammatory cytokines (115). It has been reported that the genome as well as the replicative intermediates of anellovirus are unusually rich in CpG sequences (116). The DNA of 1 genogroup of anellovirus (ViPiSAL strain) was found to provoke robust activation of TLR9 and the production of proinflammatory cytokines in *ex vivo* mouse spleen cells (117). Nevertheless, the genomes of other anellovirus strains failed to promote inflammatory responses. These findings may indicate that the effects of anelloviruses on the host's inflammatory status vary depending on genogroups.

Due to the lack of an efficient culture system to support TTV replication, the transcription profile of TTV has been largely gained from human cell lines (COS1, HEK293, and L428) transfected with TTV plasmids (87, 118). Three spliced mRNAs of TTV that produce at least 6 proteins by alternative translation initiation have been reported (85). At present, the functional role of ORF2 protein is well-characterized. Overexpression of TTV ORF2 encoded protein has been shown to suppress NF-κB activation elicited by TNFα in various human cancer cell lines, including HeLa and HepG2, and in the mouse macrophage line RAW 264.7 (86). Further analyses revealed that TTV ORF2 protein has the ability to suppress NF-κB activity *in vitro* in a dose-dependent manner, affecting translocation of NF-κB p65 and p50 subunits to the cell nucleus, thus inhibiting the transcription of downstream genes such as interleukin (IL)-6, IL-8, and cyclooxygenase-2. Together these findings indicate that TTV ORF2 protein may be involved in negative regulation of host cell inflammatory responses.

Evidence suggests that TTV encodes microRNAs (miRNA) that cooperate with viral proteins to regulate the expression of viral genes involved in replication, pathogenesis, inflammation, and immune evasion (119). The functional relevance of proteins translated from other TTV ORFs and TTV-encoded miRNAs warrant further study.

ROUTES OF TRANSMISSION

Numerous studies have suggested horizontal and vertical TTV transmission routes. Horizontal transmission includes parenteral, fecal-oral, and sexual. Vertical transmission involves the possible passage of virus from mother to fetus during pregnancy and breast feeding.

Parenteral Route

Since bone marrow cells and activated PBMCs are recognized as potential sites of TTV replication (120, 121), blood and blood products could be among possible routes of TTV transmission.

Therefore, people with blood-related diseases such as hemophilia and thalassemia (122–124), blood donors (5), patients having multiple blood transfusions (124–126), and patients who have undergone organ transplantation (73, 127–131) are more likely to have TTV colonization.

Fecal-Oral Route

To examine patterns of anellovirus shedding into the circulation and the GI tract after new infection, 2 naïve chimpanzees were injected intravenously with bacteria-free (filtered) fecal supernatant or serum from human newborns with documented acute TTV infection (132). Serum and fecal specimens obtained weekly from experimentally infected chimpanzees were tested for TTV DNA by nested PCR. In the chimpanzee that received TTV-positive human serum, TTV DNA was detected in serum starting 5 weeks post-inoculation (PI) and remained positive until 15 weeks PI. In the chimpanzee that received fecal supernatant, TTV DNA was detected in serum samples 7–12 weeks PI and peaked at 14–16 weeks PI and continued to be positive for longer than 30 weeks. TTV DNA was detected in fecal specimens from the chimpanzee inoculated with TTV-positive human fecal supernatant after 16 weeks PI (coincident with high-titer TTV DNA in the serum). However, fecal specimens obtained at 24 weeks PI (when serum titers were low) were negative for TTV DNA.

Sexual Contact

Detection of TTV DNA in semen (54), and vaginal fluid (64, 133), suggests possible TTV transmission during sexual intercourse.

Transplacental Route

The published information on transplacental TTV transmission is inconsistent. In a prospective cohort study, paired maternal and cord bloods were examined for the presence of TTV DNA (69). Among 105 participants enrolled in the study, 37 mothers were TTV DNA-positive, and 7 cord blood samples from the 37 TTV-positive mothers were also TTV-positive. All cords from TTV-negative mothers were TTV-negative. In another study (134) TTV DNA was present in the blood of 57 of 138 mothers. Among the 57 TTV-infected mothers, 19 cord sera were positive for TTV DNA. A follow-up of 3 randomly selected infants with TTV sequences in their cord blood showed positivity persisting for 8 weeks after birth. The finding of TTV in the cord blood of between 1/5 and 1/3 of colonized mothers is consistent with transplacental passage of virus, however other routes are possible, as is contamination of the cord specimens by maternal blood.

A separate study analyzed plasma samples from 54 mothers and their newborns for TTV DNA (135). Though TTV-DNA was detected in 49 of 54 mothers, only 4 (8%) infants tested positive.

By contrast, another study analyzed TTV DNA in maternal and fetal cord blood collected postpartum from 100 mother-child pairs (44). TTV DNA was detected in 84% of maternal samples, while cord blood was devoid of TTV.

The sum of these findings call into question whether transplacental transmission of TTV occurs in human pregnancy.

Breast Feeding

Several studies provide evidence of anellovirus transmission by breast feeding (9, 134, 136). In a cohort study, blood was sampled from 300 normal pregnant people (60 of whom were TTV-positive). Twenty infants born to TTV-positive women in the cohort who delivered vaginally ($n = 10$) or by C/S ($n = 10$) were sampled at both 5 days and 3 months after birth. Half the infants in each group were also tested at 6 months after birth. Additionally, breast milk was collected from 30 TTV-positive nursing women (137). All infants from TTV-positive mothers were TTV-negative at both 5 days and 3 months after birth, regardless of delivery method, arguing against TTV transmission either transplacentally or during the birth process. By 6 months after birth, 4 of the 10 infants born to TTV-positive parents were TTV-positive. TTV DNA was detected in the breast milk of 7 of 30 TTV-positive patients.

An earlier study in Germany looked for TTV in 46 women who collectively birthed 47 children. Of this cohort, 22 maternal serum samples tested positive for TTV. Notably, TTV DNA was detected in 22 of 23 serum samples of 1-week-old infants who were born to TTV-positive parents. Twenty four TTV-negative individuals gave birth to 24 TTV-negative children who remained negative throughout the study period of 28 months. TTV DNA was detected in 77% of breast milk samples from TTV-positive patients and in none from TTV-negative individuals (45).

A prospective single-center study in Russia analyzed whole blood TTV load in 98 clinically healthy breastfeeding infants of 1–12 months of age to determine TTV dynamics during the first year of life (17). The findings revealed a significant increase in TTV copy number for the first 60 days, before plateauing after 6 months, with viral loads correlating with age.

In sum, these findings suggest that newborns can acquire TTV through breast milk, but acquisition from either parents or others via alternative routes was not ruled out. There is some evidence that among infants who are breast-fed, the prevalence of TTV positivity increases with prolonged lactation (136).

Horizontal Transmission Could Be the Major Route of Anellovirus Colonization in Infants

A study determined whether the predominant route of transmission of TTV in children is horizontal, vertical, or both, by testing infants born to TTV-positive mothers (138). Serum samples were obtained from 12 mothers on the day of delivery or within 1 month after delivery. Among 12 mothers, TTV DNA was detected in 10 (83%) cases. Serum samples were obtained from infants at 0.5–3 month intervals from 1 to 12 months of age. All infants, aside from 1 born by C/S, were delivered vaginally. The prevalence of TTV in infants born to TTV-positive and TTV-negative mothers were 9/10 (90%) and 0/2 (0%) respectively. Serum TTV DNA was not detected in any infant at 1 month of age but was detected for the first time at 1.5–8 months of age, and thereafter TTV positivity persisted throughout the follow-up period. Detection of TTV in 9/10 infants born to TTV-positive mothers and 0/2 infants born to TTV-negative mothers suggests that

TTV transmission from mothers to their infants postpartum is possible.

To confirm the transmission route, a homology search was performed in 7 randomly selected TTV-positive mother-infant pairs. Although only a few clones tested for each case were sequenced, the degree of homology varied considerably in most matched mother-infant pairs. One of the 7 mother-infant pairs showed a high degree of similarity for all TTV clones (98.7–100%), 2 pairs had 88–99% homology, and the remaining 4 showed 83.6–89% nucleotide identity. While these findings indicate that colonization with maternal TTV can occur, most acquired TTV is not identical to maternal strains.

These findings suggest a predominance of horizontal, rather than vertical transmission of TTV to infants, whether from their mothers or from other sources.

HUMAN ANELLOVIRUS COLONIZATION AND PREGNANCY-RELATED COMPLICATIONS

Although the bacterial microbiota of various compartments (e.g., vagina, amniotic fluid, and placenta) have been studied in pregnancy (139–143), there has been far less emphasis on the normal or pathological viral community (144, 145). Given the prevalence of anelloviruses in various tissues and body sites of healthy asymptomatic pregnant individuals, several studies have attempted to understand what impact, if any, TTV colonization has on pregnancy, labor, and birth.

Anellovirus Colonization May Have a Role in Determining the Timing of Parturition

Evidence suggests that overt maternal viral infection with influenza (146), hepatitis (147, 148), HIV (149), and herpes (150) can lead to preterm labor and delivery. Although the mechanisms underlying these associations are not clear, it has been suggested that maternal viral infection may predispose toward an exaggerated pro-inflammatory response to a secondary inflammatory stimulus (such as bacterial infection), leading to labor through a "double-hit" mechanism (151, 152). With this premise, we examined the association of virus colonization with a preterm "initiating event of labor" [either spontaneous labor with intact membranes or premature rupture of membranes in the absence of labor (PROM)] using a prospective case-control study (153). We hypothesized that patients experiencing a preterm initiating event of labor (< 37 weeks, "cases") would be more likely to harbor viruses than patients who enter labor at term ("controls"). An initial unbiased screen for viruses performed with next-generation sequencing in serum pooled from 8 cases identified 7 unique viral sequences, all TTVs. Subsequently, 72 patient samples were analyzed individually by nested and semi-nested PCR to identify other anellovirus subtypes. Among patients experiencing spontaneous labor, TTV and TTMV were significantly more prevalent in cases than controls, while TTMDV was not different between the 2 groups. Cases were more likely to harbor at least 1 member of the anellovirus family (91% vs. 68%). In the subgroup of subjects experiencing spontaneous labor with intact membranes, the incidence of TTV was significantly higher in preterm patients (23 of 24 cases) than in controls (8 of 13), whereas there was no difference in TTMDV and TTMV. There were no significant differences in viral subtypes in serum from patients with PROM.

These observations led us to hypothesize that anelloviruses may have a role in determining parturition timing. A potential mechanism for such a phenomenon is through modulation of the inflammatory and immune landscape (154), lowering the threshold for a labor response to stimuli, such as subclinical bacterial infection or non-infectious stimuli, that on their own would be insufficient to induce parturition. It is also possible that, due to the predilection of anelloviruses for leukocytes and the changes in leukocyte populations induced by labor, premature onset of the parturition process is a cause, rather than a consequence, of increased anellovirus recovery in these subjects. Given that the findings are qualitative and were made in a small group of subjects, confirmatory studies are needed.

Anellovirus May Associate With Other Maternal Microbiomes to Precipitate Preterm Birth

A nested case-control study analyzed the vaginal eukaryotic DNA virome and its associations with the bacterial vaginal community and preterm birth (155). Viral communities were analyzed according to diversity, dynamics over time, and association with bacterial community in vaginal swabs collected longitudinally from 60 subjects across pregnancy. Overall, 6 families of human DNA viruses were detected in vaginal samples from pregnant patients, including *Papillomaviridae, Polyomaviridae, Herpesviridae, Poxviridae, Adenoviridae,* and *Anelloviridae.* Anelloviruses were the most common viruses, detected in more than 40% of the patients. Viral richness diminished through the trimesters of pregnancy in subjects who had term delivery. Changes in vaginal virome diversity were similar to changes in the vaginal bacterial microbiome over pregnancy. The 24 pregnant subjects who delivered preterm showed higher viral richness compared to term birth patients. Although higher viral richness was significantly associated with both spontaneous and indicated preterm birth subtypes, no single virus or viral community was associated with preterm birth. Nonetheless, individuals who had both high bacterial diversity [as is seen in bacterial vaginosis, itself associated with preterm birth (156)] and high viral diversity early in pregnancy had the highest risk for preterm birth.

Evidence links the composition of the vaginal microbiome with immune status and variations in cervical length in pregnant people (157, 158). Specifically, when *Lactobacillus crispatus* is dominant, the vaginal level of D-lactic acid isomer is high, matrix metalloproteinase (MMP)-8 is low, and vaginal inflammation tends to be absent. Conversely, when *Lactobacillus iners* or bacteria other than lactobacilli are dominant, D-lactic acid levels are low, and MMP-8 levels are high, which is associated with a more pro-inflammatory vaginal environment and overall shorter cervical lengths (159). A recent cohort study of 121 pregnant subjects investigated TTV presence in vaginal secretions, and how its occurrence and/or titer varies with the dominant bacteria in the vaginal microbiome (65). Vaginal secretions collected from pregnant individuals in their first trimester (≤12 weeks), third trimester (28–38 weeks), and 28–45 days postpartum were analyzed for TTV DNA by quantitative PCR. Approximately 40% of pregnant individuals who delivered a healthy baby at term had TTV detected in their vaginal secretions during at least 1 of these time points. In subjects who were tested at all time points ($n = 33$), those who were TTV-positive in the first trimester were equally likely to became negative or remain positive throughout the other sampling time points. These findings suggest that vaginal TTV colonization is most often associated with healthy gestation and normal outcomes. However, the correlation between vaginal TTV and features of bacterial vaginosis provides a mechanism by which anellovirus colonization may lead to preterm delivery. In the first trimester, *L. crispatus* was dominant in 66.7% of pregnant individuals who were negative for TTV, as opposed to 25% of those who were TTV-positive, and D-lactic acid levels were diminished in TTV-positive patients. Similarly, in the third trimester, *L. crispatus* was dominant in 50% of pregnant individuals who were TTV-negative and only 6% of those who were TTV-positive. In summary, vaginal TTV colonization appears to correlate with features of bacterial vaginosis (diminished predominance of *L. crispatus*, higher MMP-8, and lower D-lactic acid levels).

Adverse Pregnancy Outcomes May Not Be Associated With Anellovirus Presence or Quantity

A study determined the prevalence of viruses in matched maternal-infant preterm cohorts and ascertained whether viral presence or load correlates with histologic chorioamnionitis, spontaneous preterm labor, and preeclampsia (160). Preterm labor was defined as spontaneous preterm labor or preterm premature rupture of membranes that resulted in very premature delivery <31 weeks. Histological chorioamnionitis was determined by placental pathology, and preeclampsia was based on clinical diagnosis. Whole blood or plasma collected from 56 matched mothers and premature infants was analyzed for the presence and quantity of anellovirus and 8 other viruses by qPCR. Twenty-nine of the 56 maternal samples contained viral nucleic acid, of which anellovirus was most prevalent (26 samples). However, there was no association of presence or quantity of viral load in samples from mothers with or without preeclampsia, histological chorioamnionitis, or preterm labor. Taken together, this study suggests no clear relationship between TTV load and perinatal morbidity or spontaneous preterm labor, though its small size and focus only on extreme prematurity are limitations that require validation.

A MECHANISM BY WHICH ANELLOVIRUS COLONIZATION COULD INFLUENCE THE TIMING OF PARTURITION

The link between infection and preterm labor has long been recognized. In some instances, this may entail the initial presence of microorganisms (whether bacterial, viral, or fungal) which creates a favorable environment or amplifies the effect of a secondary infection. As noted above, experimental models illustrate the potential for synergy between viral and bacterial infections leading to amplification of host responses. Polyinosinic:cytidylic acid [poly(I:C)] is a TLR3 ligand and synthetic analog of double-stranded RNA, which is a replication intermediate for most viruses, including DNA viruses. Poly(I:C) induces preterm delivery when injected either into the uterus (152) or systemically (161) in mid- to late gestation and greatly amplifies the potency of bacterial products in mice when injected into the uterus (162). In a mouse model, it has been demonstrated that viral infection of the cervix during pregnancy reduces the capacity of the female reproductive tract to prevent bacterial infection of the uterus (163). Similarly, sub-clinical viral infection in pregnant mice has been shown to sensitize them to bacterial infection, leading to preterm delivery (151). These findings suggest the existence of synergism during combined viral and bacterial infection. This "2 hit" trigger and existence of synergism might be a beneficial strategy to a host, as it would blunt the maternal response to mild insults (such as subclinical infection), while providing for rapid and efficient amplification of the labor response in cases of a superimposed or more severe infection. Given the higher prevalence of circulating anellovirus in preterm than in term patients (153), and TTV's association with other bacterial communities linked to preterm birth (65, 155), we propose that anellovirus colonization during gestation might affect the onset of labor through lowering the threshold for a response to stimuli, such as subclinical bacterial infection, that on their own would be insufficient to induce parturition.

On the other hand, pregnant patients who have a normal term pregnancy and give birth to a healthy infant may harbor viral sequences or genogroups that protect against preterm labor. Functional studies have revealed that apathogenic, endogenous retroviruses (ERV), and ERV-derived proteins found in the placenta mediate cell-cell fusion, suppress maternal immunity, and protect the fetus from exogenous viruses (164). Given the evidence that TTV ORF2 protein suppresses NF-κB pathways and inhibits transcription of proinflammatory cytokine genes (86), it is possible that TTVs may act as "little helpers" in shaping the gene networks of innate and adaptive immune responses to maintain normal pregnancy.

In the majority of human body sites, microbial diversity is considered a signature of health (1). If multiple variants or genotypes of anellovirus ("anellome") found in healthy humans remain stable for a long time, they may make up the personalized and healthy part of the host microbiome (92). The gene products of anellovirus might help to maintain the composition and fitness of other (beneficial) microbial communities by preventing colonization by pathogens. At the same time, the host immune system, through immunosurveillance, may maintain a safe balance, thus protecting the body from the pathogenic effects of the virus (165). However, as noted above, microbial diversity (including anellovirus) in the pregnant vagina is associated with premature timing of delivery. In summary, under physiological conditions, human anellovirus is unlikely to be pathogenic *per se*. Nonetheless, perturbations in host defense and microbial composition may allow anellovirus to achieve an opportunistic pathogen status.

FUTURE DIRECTIONS

At present, the quality and number of studies on the association of anelloviruses with pregnancy outcomes are limited. Large cohort studies are important to clarify the role, if any, of anellovirus colonization in the timing of labor. Investigations are warranted with a focus on determining the kinetics of anellovirus colonization over the course of pregnancy, and whether certain genogroups promote or suppress preterm birth. Studying anellovirus abundance in other conditions associated with pregnancy, such as miscarriage, preeclampsia, and gestational diabetes, will provide more detailed insight in the relationship between anellovirus colonization and clinical outcomes.

CONCLUSIONS

The impact of anelloviruses on human health remains incompletely characterized. Although the possible pathogenicity of anelloviruses is still an open question, further study of anellovirus colonization during pregnancy and in mother-infant pairs will help determine whether and how these ubiquitous viruses affect microbial infection-associated preterm labor and preterm birth.

AUTHOR CONTRIBUTIONS

CK, MS, and EH contributed to the literature review and composition of the present text. All authors reviewed and approved the final version of the manuscript.

REFERENCES

1. Dekaboruah E, Suryavanshi MV, Chettri D, Verma AK. Human microbiome: an academic update on human body site specific surveillance and its possible role. *Arch Microbiol.* (2020) 202:2147–67. doi: 10.1007/s00203-020-01931-x
2. Scotti E, Boue S, Lo Sasso G, Zanetti F, Belcastro V, Poussin C, et al. Exploring the microbiome in health and disease: implications for toxicology. *Toxicol Res Appl.* (2017) 1:1–37. doi: 10.1177/2397847317741884
3. Moustafa A, Xie C, Kirkness E, Biggs W, Wong E, Turpaz Y, et al. The blood DNA virome in 8,000 humans. *PLoS Pathog.* (2017) 13:e1006292. doi: 10.1371/journal.ppat.1006292
4. Liang G, Bushman FD. The human virome: assembly, composition and host interactions. *Nat Rev Microbiol.* (2021) 19:514–27. doi: 10.1038/s41579-021-00536-5
5. Al-Qahtani AA, Alabsi ES, AbuOdeh R, Thalib L, El Zowalaty ME, Nasrallah GK. Prevalence of anelloviruses (TTV, TTMDV, and TTMV) in healthy blood donors and in patients infected with HBV or HCV in Qatar. *Virol J.* (2016) 13:208. doi: 10.1186/s12985-016-0664-6
6. De Vlaminck I, Khush KK, Strehl C, Kohli B, Luikart H, Neff NF, et al. Temporal response of the human virome to immunosuppression and antiviral therapy. *Cell.* (2013) 155:1178–87. doi: 10.1016/j.cell.2013.10.034
7. Spandole-Dinu S, Cimponeriu DG, Craciun AM, Radu I, Nica S, Toma M, et al. Prevalence of human anelloviruses in Romanian healthy subjects and patients with common pathologies. *BMC Infect Dis.* (2018) 18:334. doi: 10.1186/s12879-018-3248-9
8. Bzhalava D, Ekstrom J, Lysholm F, Hultin E, Faust H, Persson B, et al. Phylogenetically diverse TT virus viremia among pregnant women. *Virology.* (2012) 432:427–34. doi: 10.1016/j.virol.2012.06.022
9. Matsubara H, Michitaka K, Horiike N, Kihana T, Yano M, Mori T, et al. Existence of TT virus DNA and TTV-like mini virus DNA in infant cord blood: mother-to-neonatal transmission. *Hepatol Res.* (2001) 21:280–7. doi: 10.1016/S1386-6346(01)00115-2
10. Goto K, Sugiyama K, Ando T, Mizutani F, Terabe K, Tanaka K, et al. Detection rates of TT virus DNA in serum of umbilical cord blood, breast milk and saliva. *Tohoku J Exp Med.* (2000) 191:203–7. doi: 10.1620/tjem.191.203
11. Nishizawa T, Okamoto H, Konishi K, Yoshizawa H, Miyakawa Y, Mayumi M. A novel DNA virus (TTV) associated with elevated transaminase levels in posttransfusion hepatitis of unknown etiology. *Biochem Biophys Res Commun.* (1997) 241:92–7. doi: 10.1006/bbrc.1997.7765
12. Bendinelli M, Pistello M, Maggi F, Fornai C, Freer G, Vatteroni ML. Molecular properties, biology, and clinical implications of TT virus, a recently identified widespread infectious agent of humans. *Clin Microbiol Rev.* (2001) 14:98–113. doi: 10.1128/CMR.14.1.98-113.2001
13. Takahashi K, Iwasa Y, Hijikata M, Mishiro S. Identification of a new human DNA virus (TTV-like mini virus, TLMV) intermediately related to TT virus and chicken anemia virus. *Arch Virol.* (2000) 145:979–93. doi: 10.1007/s007050050689
14. Ninomiya M, Takahashi M, Shimosegawa T, Okamoto H. Analysis of the entire genomes of fifteen torque teno midi virus variants classifiable into a third group of genus Anellovirus. *Arch Virol.* (2007) 152:1961–75. doi: 10.1007/s00705-007-1046-6
15. Biagini P, Todd D, Bendinelli M, Hino S, Mankertz A, Mishiro S, et al. Anellovirus. In: Fauquet CM, Mayo MA, Maniloff J, Desselberger U, Ball LA, editors. *Virus Taxonomy.* London: Elsevier/Academic Press (2005). p. 335–41.
16. King AMQ, Adams MJ, Carstens EB, Lefkowitz EJ. Virus Taxonomy: Classification and Nomenclature of Viruses: Ninth Report of the International Committee on Taxonomy of Viruses. London; Waltham: Academic Press. Elsevier, San Diego (2012). p. 331–41.
17. Tyschik EA, Rasskazova AS, Degtyareva AV, Rebrikov DV, Sukhikh GT. Torque teno virus dynamics during the first year of life. *Virol J.* (2018) 15:96. doi: 10.1186/s12985-018-1007-6
18. Lim ES, Zhou Y, Zhao G, Bauer IK, Droit L, Ndao IM, et al. Early life dynamics of the human gut virome and bacterial microbiome in infants. *Nat Med.* (2015) 21:1228–34. doi: 10.1038/nm.3950
19. Haloschan M, Bettesch R, Gorzer I, Weseslindtner L, Kundi M, Puchhammer-Stockl E. TTV DNA plasma load and its association with age, gender, and HCMV IgG serostatus in healthy adults. *Age (Dordr).* (2014) 36:9716. doi: 10.1007/s11357-014-9716-2
20. McElvania TeKippe E, Wylie KM, Deych E, Sodergren E, Weinstock G, et al. Increased prevalence of anellovirus in pediatric patients with fever. *PLoS One.* (2012) 7:e50937. doi: 10.1371/journal.pone.0050937
21. Kazemi MJ, Yaghobi R, Saadi IM, Geramizadeh B, Moayedi J. Association between TT virus infection and cirrhosis in liver transplant patients. *Hepat Mon.* (2015) 15:e28370. doi: 10.5812/hepatmon.28370
22. Feyzioglu B, Teke T, Ozdemir M, Karaibrahimoglu A, Dogan M, Yavsan M. The presence of Torque teno virus in chronic obstructive pulmonary disease. *Int J Clin Exp Med.* (2014) 7:3461–6.

23. Abbas AA, Diamond JM, Chehoud C, Chang B, Kotzin JJ, Young JC, et al. The perioperative lung transplant virome: Torque Teno Viruses are elevated in donor lungs and show divergent dynamics in primary graft dysfunction. *Am J Transplant.* (2017) 17:1313–24. doi: 10.1111/ajt.14076
24. Maggi F, Pifferi M, Fornai C, Andreoli E, Tempestini E, Vatteroni M, et al. TT virus in the nasal secretions of children with acute respiratory diseases: relations to viremia and disease severity. *J Virol.* (2003) 77:2418–25. doi: 10.1128/JVI.77.4.2418-2425.2003
25. Liu B, Shao N, Wang J, Zhou S, Su H, Dong J, et al. An optimized metagenomic approach for virome detection of clinical pharyngeal samples with respiratory infection. *Front Microbiol.* (2020) 11:1552. doi: 10.3389/fmicb.2020.01552
26. Dodi G, Attanasi M, Di Filippo P, Di Pillo S, Chiarelli F, et al. Virome in the lungs: the role of anelloviruses in childhood respiratory diseases. *Microorganisms.* (2021) 9:1357. doi: 10.3390/microorganisms9071357
27. Camci C, Guney C, Balkan A, Buyukberber N, Buyukberber S, Kadayifci A, et al. The prevalence of TT virus in cancer patients. *New Microbiol.* (2002) 25:463–8.
28. Sawata T, Bando M, Nakayama M, Mato N, Yamasawa H, Takahashi M, et al. Clinical significance of changes in Torque teno virus DNA titer after chemotherapy in patients with primary lung cancer. *Respir Investig.* (2018) 56:173–8. doi: 10.1016/j.resinv.2017.12.004
29. Bando M, Takahashi M, Ohno S, Hosono T, Hironaka M, Okamoto H, et al. Torque teno virus DNA titre elevated in idiopathic pulmonary fibrosis with primary lung cancer. *Respirology.* (2008) 13:263–9. doi: 10.1111/j.1440-1843.2007.01217.x
30. Hettmann A, Demcsak A, Bach A, Decsi G, Dencs A, Palinko D, et al. Detection and phylogenetic analysis of torque teno virus in salivary and tumor biopsy samples from head and neck carcinoma patients. *Intervirology.* (2016) 59:123–9. doi: 10.1159/000452974
31. Garcia-Alvarez M, Berenguer J, Alvarez E, Guzman-Fulgencio M, Cosin J, Miralles P, et al. Association of torque teno virus (TTV) and torque teno mini virus (TTMV) with liver disease among patients coinfected with human immunodeficiency virus and hepatitis C virus. *Eur J Clin Microbiol Infect Dis.* (2013) 32:289–97. doi: 10.1007/s10096-012-1744-1
32. Gergely P Jr, Pullmann R, Stancato C, Otvos L Jr, Koncz A, Blazsek A, et al. Increased prevalence of transfusion-transmitted virus and cross-reactivity with immunodominant epitopes of the HRES-1/p28 endogenous retroviral autoantigen in patients with systemic lupus erythematosus. *Clin Immunol.* (2005) 116:124–34. doi: 10.1016/j.clim.2005.04.002
33. Maggi F, Andreoli E, Riente L, Meschi S, Rocchi J, Delle Sedie A, et al. Torquetenovirus in patients with arthritis. *Rheumatology (Oxford).* (2007) 46:885–6. doi: 10.1093/rheumatology/kem032
34. Yu T, Pan S, Zhang Y, Pei J, Liu J, Xie Y, et al. Occurrence and quantification of Anelloviruses and Herpesviruses in gingival tissue in Chinese Shanghai sub-population. *BMC Oral Health.* (2020) 20:196. doi: 10.1186/s12903-020-01188-2
35. Rezahosseini O, Drabe CH, Sorensen SS, Rasmussen A, Perch M, Ostrowski SR, et al. Torque-Teno virus viral load as a potential endogenous marker of immune function in solid organ transplantation. *Transplant Rev.* (2019) 33:137–44. doi: 10.1016/j.trre.2019.03.004
36. Mouton W, Conrad A, Bal A, Boccard M, Malcus C, Ducastelle-Lepretre S, et al. Torque teno virus viral load as a marker of immune function in allogeneic haematopoietic stem cell transplantation recipients. *Viruses.* (2020) 12:1292. doi: 10.3390/v12111292
37. Mrzljak A, Vilibic-Cavlek T. Torque teno virus in liver diseases and after liver transplantation. *World J Transplant.* (2020) 10:291–6. doi: 10.5500/wjt.v10.i11.291
38. Jarkasi NS, Sekawi Z, Kqueen CY, Othman Z. A review on the global widespread of TTV infection among human population. *Pertanika J Scholarly Res Rev.* (2018) 4:10–24.
39. Bzhalava D, Hultin E, Arroyo Muhr LS, Ekstrom J, Lehtinen M. Viremia during pregnancy and risk of childhood leukemia and lymphomas in the offspring: Nested case-control study. *Int J Cancer.* (2016) 138:2212–20. doi: 10.1002/ijc.29666
40. Deng X, Terunuma H, Handema R, Sakamoto M, Kitamura T, Ito M, et al. Higher prevalence and viral load of TT virus in saliva than in the corresponding serum: another possible transmission route and replication site of TT virus. *J Med Virol.* (2000) 62:531–7.
41. Gallian P, Biagini P, Zhong S, Touinssi M, Yeo W, Cantaloube JF, et al. TT virus: a study of molecular epidemiology and transmission of genotypes 1, 2 and 3. *J Clin Virol.* (2000) 17:43–9. doi: 10.1016/S1386-6532(00)00066-4
42. Matsubara H, Michitaka K, Horiike N, Yano M, Akbar SM, Torisu M, et al. Existence of TT virus DNA in extracellular body fluids from normal healthy Japanese subjects. *Intervirology.* (2000) 43:16–9. doi: 10.1159/000025018
43. Lopez-Alcorocho JM, Mariscal LF, de Lucas S, Rodriguez-Inigo E, Casqueiro M, Castillo I, et al. Presence of TTV DNA in serum, liver and peripheral blood mononuclear cells from patients with chronic hepatitis. *J Viral Hepat.* (2000) 7:440–7. doi: 10.1046/j.1365-2893.2000.00252.x
44. Tyschik EA, Shcherbakova SM, Ibragimov RR, Rebrikov DV. Transplacental transmission of torque teno virus. *Virol J.* (2017) 14:92. doi: 10.1186/s12985-017-0762-0
45. Schroter M, Polywka S, Zollner B, Schafer P, Laufs R, Feucht HH. Detection of TT virus DNA and GB virus type C/Hepatitis G virus RNA in serum and breast milk: determination of mother-to-child transmission. *J Clin Microbiol.* (2000) 38:745–7. doi: 10.1128/JCM.38.2.745-747.2000
46. Wylie KM, Wylie TN, Buller R, Herter B, Cannella MT, Storch GA. Detection of viruses in clinical samples by use of metagenomic sequencing and targeted sequence capture. *J Clin Microbiol.* (2018) 56:e01123-18. doi: 10.1128/JCM.01123-18
47. Zhang Z, Zhang Z. [Detection of transfusion transmitted virus infection and genotypes in pregnant women]. *Zhonghua Fu Chan Ke Za Zhi.* (2001) 36:325–7.
48. Okamoto H, Nishizawa T, Takahashi M, Asabe S, Tsuda F, Yoshikawa A. Heterogeneous distribution of TT virus of distinct genotypes in multiple tissues from infected humans. *Virology.* (2001) 288:358–68. doi: 10.1006/viro.2001.1097
49. Biagini P, Gallian P, Attoui H, Touinssi M, Cantaloube JF, de Micco P, et al. Genetic analysis of full-length genomes and subgenomic sequences of TT virus-like mini virus human isolates. *J Gen Virol.* (2001) 82(Pt 2):379–83. doi: 10.1099/0022-1317-82-2-379
50. Maggi F, Fornai C, Zaccaro L, Morrica A, Vatteroni ML, Isola P, et al. TT virus (TTV) loads associated with different peripheral blood cell types and evidence for TTV replication in activated mononuclear cells. *J Med Virol.* (2001) 64:190–4. doi: 10.1002/jmv.1035
51. Takahashi M, Asabe S, Gotanda Y, Kishimoto J, Tsuda F, Okamoto H. TT virus is distributed in various leukocyte subpopulations at distinct levels, with the highest viral load in granulocytes. *Biochem Biophys Res Commun.* (2002) 290:242–8. doi: 10.1006/bbrc.2001.6183
52. Martelli F, Macera L, Spezia PG, Medici C, Pistello M, Guasti D, et al. Torquetenovirus detection in exosomes enriched vesicles circulating in human plasma samples. *Virol J.* (2018) 15:145. doi: 10.1186/s12985-018-1055-y
53. Lewandowska DW, Schreiber PW, Schuurmans MM, Ruehe B, Zagordi O, Bayard C, et al. Metagenomic sequencing complements routine diagnostics in identifying viral pathogens in lung transplant recipients with unknown etiology of respiratory infection. *PLoS ONE.* (2017) 12:e0177340. doi: 10.1371/journal.pone.0177340
54. Inami T, Konomi N, Arakawa Y, Abe K. High prevalence of TT virus DNA in human saliva and semen. *J Clin Microbiol.* (2000) 38:2407–8. doi: 10.1128/JCM.38.6.2407-2408.2000
55. Okamoto H, Nishizawa T, Kato N, Ukita M, Ikeda H, Iizuka H, et al. Molecular cloning and characterization of a novel DNA virus (TTV) associated with posttransfusion hepatitis of unknown etiology. *Hepatol Res.* (1998) 10:1–16. doi: 10.1016/S1386-6346(97)00123-X
56. Ukita M, Okamoto H, Kato N, Miyakawa Y, Mayumi M. Excretion into bile of a novel unenveloped DNA virus (TT virus) associated with acute and chronic non-A-G hepatitis. *J Infect Dis.* (1999) 179:1245–8. doi: 10.1086/314716
57. Taboada B, Moran P, Serrano-Vazquez A, Isa P, Rojas-Velazquez L, Perez-Juarez H, et al. The gut virome of healthy children during the first year of life is diverse and dynamic. *PLoS ONE.* (2021) 16:e0240958. doi: 10.1371/journal.pone.0240958
58. Okamoto H, Akahane Y, Ukita M, Fukuda M, Tsuda F, Miyakawa Y, et al. Fecal excretion of a nonenveloped DNA virus (TTV) associated

with posttransfusion non-A-G hepatitis. *J Med Virol.* (1998) 56:128–32. doi: 10.1002/(SICI)1096-9071(199810)56:2<128::AID-JMV5>3.0.CO;2-A

59. Ross RS, Viazov S, Runde V, Schaefer UW, Roggendorf M. Detection of TT virus DNA in specimens other than blood. *J Clin Virol.* (1999) 13:181–4. doi: 10.1016/S1386-6532(99)00015-3
60. Burian Z, Szabo H, Szekely G, Gyurkovits K, Pankovics P, Farkas T, et al. Detection and follow-up of torque teno midi virus (small anelloviruses) in nasopharyngeal aspirates and three other human body fluids in children. *Arch Virol.* (2011) 156:1537–41. doi: 10.1007/s00705-011-1021-0
61. Mortazkar P, Karbalaie Niya MH, Javanmard D, Esghaei M, Keyvani H. Molecular epidemiology of anellovirus infection in children's urine: a cross-sectional study. *Adv Biomed Res.* (2020) 9:16. doi: 10.4103/abr.abr_169_19
62. Osiowy C, Sauder C. Detection of TT virus in human hair and skin. *Hepatol Res.* (2000) 16:155–62. doi: 10.1016/S1386-6346(99)00046-7
63. Chan PK, Tam WH, Yeo W, Cheung JL, Zhong S, Cheng AF. High carriage rate of TT virus in the cervices of pregnant women. *Clin Infect Dis.* (2001) 32:1376–7. doi: 10.1086/319983
64. Fornai C, Maggi F, Vatteroni ML, Pistello M, Bendinelli M. High prevalence of TT virus (TTV) and TTV-like minivirus in cervical swabs. *J Clin Microbiol.* (2001) 39:2022–4. doi: 10.1128/JCM.39.5.2022-2024.2001
65. Tozetto-Mendoza TR, Bongiovanni AM, Minis E, Linhares IM, Boester A, Freire WS, et al. Torquetenovirus titer in vaginal secretions from pregnant and postpartum women: association with absence of lactobacillus crispatus and levels of lactic acid and matrix metalloproteinase-8. *Reprod Sci.* (2020) 27:2075–81. doi: 10.1007/s43032-020-00227-1
66. Reyes A, Blanton LV, Cao S, Zhao G, Manary M, Trehan I, et al. Gut DNA viromes of Malawian twins discordant for severe acute malnutrition. *Proc Natl Acad Sci U S A.* (2015) 112:11941–6. doi: 10.1073/pnas.1514285112
67. Salakova M, Nemecek V, Konig J, Tachezy R. Age-specific prevalence, transmission and phylogeny of TT virus in the Czech Republic. *BMC Infect Dis.* (2004) 4:56. doi: 10.1186/1471-2334-4-56
68. Zhong S, Yeo W, Lin CK, Lin XR, Tang MW, Johnson PJ. Quantitative and genotypic analysis of TT virus infection in Chinese blood donors. *Transfusion.* (2001) 41:1001–7. doi: 10.1046/j.1537-2995.2001.41081001.x
69. Saback FL, Gomes SA, de Paula VS, da Silva RR, Lewis-Ximenez LL, Niel C. Age-specific prevalence and transmission of TT virus. *J Med Virol.* (1999) 59:318–22. doi: 10.1002/(sici)1096-9071(199911)59:3<318::aid-jmv10>3.0.co;2-q
70. Focosi D, Spezia PG, Macera L, Salvadori S, Navarro D, Lanza M, et al. Assessment of prevalence and load of torquetenovirus viraemia in a large cohort of healthy blood donors. *Clin Microbiol Infect.* (2020) 26:1406–10. doi: 10.1016/j.cmi.2020.01.011
71. Mushahwar IK, Erker JC, Muerhoff AS, Leary TP, Simons JN, Birkenmeyer LG, et al. Molecular and biophysical characterization of TT virus: evidence for a new virus family infecting humans. *Proc Natl Acad Sci U S A.* (1999) 96:3177–82. doi: 10.1073/pnas.96.6.3177
72. Touinssi M, Gallian P, Biagini P, Attoui H, Vialettes B, Berland Y, et al. TT virus infection: prevalence of elevated viraemia and arguments for the immune control of viral load. *J Clin Virol.* (2001) 21:135–41. doi: 10.1016/S1386-6532(01)00157-3
73. Burra P, Masier A, Boldrin C, Calistri A, Andreoli E, Senzolo M, et al. Torque Teno Virus: any pathological role in liver transplanted patients? *Transpl Int.* (2008) 21:972–9. doi: 10.1111/j.1432-2277.2008.00714.x
74. Gorzer I, Jaksch P, Kundi M, Seitz T, Klepetko W, Puchhammer-Stockl E. Pre-transplant plasma Torque Teno virus load and increase dynamics after lung transplantation. *PLoS One.* (2015) 10:e0122975. doi: 10.1371/journal.pone.0122975
75. Maggi F, Ricci V, Bendinelli M, Nelli LC, Focosi D, Papineschi F, et al. Changes In CD8+57+ T lymphocyte expansions after autologous hematopoietic stem cell transplantation correlate with changes in torquetenovirus viremia. *Transplantation.* (2008) 85:1867–8. doi: 10.1097/TP.0b013e31817615e6
76. Masouridi-Levrat S, Pradier A, Simonetta F, Kaiser L, Chalandon Y, Roosnek E. Torque teno virus in patients undergoing allogeneic hematopoietic stem cell transplantation for hematological malignancies. *Bone Marrow Transplant.* (2016) 51:440–2. doi: 10.1038/bmt.2015.262
77. Gorzer I, Haloschan M, Jaksch P, Klepetko W, Puchhammer-Stockl E. Plasma DNA levels of Torque teno virus and immunosuppression after lung transplantation. *J Heart Lung Transplant.* (2014) 33:320–3. doi: 10.1016/j.healun.2013.12.007
78. Thom K, Petrik J. Progression towards AIDS leads to increased Torque teno virus and Torque teno minivirus titers in tissues of HIV infected individuals. *J Med Virol.* (2007) 79:1–7. doi: 10.1002/jmv.20756
79. Walton AH, Muenzer JT, Rasche D, Boomer JS, Sato B, Brownstein BH, et al. Reactivation of multiple viruses in patients with sepsis. *PLoS One.* (2014) 9:e98819. doi: 10.1371/journal.pone.0098819
80. Shibayama T, Masuda G, Ajisawa A, Takahashi M, Nishizawa T, Tsuda F, et al. Inverse relationship between the titre of TT virus DNA and the CD4 cell count in patients infected with HIV. *AIDS.* (2001) 15:563–70. doi: 10.1097/00002030-200103300-00004
81. Blatter JA, Sweet SC, Conrad C, Danziger-Isakov LA, Faro A, Goldfarb SB, et al. Anellovirus loads are associated with outcomes in pediatric lung transplantation. *Pediatr Transplant.* (2018) 22:10.1111/petr.13069. doi: 10.1111/petr.13069
82. Itoh Y, Takahashi M, Fukuda M, Shibayama T, Ishikawa T, Tsuda F, et al. Visualization of TT virus particles recovered from the sera and feces of infected humans. *Biochem Biophys Res Commun.* (2000) 279:718–24. doi: 10.1006/bbrc.2000.4013
83. Leppik L, Gunst K, Lehtinen M, Dillner J, Streker, de Villiers EM, et al. *In vivo* and *in vitro* intragenomic rearrangement of TT viruses. *J Virol.* (2007) 81:9346–56. doi: 10.1128/JVI.00781-07
84. Hallett RL, Clewley JP, Bobet F, McKiernan PJ, Teo CG. Characterization of a highly divergent TT virus genome. *J Gen Virol.* (2000) 81:2273–9. doi: 10.1099/0022-1317-81-9-2273
85. Qiu J, Kakkola L, Cheng F, Ye C, Soderlund-Venermo M, Hedman K, et al. Human circovirus TT virus genotype 6 expresses six proteins following transfection of a full-length clone. *J Virol.* (2005) 79:6505–10. doi: 10.1128/JVI.79.10.6505-6510.2005
86. Zheng H, Ye L, Fang X, Li B, Wang Y, Xiang X, et al. Torque teno virus (SANBAN isolate) ORF2 protein suppresses NF-kappaB pathways via interaction with IkappaB kinases. *J Virol.* (2007) 81:11917–24. doi: 10.1128/JVI.01101-07
87. Kakkola L, Hedman K, Qiu J, Pintel D, Soderlund-Venermo M. Replication of and protein synthesis by TT viruses. *Curr Top Microbiol Immunol.* (2009) 331:53–64. doi: 10.1007/978-3-540-70972-5_4
88. Kooistra K, Zhang YH, Henriquez NV, Weiss B, Mumberg D, Noteborn MHM. TT virus-derived apoptosis-inducing protein induces apoptosis preferentially in hepatocellular carcinoma-derived cells. *J Gen Virol.* (2004) 85:1445–50. doi: 10.1099/vir.0.79790-0
89. Nishizawa T, Okamoto H, Tsuda F, Aikawa T, Sugai Y, Konishi K, et al. Quasispecies of TT virus (TTV) with sequence divergence in hypervariable regions of the capsid protein in chronic TTV infection. *J Virol.* (1999) 73:9604–8. doi: 10.1128/JVI.73.11.9604-9608.1999
90. Cebria-Mendoza M, Arbona C, Larrea L, Diaz W, Arnau V, Pena C, et al. Deep viral blood metagenomics reveals extensive anellovirus diversity in healthy humans. *Sci Rep.* (2021) 11:6921. doi: 10.1038/s41598-021-86427-4
91. Biagini P. Human circoviruses. *Vet Microbiol.* (2004) 98:95–101. doi: 10.1016/j.vetmic.2003.10.004
92. Arze CA, Springer S, Dudas G, Patel S, Bhattacharyya A, Swaminathan H, et al. Global genome analysis reveals a vast and dynamic anellovirus landscape within the human virome. *Cell Host Microbe.* (2021) 29:1305–15 e6. doi: 10.1016/j.chom.2021.07.001
93. Maggi F, Andreoli E, Lanini L, Fornai C, Vatteroni M, Pistello M, et al. Relationships between total plasma load of torquetenovirus (TTV) and TTV genogroups carried. *J Clin Microbiol.* (2005) 43:4807–10. doi: 10.1128/JCM.43.9.4807-4810.2005
94. de Castro Amarante MF, Kashima S, Covas DT. TT virus (TTV) genotyping in blood donors and multiple transfused patients in Brazil. *Virus Genes.* (2007) 35:503–9. doi: 10.1007/s11262-007-0124-x
95. Okamoto H, Takahashi M, Nishizawa T, Ukita M, Fukuda M, Tsuda F, et al. Marked genomic heterogeneity and frequent mixed infection of TT virus demonstrated by PCR with primers from coding and noncoding regions. *Virology.* (1999) 259:428–36. doi: 10.1006/viro.1999.9770
96. Devalle S, Niel C. Distribution of TT virus genomic groups 1-5 in Brazilian blood donors, HBV carriers, HIV-1-infected patients. *J Med Virol.* (2004) 72:166–73. doi: 10.1002/jmv.10564

97. Ninomiya M, Takahashi M, Nishizawa T, Shimosegawa T, Okamoto H. Development of PCR assays with nested primers specific for differential detection of three human anelloviruses and early acquisition of dual or triple infection during infancy. *J Clin Microbiol.* (2008) 46:507–14. doi: 10.1128/JCM.01703-07
98. Najafimemar Z, Tabarraei A, Talei G, Moradi A. Prevalence and genotyping of Torque Teno Virus in HBV/HIV and chronic HBV patients in Iran. *Iran Biomed J.* (2018) 22:338–44. doi: 10.29252/ibj.22.5.338
99. Peng J, Fang Y, Zhao X, Peng Y. New prevalence estimate of Torque Teno virus (TTV) infection in healthy population and patients with chronic viral hepatitis in Jiujiang, China. *Virol Sin.* (2015) 30:218–20. doi: 10.1007/s12250-014-3531-x
100. Kenar Koohi A, Ravanshad M, Rasouli M, Falahi S, Baghban A. Phylogenetic analysis of torque teno virus in hepatitis C virus infected patients in shiraz. *Hepat Mon.* (2012) 12:437–41. doi: 10.5812/hepatmon.6133
101. Hsiao KL, Wang LY, Lin CL, Liu HF. New phylogenetic groups of Torque teno virus identified in Eastern Taiwan Indigenes. *PLoS One.* (2016) 11:e0149901. doi: 10.1371/journal.pone.0149901
102. Hu YW, Al-Moslih MI, Al Ali MT, Khameneh SR, Perkins H, Diaz-Mitoma F, et al. Molecular detection method for all known genotypes of TT virus (TTV) and TTV-like viruses in thalassemia patients and healthy individuals. *J Clin Microbiol.* (2005) 43:3747–54. doi: 10.1128/JCM.43.8.3747-3754.2005
103. Mankotia DS, Irshad M. Cloning and expression of N22 region of Torque Teno virus (TTV) genome and use of peptide in developing immunoassay for TTV antibodies. *Virol J.* (2014) 11:96. doi: 10.1186/1743-422X-11-96
104. Okamoto H, Takahashi M, Kato N, Fukuda M, Tawara A, Fukuda S, et al. Sequestration of TT virus of restricted genotypes in peripheral blood mononuclear cells. *J Virol.* (2000) 74:10236–9. doi: 10.1128/JVI.74.21.10236-10239.2000
105. Okamura A, Yoshioka M, Kubota M, Kikuta H, Ishiko H, Kobayashi K. Detection of a novel DNA virus (TTV) sequence in peripheral blood mononuclear cells. *J Med Virol.* (1999) 58:174–7. doi: 10.1002/(sici)1096-9071(199906)58:2<174::aid-jmv12>3.0.co;2-x
106. Schiemann M, Puchhammer-Stockl E, Eskandary F, Kohlbeck P, Rasoul-Rockenschaub S, Heilos A. Torque Teno Virus Load-Inverse Association with antibody-mediated rejection after kidney transplantation. *Transplantation.* (2017) 101:360–7. doi: 10.1097/TP.0000000000001455
107. Kosulin K, Kernbichler S, Pichler H, Lawitschka A, Geyeregger R, Witt V, et al. Post-transplant replication of Torque Teno Virus in Granulocytes. *Front Microbiol.* (2018) 9:2956. doi: 10.3389/fmicb.2018.02956
108. Kikuchi K, Miyakawa H, Abe K, Kako M, Katayama K, Fukushi S, et al. Indirect evidence of TTV replication in bone marrow cells, but not in hepatocytes, of a subacute hepatitis/aplastic anemia patient. *J Med Virol.* (2000) 61:165–70.
109. Desai M, Pal R, Deshmukh R, Banker D. Replication of TT virus in hepatocyte and leucocyte cell lines. *J Med Virol.* (2005) 77:136–43. doi: 10.1002/jmv.20426
110. Okamoto H, Ukita M, Nishizawa T, Kishimoto J, Hoshi Y, Mizuo H, et al. Circular double-stranded forms of TT virus DNA in the liver. *J Virol.* (2000) 74:5161–7. doi: 10.1128/JVI.74.11.5161-5167.2000
111. Young JC, Chehoud C, Bittinger K, Bailey A, Diamond JM, Cantu E, et al. Viral metagenomics reveal blooms of anelloviruses in the respiratory tract of lung transplant recipients. *Am J Transplant.* (2015) 15:200–9. doi: 10.1111/ajt.13031
112. Maggi F, Pistello M, Vatteroni M, Presciuttini S, Marchi S, Isola P, et al. Dynamics of persistent TT virus infection, as determined in patients treated with alpha interferon for concomitant hepatitis C virus infection. *J Virol.* (2001) 75:11999–2004. doi: 10.1128/JVI.75.24.11999-12004.2001
113. de Villiers EM, Borkosky SS, Kimmel R, Gunst K, Fei JW. The diversity of torque teno viruses: *in vitro* replication leads to the formation of additional replication-competent subviral molecules. *J Virol.* (2011) 85:7284–95. doi: 10.1128/JVI.02472-10
114. Galmes J, Li Y, Rajoharison A, Ren L, Dollet S, Richard N, et al. Potential implication of new torque teno mini viruses in parapneumonic empyema in children. *Eur Respir J.* (2013) 42:470–9. doi: 10.1183/09031936.00107212
115. Krieg AM. CpG motifs in bacterial DNA and their immune effects. *Annu Rev Immunol.* (2002) 20:709–60. doi: 10.1146/annurev.immunol.20.100301.064842
116. Freer G, Maggi F, Pifferi M, Di Cicco ME, Peroni DG, Pistello M. The virome and its major component, anellovirus, a convoluted system molding human immune defenses and possibly affecting the development of asthma and respiratory diseases in childhood. *Front Microbiol.* (2018) 9:686. doi: 10.3389/fmicb.2018.00686
117. Rocchi J, Ricci V, Albani M, Lanini L, Andreoli E, Macera L, et al. Torquetenovirus DNA drives proinflammatory cytokines production and secretion by immune cells via toll-like receptor 9. *Virology.* (2009) 394:235–42. doi: 10.1016/j.virol.2009.08.036
118. Kamahora T, Hino S, Miyata H. Three spliced mRNAs of TT virus transcribed from a plasmid containing the entire genome in COS1 cells. *J Virol.* (2000) 74:9980–6. doi: 10.1128/JVI.74.21.9980-9986.2000
119. Vignolini T, Macera L, Antonelli G, Pistello M, Maggi F, Giannecchini S. Investigation on torquetenovirus (TTV) microRNA transcriptome in vivo. *Virus Res.* (2016) 217:18–22. doi: 10.1016/j.virusres.2016.03.003
120. Okamoto H, Takahashi M, Nishizawa T, Tawara A, Sugai Y, Sai T, et al. Replicative forms of TT virus DNA in bone marrow cells. *Biochem Biophys Res Commun.* (2000) 270:657–62. doi: 10.1006/bbrc.2000.2481
121. Mariscal LF, Lopez-Alcorocho JM, Rodriguez-Inigo E, Ortiz-Movilla N, de Lucas S, Bartolomé J, et al. TT virus replicates in stimulated but not in non-stimulated peripheral blood mononuclear cells. *Virology.* (2002) 301:121–9. doi: 10.1006/viro.2002.1545
122. Takayama S, Miura T, Matsuo S, Taki M, Sugii S. Prevalence and persistence of a novel DNA TT virus (TTV) infection in Japanese haemophiliacs. *Br J Haematol.* (1999) 104:626–9. doi: 10.1046/j.1365-2141.1999.01207.x
123. Yokozaki S, Toyoda H, Nakano I, Katano Y, Ebata M, Fukuda Y, et al. Infection with TT virus, a novel transfusion-transmissible DNA virus, in haemophiliacs and in blood products. *Br J Haematol.* (1999) 105:1114–9. doi: 10.1046/j.1365-2141.1999.01452.x
124. Jalali H, Mahdavi MR, Zaeromali N. Torque teno virus (TTV) among beta-thalassemia and haemodialysis patients in Mazandaran Province (North of Iran). *Int J Mol Cell Med.* (2017) 6:56–60.
125. El-Taher SM, Fouad NA, Fouad MA, Mahedy AW, Elnazi AK. Transfusion-transmitted virus infection in hemodialysis patients in Arar, Saudi Arabia: prevalence, predictors and genotyping. *Saudi J Kidney Dis Transpl.* (2015) 26:1215–22. doi: 10.4103/1319-2442.168643
126. Konishi K, Ueyama T. [Involvement of TTV, a new infectious factor in post-transfusion hepatitis, non A-non G]. *Nihon Rinsho.* (1999) 57:1279–84.
127. Wolff C, Diekmann A, Boomgaarden M, Korner MM, Kleesiek K. Viremia and excretion of TT virus in immunosuppressed heart transplant recipients and in immunocompetent individuals. *Transplantation.* (2000) 69:351–6. doi: 10.1097/00007890-200002150-00007
128. Akbari H, Piroozmand A, Dadgostar E, Nikoueinejad H, Chitsazian Z, B., et al. Prevalence of transfusion-transmitted virus (TTV) infection and its association with renal post-transplantation complications in Iran. *Int J Organ Transplant Med.* (2018) 9:126–31.
129. Takemoto AY, Okubo P, Saito PK, Yamakawa RH, Watanabe MA W, et al. Torque teno virus among dialysis and renal-transplant patients. *Braz J Microbiol.* (2015) 46:307–311. doi: 10.1590/S1517-838246120131195
130. Kanda Y, Tanaka Y, Kami M, Saito T, Asai T, Izutsu K, et al. TT virus in bone marrow transplant recipients. *Blood.* (1999) 93:2485–90. doi: 10.1182/blood.V93.8.2485.408k06_2485_2490
131. Thijssen M, Tacke F, Beller L, Deboutte W, Yinda KC, Nevens F, et al. Clinical relevance of plasma virome dynamics in liver transplant recipients. *EBioMedicine.* (2020) 60:103009. doi: 10.1016/j.ebiom.2020.103009
132. Tawara A, Akahane Y, Takahashi M, Nishizawa T, Ishikawa T, Okamoto H. Transmission of human TT virus of genotype 1a to chimpanzees with fecal supernatant or serum from patients with acute TTV infection. *Biochem Biophys Res Commun.* (2000) 278:470–6. doi: 10.1006/bbrc.2000.3825
133. Wylie KM, Mihindukulasuriya KA, Zhou Y, Sodergren E, Storch GA, Weinstock GM. Metagenomic analysis of double-stranded DNA viruses in healthy adults. *BMC Biol.* (2014) 12:71. doi: 10.1186/s12915-014-0071-7
134. Gerner P, Oettinger R, Gerner W, Falbrede J, Wirth S. Mother-to-infant transmission of TT virus: prevalence, extent and mechanism of vertical transmission. *Pediatr Infect Dis J.* (2000) 19:1074–7. doi: 10.1097/00006454-200011000-00009

135. Mutlu D, Abacioglu H, Altunyurt S. [Investigation of transplacental transmission of TT virus in mother–newborn pairs]. *Mikrobiyol Bul.* (2007) 41:71–7.
136. Inaba N, Oshima K, Okajima Y, Nagase T. [TTV materno-infantile infection–a study on the TTV frequency in Japanese pregnant women and the natural history of TTV mother-to-infant infection]. *Nihon Rinsho.* (1999) 57:1406–9.
137. Iso K, Suzuki Y, Takayama M. Mother-to-infant transmission of TT virus in Japan. *Int J Gynaecol Obstet.* (2001) 75:11–9. doi: 10.1016/S0020-7292(01)00450-7
138. Sugiyama K, Goto K, Ando T, Mizutani F, Terabe K, Yokoyama T. Highly diverse TTV population in infants and their mothers. *Virus Res.* (2001) 73:183–188. doi: 10.1016/S0168-1702(00)00242-2
139. Aagaard K, Riehle K, Ma J, Segata N, Mistretta TA, Coarfa C, et al. A metagenomic approach to characterization of the vaginal microbiome signature in pregnancy. *PLoS ONE.* (2012) 7:e36466. doi: 10.1371/journal.pone.0036466
140. Parnell LA, Briggs CM, Cao B, Delannoy-Bruno O, Schrieffer AE, Mysorekar IU. Microbial communities in placentas from term normal pregnancy exhibit spatially variable profiles. *Sci Rep.* (2017) 7:11200. doi: 10.1038/s41598-017-11514-4
141. Stinson LF, Boyce MC, Payne MS, Keelan JA. The Not-so-Sterile Womb: evidence that the human fetus is exposed to bacteria prior to birth. *Front Microbiol.* (2019) 10:1124. doi: 10.3389/fmicb.2019.01124
142. Payne MS, Newnham JP, Doherty DA, Furfaro LL, Pendal NL, Loh DE, et al. A specific bacterial DNA signature in the vagina of Australian women in midpregnancy predicts high risk of spontaneous preterm birth (the Predict1000 study). *Am J Obstet Gynecol.* (2021) 224:206.e1–e23. doi: 10.1016/j.ajog.2020.08.034
143. Khoudia D, Jean-Charles D, Anthony L, Florence F. Exhaustive repertoire of human vaginal microbiota. *Human Microbiome J.* (2019) 11:100051. doi: 10.1016/j.humic.2018.11.002
144. Silasi M, Cardenas I, Kwon JY, Racicot K, Aldo P, Mor G. Viral infections during pregnancy. *Am J Reprod Immunol.* (2015) 73:199–213. doi: 10.1111/aji.12355
145. Racicot K, Mor G. Risks associated with viral infections during pregnancy. *J Clin Invest.* (2017) 127:1591–9. doi: 10.1172/JCI87490
146. Michaan N, Amzallag S, Laskov I, Cohen Y, Fried M, Lessing JB, et al. Maternal and neonatal outcome of pregnant women infected with H1N1 influenza virus (swine flu). *J Matern Fetal Neonatal Med.* (2012) 25:130–2. doi: 10.3109/14767058.2011.562569
147. Reddick KL, Jhaveri R, Gandhi M, James AH, Swamy GK. Pregnancy outcomes associated with viral hepatitis. *J Viral Hepat.* (2011) 18:e394–8. doi: 10.1111/j.1365-2893.2011.01436.x
148. Liu J, Zhang S, Liu M, Wang Q, Shen H, Zhang Y. Maternal pre-pregnancy infection with hepatitis B virus and the risk of preterm birth: a population-based cohort study. *Lancet Glob Health.* (2017) 5:e624–32. doi: 10.1016/S2214-109X(17)30142-0
149. Xiao PL, Zhou YB, Chen Y, Yang MX, Song XX, Shi Y, et al. Association between maternal HIV infection and low birth weight and prematurity: a meta-analysis of cohort studies. *BMC Pregnancy Childbirth.* (2015) 15:246. doi: 10.1186/s12884-015-0684-z
150. Li DK, Raebel MA, Cheetham TC, Hansen C, Avalos L, Chen H, et al. Genital herpes and its treatment in relation to preterm delivery. *Am J Epidemiol.* (2014) 180:1109–17. doi: 10.1093/aje/kwu242
151. Cardenas I, Mor G, Aldo P, Lang SM, Stabach P, Sharp A, et al. Placental viral infection sensitizes to endotoxin-induced pre-term labor: a double hit hypothesis. *Am J Reprod Immunol.* (2011) 65:110–7. doi: 10.1111/j.1600-0897.2010.00908.x
152. Ilievski V, Hirsch E. Synergy between viral and bacterial toll-like receptors leads to amplification of inflammatory responses and preterm labor in the mouse. *Biol Reprod.* (2010) 83:767–73. doi: 10.1095/biolreprod.110.085464
153. Shah AA, Wang D, Hirsch E. Nucleic acid-based screening of maternal serum to detect viruses in women with labor or PROM. *Reprod Sci.* (2020) 27:537–44. doi: 10.1007/s43032-019-00051-2
154. Focosi D, Antonelli G, Pistello M, Maggi F. Torquetenovirus: the human virome from bench to bedside. *Clin Microbiol Infect.* (2016) 22:589–93. doi: 10.1016/j.cmi.2016.04.007
155. Wylie KM, Wylie TN, Cahill AG, Macones GA, Tuuli MG, Stout MJ. The vaginal eukaryotic DNA virome and preterm birth. *Am J Obstet Gynecol.* (2018) 219:189.e1–12. doi: 10.1016/j.ajog.2018.04.048
156. Shimaoka M, Yo Y, Doh K, Kotani Y, Suzuki A, Tsuji I, et al. Association between preterm delivery and bacterial vaginosis with or without treatment. *Sci Rep.* (2019) 9:509. doi: 10.1038/s41598-018-36964-2
157. Witkin SS, Moron AF, Ridenhour BJ, Minis E, Hatanaka A, Sarmento SGP, et al. Vaginal biomarkers that predict cervical length and dominant bacteria in the vaginal microbiomes of pregnant women. *mBio.* (2019) 10:e02242–19. doi: 10.1128/mBio.02242-19
158. Elovitz MA, Gajer P, Riis V, Brown AG, Humphrys MS, Holm JB, et al. Cervicovaginal microbiota and local immune response modulate the risk of spontaneous preterm delivery. *Nat Commun.* (2019) 10:1305. doi: 10.1038/s41467-019-09285-9
159. Witkin SS, Linhares IM. Why do lactobacilli dominate the human vaginal microbiota? *BJOG.* (2017) 124:606–11. doi: 10.1111/1471-0528.14390
160. Sloan P, Rodriguez C, Bedell BA, Murray J, Dagle J, Ryckman K, et al. Alphatorquevirus is the most prevalent virus identified in blood from a matched maternal-infant preterm cohort. *J Matern Fetal Neonatal Med.* (2020) 2020:1–7. doi: 10.1080/14767058.2020.1763298
161. Koga K, Cardenas I, Aldo P, Abrahams VM, Peng B, Fill S, et al. Activation of TLR3 in the trophoblast is associated with preterm delivery. *Am J Reprod Immunol.* (2009) 61:196–212. doi: 10.1111/j.1600-0897.2008.00682.x
162. Jaiswal MK, Agrawal V, Mallers T, Gilman-Sachs A, Hirsch E, Beaman KD. Regulation of apoptosis and innate immune stimuli in inflammation-induced preterm labor. *J Immunol.* (2013) 191:5702–13. doi: 10.4049/jimmunol.1301604
163. Racicot K, Cardenas I, Wunsche V, Aldo P, Guller S, Means RE, et al. Viral infection of the pregnant cervix predisposes to ascending bacterial infection. *J Immunol.* (2013) 191:934–41. doi: 10.4049/jimmunol.1300661
164. Chuong EB. The placenta goes viral: retroviruses control gene expression in pregnancy. *PLoS Biol.* (2018) 16:e3000028. doi: 10.1371/journal.pbio.3000028
165. Reshetnyak VI, Maev IV, Burmistrov AI, Chekmazov IA, Karlovich TI. Torque teno virus in liver diseases: on the way towards unity of view. *World J Gastroenterol.* (2020) 26:1691–707. doi: 10.3748/wjg.v26.i15.1691

21

Placental Autophagy and Viral Replication Co-localize in Human and Non-human Primate Placentae Following Zika Virus Infection: Implications for Therapeutic Interventions

Jennifer R. McKinney[1], *Maxim D. Seferovic*[1], *Angela M. Major*[2], *Melissa A. Suter*[1], *Suzette D. Tardif*[3], *Jean L. Patterson*[4], *Eumenia C. C. Castro*[2] *and Kjersti M. Aagaard*[1,2,5*]

[1] *Departments of Obstetrics and Gynecology, Division of Maternal-Fetal Medicine, Baylor College of Medicine and Texas Children's Hospital, Houston, TX, United States,* [2] *Pathology and Laboratory Medicine, Baylor College of Medicine and Texas Children's Hospital, Houston, TX, United States,* [3] *Southwest National Primate Research Center, Texas Biomedical Research Institute, San Antonio, TX, United States,* [4] *Department of Virology and Immunology, Texas Biomedical Research Institute, San Antonio, TX, United States,* [5] *Molecular and Human Genetics, Baylor College of Medicine, Houston, TX, United States*

Correspondence:
Kjersti M. Aagaard
aagaardt@bcm.edu

Background: Multiple studies have shown both induction and inhibition of autophagy during Zika virus (ZIKV) infection. While some have proposed mechanisms by which autophagic dysregulation might facilitate ZIKV vertical transmission, there is a lack of *in situ* data in human and non-human primate models. This is an especially pertinent question as autophagy-inhibitors, such as hydroxychloroquine, have been proposed as potential therapeutic agents aimed at preventing vertical transmission of ZIKV and other RNA viruses.

Objectives: Given the paucity of pre-clinical data in support of either autophagic enhancement or inhibition of placental ZIKV viral infection, we sought to assess cellular, spatial, and temporal associations between placental ZIKV infection and measures of autophagy in human primary cell culture and congenital infection cases, as well as an experimental non-human primate (marmoset, *Callithrix jacchus*) model.

Study Design: Primary trophoblast cells were isolated from human placentae ($n = 10$) and infected *in vitro* with ZIKV. Autophagy-associated gene expression (*ULK-1, BECN1, ATG5, ATG7, ATG12, ATG16L1, MAP1LC3A, MAP1LC3B, p62/SQSTM1*) was then determined by TaqMan qPCR to determine fold-change with ZIKV-infection. In *in vivo* validation experiments, autophagy genes *LC3B* and *p62/SQSTM1* were probed using *in situ* hybridization (ISH) in the placentae of human Congenital Zika Syndrome (CZS) cases ($n = 3$) and ZIKV-infected marmoset placenta ($n = 1$) and fetal tissue ($n = 1$). Infected and uninfected villi were compared for mean density and co-localization of autophagic protein markers.

Results: Studies of primary cultured human trophoblasts revealed **decreased** expression of autophagy genes *ATG5* and *p62/SQSTM1* in ZIKV-infected trophoblasts [*ATG5* fold change (±SD) 0.734-fold (±0.722), $p = 0.036$; p62/SQSTM1 0.661-fold (±0.666), $p = 0.029$]. Histologic examination by ISH and immunohistochemistry confirmed spatial association of autophagy and ZIKV infection in human congenital infection cases, as well as marmoset placental and fetal tissue samples. When quantified by densitometric data, autophagic protein LC3B, and p62/SQSTM1 expression in marmoset placenta were significantly *decreased* in *in situ* ZIKV-infected villi compared to less-infected areas [LC3B mean 0.951 (95% CI, 0.930–0.971), $p = 0.018$; p62/SQSTM1 mean 0.863 (95% CI, 0.810–0.916), $p = 0.024$].

Conclusion: In the current study, we observed that in the non-transformed human and non-human primate placenta, disruption (specifically down-regulation) of autophagy accompanies later ZIKV replication *in vitro, in vivo,* and *in situ*. The findings collectively suggest that dysregulated autophagy spatially and temporally accompanies placental ZIKV replication, providing the first *in situ* evidence in relevant primate pre-clinical and clinical models for the importance of timing of human therapeutic strategies aimed at agonizing/antagonizing autophagy. These studies have likely further implications for other congenitally transmitted viruses, particularly the RNA viruses, given the ubiquitous nature of autophagic disruption and dysregulation in host responses to viral infection during pregnancy.

Keywords: autophagy, congenital Zika syndrome, placental viral infection, autophagy and viral infection, viral transmission, Zika virus

HIGHLIGHTS

- Given the contradictory nature of pre-clinical data supporting both autophagic enhancement and inhibition of placental ZIKV viral infection, we sought to assess cellular, spatial, and temporal associations between human and non-human primate placental ZIKV replication and measures of autophagy.
- Dysregulated autophagy spatially and temporally co-localizes with placental ZIKV replication in human placentae and non-human primate placental and fetal tissue from congenital infection cases.
- Demonstrating the relationship between dysregulated autophagy and placental ZIKV infection provides the first *in situ* evidence in relevant pre-clinical models for human therapeutic strategies aimed at agonizing/antagonizing autophagy, potentially suggesting a means for mediating vertical transmission of ZIKV.

INTRODUCTION

Autophagy is a critical cytoplasmic process of degradation, which is felt to be crucial in the maintenance of cellular and tissue integrity. It occurs at a basal level in eukaryotic cells, in which cytoplasmic contents are partitioned into a double membrane-enclosed autophagosome (AP). This AP complex can then fuse with lysosomes to participate in cellular degradation and recycling. Every step of the process (initiation, vesicle elongation, maturation, docking and fusion, vesicle degradation) is controlled by a complex set of regulatory proteins (1–3). Over the past decade, interest in the role of autophagy in many areas of the pathophysiology of human disease has increased, including cellular response to infection.

There are several examples of co-evolution of viral mechanisms that take advantage of (or co-opt) host clearance mechanisms to accentuate their virulence. For example, recognition of viral antigens and the subsequent triggering of interferons and neutralizing antibodies limit viral replication, and thus viruses have co-opted key aspects of immune recognition and interferon production to instead facilitate their replication with enhanced cell entry and suppressed immunoreactivity (1, 4). Autophagic mechanisms that clear viruses, as obligate intracellular organisms, are no exception. Japanese encephalitis (5), HIV (6), Dengue (7, 8), Ebola (9), Parvo, Polio, Coxsackie, Hepatitis B, and Hepatitis C (10) viruses are all examples of viruses that exploit autophagy to enhance their replication and trigger host pathogenesis in the process (11).

Zika virus (ZIKV), a positive-strand RNA arbovirus in the *Flaviviridae* family initially identified in Uganda in 1947, evolved an Asian clade that then was identified as causing birth anomalies after emerging in the Caribbean and South America in late 2014 and early 2015 (12, 13). The latest pathological Asian strain has since become endemic, not only regionally, but has re-emerged in Africa and Asia in a largely immuno-naïve population (14). Recognition of congenital Zika syndrome (CZS), a phenotype that includes severe fetal neural anomalies (12, 15) during the last epidemic in South America, spurred a wave of research into mechanism and route of ZIKV infection and perinatal transmission (13, 16–23). Through this research, autophagy was identified as a potential key interrupted process rendering CZS. This was not entirely surprising, as dysregulation of autophagy has been previously linked to neural pathogenesis in neurodegenerative conditions (24), is known to be important for normal neurogenesis in human fetal neural stem cells (25, 26), and has been shown to affect central nervous system consequences of ZIKV infection in a pregnant mouse model (27). Moreover, *in vitro* infection models demonstrate that some degree of dysregulation of autophagy accompanied ZIKV infection of cell lines, including human umbilical vein endothelial cells (28), fetal neural stem cells (25, 29), and human skin fibroblasts (30). Several potential genes and pathways involved in the process have been identified in non-human or primate models (29, 31–35). However, the exact manner of and mechanisms by which autophagy dysregulation might facilitate ZIKV vertical transmission is still under investigation, especially regarding avoidance of clearance through the normal anti-viral autophagic processes after initial induction. This is crucial, as pharmacologic autophagy inhibitors are both available and have historical use with safety data for other indications in pregnancy (36–38). Specifically, anti-autophagic drugs such as mefloquine (37) or chloroquine (38, 39) have been proposed as potentially effective treatment to prevent maternal-fetal transmission in ZIKV-exposed pregnancies.

Autophagic processes have previously been shown to affect resistance to infection in human placentae [for example Cao et al. (40)]. Biologically plausible candidates for autophagy dysregulation facilitating vertical transmission include several of the cells of the human placenta. Indeed, we and others previously demonstrated *in vivo*, *in vitro*, and *in situ* replication of ZIKV in primary human and primate placental cells (cyto- and syncytiotrophoblasts, Hofbauer cells, endothelial cells, fibroblasts) (13, 19), as well as cells in the chorioamniotic membrane (epithelial cells and trophoblast progenitors) (41). We demonstrated previously that even small focal infections of the villous tissue are sufficient for vertical transmission of the virus, even with asymptomatic maternal infection (16). Experimental infections in animals (primates and manipulated murine models) demonstrated that placental trophoblast replication preceded fetal infection (18, 42). Collectively, these data document varying degrees of placental cellular infection in both the absence and presence of fetal infection and pathogenesis, leading to the conclusion that the placenta potentially seeds and serves as a reservoir for subsequent diffuse fetal infection.

These observations inspired our current study. Because the placenta is a highly active in autophagic flux throughout pregnancy (43), we and a few others have hypothesized that the interaction of autophagy and ZIKV infection in the placenta may contribute to pathogenesis. For example, impairment of autophagy through use of knock out mouse models reduces vertical transmission and fetal and placental damage following ZIKV infection (40). Results were echoed in studies of human neuronal precursors and glial cells in culture in which ZIKV seems to induce autophagy early on during infection, but then downregulates autophagy through induction of mTOR in order to facilitate ZIKV replication (44).

Given the paucity of human clinical (observational cases) or pre-clinical experimental animal data in support of either autophagic enhancement or inhibition of placental viral infection, we sought to leverage our previous human translation and non-human experimental infection research to assess cellular, spatial, and temporal associations between placental ZIKV replication and measures of macroautophagy. The objectives were therefore to first directly assess autophagic gene expression changes in primary syncytiotrophoblast cell culture infected *in vitro*. We then aimed to provide detailed histopathology *in vivo* employing human placental tissue and our non-human primate model (*Callithrix jacchus*, common marmoset) that, unlike other mammalian models, is naturally susceptible to infection and vertical viral transmission.

MATERIALS AND METHODS

ZIKV-Associated Autophagy Gene Expression Changes in Primary Human Trophoblasts by qPCR

Placental donors were comprised of primarily white Hispanic women with uncomplicated term deliveries, without major maternal or fetal comorbidities or anomalies, and high integrity placental tissue samples. Subjects and their samples were recruited via methods described previously in the index study for the current report (13). The clinical characteristics of the donor pregnancies are summarized in **Supplementary Table 1**. Briefly, placental tissue was dissected, then enzymatically digested, then Percoll separated to isolate cytotrophoblasts, which then syncytialized *in vitro*. After 2–5 days, syncytiotrophoblasts were infected with 1×10^5 RNA copies of first passage clinically isolated ZIKV FLR [10 Tissue Culture Infectious Dose (TCID) or mock]. Active replication was confirmed as described in our previously published work (13). After 4–5 days cells were scraped and flash-frozen in RNA*later* (ThermoFisher Scientific). Exosomal RNA was isolated from ZIKV-infected trophoblast cultures using TRIzol LS (Invitrogen) purification as previously described (13). Levels of specific mRNAs for autophagy-associated genes (*ULK1, BECN1, ATG5, ATG7, ATG12, ATG16L1, MAP1LC3A, MAP1LC3B, p62/SQSTM1*) were assessed against GAPDH as the endogenous control, using TaqMan qPCR assays (ThermoFisher Scientific) (assay IDs are listed in **Supplementary Table 2**). Template cDNA was generated using High Capacity cDNA reverse transcription Kit (Applied Biosystems) per manufacturer's instructions. Triplicate reactions were then prepared using 1 ug template cDNA per well. TaqMan assays were performed with a StepOnePlus platform (Applied Biosystems) according to standard conditions of 60°C annealing temperature for 40 cycles. Delta C_t data was filtered for outliers with a $Q = 0.01$. Differences were determined using paired t-tests within donors compared to mock. Fold change was calculated by delta delta C_t method. All statistics were performed with Prism software (GraphPad, v8.4.3, La Jolla, CA).

Co-localization of ZIKV Replication and Autophagy Activity in Human and Marmoset Placentae via *In situ* Hybridization and Immunohistochemistry

No new samples were obtained for this current work. Histological sections from human case reports as well as experimental non-human primate infections were obtained from two separate studies that have been previously published (16, 19) [human studies were approved by Baylor College of Medicine IRB H-25735; non-human primate studies were performed at Southwest National Primate Research Center and approved by local Institutional Animal Care and Use Committee (IACUC) and Biohazard Committee]. For the human study, subjects with risk for, or suspected, CZS were recruited and consented as described in the previous publication (16). A clinical description of the cases is summarized in **Supplementary Table 3**. Immediately following delivery, a full cross section of placental tissue was removed 4 cm from the cord insertion site for three suspected CZS cases, and one healthy neonate. Tissue was then further dissected and fixed in formalin for ~8 h then processed into paraffin blocks.

Under IACUC approval, two pregnant common marmosets were experimentally infected with an injection of 2.5×10^5 plaque forming units (PFU) of the first passage contemporaneous Brazil ZIKV strain SPH2015 (GenBank accession number KU321639) twice 4 days apart, on estimated gestational days 79/83 and 68/72, respectively, as previously published (19). After 16 days (dam 1) and 18 days (dam 2) of asymptomatic infection, both pregnancies spontaneously aborted, from which tissue was obtained and formalin fixed prior to processing. Because of tissue destruction prior to initial collection, sections of collected tissue from only dam 2 were paraffin-embedded into blocks and used for the current work: marmoset fetus [full sagittal ($n = 1$) and frontal/coronal ($n = 1$)] and placenta ($n = 1$). Detailed examination of the tissues as previously described revealed focal infection and viral replication in diverse placental and fetal tissues.

In the current study, for all tissues, serial sections were meticulously prepared in parallel to allow for cross-comparison using different stains to label viral replication and markers of autophagy. To assess for viral infection, *in situ* hybridization (ISH) was carried out against the ZIKV positive strand viral genome using a ZIKV-specific probe set largely according to manufacturer's instructions. An additional pretreatment with Protease Plus for 15 min and Target Retrieval Reagent for 15 min (RNAscope, ACD Biosciences) was performed for optimal retrieval. To assess for the levels of autophagy-associated proteins LC3B and p62/SQSTM1, immunohistochemistry was employed. Serial sections of the human placental blocks were deparaffinized and rehydrated, then probed with antibodies against LC3B (#3868, Cell Signaling Technology, Danvers, MA, USA) or p62/SQSTM1 (#H00008878-M01, Abnova, Walnut, CA, USA). It was determined that these were non-cross reacting antibodies with testing, and therefore LC3B (NB100-2220) and p62/SQSTM1(NBP1-49956) (Novus, Centennial, CO, USA) were alternatively used for non-human primate tissue sections.

Bright field slides were examined under low (4x), medium (20x), medium-high (40x), and high power (60x) using a Nikon Eclipse 90i microscope (Nikon Instruments, Melville, NY, USA). As a first pass, areas of active ZIKV infection were identified and marked. The same villi and areas were then identified on each serial immunohistochemistry section by comparing those markings and confirmed by comparing landmarks within the microanatomy of those areas. In this way, precise co-localization could be confidently determined. Images were captured using NIS Elements 4.20 (Nikon). Staining within areas of interest was assessed visually and using metrics within the software as described below. Minor adjustment for contrast and background levels were made using NIS Elements 4.20 for publication (Nikon).

Quantitative Measures of Autophagy Activity in Marmoset Placentae

Sections were inspected for focal areas of infected villi. Four such areas per slide in the marmoset placental tissue were selected, where heavily ZIKV-infected villi were adjacent to apparently un-stained, and uninfected villi. Densitometry was then performed within these villi to establish and compare the levels of autophagic marker proteins. Standard colorimetric thresholds were established for each of the three stains (ZIKV, LC3B, and p62 antibodies) using NIS Elements 4.20 (Nikon). To do this, the most densely stained area of the highest power image was selected, and serial areas of staining were selected until all apparent staining was captured as assessed visually. Villi of interest were then manually traced using the inside of the syncytiotrophoblast as the perimeter. From the ZIKV stained slides, densitometry was used to systematically establish the placental villi within the captured fields with the most ($n = 2$) and least ($n = 2$) ZIKV infection. The most and least infected villi were then set as our regions of interest in the serially stained autophagy marker protein slides.

Areas were then traced to the same villi in the probed serial sections. The established thresholds for each antibody were then applied to each region of interest across all the slides, and densitometric measurements were made. Mean area density of the stain (as defined by previously-set colorimetric thresholds) was calculated for each region of interest and used as the basis of comparison. Differences between the most and least infected areas on all marmoset placental slides were determined using paired t-tests. All statistics were performed with Prism software (GraphPad, v8.4.3, La Jolla, CA).

RESULTS

Autophagy-Related Gene Expression Changes in ZIKV-Infected Primary Human Trophoblasts

To determine whether transcription of autophagic genes were altered (either up or down regulated, shown as fraction of mock-infected same subject controls) with cellular ZIKV infection, we analyzed *in vitro* infection of primary human trophoblasts.

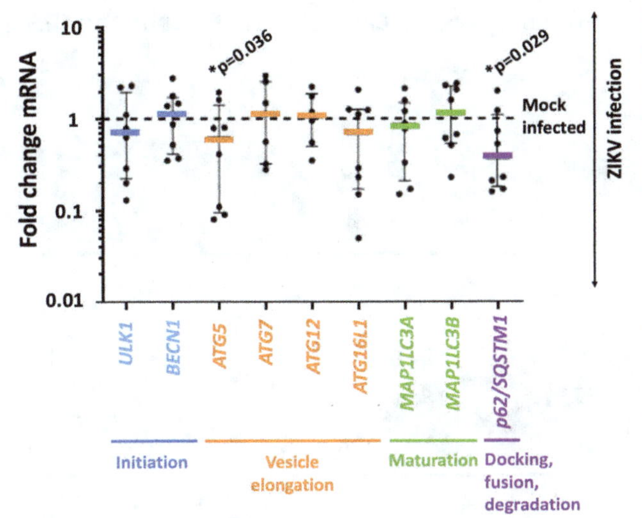

FIGURE 1 | ZIKV infection is accompanied by decreased gene expression in autophagy-related genes *ATG5* and *p62/SQSTM1* in primary human trophoblasts. Primary human trophoblasts were infected with 10^5 RNA copies of first passage clinically isolated ZIKV FLR or mock, and autophagic gene expression was assessed. Genes were selected based on involvement in multiple phases of autophagy (stage noted in colored text underlying the *x* axis). Expression of *ATG5* and *p62/SQSTM1* were significantly decreased (*ATG5* mean fold change expression 0.734 ± 0.722 SD; *p*-value 0.036, *p62/SQSTM1* mean fold change expression 0.661 ± 0.666 SD, *p*-value 0.029) following infection 2–5 days post-isolation. Fold change in expression was calculated by delta delta Ct method, normalizing first to GAPDH and then mean delta Ct of mock-infected controls. Data was filtered for outliers with $Q = 0.01$. Significance was determined using *t*-tests of *Ct*-values with a *p*-value < 0.05 denoting significance (*).

Placentas from normal, healthy term pregnancies were collected, dissected, and cytotrophoblasts isolated. *In vitro* syncytialization was monitored by assessing the βhCG levels in the conditioned media, and cell purity was assessed on a subset by subjecting the cells to flow cytometry as we have previously published (13). The syncytiotrophoblasts were then infected with first passage ZIKV FLR or a mock. The infection was confirmed by daily monitoring of the conditioned media for ZIKV RNA. After 3–5 days cells were then collected, and RNA purified to measure for gene changes of interest.

Autophagy-related genes *ULK1, BECN1, ATG5, ATG7, ATG12, ATG16L1, MAP1LC3A, MAP1LC3B*, and *p62/SQSTM1* were assessed by TaqMan qPCR. Two significant changes in gene expression were observed by *t*-test. The expression of *ATG5* was decreased by 27% (mean fold change expression 0.734 ± 0.722; *p*-value 0.036), and *p62/SQSTM1* was decreased by 33% (mean fold change expression 0.661 ± 0.666, *p*-value 0.029) compared to mock infected placental trophoblasts (**Figure 1**).

Spatial Association of ZIKV Replication and Autophagy in Human Placental Tissue

Given the observed changes to key autophagy genes with *in vitro* ZIKV infection, we set out to examine known ZIKV-infected human placentae (with CZS-affected fetuses) for similar changes in protein *in situ*. Specifically, we chose LC3B as the primary marker of autophagy, as it directly interacts with our gene products of interest, as well as p62 protein. However, we first assessed the placenta for ZIKV presence via +strand RNA detection, so as to identify areas of interest with autophagic activity for examination.

Histologic examination of cases of CZS alongside uninfected, unaffected controls demonstrated the presence of replicating ZIKV in cases but not controls (brown staining, black arrowheads, **Figure 2A**). The virus was noted in multiple areas of placental villi including multinucleated syncytiotrophoblasts at the maternal–fetal interface. Histologic examination of serial placental sections stained with autophagy markers LC3B and p62/SQSTM1 was performed with careful identification of exact areas of ZIKV. Co-localization of autophagy and ZIKV infection were noted in all three cases of CZS. **Figure 2B** demonstrates colocalization of LC3B with red-brown staining, while **Figure 2C** demonstrates colocalization of p62/SQSTM1 with bright red staining. Black arrowheads identify areas of ZIKV infection noted in prior sections. The small amount of visible ZIKV infection at time of tissue harvesting is likely due to the inclusion criteria of the initial study which was for infants suspected with CZS, allowing for maternal serum IgM seronegativity for ZIKV at the time of delivery.

ZIKV and Autophagy Co-localize in Marmoset Placental Tissue as Well as Marmoset Fetal Neuro-Ophthalmic Structures

Unsurprisingly, examination of placental tissue from timed experimental infections in non-human primates showed a very high degree of ZIKV infection compared to the human cases. Dense dark brown staining was most apparent in the parenchyma of the tissue, while some staining was also apparent in the syncytiotrophoblasts. The darkest staining is most likely attributed to ZIKV infection of Hofbauer cells. Histologic examination of the placental tissue demonstrated focal areas of infection, with highly infected villi adjacent to villi without evidence of apparent ZIKV (**Figure 3A**, brown labeling). By comparing serial sections for morphological markers within the villous shapes, autophagy markers could be compared between infected and non-infected areas. Again, autophagy-related proteins LC3B and p62/SQSTM1 were selected as the markers of autophagy for these studies. At first glance, the staining appears universal for the constitutively expressed proteins, however co-localization within the same areas as ZIKV revealed spatial distinction (**Figure 3B**: LC3B, red/brown labeling; **Figure 3C**: p62/SQSTM1, red/brown labeling).

Examination was also made of marmoset fetal tissue from a second pregnancy with experimental infection that was spontaneously aborted. A frontal cross-section immediately posterior to the fetal eye was examined. ZIKV infection was noted within the neural tissue of the developing visual cortex, within the cortical plate of the developing frontal brain, and within the periorbital musculature. Co-localization of autophagic activity via autophagy markers LC3B (red/brown labeling) and

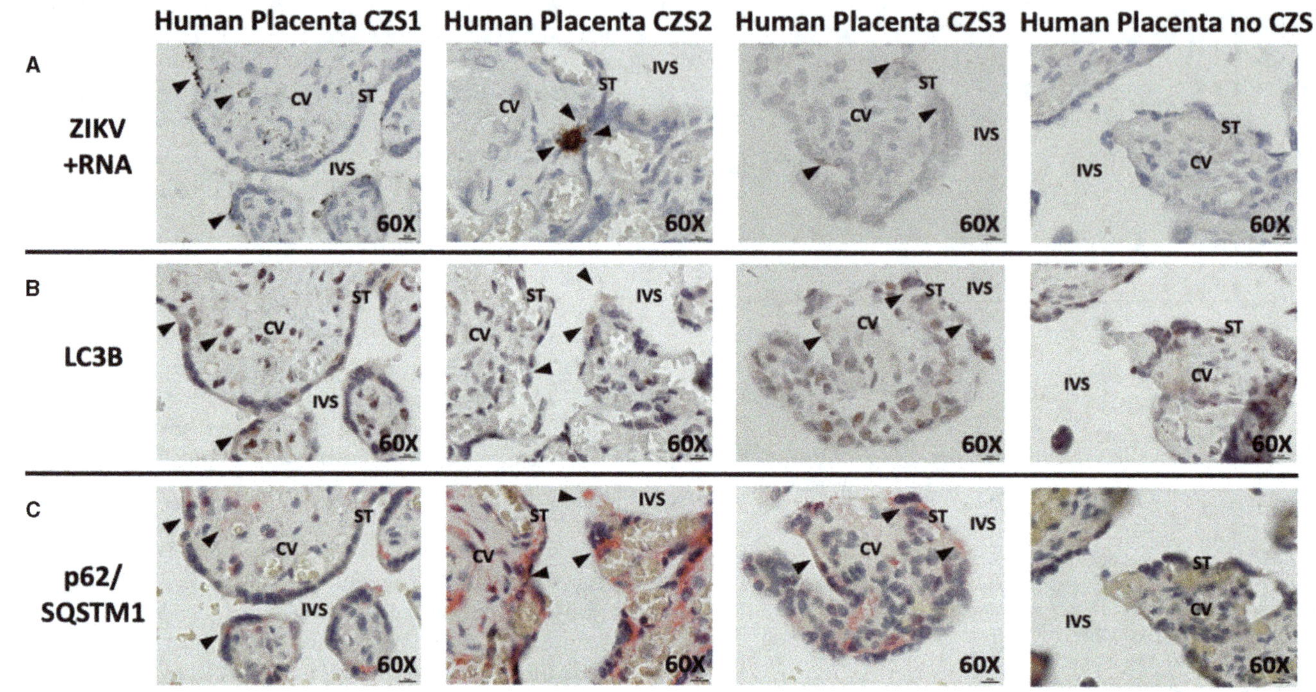

FIGURE 2 | *In situ* hybridization and immunohistochemistry staining demonstrate autophagy and ZIKV replication co-localize in human placentae of neonates affected by CZS. *In situ* hybridization with positive-strand ZIKV RNA probe set demonstrates ZIKV replication within villi from confirmed CZS cases but not in the placenta from the unaffected neonate (**A**: brown labeling, black arrowheads). Immunohistochemical staining for autophagic markers LC3B (**B**: dark red-brown labeling, black arrowheads) and SQSTM1/p62 (**C**: bright red labeling, black arrowheads) was noted in the same area of the villi where ZIKV replication was present. Probe-free controls confirm no non-specific binding in the absence of ZIKV, LC3B, SQSTM1/P62 probes, respectively. All images shown were obtained at 60X magnification. Micron bar scale in bottom right corner of images = 10 μm. CV, chorionic villus; IVS, intervillous space; ST, syncytiotrophoblast.

p62/SQSTM1 (red/brown labeling) was again noted within these same fetal neuro-ophthalmic structures (**Figures 4A–C**). Due to the breadth of tissue types present within these sections, analysis was limited to noting co-localization of ZIKV and autophagic activity rather than allowing quantification of autophagic activity.

Quantitative Comparison of Autophagy Protein Markers Between Infected and Uninfected Marmoset Placental Villi

To assess for a direct association between the viral infection and changing autophagy in an experimental *in vivo* primate model, post-imaging densitometric analysis of the bright field images was used to compare the levels of the autophagy proteins LC3B and p62/SQSTM1. Areas where infected and uninfected villous tissue was in close proximity were carefully chosen for comparison studies. **Figure 5A** labels ZIKV replication employing ISH. Stain thresholds were then set via post-processing densitometry to quantify the mean area of staining in each villi (defined as a region of interest) (**Figure 5B**). This allowed selection of villi with evidence of the most dense staining for ZIKV infection (**Figures 5A,B**: regions Z1–Z2) and least dense staining for ZIKV infection (**Figures 5A,B**: regions N1–N2). The same most ZIKV-infected and least infected villous regions of interest were identified in subsequent sections for LC3B and p62/SQSTM1 studies. Densitometry was again used to define autophagic protein stain area in each region for LC3B and p62/SQSTM1, respectively (**Figure 5B**, bright green color). Defined densitometric thresholds did not identify any stain in probe-free control images for ZIKV infection, LC3B, or p62/SQSTM1 (data not shown). Using the densitometric data, mean area density of staining was compared between ZIKV-infected and less-infected villi. Mean density of both LC3B and p62/SQSTM1 were significantly decreased in ZIKV-infected villi compared to less-infected areas [**Figure 5C**; LC3B mean (95%CI) 0.951 (0.930–0.971), $p = 0.018$; p62/SQSTM1 mean (95%CI) 0.863 (0.810–0.916), $p = 0.024$].

DISCUSSION

Principal Findings

In the current study, we observed that in the placenta, disruption of autophagy accompanies ZIKV replication *In vitro, In vivo,* and *In situ* in human and non-human primate infections. Specifically, we observed changes in gene expression of key autophagy genes *Atg5* and *p62/SQSTM1* accompanying ZIKV-infection and replication in human primary placental trophoblasts when compared to mock-infected controls. Similar reduction in autophagic gene expression has been shown to affect viral replication and infectivity in other models (45). When we additionally assessed measures of autophagy in experimental

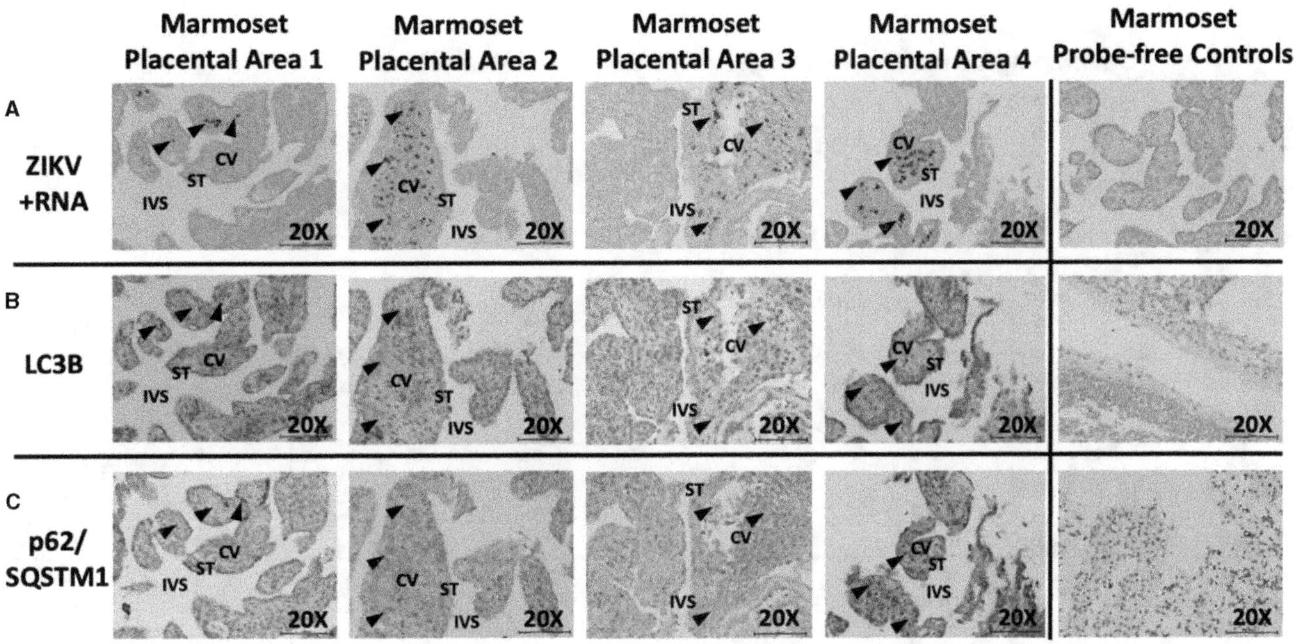

FIGURE 3 | *In situ* hybridization and immunohistochemistry staining demonstrates autophagy and ZIKV replication co-localize in ZIKV-infected marmoset placenta. *In situ* hybridization with positive-strand ZIKV RNA probe set demonstrates ZIKV replication (first passage Brazil ZIKV strain SPH2015) within some villi of the placenta from a ZIKV-infected marmoset (**A**: brown labeling, black arrowheads). Immunohistochemical staining for autophagic markers LC3B (**B**: red-brown labeling, black arrowheads) and SQSTM1/p62 (**C**: red-brown labeling, black arrowheads) was noted in the same areas of the villi where ZIKV replication was present. Probe-free controls confirm no non-specific binding in the absence of ZIKV, LC3B, SQSTM1/P62 probes, respectively. All images shown were obtained at 20X magnification. Micron bar scale in bottom right corner of images = 100 μm. CV, chorionic villus; IVS, intervillous space; ST, syncytiotrophoblast.

in vivo primate model and human cases of CZS, we observed significant spatial co-localization with the presence of key autophagic protein markers LC3B and p62/SQSTM1 proximal to ZIKV replication. When immunohistochemical staining in human and non-human primate placentae is quantified by densitometry, p62/SQSTM1, and to a lesser extent LC3B, are both significantly decreased in ZIKV infected placental cells when measured with an unbiased algorithmic method. These findings collectively suggest that dysregulated autophagy spatially and temporally accompanies placental ZIKV replication, providing the first *in situ* evidence in relevant pre-clinical models for human molecular therapeutic strategies aimed at agonizing/antagonizing autophagy. These studies have likely implications for other congenitally transmitted viruses, given the ubiquitous nature of autophagic disruption and dysregulation in host responses to viral infection during pregnancy.

Results

Our findings provide key evidence which reconciles seeming disparate prior studies demonstrating ZIKV-related induction of autophagic activity and seemingly pro-viral effects of autophagy. Specifically, we demonstrate that key autophagy gene transcription and protein translation are actually significantly **decreased** in foci of ZIKV-infected normal primary (i.e., non-transformed) human and primate cells with evidence of active replication. Prior suggestions for induction of autophagy and pro-viral effect of autophagy arose from transformed (i.e., high passage placental cancer) cell lines, where a marked increase in autophagy activity was found to accompany ZIKV infection (25, 28, 30). Induction of autophagy in these transformed cell lines seems to have pro-viral effects. In addition, inhibition of autophagy, via knock-out mouse models (40) or with use of pharmacologic inhibitors (28, 30), decreases viral infection. This is in contrast to the general tenet that induction of autophagy tends to confer placental cells with high resistance to viral infection, while inhibition of autophagy confers permissivity to viral infection (46, 47). Findings supporting an anti-viral role of autophagy have been seen in human neuroprogenitor and glial cells in culture (44) and Drosophila (48), where autophagy induction is associated with restricted ZIKV infection, and inhibition is associated with promotion of ZIKV infection.

Clinical Implications

In this current study, we demonstrate downregulation of autophagy in the endogenous setting of placental infection (e.g., *in vitro* infection of primary human trophoblasts or *in situ* measures of CZS-affected cases). Our observations reported herein show that key autophagy gene transcription and protein translation are actually significantly **decreased** in non-transformed placentae. This is further consistent with clinical observations of human cases. Namely, placental infection is not always (and even rarely) associated with either histologic nor molecular evidence of placental inflammation (49–51), but does

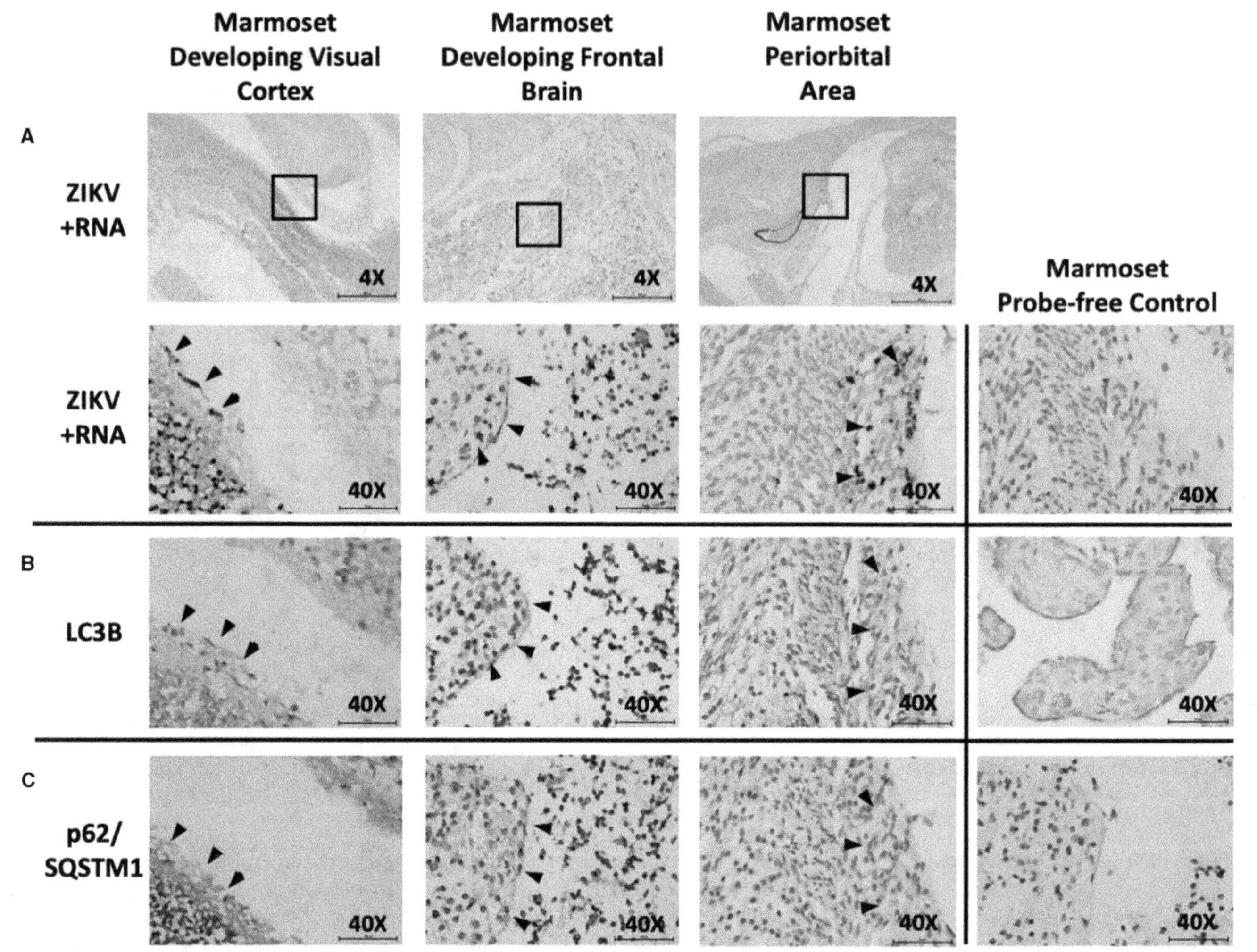

FIGURE 4 | *In situ* hybridization and immunohistochemistry staining demonstrate co-localization of autophagy and ZIKV replication in neuro-ophthalmic structures of ZIKV-infected marmoset abortus. *in situ* hybridization with positive-strand ZIKV RNA probe set demonstrates ZIKV replication within the developing visual cortex, frontal brain, and periocular structures in marmoset fetus (**A**: brown labeling, black arrowheads). Boxes indicate areas imaged further at 40X. Immunohistochemical staining for autophagic markers LC3B (**B**: red-brown labeling, black arrowheads) and SQSTM1/p62 (**C**: red-brown labeling, black arrowheads) was noted in the same neuro-ophthalmic structures where ZIKV replication was present. Probe-free controls confirm no non-specific binding in the absence of ZIKV, LC3B, SQSTM1/P62 probes, respectively. Images shown were obtained at 4X magnification (top row, **A**) or 40X magnification (all other images). Micron bar scale in bottom right corner of images = 500 μm (4X) or 50 μm (40X).

accompany pregnancy loss and fetal infection. There may be several biological reasons for our observations.

One explanation for these seemingly contradictory findings is suggested by Sahoo et al. (44), who similarly found evidence of a temporal relationship between diminished autophagy and persistence of infection. Initial autophagy induction (with limited viral replication during a brief period of <24 h post infection) was followed by mTOR activation and subsequent down regulation of autophagy with associated increased viral replication later in the course of ZIKV infection. Initial autophagic activation may serve to provide the substrates needed for initial viral replication resulting in the decreased p62/SQSTM1 levels (signal of autophagic flux) seen in this work. Subsequent autophagic downregulation prior to viral clearance may allow continued infection and is supported by the decreased p62/SQSTM1 gene expression and decreased LC3B presence seen in our non-human primate samples.

Second, support for subsequent downregulation of autophagy with ZIKV infection also arises from experiments conducted in primary human epithelial cells, primary skin fibroblasts, and non-transformed astrocytes where an alternate pathway for ZIKV-induced cell death was identified, making it unlikely that ZIKV requires autophagy later in infection for viral spread (52). This concept is not unheard of for flaviviruses, with DENV seemingly following a similar pattern of initial induction of autophagy with primary infection, followed by inhibition of autophagy with persistent infection (7). Our results are likely most consistent with downregulation of autophagy later in course

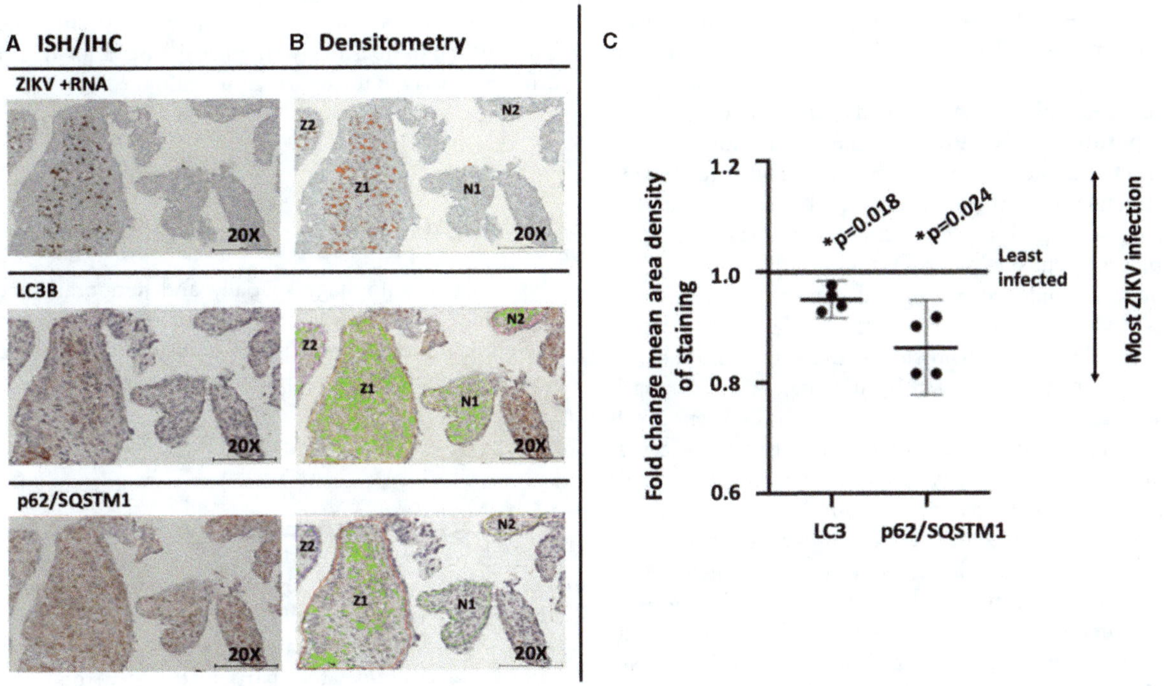

FIGURE 5 | Mean density of autophagic proteins LC3B and p62/SQSTM1 is significantly decreased in the greatest compared to the least ZIKV-infected marmoset placental villi. Villi with the greatest (regions Z1–2) and least (regions N1–2) dense staining for ZIKV infection were identified using stain thresholds and defined as regions of interest **(A)**. The same greatest and least infected regions of interest were identified in subsequent sections for LC3B and p62/SQSTM1 studies, and densitometry was again used to define autophagic protein stain area in each region (**B**, bright green color). Mean area density of staining was then compared between regions of interest. Mean density of both LC3B and p62/SQSTM1 were significantly decreased in the most ZIKV-infected villi compared to the least-infected areas [**C**; LC3B mean (95%CI) 0.951 (0.930–0.971), $p = 0.018$; p62/SQSTM1 mean (95%CI) 0.863 (0.810–0.916), $p = 0.024$]. All images shown were obtained at 20X magnification. Micron bar scale in bottom right corner of images = 100 μm. Statistical significance was determined using a p-value < 0.05 (*).

of the infection and disease process, since we observed that both the RNA from the primary human trophoblasts, and the human and non-human primate tissues were isolated past the 24 h of initial autophagy induction demonstrated by Sahoo et al. (44). p62/SQSTM1 as a pathogen recognition reception (PRR), and Atg5 which has been proposed to downregulate some PRRs, are both logical candidates for downregulation of autophagy by a virus trying to avoid normal anti-viral degradative pathways (3, 53), findings supported by this study. Put another way, if we could have sampled the same human and non-human primate placentae much earlier in infection (h), rather than days, weeks, or months later, we may have observed transient initial induction of autophagy, with subsequent downmodulation of autophagy. Such experiments will be the focus of future *in vivo* work, and our conclusions remain speculative.

Research Implications

While this study does demonstrate spatial and temporal co-localization between autophagy and ZIKV infection at a discrete point in time, further studies are necessary to define exactly when and how autophagy is induced and/or down-modulated during the entire course of ZIKV infection, especially within human placentae. This information will better inform the timing and pharmacologic basis (if any) of potential therapeutic options. In addition, it may help identify mechanisms and pathways by which viral persistence in the placenta might occur in some, but not all, cases of congenital Zika infection and resultant fetal disease.

Strengths and Limitations

Strengths of this study include the use of a highly relevant non-human primate model of congenital infection, with confirmation in human placental samples, both *in vitro* and *in vivo*. Limitations of this study include a small chance of cross-reactivity of the LC3B antibodies to other LC3 isoforms. In addition, the static nature of these experiments does not enable us to assess for longitudinal changes. Therefore, we cannot draw conclusions about autophagy in the initial phases of infection given our non-human primate model spontaneously aborted at 2 weeks with a highly advanced placental infection.

In general, reliance on specimens from other index studies constrained our experimental design and limited our biologic replicates. This is notably true in our *in vivo* infected marmosets (19). In the initial study, as we have previously published, we infected two pregnant marmoset dams with Brazil ZIKV at estimated gestational days 79 and 68, with a second inoculation 4 days later. As we initially detailed in the primary index study (19), spontaneous expulsion of intrauterine demised fetuses at post-inoculation day 16 (dam 1, dizygotic twins) and 18 (dam 2, singleton) occurred. The placenta from dam 1 was unavailable for analysis, as it was mauled by the dam post-delivery. The second dam's expulsed singleton fetus and placenta were both collected and retained for analyses, and because they constituted a single exposure they were used in the current analysis (19). Recognizing the limitations of drawing meaningful conclusions based on a single pregnancies placenta and fetus, we attempted to mitigate these limitations with technical replicates by sampling different placental subsites and rigorous use of internal controls. In addition, we employed orthogonal approaches with use of human tissue specimens and primary trophoblasts in the current study. Nonetheless, we acknowledge the constraints in our primate specimens being derived from a single dam. Similarly, we acknowledge that architectural and histologic differences exist when comparing human and non-human primate placentae. However, the notable similarity of consequence for the current study is the hemochorial nature common to both human and non-human primate placentae whereby (unlike other species) the villi bathe in the maternal intervillous space. As such we feel that the marmoset is a highly appropriate model despite some anatomical differences. Moreover, we are further buoyed in the confidence of our findings and conclusions by the consistency of observations among our human and non-human primate subject's specimens.

CONCLUSIONS

Although the exact role of autophagy in ZIKV pathogenesis is still being determined, autophagy inhibitors, such as hydroxychloroquine (38), are being proposed as potential therapeutic agents to prevent vertical transmission and mitigate adverse fetal effects of the virus. Our results shed key light on this topic, and herald warning that such therapeutic approaches must be approached with thoughtful consideration of both timing and duration of therapy. Since our findings show that diminished autophagy later in the infection temporally and spatially co-localizes with ZIKV replication in non-human primate placentae from congenital infection cases, it cannot be concluded *de facto* that inhibition of autophagy will be of benefit. Conversely, we cannot assume that it would be of harm as our observations could be evidence of an adaptive response for maternal benefit. Rather, the appropriate interpretation and application of our findings suggest that future experimentation with anti-autophagic drugs as potentially effective in mitigating vertical transmission of ZIKV must consider the timing of administration with respect to infection. Likely subsequent downregulation of autophagic processes does not negate the benefits that such therapy may have, although does likely support the need for treatment to be limited to early in the course of infection.

SUMMARY

Dysregulated autophagy spatially and temporally accompanies placental ZIKV replication, providing *in situ* evidence in relevant pre-clinical models for human molecular therapeutic strategies aimed at agonizing/antagonizing autophagy.

ETHICS STATEMENT

The studies involving human participants were reviewed and approved by Baylor College of Medicine IRB H-257. The patients/participants provided their written informed consent to participate in this study. The animal study was reviewed and approved by Southwest National Primate Research Center and approved by local Institutional Animal Care and Use Committee (IACUC) and Biohazard Committee.

AUTHOR'S NOTE

Poster presentation at Society for Maternal Fetal Medicine, the 41st Annual Pregnancy Meeting, January 25-30, 2021.

AUTHOR CONTRIBUTIONS

JM, MDS, MAS, and KA contributed to the conception and design of the study. JM, MDS, AM, ST, JP, EC, and KA performed the experiments. JM, MDS, AM, ST, JP, EC, and KA analyzed and interpreted the data. JM, MDS, and KA wrote the manuscript. All authors contributed to the article and approved the submitted version.

REFERENCES

1. Choi AM, Ryter SW, Levine B. Autophagy in human health and disease. *N Engl J Med.* (2013) 368:1845–6. doi: 10.1056/NEJMc1303158
2. Fullgrabe J, Ghislat G, Cho DH, Rubinsztein DC. Transcriptional regulation of mammalian autophagy at a glance. *J Cell Sci.* (2016) 129:3059–66. doi: 10.1242/jcs.188920
3. Chiramel AI, Best SM. Role of autophagy in Zika virus infection and pathogenesis. *Virus Res.* (2018) 254:34–40. doi: 10.1016/j.virusres.2017.09.006
4. Levine B, Mizushima N, Virgin HW. Autophagy in immunity and inflammation. *Nature.* (2011) 469:323–35. doi: 10.1038/nature09782
5. Li JK, Liang JJ, Liao CL, Lin YL. Autophagy is involved in the early step of Japanese encephalitis virus infection. *Microbes Infect.* (2012) 14:159–68. doi: 10.1016/j.micinf.2011.09.001

6. Wang X, Gao Y, Tan J, Devadas K, Ragupathy V, Takeda K, et al. HIV-1 and HIV-2 infections induce autophagy in Jurkat and CD4+ T cells. *Cell Signal.* (2012) 24:1414–9. doi: 10.1016/j.cellsig.2012.02.016
7. Metz P, Chiramel A, Chatel-Chaix L, Alvisi G, Bankhead P, Mora-Rodriguez R, et al. Dengue virus inhibition of autophagic flux and dependency of viral replication on proteasomal degradation of the autophagy receptor p62. *J Virol.* (2015) 89:8026–41. doi: 10.1128/JVI.00787-15
8. Heaton NS, Randall G. Dengue virus-induced autophagy regulates lipid metabolism. *Cell Host Microbe.* (2010) 8:422–32. doi: 10.1016/j.chom.2010.10.006
9. Shtanko O, Reyes AN, Jackson WT, Davey RA. Autophagy-associated proteins control ebola virus internalization into host cells. *J Infect Dis.* (2018) 218(Suppl_5):S346–54. doi: 10.1093/infdis/jiy294
10. Sir D, Kuo CF, Tian Y, Liu HM, Huang EJ, Jung JU, et al. Replication of hepatitis C virus RNA on autophagosomal membranes. *J Biol Chem.* (2012) 287:18036–43. doi: 10.1074/jbc.M111.320085
11. Dreux M, Chisari FV. Viruses and the autophagy machinery. *Cell Cycle.* (2010) 9:1295–307. doi: 10.4161/cc.9.7.11109
12. Rasmussen SA, Jamieson DJ, Honein MA, Petersen LR. Zika virus and birth defects–reviewing the evidence for causality. *N Engl J Med.* (2016) 374:1981–7. doi: 10.1056/NEJMsr1604338
13. Aagaard KM, Lahon A, Suter MA, Arya RP, Seferovic MD, Vogt MB, et al. Primary human placental trophoblasts are permissive for Zika Virus (ZIKV) replication. *Sci Rep.* (2017) 7:41389. doi: 10.1038/srep41389
14. Musso D, Ko AI, Baud D. Zika virus infection - after the pandemic. *N Engl J Med.* (2019) 381:1444–57. doi: 10.1056/NEJMra1808246
15. Mlakar J, Korva M, Tul N, Popovic M, Poljsak-Prijatelj M, Mraz J, et al. Zika virus associated with microcephaly. *N Engl J Med.* (2016) 374:951–8. doi: 10.1056/NEJMoa1600651
16. Seferovic MD, Turley M, Valentine GC, Rac M, Castro ECC, Major AM, et al. Clinical importance of placental testing among suspected cases of congenital Zika syndrome. *Int J Mol Sci.* (2019). 20:712. doi: 10.3390/ijms20030712
17. Dudley DM, Van Rompay KK, Coffey LL, Ardeshir A, Keesler RI, Bliss-Moreau E, et al. Miscarriage and stillbirth following maternal Zika virus infection in nonhuman primates. *Nat Med.* (2018) 24:1104–7. doi: 10.1038/s41591-018-0088-5
18. Valentine GC, Seferovic MD, Fowler SW, Major AM, Gorchakov R, Berry R, et al. Timing of gestational exposure to Zika virus is associated with postnatal growth restriction in a murine model. *Am J Obstet Gynecol.* (2018). 219:403.e1–9. doi: 10.1016/j.ajog.2018.06.005
19. Seferovic M, Sanchez-San Martin C, Tardif SD, Rutherford J, Castro ECC Li T, et al. Experimental Zika virus infection in the pregnant common marmoset induces spontaneous fetal loss and neurodevelopmental abnormalities. *Sci Rep.* (2018) 8:6851. doi: 10.1038/s41598-018-25205-1
20. Sanz Cortes M, Rivera AM, Yepez M, Guimaraes CV, Diaz Yunes I, Zarutskie A, et al. Clinical assessment and brain findings in a cohort of mothers, fetuses and infants infected with ZIKA virus. *Am J Obstet Gynecol.* (2018). 218:440.e1–36. doi: 10.1016/j.ajog.2018.01.012
21. Eppes C, Rac M, Dunn J, Versalovic J, Murray KO, Suter MA, et al. Testing for Zika virus infection in pregnancy: key concepts to deal with an emerging epidemic. *Am J Obstet Gynecol.* (2017) 216:209–25. doi: 10.1016/j.ajog.2017.01.020
22. Murray KO, Gorchakov R, Carlson AR, Berry R, Lai L, Natrajan M, et al. Prolonged detection of Zika virus in vaginal secretions and whole blood. *Emerg Infect Dis.* (2017) 23:99–101. doi: 10.3201/eid2301.161394
23. Suter MA, Aagaard KM. Disease watch: Zika virus - placental passage and permissivity for infection. *Nat Rev Endocrinol.* (2016) 12:437–8. doi: 10.1038/nrendo.2016.101
24. Menzies FM, Fleming A, Rubinsztein DC. Compromised autophagy and neurodegenerative diseases. *Nat Rev Neurosci.* (2015) 16:345–57. doi: 10.1038/nrn3961
25. Liang Q, Luo Z, Zeng J, Chen W, Foo SS, Lee SA, et al. Zika virus NS4A and NS4B proteins deregulate Akt-mTOR signaling in human fetal neural stem cells to inhibit neurogenesis and induce autophagy. *Cell Stem Cell.* (2016) 19:663–71. doi: 10.1016/j.stem.2016.07.019
26. Christian KM, Song H, Ming GL. Pathophysiology and mechanisms of zika virus infection in the nervous system. *Annu Rev Neurosci.* (2019) 42:249–69. doi: 10.1146/annurev-neuro-080317-062231
27. Karuppan MKM, Ojha CR, Rodriguez M, Lapierre J, Aman MJ, Kashanchi F, et al. Reduced-Beclin1-expressing mice infected with Zika-R103451 and viral-associated pathology during pregnancy. *Viruses.* (2020). 12:608. doi: 10.3390/v12060608
28. Peng H, Liu B, Yves TD, He Y, Wang S, Tang H, et al. Zika virus induces autophagy in human umbilical vein endothelial cells. *Viruses.* (2018). 10:259. doi: 10.3390/v10050259
29. Tiwari SK, Dang JW, Lin N, Qin Y, Wang S, Rana TM. Zika virus depletes neural stem cells and evades selective autophagy by suppressing the *Fanconi anemia* protein FANCC. *EMBO Rep.* (2020) 21:e49183. doi: 10.15252/embr.201949183
30. Hamel R, Dejarnac O, Wichit S, Ekchariyawat P, Neyret A, Luplertlop N, et al. Biology of Zika virus infection in human skin cells. *J Virol.* (2015) 89:8880–96. doi: 10.1128/JVI.00354-15
31. He J, Yang L, Chang P, Yang S, Lin S, Tang Q, et al. Zika virus NS2A protein induces the degradation of KPNA2 (karyopherin subunit alpha 2) via chaperone-mediated autophagy. *Autophagy.* (2020) 16:2238–51. doi: 10.1080/15548627.2020.1823122
32. Lin Q, Zhou S, Huang Y, Huo Z, Chen C, Luo X, et al. ANKS4B restricts replication of Zika virus by downregulating the autophagy. *Front Microbiol.* (2020) 11:1745. doi: 10.3389/fmicb.2020.01745
33. Huang Y, Wang Y, Meng S, Chen Z, Kong H, Pan T, et al. Autophagy contributes to host immunity and protection against Zika virus infection via type I IFN signaling. *Mediators Inflamm.* (2020) 2020:9527147. doi: 10.1155/2020/9527147
34. Evans AS, Lennemann NJ, Coyne CB. BPIFB3 regulates endoplasmic reticulum morphology to facilitate flavivirus replication. *J Virol.* (2020). 94:e00029-20. doi: 10.1128/JVI.00029-20
35. Sun P, Nie K, Zhu Y, Liu Y, Wu P, Liu Z, et al. A mosquito salivary protein promotes flavivirus transmission by activation of autophagy. *Nat Commun.* (2020) 11:260. doi: 10.1038/s41467-019-14115-z
36. Munjal A, Khandia R, Dhama K, Sachan S, Karthik K, Tiwari R, et al. Advances in developing therapies to combat Zika virus: current knowledge and future perspectives. *Front Microbiol.* (2017) 8:1469. doi: 10.3389/fmicb.2017.01469
37. Barrows NJ, Campos RK, Powell ST, Prasanth KR, Schott-Lerner G, Soto-Acosta R, et al. A screen of FDA-approved drugs for inhibitors of zika virus infection. *Cell Host Microbe.* (2016) 20:259–70. doi: 10.1016/j.chom.2016.07.004
38. Delvecchio R, Higa LM, Pezzuto P, Valadao AL, Garcez PP, Monteiro FL, et al. Chloroquine, an endocytosis blocking agent, inhibits Zika virus infection in different cell models. *Viruses.* (2016). 8:322. doi: 10.3390/v8120322
39. Cao B, Sheth MN, Mysorekar IU. To Zika and destroy: an antimalarial drug protects fetuses from Zika infection. *Future Microbiol.* (2018) 13:137–9. doi: 10.2217/fmb-2017-0213
40. Cao B, Parnell LA, Diamond MS, Mysorekar IU. Inhibition of autophagy limits vertical transmission of Zika virus in pregnant mice. *J Exp Med.* (2017) 214:2303–13. doi: 10.1084/jem.20170957
41. Tabata T, Petitt M, Puerta-Guardo H, Michlmayr D, Wang C, Fang-Hoover J, et al. Zika virus targets different primary human placental cells, suggesting two routes for vertical transmission. *Cell Host Microbe.* (2016) 20:155–66. doi: 10.1016/j.chom.2016.07.002
42. Miner JJ, Cao B, Govero J, Smith AM, Fernandez E, Cabrera OH, et al. Zika virus infection during pregnancy in mice causes placental damage and fetal demise. *Cell.* (2016) 165:1081–91. doi: 10.1016/j.cell.2016.05.008
43. Hung TH, Hsieh TT, Chen SF Li MJ, Yeh YL. Autophagy in the human placenta throughout gestation. *PLoS ONE.* (2013) 8:e83475. doi: 10.1371/journal.pone.0083475
44. Sahoo BR, Pattnaik A, Annamalai AS, Franco R, Pattnaik AK. Mechanistic target of rapamycin signaling activation antagonizes autophagy to facilitate Zika virus replication. *J Virol.* (2020). 94:e01575-20. doi: 10.1128/JVI.01575-20
45. Guo L, Yu H, Gu W, Luo X, Li R, Zhang J, et al. Autophagy negatively regulates transmissible gastroenteritis virus replication. *Sci Rep.* (2016) 6:23864. doi: 10.1038/srep23864
46. Delorme-Axford E, Donker RB, Mouillet JF, Chu T, Bayer A, Ouyang Y, et al. Human placental trophoblasts confer viral resistance to recipient cells. *Proc Natl Acad Sci USA.* (2013) 110:12048–53. doi: 10.1073/pnas.1304718110

47. Delorme-Axford E, Sadovsky Y, Coyne CB. The placenta as a barrier to viral infections. *Annu Rev Virol.* (2014) 1:133–46. doi: 10.1146/annurev-virology-031413-085524
48. Liu Y, Gordesky-Gold B, Leney-Greene M, Weinbren NL, Tudor M, Cherry S. Inflammation-induced, STING-dependent autophagy restricts Zika virus infection in the drosophila brain. *Cell Host Microbe.* (2018). 24:57–68.e3. doi: 10.1016/j.chom.2018.05.022
49. Roberts DJ, Frosch MP. Zika and histopathology in first trimester infections. *Lancet.* (2016) 388:847–9. doi: 10.1016/S0140-6736(16)30930-8
50. de Noronha L, Zanluca C, Burger M, Suzukawa AA, Azevedo M, Rebutini PZ, et al. Zika virus infection at different pregnancy stages: anatomopathological findings, target cells and viral persistence in placental tissues. *Front Microbiol.* (2018) 9:2266. doi: 10.3389/fmicb.2018.02266
51. Schwartz DA. Viral infection, proliferation, and hyperplasia of Hofbauer cells and absence of inflammation characterize the placental pathology of fetuses with congenital Zika virus infection. *Arch Gynecol Obstet.* (2017) 295:1361–8. doi: 10.1007/s00404-017-4361-5
52. Monel B, Compton AA, Bruel T, Amraoui S, Burlaud-Gaillard J, Roy N, et al. Zika virus induces massive cytoplasmic vacuolization and paraptosis-like death in infected cells. *EMBO J.* (2017) 36:1653–68. doi: 10.15252/embj.2016 95597
53. Gratton R, Agrelli A, Tricarico PM, Brandao L, Crovella S. Autophagy in Zika virus infection: a possible therapeutic target to counteract viral replication. *Int J Mol Sci.* (2019). 20:1048. doi: 10.3390/ijms20051048

Permissions

All chapters in this book were first published by Frontiers; hereby published with permission under the Creative Commons Attribution License or equivalent. Every chapter published in this book has been scrutinized by our experts. Their significance has been extensively debated. The topics covered herein carry significant findings which will fuel the growth of the discipline. They may even be implemented as practical applications or may be referred to as a beginning point for another development.

The contributors of this book come from diverse backgrounds, making this book a truly international effort. This book will bring forth new frontiers with its revolutionizing research information and detailed analysis of the nascent developments around the world.

We would like to thank all the contributing authors for lending their expertise to make the book truly unique. They have played a crucial role in the development of this book. Without their invaluable contributions this book wouldn't have been possible. They have made vital efforts to compile up to date information on the varied aspects of this subject to make this book a valuable addition to the collection of many professionals and students.

This book was conceptualized with the vision of imparting up-to-date information and advanced data in this field. To ensure the same, a matchless editorial board was set up. Every individual on the board went through rigorous rounds of assessment to prove their worth. After which they invested a large part of their time researching and compiling the most relevant data for our readers.

The editorial board has been involved in producing this book since its inception. They have spent rigorous hours researching and exploring the diverse topics which have resulted in the successful publishing of this book. They have passed on their knowledge of decades through this book. To expedite this challenging task, the publisher supported the team at every step. A small team of assistant editors was also appointed to further simplify the editing procedure and attain best results for the readers.

Apart from the editorial board, the designing team has also invested a significant amount of their time in understanding the subject and creating the most relevant covers. They scrutinized every image to scout for the most suitable representation of the subject and create an appropriate cover for the book.

The publishing team has been an ardent support to the editorial, designing and production team. Their endless efforts to recruit the best for this project, has resulted in the accomplishment of this book. They are a veteran in the field of academics and their pool of knowledge is as vast as their experience in printing. Their expertise and guidance has proved useful at every step. Their uncompromising quality standards have made this book an exceptional effort. Their encouragement from time to time has been an inspiration for everyone.

The publisher and the editorial board hope that this book will prove to be a valuable piece of knowledge for researchers, students, practitioners and scholars across the globe.

List of Contributors

Perri C. Callaway
Infectious Diseases and Immunity Graduate Group, University of California, Berkeley, Berkeley, CA, United States
Department of Medicine, University of California, San Francisco, San Francisco, CA, United States

Lila A. Farrington
Department of Medicine, University of California, San Francisco, San Francisco, CA, United States

Margaret E. Feeney
Department of Medicine, University of California, San Francisco, San Francisco, CA, United States
Department of Pediatrics, University of California, San Francisco, San Francisco, CA, United States

Koko Vanda, Naveen Bobbili and Diane Wallace Taylor
Department of Tropical Medicine, Medical Microbiology and Pharmacology, John A. Burns School of Medicine, University of Hawaii, Honolulu, HI, United States

Masako Matsunaga and John J. Chen
Department of Quantitative Health Sciences, John A. Burns School of Medicine, University of Hawaii, Honolulu, HI, United States

Ali Salanti
Centre for Medical Parasitology, Department for Immunology and Microbiology, Faculty of Health and Medical Sciences, University of Copenhagen and Department of Infectious Disease, Copenhagen University Hospital, Copenhagen, Denmark

Rose F. G. Leke
Faculty of Medicine and Biomedical Research, The Biotechnology Center, University of Yaoundé 1, Yaoundé, Cameroon

Geraldo Magela de Faria Junior, Letícia Carolina Paraboli Assoni, Christiane Maria Ayo, Cinara Cássia Brandão and Luiz Carlos de Mattos
Immunogenetics Laboratory, Molecular Biology Department, Faculdade de Medicina de São José do Rio Preto (FAMERP), São José do Rio Preto, Brazil

Fernando Henrique Antunes Murata
Beltsville Agricultural Research Center, Animal Parasitic Diseases Laboratory, United States Department of Agriculture, Agricultural Research Service, Beltsville, MD, United States

Hernan Alejandro Lorenzi
Department of Infectious Diseases, J. Craig Venter Institute, Rockville, MD, United States

Bruno Bello Pede Castro
Department of Preventive Veterinary Medicine and Animal Health, Faculty of Veterinary Medicine, University of São Paulo, São Paulo, Brazil

Caroline L. L. Chua
School of Biosciences, Taylor's University, Subang Jaya, Malaysia

Wina Hasang and Stephen J. Rogerson
Department of Medicine at Royal Melbourne Hospital, Peter Doherty Institute, University of Melbourne, Melbourne, VIC, Australia

Andrew Teo
Department of Medicine at Royal Melbourne Hospital, Peter Doherty Institute, University of Melbourne, Melbourne, VIC, Australia
Lee Kong Chian School of Medicine, Nanyang Technological University, Singapore, Singapore

Edward R. Kabyemela
Mother Offspring Malaria Studies (MOMS) Project, Seattle Biomedical Research Institute, Seattle, WA, United States
School of Medicine, Muhimbili University of Health and Allied Sciences, Dar es Salaam, Tanzania

Michal Fried and Patrick E. Duffy
Mother Offspring Malaria Studies (MOMS) Project, Seattle Biomedical Research Institute, Seattle, WA, United States
Laboratory of Malaria Immunology and Vaccinology, National Institutes of Allergy and Infectious Diseases, National Institutes of Health (NIH), Bethesda, MD, United States

Jonathan D. Kurtis
Department of Pathology and Laboratory Medicine, Center for International Health Research, Rhode Island Hospital, Brown University, Providence, RI, United States

Gwamaka Moses
Mother Offspring Malaria Studies (MOMS) Project, Seattle Biomedical Research Institute, Seattle, WA, United States
Mbeya College of Health and Allied Sciences, University of Dar es Salaam, Mbeya, Tanzania

J. Patrick Gorres
Laboratory of Malaria Immunology and Vaccinology, National Institutes of Allergy and Infectious Diseases, National Institutes of Health (NIH), Bethesda, MD, United States

Atis Muehlenbachs
Mother Offspring Malaria Studies (MOMS) Project, Seattle Biomedical Research Institute, Seattle, WA, United States

Luiz Carlos De Mattos, Ana Iara Costa Ferreira, Karina Younan de Oliveira and Fabiana Nakashima
Immunogenetics Laboratory, Molecular Biology Department, Faculty of Medicine - FAMERP, São José do Rio Preto, Brazil

Cinara Cássia Brandão
Immunogenetics Laboratory, Molecular Biology Department, Faculty of Medicine - FAMERP, São José do Rio Preto, Brazil
FAMERP Toxoplasma Research Group, Molecular Biology Department, Faculty of Medicine - FAMERP, São José do Rio Preto, Brazil

Demba Sarr and Balázs Rada
Department of Infectious Diseases, College of Veterinary Medicine, University of Georgia, Athens, GA, United States

Lilian J. Oliveira
Department of Pathology, College of Veterinary Medicine, University of Georgia, Athens, Georgia, United States
Department of Infectious Diseases and Immunology, College of Veterinary Medicine, University of Florida, Gainesville, FL, United States

Brittany N. Russ
Department of Infectious Diseases and Immunology, College of Veterinary Medicine, University of Florida, Gainesville, FL, United States

Simon O. Owino
Department of Infectious Diseases and Immunology, College of Veterinary Medicine, University of Florida, Gainesville, FL, United States
Vector Biology and Control Research Centre, Kenya Medical Research Institute, Kisian, Kenya
University of Georgia/Kenya Medical Research Institute Placental Malaria Study, Siaya District Hospital, Siaya, Kenya
Faculty of Science, Department of Zoology, Maseno University, Maseno, Kenya

Joab D. Middii
Vector Biology and Control Research Centre, Kenya Medical Research Institute, Kisian, Kenya
University of Georgia/Kenya Medical Research Institute Placental Malaria Study, Siaya District Hospital, Siaya, Kenya
Kisumu Specialists Hospital Laboratory, Kisumu, Kenya

Stephen Mwalimu
Vector Biology and Control Research Centre, Kenya Medical Research Institute, Kisian, Kenya
University of Georgia/Kenya Medical Research Institute Placental Malaria Study, Siaya District Hospital, Siaya, Kenya
Animal and Human Health Program, International Livestock Research Institute, Nairobi, Kenya

Linda Ambasa
Vector Biology and Control Research Centre, Kenya Medical Research Institute, Kisian, Kenya
University of Georgia/Kenya Medical Research Institute Placental Malaria Study, Siaya District Hospital, Siaya, Kenya
#1 Heartsaved Adult Family Care, Marysville, WA, United States

Faris Almutairi
Department of Infectious Diseases, College of Veterinary Medicine, University of Georgia, Athens, GA, United States
Department of Pharmaceutical and Biomedical Sciences, College of Pharmacy, University of Georgia, Athens, GA, United States

John Vulule
Vector Biology and Control Research Centre, Kenya Medical Research Institute, Kisian, Kenya,

Julie M. Moore
Department of Infectious Diseases and Immunology, College of Veterinary Medicine, University of Florida, Gainesville, FL, United States
Vector Biology and Control Research Centre, Kenya Medical Research Institute, Kisian, Kenya
University of Georgia/Kenya Medical Research Institute Placental Malaria Study, Siaya District Hospital, Siaya, Kenya

Madeleine C. Wiebe
Department of Medical Microbiology and Immunology, University of Alberta, Edmonton, AB, Canada

Stephanie K. Yanow
Department of Medical Microbiology and Immunology, University of Alberta, Edmonton, AB, Canada
School of Public Health, University of Alberta, Edmonton, AB, Canada

William Robert Pownall and Franck Forterre
Division of Small Animal Surgery, Department of Clinical Veterinary Sciences, Vetsuisse Faculty, University of Bern, Bern, Switzerland

Dennis Imhof and Andrew Hemphill
Institute of Parasitology, DIP, Vetsuisse Faculty, University of Bern, Bern, Switzerland

Nerea Fernandez Trigo and Stephanie C. Ganal-Vonarburg
Department for BioMedical Research (DBMR), Universitätsklinik für Viszerale Chirurgie und Medizin, Inselspital, Bern University Hospital, University of Bern, Bern, Switzerland

Philippe Plattet, Camille Monney and Anna Oevermann
Division of Neurological Sciences, DCR-VPH, Vetsuisse Faculty, University of Bern, Bern, Switzerland

Benoît Gamain
Université de Paris, Inserm, Biologie Intégrée du Globule Rouge, Paris, France
Institut National de la Transfusion Sanguine, Paris, France

Nicola K Viebig
European Vaccine Initiative, UniversitätsKlinikum Heidelberg, Heidelberg, Germany

Nicaise Tuikue Ndam
Université de Paris, MERIT, IRD, Paris, France

Morten A Nielsen
Centre for Medical Parasitology at Department of Immunology and Microbiology, Faculty of Health and Medical Sciences, University of Copenhagen, Copenhagen, Denmark
Department of Infectious Diseases, Rigshospitalet, Copenhagen, Denmark

Alice Tomlinson, Jean-Philippe Semblat, Benoît Gamain and Arnaud Chêne
Université de Paris, Biologie Intégrée du Globule Rouge, UMR_S1134, BIGR, INSERM, Paris, France
Institut National de la Transfusion Sanguine, Paris, France
Laboratory of Excellence GR-Ex, Paris, France

Marta García-Sánchez, Laura Jiménez-Pelayo, Patricia Vázquez, Pilar Horcajo, Javier Regidor-Cerrillo, Alejandro Jiménez-Meléndez, Luis Miguel Ortega-Mora and Esther Collantes-Fernández
Saluvet, Animal Health Department, Complutense University of Madrid, Madrid, Spain

Koldo Osoro
Regional Service for Research and Agri-Food Development (SERIDA), Villaviciosa, Spain

Alistair R. D. McLean
Burnet Institute, Melbourne, VIC, Australia
Centre for Tropical Medicine and Global Health, Nuffield Department of Medicine, University of Oxford, Oxford, United Kingdom

D. Herbert Opi
Burnet Institute, Melbourne, VIC, Australia
Department of Immunology and Pathology, Monash University, Melbourne, VIC, Australia
Papua New Guinea Institute of Medical Research, Madang, Papua New Guinea

Danielle I. Stanisic
Papua New Guinea Institute of Medical Research, Madang, Papua New Guinea
Institute for Glycomics, Griffith University, Southport, QLD, Australia

Julia C. Cutts and Gaoqian Feng
Burnet Institute, Melbourne, VIC, Australia
Department of Medicine at the Doherty Institute, University of Melbourne, Melbourne, VIC, Australia

Alice Ura
Papua New Guinea Institute of Medical Research, Madang, Papua New Guinea

Ivo Mueller
Papua New Guinea Institute of Medical Research, Madang, Papua New Guinea
Population, Health and Immunity Division, Walter and Eliza Hall Institute of Medical Research, Parkville, VIC, Australia
Département Parasites et Insectes Vecteurs, Institute Pasteur, Paris, France

Stephen J. Rogerson
Department of Medicine at the Doherty Institute, University of Melbourne, Melbourne, VIC, Australia

Freya J. I. Fowkes
Burnet Institute, Melbourne, VIC, Australia
Department of Infectious Diseases, Central Clinical School, Monash University, Melbourne, VIC, Australia
Centre for Epidemiology and Biostatistics, University of Melbourne, Melbourne, VIC, Australia
Department of Epidemiology and Preventive Medicine, Monash University, Melbourne, VIC, Australia

James G. Beeson
Burnet Institute, Melbourne, VIC, Australia
Department of Medicine at the Doherty Institute, University of Melbourne, Melbourne, VIC, Australia
Department of Microbiology, Monash University, Clayton, VIC, Australia

Mariana Barros and Daniela Teixeira
Departamento de Ciências Biológicas, Faculdade de Farmácia, Universidade do Porto, Porto, Portugal

Manuel Vilanova and Alexandra Correia
Immunobiology Group, Instituto de Investigação e Inovação em Saúde (i3S), Universidade do Porto, Porto, Portugal
Instituto de Biologia Molecular e Celular (IBMC), Universidade do Porto, Porto, Portugal
Departamento de Imuno-Fisiologia e Farmacologia, Instituto de Ciências Biomédicas Abel Salazar (ICBAS), Universidade do Porto, Porto, Portugal

Natercia Teixeira and Margarida Borges
Applied Molecular Biosciences Unit/Rede de Química e Tecnologia (UCIBIO/REQUIMTE), Departamento de Ciências Biológicas, Faculdade de Farmácia, Universidade do Porto, Porto, Portugal

David Arranz-Solís and Jeroen P. J. Saeij
Pathology, Microbiology and Immunology Department, Veterinary Medicine School 3A, University of California Davis, Davis, CA, United States

Cristina G. Carvalheiro
Laboratory of Parasitic Diseases, Molecular Parasitology Section, National Institute of Allergy and Infectious Diseases, National Institutes of Health, Bethesda, MD, United States
Department of Pediatrics, Ribeirão Preto Medical School, University of São Paulo, Ribeirão Preto, Brazil

Elizabeth R. Zhang and Michael E. Grigg
Laboratory of Parasitic Diseases, Molecular Parasitology Section, National Institute of Allergy and Infectious Diseases, National Institutes of Health, Bethesda, MD, United States

Bernard Tornyigah and Nicaise Tuikue Ndam
Université de Paris, MERIT, IRD, Paris, France
Department of Immunology, Noguchi Memorial Institute for Medical Research, College of Health Sciences, University of Ghana, Legon, Ghana

Tania d'Almeida
Université de Paris, MERIT, IRD, Paris, France
Université Pierre et Marie Curie, Ecole doctorale 393 Pierre Louis de Santé publique, Paris, France

Guillaume Escriou and Philippe Deloron
Université de Paris, MERIT, IRD, Paris, France

Firmine Viwami
Centre d'Etude et de Recherche sur le Paludisme Associé à la Grossesse et à l'Enfance, Cotonou, Benin

Nadine Fievet and Adrian J. F. Luty
Université de Paris, MERIT, IRD, Paris, France
Centre d'Etude et de Recherche sur le Paludisme Associé à la Grossesse et à l'Enfance, Cotonou, Benin

Achille Massougbodji
Centre d'Etude et de Recherche sur le Paludisme Associé à la Grossesse et à l'Enfance, Cotonou, Benin

Morten A. Nielsen
Centre for Medical Parasitology, University of Copenhagen, Copenhagen, Denmark

Lisvaneth Medina, Christian Castillo, Ana Liempi, Jesús Guerrero-Muñoz and Ulrike Kemmerling
Programa de Anatomía y Biología del Desarrollo, Facultad de Medicina, Instituto de Ciencias Biomédicas, Universidad de Chile, Santiago, Chile

Maura Rojas-Pirela
Instituto de Biología, Pontificia Universidad Católica de Valparaíso, Valparaíso, Chile

Juan Diego Maya
Programa de Farmacología Molecular y Clínica, Facultad de Medicina, Instituto de Ciencias Biomédicas, Universidad de Chile, Santiago, Chile

Humberto Prieto
Instituto de Investigaciones Agropecuarias, Ministerio de Agricultura, Santiago, Chile

Yu-Chao Zhu, Ji-Li Zhang and Yong He
Department of Radiology, The Affiliated Hospital of Medical School of Ningbo University, Ningbo University School of Medicine, Ningbo, China

Li-Juan Ma
Department of Integrated Chinese and Western Medicine Oncology, The Affiliated People's Hospital of Ningbo University, Ningbo, China

Jian-Fa Liu
Immunology Innovation Team, Ningbo University School of Medicine, Ningbo, China

Ji-Ye Feng
Department of Hepatobiliary Surgery, The Affiliated People's Hospital of Ningbo University, Ningbo, China

Jia Chen
Department of Radiology, The Affiliated Hospital of Medical School of Ningbo University, Ningbo University School of Medicine, Ningbo, China
Immunology Innovation Team, Ningbo University School of Medicine, Ningbo, China

Ana Espino, Hicham El Costa, Julie Tabiasco and Nabila Jabrane-Ferrat
Infinity, Université de Toulouse - CNRS – Inserm, CHU Purpan, Toulouse, France

Reem Al-Daccak
Inserm UMRS976 - Université de Paris - Hôpital Saint-Louis, Paris, France

Chandrashekara Kyathanahalli and Emmet Hirsch
Department of Obstetrics and Gynecology, NorthShore University HealthSystem, Evanston, IL, United States
Department of Obstetrics and Gynecology, Pritzker School of Medicine, University of Chicago, Chicago, IL, United States

Madeline Snedden
Department of Obstetrics and Gynecology, NorthShore University HealthSystem, Evanston, IL, United States

Jennifer R. McKinney, Maxim D. Seferovic and Melissa A. Suter
Departments of Obstetrics and Gynecology, Division of Maternal-Fetal Medicine, Baylor College of Medicine and Texas Children's Hospital, Houston, TX, United States

Angela M. Major
Pathology and Laboratory Medicine, Baylor College of Medicine and Texas Children's Hospital, Houston, TX, United States

Suzette D. Tardif
Southwest National Primate Research Center, Texas Biomedical Research Institute, San Antonio, TX, United States

Jean L. Patterson
Department of Virology and Immunology, Texas Biomedical Research Institute, San Antonio, TX, United States

Eumenia C. C. Castro
Pathology and Laboratory Medicine, Baylor College of Medicine and Texas Children's Hospital, Houston, TX, United States

Kjersti M. Aagaard
Departments of Obstetrics and Gynecology, Division of Maternal-Fetal Medicine, Baylor College of Medicine and Texas Children's Hospital, Houston, TX, United States
Pathology and Laboratory Medicine, Baylor College of Medicine and Texas Children's Hospital, Houston, TX, United States
Molecular and Human Genetics, Baylor College of Medicine, Houston, TX, United States

Index

www.ingramcontent.com/pod-product-compliance
Lightning Source LLC
LaVergne TN
LVHW080946210926
848485LV00004B/786